AF333994

Core Curriculum
for the Nursing Care
of Children and Their Families

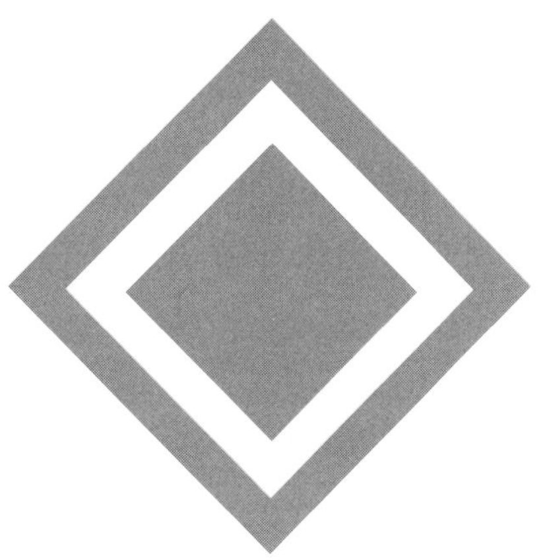

Marion E. Broome, PhD, RN, FAAN
Judy A. Rollins, MS, RN
Editors

ISBN 0-9655310-3-1

Copyright © 1999
Jannetti Publications, Inc.
East Holly Avenue/Box 56, Pitman, New Jersey 08071

Statement of Endorsement

◆◆

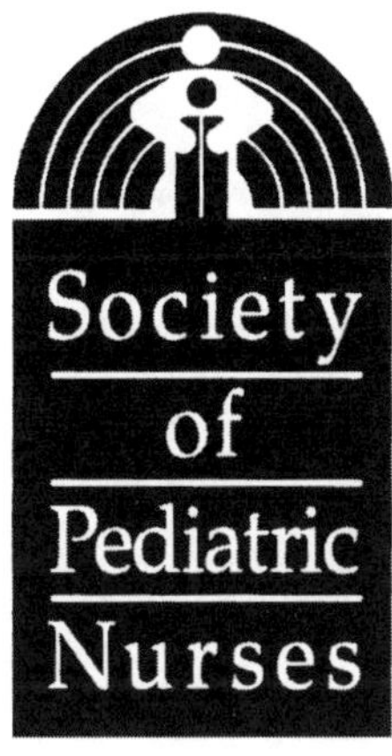

The *Core Curriculum for the Nursing Care of Children and Their Families* is endorsed by The Society of Pediatric Nurses (SPN). The SPN represents more than 2,200 nurses who support the mission of promoting optimal health of children and excellence in nursing care of children and their families.

The goals of the Society are:

◆ To advocate for accessible, affordable, comprehensive health care services for children.

◆ To advance the art and science of pediatric nursing through interactive efforts among all nurses in clinical practice, research, education, and administration.

◆ To establish position statements and standards of practice.

◆ To collaborate with other health care professionals, child health advocates, and related organizations.

Jannetti Publications, Inc. would like to acknowledge and thank the SPN reviewers who reviewed the *Core Curriculum for the Nursing Care of Children and Their Families*: Susan D. Beyer, BSN, RN, and Marilyn R. Breuer, MS, RN. We would also like to thank Jody Foss, MS, RN, DAE, SPN's Executive Director, and Brenda Woodard, Association Coordinator, for their support and cooperation.

Contents

◆ ◆

Contents

Preface

In January 1994, a group of nurse educators from academic and clinical settings gathered in Chicago, IL, to draft guidelines for pediatric nursing education. The project, directed by Karen F. Pridham, PhD, RN, FAAN, was a joint venture between the Maternal and Child Health Bureau and the Society of Pediatric Nurses.

Members of this working conference acknowledged the fact that the nature of care and where it is delivered has shifted and that (a) education for pediatric nursing must be reoriented to family-centered, community-based, and coordinated care that is sensitive and responsive to the beliefs, practices, and strengths of cultural groups; and (b) much of the care of children with an acute or chronic illness or disability has shifted from the hospital to community settings, including homes, schools, child care centers, and primary care clinics. The result of that meeting was a document entitled *Standards and Guidelines for Pre-licensure and Early Professional Education for the Nursing Care of Children and Their Families.*

It is upon that document that *Core Curriculum for the Nursing Care of Children and Their Families* is based. Intended as a reference source for pediatric nurse educators, clinicians, and students, the Core Curriculum has 31 chapters divided into three sections:

- ◆ **Section 1: Child, Family, and Societal Factors**, covers the concepts of (a) anatomic structures and physiologic, psychologic, and spiritual processes in neonates, infants, children, and adolescents; (b) health behavior; (c) separation, loss, and bereavement; and (d) economic, social, and political influences.
- ◆ **Section 2: Clinical Problems or Areas**, covers the concepts of (a) safety and injury prevention; (b) children with acute illness or injuries and their families; and (c) children with a chronic condition, disability, or special health need and their families.
- ◆ **Section 3: Care Delivery**, covers the concepts of (a) family-centered care; (b) cultural competence; (c) communication; and (d) values and moral and ethical reasoning.

A project of this nature and scope requires smooth teamwork. Associate Editors Barbara Woodring, EdD, RN; Richard E. Harbin, MSN, MEd, RN, CPNP; and Mary Kachoyeanos, EdD, RN, were with us from the book's conception, helping us to determine essential content and identify experts in that content as chapter authors. We thank them for the endless hours they spent reviewing manuscripts and working with authors to help assure sound and relevant content. We truly appreciate all 31 contributors for sharing their expertise; it was an honor to work with so many talented individuals. We acknowledge and are most grateful for the wisdom of Gus Ostrum, Director of Editorial Services, for choosing Claudia Cuddy, Managing Editor, and Janet D'Alesandro, Editorial Coordinator, for our publication team. Their professionalism and attention to detail kept the project humming and on track, and their constant support and enthusiasm made working together a true delight. And finally, we sincerely appreciate Susan D. Beyer, BSN, RN, and Marilyn R. Breuer, MS, RN, for serving as manuscript reviewers on behalf of the Society of Pediatric Nurses. They kept us true to our mission to attempt to articulate the standards and guidelines born of that 1994 meeting in Chicago.

We hope that this resource, by taking a fresh approach to outlining what nurses need to know, will help those who use it make a significant contribution to improving care for children and their families across the health care continuum.

Marion E. Broome, PhD, RN, FAAN
Judy A. Rollins, MS, RN

 EDITORS

Marion E. Broome, PhD, RN, FAAN
Professor and Associate Dean for Research
University of Wisconsin–Milwaukee and
Research Chair
Children's Hospital of Wisconsin
Milwaukee, Wisconsin
Editor, *Journal of Child and Family Nursing*

Judy A. Rollins, MS, RN
Child Health Consultant, Rollins & Associates, Inc.
Washington, DC
Adjunct Instructor, Georgetown University School of Medicine
Washington, DC
Coordinator, Studio G
Georgetown University Medical Center
Washington, DC
Associate Editor, *Pediatric Nursing,* Pitman, NJ

 ASSOCIATE EDITORS

Barbara C. Woodring, EdD, RN
Associate Professor and Chair
Parent-Child Nursing
School of Nursing
Medical College of Georgia
Augusta, Georgia

Mary Kachoyeanos, EdD, RN, FAAN
Director of Research
Children's Hospital of Wisconsin
Milwaukee, Wisconsin

Richard E. Harbin, MSN, MEd, RN, CPNP
Advanced Registered Nurse Practitioner
University of Central Florida
School of Nursing
Orlando, Florida

 CONTRIBUTORS

Elizabeth Ahmann, ScD, RN
Senior Lecturer
Columbia University School of Nursing
Consultant, Child and Family Health
Washington, DC
Section Editor: "Family Matters"
Pediatric Nursing, Pitman, New Jersey

Mary A. Baroni, PhD, RN, CPNP
Associate Professor
Marquette University College of Nursing
Milwaukee, Wisconsin

Carol C. Beausang, PhD, RN
Assistant Professor
Indiana University
Indianapolis, Indiana

Judy Benka, MS, RN, PNP
Practitioner–Teacher
Rush University College of Nursing
Chicago, Illinois
Pediatric Nurse Practitioner
Elmhurst Clinic
Elmhurst, Illinois

Ruth Bindler, MS, RN,C
Associate Professor
Intercollegiate Center for Nursing
    Education
Washington State University
Spokane, Washington

Elizabeth A. Bossert, DNS, RN
Professor
Loma Linda University
Loma Linda, California

Jeanne Braby, MSN, RN, CCRN
ECMO Clinician
Children's Hospital of Wisconsin
Milwaukee, Wisconsin

Martha J. Bradshaw, PhD, RN
Assistant Professor, Parent-Child Nursing
Medical College of Georgia
Augusta, Georgia

Marion E. Broome, PhD, RN, FAAN
Professor and Associate Dean for Research
University of Wisconsin–Milwaukee
Milwaukee, Wisconsin
Research Chair
Children's Hospital of Wisconsin
Milwaukee, Wisconsin

Marion L. Donohoe, MSN, RN, PNP
Pediatric Nurse Practitioner
St. Jude Children's Research Hospital
Memphis, Tennessee

Mary Lou Gostisha, MSN, RN
Patient Care Manager, PICU
Children's Hospital of Wisconsin
Milwaukee, Wisconsin

Dynnette E. Hart, DrPH, RN
Assistant Professor, Child Health Nursing
Loma Linda University School of Nursing
Loma Linda, California

Sandra M. Hicks, MSN, RN
Lower Division Coordinator/Lecturer
North Carolina A & T State University
    School of Nursing
Greensboro, North Carolina

Myra Martz Huth, MSN, RN
Doctoral Student
Case Western Reserve University
Frances Payne Bolton School of Nursing
Cleveland, Ohio

Francine Clark Jones, PhD, RN
Assistant Professor
Medical College of Wisconsin
Department of Pediatrics
Milwaukee, Wisconsin

Deborah G. Loman, PhD, RN, CPNP
Assistant Professor
St. Louis University
St. Louis, Missouri

Maureen C. Maguire, MSN, RN, PNP
Clinical Nurse Specialist
Kennedy–Krieger Institute
Baltimore, Maryland

Carmel C. Mahan, MSEd, CCLS
Child Life Coordinator
Georgetown University Medical Center
Washington, DC

Virginia E. Maikler, PhD, RN
Acting Chairperson
Department of MCN
Rush University
Chicago, Illinois

Patricia A. Moloney-Harmon, MS, RN, CCRN
Advanced Practice Nurse/Clinical Nurse
  Specialist, Children's Services
Sinai Hospital of Baltimore
Baltimore, Maryland

Sandra R. Mott, PhD(c), MS, RN,C
Associate Professor
Boston College School of Nursing
Chestnut Hill, Massachusetts

Beth S. Nachtsheim, MS, RN, PCCNP
Pediatric Critical Care Nurse Practitioner
Rush Children's Hospital
Rush Presbyterian–St. Luke's Medical
  Center
Chicago, Illinois

Wendy M. Nehring, PhD, RN, FAAMR
Associate Professor, School of Nursing
Southern Illinois University–Edwardsville
Edwardsville, Illinois

Maureen E. O'Brien, PhD, RN
Assistant Professor
Marquette University College of Nursing
Milwaukee, Wisconsin

Christine K. Olson, MSN, RN
Director of Patient Care Services
St. Luke's Medical Center
Milwaukee, Wisconsin

Lois J. Pearson, MEd, CCLS
Child Life Specialist
Children's Hospital of Wisconsin
Milwaukee, Wisconsin
Children's Grief Group Facilitator
Consultant, Community Memorial Hospital
Menomonee Falls, Wisconsin
Lecturer in Child Life
Department of Education, Edgewood College
Madison, Wisconsin

Teresa A. Savage, PhD, RN
Post-Doctoral Research Fellow
Primary Health Care/Social Ethics
University of Illinois at Chicago College
  of Nursing
Chicago, Illinois

Judith Schurr Salzer, MS, RN, CPNP
Assistant Professor
Medical College of Georgia
Augusta, Georgia

Janice Selekman, DNSc, RN
Professor and Chairman
Department of Nursing
University of Delaware
Newark, Delaware

Joan P. Totka, MSN, RN, CDE
Clinical Nurse Specialist – Diabetes
Children's Hospital of Wisconsin
Milwaukee, Wisconsin

Lois Van Cleve, PhD, RN
Professor, Associate Dean
Loma Linda University School of Nursing
Loma Linda, California

Barbara Velsor-Friedrich, PhD, RN
Associate Professor
Department of Maternal Child Health
  Nursing
Loyola University
Chicago, Illinois

Judith A. Vessey, PhD, RN, CRNP, FAAN
Professor, Johns Hopkins University
School of Nursing
Baltimore, Maryland

Carolyn L. Walker, PhD, RN, CPON
Professor and Graduate Advisor
San Diego State University–School of
  Nursing
San Diego, California

Jenifer M. Wincek, MSN, RN, CPNP
Director, Maternal-Child Health
Goshen General Hospital
Goshen, Indiana

Barbara C. Woodring, RN, EdD
Associate Professor and Chair
Parent-Child Nursing
School of Nursing
Medical College of Georgia
Augusta, Georgia

◆ Reviewers from the Society of Pediatric Nurses

Susan D. Beyer, BSN, RN
Nursing Administrative Specialist
Texas Children's Hospital
Houston, Texas

Marilyn R. Breuer, MS, RN
Assistant Professor, Division of Nursing
American International College
Springfield, Massachusetts

◆ Publication Management by Anthony J. Jannetti, Inc.

Managing Editor
Claudia Cuddy

Editorial Coordinator
Janet Perrella D'Alesandro

Director, Editorial Services
Gus Ostrum

Art Director
Jack Bryant

Layout Consultant
Darin Peters

Production Assistant
Conni Bernosky

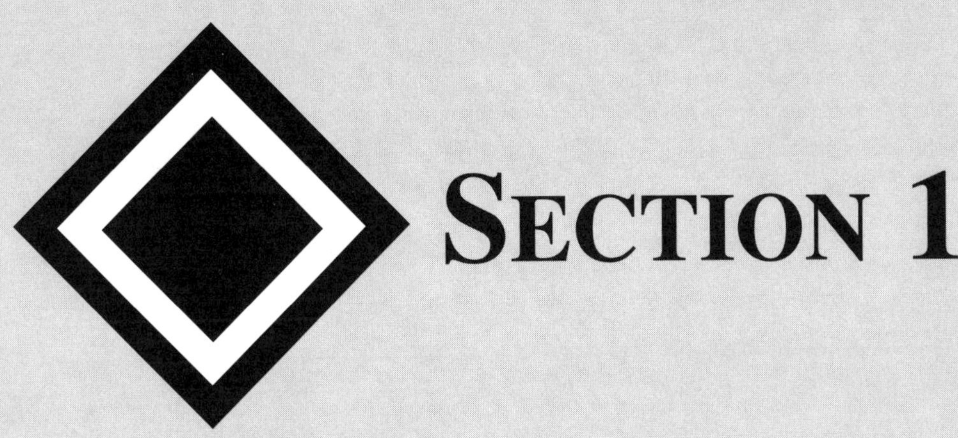

SECTION 1

Child, Family, and Societal Factors

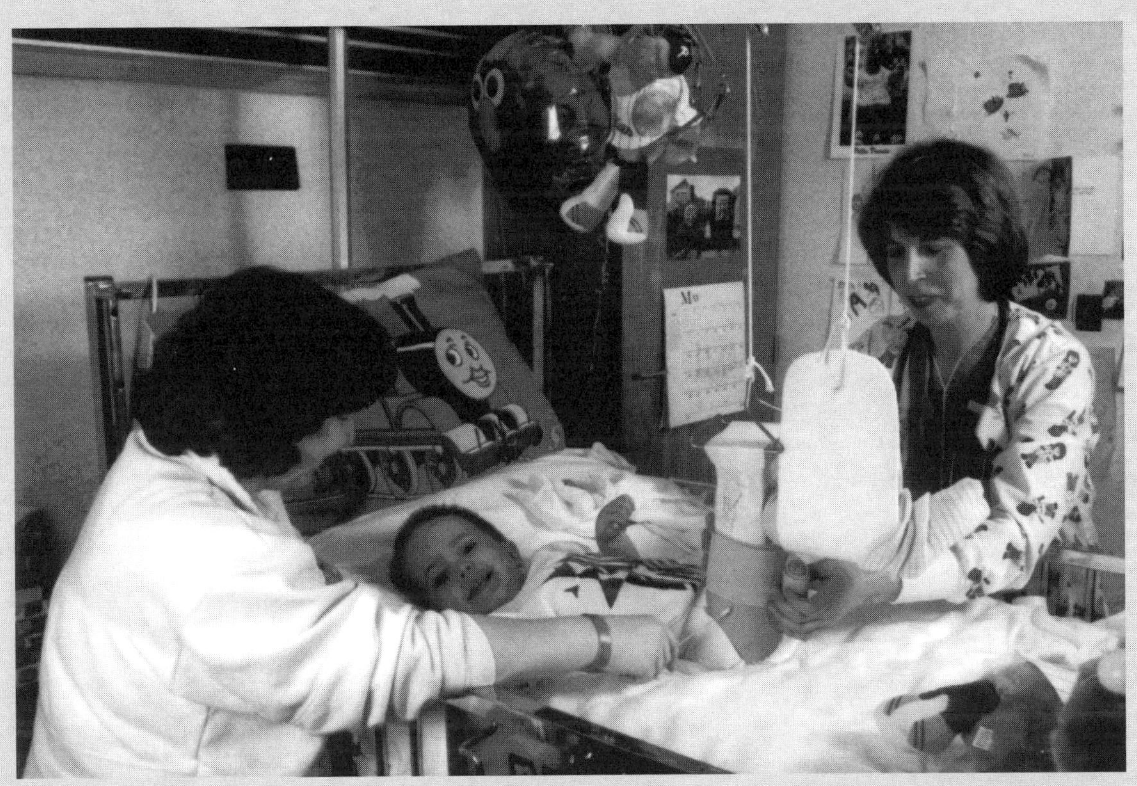

Chapter 1

Biologic Development

Sandra M. Hicks, MSN, RN

Concept

◆◆◆◆◆◆◆◆◆◆◆◆◆◆◆◆◆◆◆◆◆◆◆◆◆◆

◆ Anatomic structures and physiologic, psychologic, and spiritual processes in neonates, infants, children, and adolescents.

Objectives

◆◆◆◆◆◆◆◆◆◆◆◆◆◆◆◆◆◆◆◆◆◆◆◆◆◆

At the completion of this chapter, the reader will be able to:

◆ Discuss basic principles of growth and development.

◆ Analyze the effects of growth and development parameters on body systems.

◆ Recognize biologic factors that influence a child's growth and development.

◆ Identify anatomic and structural differences unique to children.

◆ Identify biologic and physiologic processes that influence nursing care delivery.

◆ Use growth parameters and developmental characteristics to plan care for children.

Key Points

◆◆◆◆◆◆◆◆◆◆◆◆◆◆◆◆◆◆◆◆◆◆◆◆◆◆

◆ Internal and external factors influence the acquisition of fine and gross motor skills, cephalocaudal-proximodistal growth and development, and differentiation of the nervous system.

◆ Locomotion, the major gross motor skill acquired during toddlerhood, allows the child to master a wide variety of activities.

◆ Biologic development in the preschool period is characterized by mature body systems and refinement in gross and fine motor behavior as evidenced by participation in activities such as running, riding, and drawing.

◆ Physiologically, the school age period begins with shedding the deciduous teeth and ends at puberty with acquisition of final permanent teeth.

◆ The major hormonal changes during adolescence result in the development of primary and secondary sex characteristics.

Biologic Development

I. OVERVIEW OF THE PRINCIPLES OF GROWTH AND DEVELOPMENT

The study of biologic development generally involves the finding of patterns or general principles that apply to children from infancy through adolescence. Patterns and general principles of biologic development can be used to guide health promotion, maintenance and restoration. Health promotion, maintenance and restoration, standards, and expectations vary according to a number of internal and external influences. The internal and external influences affect growth and development across the life span.

A. Definitions.
1. Growth: an increase in physical attributes, which results from biologic changes such as body cell content, and metabolic and biochemical processes; growth may be objectively evaluated in quantitative measures.
   a. Incremental growth refers to maintaining an excess in growth over normal daily losses (e.g., height and weight).
   b. Replacement growth refers to normal refills of essential body components necessary for survival (e.g., erythrocytes, which circulate an average of 120 days before disintegrating and new red blood cells take over).
2. Development: the progression in skill and complexity of function; development occurs as a result of growth and embraces all the physical, psychologic, intellectual, and social changes that occur throughout the life span.
3. Maturation: a term often used interchangeable with development but actually refers to qualitative changes genetically programmed.
   a. Maturation typically parallels growth and theoretically may occur in the absence of learning.
   b. Learning indicates that changes are produced by outside influences.
4. Physical competency: the child's ability to apply various motor and neurologic capacities to steadily achieve more mature self-care abilities requiring mobility and manipulative skills; aspects of this competency include:
   a. Physical health.
   b. Body build and configuration.
   c. Symmetry and strength of extremities.
   d. Rate of motor, neurologic, and biologic maturation.
   e. Motor skill performance.
5. "Growth and development": the process toward maturation and the assumption that learning has taken place; Age/Stages of growth and development may be conceptualized in many ways, but generally changes in characteristics and behaviors are linked to the age at which differences are expected.
   a. Parental: conception to birth.
   b. Neonatal: birth through 1 month.
   c. Infancy: 1 month to 1 year.
   d. Toddler: 1 to 3 years.
   e. Preschool: 3 to 6 years.
   f. School-age: 6 to 11 years.
   g. Adolescent: 12 to 19 years.

II. CHARACTERISTICS OF GROWTH

A. Directional pattern.
1. Cephalocaudal.
   a. Growth and development proceeds from head to toe.
   b. Structures and functions originating in the head develop before those in the lower parts of the body.
   c. This pattern is readily observed as the head is the largest part of the body at birth and an infant can raise the head before sitting.
2. Proximodistal.
   a. A Latin term, "proximodistal," translates as "near to far."
   b. Growth and development progression is from center outward or from the midline to the periphery.
   c. An example of normal proximodistal pattern can be seen as motor control develops; the infant gains control of the arms before the ability to control the hands and then fingers.

Table 1-1
Numerical Formula to Present
Observed Postnatal Changes

Growth specialists have identified an overall numerical formula to present postnatal changes observed in the human body: 2 – 3 – 4 – 5

2 – indicates that between birth and adulthood, an individual's head and neck dimensions will increase by two times.

3 – refers to the trunk increasing three times.

4 – indicates the arms grow four times

5 – signifies the legs will increase five times.

---

3. General to specific.
   a. Activities of the infant become less generalized and more focused.
   b. In motor development, reaching for an object with the whole hand is replaced by the pincer grasp at about nine months of age.
4. Simple to complex.
   a. This pattern may best be observed in young children through language development.
   b. The infant makes a request using one word, the toddler may string two or three words together, and the preschool child will begin to use grammatically correct sentences with assistance.

B. Pace.
   1. Growth and development have sequential trends, which are fixed and precise.
      a. The pace or timely movement toward maturation is inconsistent.
      b. At times children demonstrate tremendous spurts in growth or development, and at other times plateaus occur when little change is apparent.
      c. Examples of sequence of growth and development have been identified, but the uniqueness for each child is within the pace. Pace is unique to the child as an individual and is influenced by external and internal stimuli. The general expected pace is:
         (1) Rapid – from birth to 2 years
         (2) Slower – from 2 years to puberty
         (3) Rapid – from puberty to 15 years of age
         (4) A sharp decline – from 16 to about 24 years of age
   2. Over the past century, secular trends in physical growth change in body size from one generation to the next have been noted.

   a. The pattern of secular trends is mostly due to the faster rate of physical maturation and improved nutrition.
   b. This pattern is not as great among low-income groups.

C. Anatomic/structural changes.
   1. Growth specialists have identified an overall numerical formula to present postnatal changes observed in the human body (see Table 1-1)
   2. Linear growth or height.
      a. The cephalocaudal trend of growth and development is evident in linear growth or height that occurs as a result of skeletal growth.
      b. Maximum growth in length occurs before birth.
      c. During fetal development the head is the fastest growing part of the body; at 2 months of gestation, the head represents 50% of the total body length.
      d. At birth the average length of a European-American neonate is about 50 cm (20 inches); African-American neonates tend to be shorter, ranging from 47.5 to 52.5 cm (19 to 21 inches).
      e. During infancy, growth of the trunk predominates and by 6 months, the infant gains another 13.75 cm (5.5 inches) of height.
      f. During childhood the legs are the most rapidly growing part of the body.
         (1) At 2 years of age, children normally have achieved 50% of their adult height.
         (2) Children usually double their birth length by age 4 years.
      g. During adolescence the trunk again is the predominant area of growth.
         (1) Other proportional changes are also noted in the shoulder and hip breadth.
         (2) Hormone secretions in both sexes during the adolescent period are responsible for these changes.
      h. As growth proceeds, the midpoint in head-to-toe measurement gradually descends from the level even with the umbilicus at birth to the level of the symphysis pubis at maturity.
   3. Metabolism.
      a. Basal metabolic rate (BMR) is the rate of metabolism when the body is at rest.
      b. The BMR is, therefore, highest in the newborn infant and decreases with maturity as energy requirements to build tissue decrease.
      c. The energy needs of children vary greatly due to age and biologic changes.
      d. The rate of metabolism also determines the caloric requirements of the child.

4. Temperature.
   a. Body temperature also reflects metabolism and displays the same decrement from infancy to maturity.
   b. Infants and young children are highly susceptible to temperature fluctuation as the body responds to environment changes, activity, and emotional upset.
   c. In relation to body weight, infants produce more heat per unit than older children; thus infants are more prone to become overheated.

D. Skeletal and neurologic maturation.
  1. Skeletal growth.
    a. Bone formation begins during the second month of fetal life.
    b. Bone formation can be used as indicators of age throughout the life span.
  2. Neurologic maturation.
    a. The nervous system, in contrast to other body systems, grows proportionally more rapidly before birth.
    b. Although, it is believed that no new nerve cells appear after the 6th month of fetal life, rapid brain cell growth continues during early childhood.
    c. Neurophysiologic changes provide the foundation for language, learning, and behavior development.

E. Functional changes.
  1. Lymphoid tissue.
    a. The lymph tissue follows a pattern different from other body tissue.
    b. Tissue increases rapidly to adult size by 6 years of age and continues to grow.
    c. By the end of adolescence, the lymph tissue declines to adult dimensions.
  2. Hormonal function.
    a. The pituitary and thyroid glands play a significant role in promoting a young child's growth.
    b. The thyroid gland helps the child's bones, teeth, and brain to mature; it also plays an essential role in controlling metabolism.
    c. The most important hormones for human growth are released by the pituitary gland, growth hormone and thyroid stimulating hormone.
  3. Sex hormones.
    a. Sex hormones are secreted by the ovaries, testes, and adrenals.
    b. They are produced in varying amounts by both sexes throughout the life span.
    c. The adrenal cortex is responsible for the small amounts secreted before pubescent years, but the sex hormone production that accompanies maturation of the glands is responsible for the variety of biologic changes observed during puberty.
    d. Estrogen, the feminizing hormone:
     (1) Is found in low quantities during childhood.
     (2) Is secreted in slowly increasing amounts starting at about age 11 years.
    e. Androgen, the masculinizing hormone:
     (1) Is secreted in small and gradually increasing amounts up to about 7 or 9 years of age, at which time there is a more rapid increase in both sexes, especially boys, until about age 15 years.
     (2) Appears to be responsible for most of the rapid growth changes of early adolescence.
  4. Sleep and rest.
    a. Sleep and rest are protective functions that allow tissues to repair and recover following activity.
    b This human need varies in individual children, but generally changes in quality with age.
    c. Infants spend as much 50% of sleep time in what is called active sleep.
     (1) Active sleep is often identified by rapid eye movement.
     (2) Rapid eye movement exercises the brain, possibly helping it to mature.
    d. During the latter part of the first year, most children sleep through the night, and daytime sleep begins to decrease in length.
    e. By 5 years of age, 20% of sleep time is in the rapid eye movement phase; the remainder is in deep quiet slumber.

III. Influences Affecting Growth and Development

◆ ◆ ◆ ◆ ◆ ◆ ◆ ◆ ◆ ◆ ◆ ◆ ◆ ◆ ◆ ◆ ◆ ◆

A. Internal influences.
  1. Heredity.
    a. Genetic characteristics are transmitted from parent to child.
    b. Biologic inheritance is an active influence on human development throughout life.
     (1) Different forms of genes are inherited in pairs from each parent.
     (2) They work together in a dominant (controlling) or recessive (yielding) relationship.
    c. Genes have been shown to be responsible for certain diseases and physical characteristics in children. For example:
     (1) Cystic fibrosis is carried by a recessive gene.
     (2) Full lips are an example of a physical

Table 1-2
Physical Characteristics Inherited as Dominant or Recessive Traits

Dominant
Brown eyes
Long eye lashes
Narrow nose bridge
Full lips
Dark hair
Curly hair
2nd toe longer than big toe
Right handed
Dark skin color

Recessive
Blue eyes
Short eye lashes
Broad nose bridge
Thin lips
Blond hair
Straight hair
Big toe the longest toe
Left handed
Light skin

Table 1-3
Common Conditions Inherited as Dominant or Recessive Traits: Chance of Occurrence

Dominant
Neurofibromatosis
50% chance of having
50% chance of not having

Recessive
Cystic Fibrosis
25% chance of having
50% chance of carrying
25% chance of not having

Sickle Cell Anemia
25% chance of having
50% chance of carrying
25% chance of not having

Autosomal recessive disorders or characteristics will occur only when both genes of the pair are abnormal. Parents with autosomal recessive disorder (carrier state) have a 25% chance of passing the defect on to each child, a 50% chance of passing on the carrier state, and a 25% chance of passing on normal genes.

characteristic that demonstrates the dominant relationship (see Tables 1-2 and 1-3).

2. Gender.
   a. Differences in abilities, strength, and temperament have been attributed to gender.
   b. However, recent research studies conducted by Jacklin and Maccoby (1992) conclude that predicting an individual's ability on gender is impossible.

B. External influences. *See Chapter 7: Home and Family.*
   1. Cultural patterns. *See Chapter 29: Cultural Influences.*
      a. Culture is the way of life of a people.
      b. It is significant in the development of motor skills, speech patterns, and play.
      c. These, in turn, influence the growth and development of a child.
   2. Socioeconomic status.
      a. The socioeconomic level of a family depends on the income, education, and social status of its members.
      b. Resources available and stimulation provided may influence the child's ability to reach potentials.
      c. These resources may be more of an influence than actual socioeconomic status.
   3. Family structure.
      a. The family structure is the actual physical composition of the family.
      b. The structure of the American family is frequently cited as a source of emotional or criminal behavior in children.
      c. Current research, however, seems to indicate family functioning has a greater influence on growth and development (Hetherington, Law, & O'Conner, 1993).
   4. Family functioning.
      a. Family relationships, interaction, and child rearing practices are some components of family functioning.
      b. These factors are major determinants of how children grow and progress.
      c. Lack of nurturing and abuse are major outcomes of the dysfunctional family.
   5. Nutrition.
      a. Adequate nutrition is necessary for prenatal brain growth.
      b. Throughout childhood, adequate nutrition is needed for normal body functioning, growth, and energy.

IV. GROWTH PARAMETERS

A. Classification of infants at birth according to weight and gestational age.
1. Appropriate for gestational age (AGA): between the 10th and 90th percentile of weight 2700-4000g (6–9 lbs.); can presume that the neonate has grown at a normal weight regardless of the time of birth.
2. Large for gestational age (LGA): above the 90th percentile; can presume that the neonate has grown at an accelerated rate during fetal life.
3. Small for gestational age (SGA): below the 10th percentile or less than 2500 g (5 lbs., 8 oz.); can presume that the neonate has grown at a retarded rate during intrauterine life.

B. The American Academy of Pediatrics classification (1996).
1. Preterm: any infant less than 37 weeks of gestation.
2. Term: an infant born between the 38th week and the end of the 42nd week of gestation.
3. Postterm: an infant born after completion of the 42nd week of gestation regardless of the birth weight.

C. Other general measurements.
1. Several other general measures are sometimes used.
   a. New Ballad Maturational Assessment of Gestational Age: a valid and reliable instrument for assessing infant functioning.
   b. Brazelton Neonatal Behavioral Assessment Scale: an interactive exam measuring some aspects of a neurologic test.
   c. Dubowitz Scoring System: a measure based on external and neurologic development.
2. These measures, when compared with each other and plotted on a growth chart over time, give important information relative to the expected growth and overall health during infancy.

V. AGE-RELATED CHARACTERISTICS

A. Infant.
1. Physical growth.
   a. Weight averages 2700–4000 g (6–9 lbs.) at birth and is expected to:
      (1) Increase by 680 g (1½ lbs.) per month the first 5 months.
      (2) Double the birth weight at 6 months.
      (3) Triple the birth weight at 1 year of age.
   b. Height or the average length at birth is 48–55 cm (19–21 inches) and is expected to:
      (1) Increase by 2.5 cm (1 inch) per month during the first 6 months.
      (2) Increase by 50% by 1 year of age.
   c. Head circumference, an indirect measurement of cerebral growth:
      (1) Ranges between 33 and 35.5 cm (13–14 inches) at birth.
      (2) Increases 0.64 cm (¼ inch) per month for the first year.
      (3) Fontanels are open at birth.
         (a) Posterior fontanel fuses by 6–8 weeks.
         (b) Anterior fontanel closed between 12 and 18 months.
   d. Chest circumferences averages 30.3–33 cm (12–13 inches) and is expected to be:
      (1) 1 inch less than the head circumference.
      (2) Relatively equal to head circumference between 12 and 16 months.
   e. Appearance.
      (1) The body proportions of the infant are rapidly changing.
      (2) The head is largest and most developed at birth.
      (3) The trunk and legs slowly catch up during the first year.
   f. Dentition.
      (1) The age of tooth eruption shows a considerable variation among infants.
      (2) The order of their appearance is predictable.
         (a) Lower central incisors 6 to 8 months.
         (b) Upper central incisors 8 to 12 months.
         (c) A quick guide to assessment of deciduous (primary) teeth during the first 2 years of life is the age of the child in months minus 6 equals the expected number of teeth.
2. Maturation of systems.
   a. The brain, heart, and lungs of the neonate are mature enough to make the transitional changes that occur at birth.
   b. Survival of the neonate requires the exchange of oxygen and carbon dioxide to be transferred from the placenta to the lungs.
   c. Reflexes.
      (1) Respiratory reflexes become activated within seconds after birth.
      (2) Several other reflex behaviors with life preserving functions (e.g., sucking, swallowing, and crying) are also elicited in the healthy neonate and are readily observed.
      (3) For other reflexes elicited during infancy, see Table 1-4.
   d. Respiratory.

Table 1-4
Selected Reflexes Elicited During Infancy

Reflex	Stimulation	Behavior	Importance	Age Elicited
Babinski	Stroke the bottom of the infant's foot from heel to the toe.	Toes should fan out as foot turns in.	Lack of this reflex has been associated with brain damage.	6 to 9 months
Moro	Elicited by sudden movement of the crib or change in equilibrium.	The infant will swing arms and legs out, fanning of fingers with the index and thumb forming a "c" shape.	Absence of this reflex has been associated with brain damage.	3 months
Grasp (Palmar or Plantar)	Place a finger or object in the infant's palm or sole of the foot near the toes.	Very tight contractions of the hand muscles or toes around the object allow the infant to support his or her own weight.	This reflex provides protection from falling.	3 to 4 months
Rooting	Stroke the infant's cheek lightly from the corner of the mouth toward the ear.	The infant will turn the head, mouth, and tongue toward the stimulus.	This reflex helps the infant find food.	3 weeks
Tonic Neck Reflex	Elicited when the infant lies on his or her back with head turned to one side.	The infant will extend the arm and leg on the side and flex the opposite arm and leg to assume a fencing position.	This reflex is the first step in acquiring the ability to rotate the head toward a visual target.	3 to 4 months

(1) During the first year of life, the lungs increase three times their weight and six times their volume.

(2) The respiratory rate decreases from 60 to 30, and rhythm becomes more regular.

(3) The eustachian tube is short and relatively horizontal, placing the infant at risk of middle ear infections.

(4) The diameter and length of the small bronchi and bronchiolus leave the infant vulnerable to respiratory infections.

  e. Cardiovascular.

(1) Two unique prenatal shunts, which relate to the circulatory system, close at birth.

(2) The foramen ovale, which is the connection between the right and left atria of the heart closes.

(3) The ductus arteriosus, which allows blood to bypass the lung prior to birth closes.

  f. Gastrointestinal.

(1) The stomach capacity rapidly increases during infancy.

(2) The capacity increases from 90 cc as a neonate to 200 cc by 1 year of age.

(3) Gastric emptying time is unpredictable, peristalsis is increased, and the small intestine is immature, leading to the frequent soft and liquid stools of infancy.

(4) The gastrointestinal system is unable to handle complex nutrients until 4–6 months when solid food may be introduced.

(5) The ability to digest proteins is followed by digestion and absorption of fats by 6 to 9 months.

(6) The immature cardiac sphincter is responsible for regurgitation frequently seen in the infant.

  g. Renal.

(1) Kidney mass increases threefold during the first year of life.

(2) However, the kidney is not effective as a filtration organ or in concentrating urine.

(3) The combinations of the immature GI system and renal system create vulnerability to dehydration, which is a major

concern during infancy.

h. Musculoskeletal.
(1) An infant has all muscle fibers at birth, but they are immature.
(2) The first muscles to develop are in the head and neck, which demonstrates the cephalocaudal principle.
(3) Head control is the first motor skill an infant develops.
  (a) At 1 month the infant can lift the head briefly.
  (b) At 2 to 3 months the infant can lift the head 90 degrees from the prone position.
  (c) At 3 to 4 months head control is established.
(4) Proximodistal characteristic is seen in fine motor development.
  (a) At 2 to 3 months the infant has the grasp reflex using the whole hand.
  (b) At 8 to 9 months the infant has a voluntary, but crude pincer grasp (using the thumb and index finger).
  (c) At 11 months the infant has a neat pincer grasp, which allows voluntary handling of objects.

i. Sleep and rest.
(1) Sleep patterns change during infancy.
(2) The neonate sleeps an average of 18 hours in a 24-hour period.
(3) By 6 months, 15–16 hours of sleep are required.
(4) By 1 year, only 12–14 hours are required in the 24-hour period.

B. Toddler.
1. Physical growth.
a. Weight gain averages 1.8 to 2.7 kg (4 to 6 lbs.) per year.
b. Height increases an average of 7.5 cm (3 inches) per year.
c. Appearance.
(1) The chest circumference exceeds the head and abdominal circumferences.
(2) This increase in chest circumference, when combined with the growth of the lower extremities, gives the child a taller leaner appearance.
d. Dentition.
(1) The remainder of the primary teeth appear during this stage.
(2) The child has 20 teeth by 3 years of age.
2. Maturation of systems.
a. Respiratory.
(1) Respiration continues to be abdominal.
(2) The respiratory rate slows.

b. Cardiovascular.
(1) The blood pressure increases.
(2) The heart rate slows.
c. Gastrointestinal.
(1) The stomach capacity increases.
(2) This increase in size allows the three meals per day schedule.
d. Renal.
(1) Bladder capacity increases along with the physiologic ability to control the urethral sphincter.
(2) By 14 to 18 months of age, the child is able to retain urine approximately 2 hours before voluntarily letting go of it.
e. Musculoskeletal.
(1) Unsteady gait disappears as muscles develop and long bones grow rapidly.
(2) Muscle tissue begins to replace the high proportion of adipose tissue.
(3) Fine motor and gross motor skills increase during the toddler stage.
  (a) The 1 year old:
    [1] Builds a tower with two to three blocks.
    [2] Holds crayon with whole hand.
    [3] Walks with a wide stance or toddling gait.
    [4] Pulls or pushes large toys.
  (b) The 3 year old:
    [1] Builds a tower with eight to nine blocks.
    [2] Holds crayon with fingers.
    [3] Runs with few falls.
    [4] Manipulates pedals.
f. Lymph.
(1) Lymphatic tissue increases in size.
(2) This accounts for the presence of peripheral lymph nodes, enlarged tonsils, and adenoids.
g. Sleep and rest.
(1) The toddler sleeps 10 to 12 hours per night.
(2) One nap during the day is the norm.

C. Preschooler.
1. Physical characteristics.
a. Weight gain average remains 2.3 kg (5 lbs.) per year.
b. Height remains steady with a gain of 7.5 cm (2 ½ to 3 inches) per year.
c. Appearance is transformed as the potbellied toddler now becomes better proportioned.
d. Dentition.
(1) A few children begin to lose deciduous teeth.
(2) This may occur by age 5 years.
2. Maturation of systems.

a. Respirations remain primarily diaphragmatic until 5 to 6 years of age.
b. Cardiovascular.
   (1) Chest walls are thin.
   (2) Changing relationship between the cardiac and thoracic structures allow cardiac murmurs to be heard.
   (3) Heart rate decreases and blood pressure increases.
c. Gastrointestinal.
   (1) The stomach is positioned more vertically so it empties upward more easily leading to frequent vomiting during illness.
   (2) The gastrointestinal tract is functionally mature with gastric acids and enzymes at adult level.
   (3) This maturity allows the preschooler to tolerate most foods.
d. Genitourinary.
   (1) The sex organs continue to grow but remain dormant functionally.
   (2) Bladder control is established and kidney function is similar to adults.
e. Skeletal.
   (1) Ossification and calcification continue.
   (2) The amount of red bone marrow decreases.
f. Muscular.
   (1) Both gross and fine motor skills are used in everyday activities.
   (2) Gross motor skills are important for everyday activities such as moving from room to room and climbing stairs at this age. Gross motor accomplishments include:
       (a) Runs well.
       (b) Walks backward.
       (c) Walks up and down stairs without use of hand rail.
   (3) Fine motor skills provide information to and creative expressions for the mind, e.g., everyday tasks such as turning doorknobs and unbuttoning shirts. Fine motor accomplishments include:
       (a) Cuts out paper.
       (b) Puts together puzzles.
       (c) Makes recognizable letters.
g. Sleep and rest.
   (1) Averages 11 to 13 hours of sleep per night.
   (2) Usually eliminates nap during this stage.

D. School-age.
1. Physical growth.
   a. Weight gain averages 1.4 to 2.2 kg (3 to 5 lbs.) per year.
   b. Height increases by 4 to 6 cm (1½ to 2½ in) per year.

c. Appearance.
   (1) The child is now more graceful, takes on a slimmer look, with long legs.
   (2) Posture improves.
   (3) Facial proportions also change as the face grows faster in relation to the remainder of the cranium.
d. Dentition.
   (1) The loss of the first deciduous teeth and eruption of permanent teeth usually occurs at the beginning of this stage (about 6 years of age).
   (2) 22–26 of the permanent teeth erupt by end of this stage (12 years of age).
2. Maturation of systems.
   a. Respiratory.
      (1) The lungs and alveoli are fully developed, and the eustachian tube assumes a more downward position.
      (2) Therefore, fewer respiratory infections occur.
   b. Gastrointestinal.
      (1) The stomach capacity increases.
      (2) This permits retention of food for longer periods.
      (3) Blood glucose level is also better maintained.
   c. Musculoskeletal.
      (1) Bones continue to ossify but still yield to pressure and muscle pull more than mature bones.
      (2) The four basic motor capacities gained during this period are flexibility, balance, agility, and force.
      (3) Gross motor accomplishments include:
          (a) The 6-year-old skips, jumps, and rides a bicycle.
          (b) The 7-year-old jumps rope well.
          (c) The 8-year-old rides a bicycle well.
          (d) The 9- to 10-year-old has improved coordination and can participate in team sports.
      (4) Fine motor accomplishments include:
          (a) The 6-year-old can tie shoes, print, and cut with scissors.
          (b) The 7-year-old draws a person with 16 parts.
          (c) The 8-year-old writes in cursive.
          (d) The 9- to 10-year-old has good hand/eye coordination and can work with crafts.
      (5) The growth of this system leads to greater coordination and strength.
   d. Sleep and rest requirements for the 6- to 9-year-old is 11 to 12 hours of sleep in a 24-hour period.

Table 1-5
Sequence of Major Maturational Changes with Age Ranges (In Years)

Boys		Girls	
9.5 to 13.5	Testes begins to enlarge	9 to 13	Thelarche (appearance of breast)
8 to 14	Appearance of pubic hair	10 to 15	Pubarche (appearance of pubic hair)
10.5 to 14.5	Penis begins to enlarge	10 to 14	Adrenarche (dark thick hair covering the mons pubis)
12.5 to 15.5	Facial hair begins to grow	10.5 to 15	Menarche (first menstruation)
12 to 15	Spermarche (first ejaculation)	12 to 17	Ovulation

E. Adolescence.
1. Physical growth.
   a. Weight gains vary regarding timing between girls and boys.
      (1) Girls gain 7–25 kg (15-55 lbs).
      (2) Boys gain 7–30 kg (15-65) between 12.5 and 15 years of age.
   b. Height growth rates vary regarding amount and timing between girls and boys.
      (1) Girls grow 5–20 cm (2–8 inches).
      (2) Boys grow 10–30 cm (4–12 inches).
   c. Appearance.
      (1) A long legged, gawky appearance is characteristic.
      (2) This is due to the growth of extremities, and increases in hip and chest breadth and shoulder width.
   d. Dentition changes involve gaining second and third molars (wisdom teeth).
2. Puberty.
   a. Puberty encompasses the 1 to 2 years of rapid growth, a predictable sequence of hormonal and physical changes during which individuals become capable of sexual reproduction.
   b. The age of onset varies widely.
      (1) Onset for girls usually occurs at 8–10 years old.
      (2) Onset for boys usually occurs at 10–12 years old, 2 years later than for girls.
   c. Tanner (1969) uses five stages based on pubic hair and breast development in girls or pubic hair and genital development in boys to evaluate maturation (see Table 1-5).
   d. Pubertal delays are evaluated by the following factors:
      (1) No breast development by 13 years of age in females.
      (2) No enlargement of testes or scrotal changes by 13.5 to 14 years of age in males.
3. Reproductive development.
   a. Girls: menarche, the first menstruation, usually occurs at 10.5 to 15 years of age, with ovulation occurring 6 to 14 months later.
   b. Boys: spermarche, the first sperm production, usually occurs between 12 and 15 years of age.
   c. See Table 1-5 for the sequences of major maturational changes with age ranges.
4. Maturation of systems.
   a. Respiratory.
      (1) The rate reaches adult level.
      (2) However, respiratory volume, vital capacity and other physiologic properties related to the respiratory function are increased.
   b. Cardiovascular.
      (1) Size and strength of the heart, blood volume, hemoglobin, and blood pressure increase.
      (2) Pulse and basal heat production decrease.
   c. Genitourinary.
      (1) The hypothalamus induced pituitary output of sex hormones causes growth of gonads and production of sex specific hormones.
      (2) Girls grow pubic hair, the clitoris develops, and the ovaries grow.
      (3) Boys have an increase in genital size, then the appearance of pubic, facial, axillary, and chest hair.
   d. Musculoskeletal.
      (1) Growth of lean body mass, primarily muscles, tends to occur during adolescence after the bone growth spurt.
      (2) Epiphyseal (growth plate) closes.
   e. Integumentary.
      (1) The increase of sweat gland activity in both sexes is evident.
      (2) This change underlines the need for good personal hygiene.
      (3) The apocrine glands, mainly located in the axillae, anogenital, and nipples, become active sweat glands during adolescence.
      (4) The sebaceous glands in adolescence also create an increased skin oiliness and acne.
   f. Sleep and rest requirement for the adolescent is 8 hours per night of sleep.

BIBLIOGRAPHY

◆ ◆ ◆ ◆ ◆ ◆ ◆ ◆ ◆ ◆ ◆ ◆ ◆ ◆ ◆ ◆ ◆ ◆

American Academy of Pediatrics, Committee on Genetics. (1996). Newborn screening fact sheet. *Pediatrics, 97*(5), 758–760.

Ashwell, J.W., & Draske, S.C. (1997). *Nursing care of children.* Philadelphia: Saunders.

Ballad, J.L., Khourg, J.C., Wedig, K., Way, L., Eilers-Watsmon, B., & Lipp, R. (1991). New Ballad score expanded to include extremely premature neonates. *Journal of Pediatrics, 119,* 417–423.

Berk, L.E. (1996). *Infants, children and adolescents.* Boston: Allyn and Bacon.

Hetherington, E., Law, T., & O'Conner, T. (1993). Divorce: Challenges, changes and new chances. In F. Walsh (Ed.), *Normal family processes* (pp. 208–234). New York: Guilford Press.

Jacklin, C., & Maccoby, E. (1992). Issues of gender differentiation. In M.D. Levine, W.B. Carey, & A.C. Crocker (Eds.), *Developmental-behavioral pediatrics* (pp. 175–184). Philadelphia: Saunders.

Jackson, D.B., & Saunders, R.B. (1993). *Child health nursing.* Philadelphia: Lippincott.

Marshall, W. A., & Tanner, J. M. (1969). Variation in the pattern of pubertal changes in girls. *Archives of Disease in Childhood, 44,* 291.

Wong, D. (1995). *Whaley & Wong's Nursing care of infants and children* (5th ed.). St. Louis: Mosby.

Zaichowsky, L.D., & Larson, G.A. (1995.) Physical, motor, and fitness development in children and adolescence. *Journal of Education, 177*(2), 55–79.

STUDY QUESTIONS

1. The term "growth" can best be defined as:
   a. an increase in physical skills.
   b. observable increase in size or structure.
   c. progression toward adult levels of functioning.
   d. advancements in physiologic domains.

2. The terms "growth" and "development" are often used interchangeably. In reality, however, development refers to:
   a. linear growth.
   b. an increase in skills.
   c. a quantitative change.
   d. changes in body composition with maturity.

3. Infant growth and development:
   a. progresses through the same pattern of development or sequence.
   b. progresses steadily forward in a smooth uninterrupted fashion.
   c. progresses in one system at a time (for example, the respiratory system).
   d. progresses independently of environmental influence.

4. In describing the normal pace of physical growth, which would be the most accurate statement?
   a. Growth is rapid during infancy and childhood, then slows down.
   b. Growth is rapid in early infancy, then slows to a steady pace until just before puberty, when it speeds up again.
   c. Growth is slow at first, then accelerates until the completion of puberty, when it slows down again.
   d. Growth is so individualized that a so-called normal pattern really does not exist.

5. The cephalocaudal principle states that development proceeds:
   a. from simple to more complex forms of behavior.
   b. from the central part of the body to the peripheral parts.
   c. from the head to the lower part of the body.
   d. in an irreversible, cumulative manner.

6. In assessing a child's growth, a nurse should be aware that normal infants usually triple their birth weights by:
   a. 4 months of age.
   b. 6 months of age.
   c. 10 months of age.
   d. 12 months of age.

7. A 3-month-old infant appears to spit out cereal when being fed. What is this normal reflex called?
   a. Tonic neck reflex
   b. Babinski reflex
   c. Rooting reflex
   d. Extrusion reflex

8. The expected dentition for a 3-year-old child is:
   a. 6 deciduous and 12 permanent teeth.
   b. 12 deciduous teeth.
   c. 16 deciduous teeth and 2 permanent teeth.
   d. 20 deciduous teeth.

9. Physical characteristics of the school-age child include:
   a. slimmer, more coordinated and graceful.
   b. increase in baby fat.
   c. short legs with potbelly.
   d. poor eye/hand coordination.

10. Which of the changes below occurs first in girls?
    a. Menarche
    b. Thelarche
    c. Adrenarche
    d. Leukorrhea

ANSWERS

1.b 2.b 3.a 4.b 5.c 6.a 7.d 8.d 9.a 10.b

Chapter 2

Physiologic Principles Unique to Children

Mary Lou Gostisha, MSN, RN
Jeanne Braby, MSN, RN, CCRN

Concept

◆◆◆◆◆◆◆◆◆◆◆◆◆◆◆◆◆◆◆◆◆◆◆◆◆◆◆◆◆

◆ Anatomic structures and physiologic, psychologic, and spiritual processes in neonates, infants, children, and adolescents

Objectives

◆◆◆◆◆◆◆◆◆◆◆◆◆◆◆◆◆◆◆◆◆◆◆◆◆◆◆◆◆

At the completion of this chapter, the reader will be able to:

◆ Identify key differences in fluid status in children.

◆ Identify essential components of an assessment for fluid volume status in a child.

◆ Identify the key components of a healthy child's diet.

◆ Identify the age-related differences that occur affecting the absorption, distribution, metabolism, and excretion of drugs.

◆ Discuss problems associated with drug monitoring in children.

Key Points

◆◆◆◆◆◆◆◆◆◆◆◆◆◆◆◆◆◆◆◆◆◆◆◆◆◆◆◆◆

◆ Infants and children are more susceptible to changes in fluid volume status than are adults.

◆ Careful assessment of multiple parameters can detect changes in fluid volume status before the child is in acute distress.

◆ Nutrition during the first 12 months of life has an impact on the future growth, health, and development of the child.

◆ Breast milk provides essential nutrients and is ideal for absorption and utilization by the infant.

◆ Drug absorption, distribution, metabolism, and excretion are affected by various physical and chemical properties of medications, as well as by changes in physical growth and development.

2

Physiologic Principles Unique to Children

I. DIFFERENCES IN FLUID BALANCE

A. Overview.
Maintaining a balance of fluid is an important aspect of care for all infants and children. Physiologic differences in children make them more vulnerable to changes in their fluid status. Infants have higher metabolic rates, less mature kidney function, a larger portion of extracellular body fluid, and a greater body surface area than older children or adults. Understanding these differences and how they impact assessment and interventions is critical for all caregivers.
1. Definitions: fluid balance is the maintenance of fluid and electrolyte balance while accounting for variables that affect this balance such as dietary intake, fluid intake, metabolic rate, and kidney function.
2. Considerations across the life span.
   a. Total body water and its distribution varies with age.
      (1) At gestational week 28, 80% of the body weight is water.
      (2) At birth, 70% of the body weight is water.
      (3) Water percentage decreases until age 2 when it is 60%, the same as adulthood.
   b. Water distribution changes as we age.
      (1) There are two body fluid compartments.
         (a) Extracellular fluid (ECF) is composed of intravascular fluid (plasma) and intravascular fluid (lymph and spinal fluid). The main electrolyte in ECF is sodium.
         (b) Intracellular fluid (ICF) includes fluid contained within the cellular walls. The main electrolyte in ICF is potassium.
      (2) At birth, ECF volume exceeds ICF volume; 35% to 45% of body water is in the ECF.
      (3) By the age of 2, 24% of body water is in the ECF, approximately equal to that of an adult.
      (4) 50% of the ECF in an infant is exchanged daily. This results in a higher daily fluid requirement.

      (5) Infants are more susceptible to fluid overloads and dehydration, due to the accessibility of body fluid in the extracellular space.
   c. The metabolic rate of the child is 2–3 times greater than that of an adult. This higher rate requires greater fluid volumes to remove waste from the body.
   d. The body surface area (BSA) in infants and children per weight is greater than that of adults.
      (1) Greater BSA results in greater potential for evaporative fluid loss.
      (2) Fever and increased respiratory rate can further increase evaporative fluid loss.
   e. Infants have immature kidney function. Maturation continues for the first 2 years of life.
      (1) Decreased levels of antidiuretic hormone (ADH) and a decreased response to ADH in the renal system result in decreased ability to concentrate urine, excrete waste, or conserve fluid.
      (2) Blood flow to the kidneys is decreased due to increased vascular resistance within the renal structures.
      (3) Sodium regulation functions are immature, and unable to excrete excess sodium.
      (4) Adequate fluid intake is essential to avoid severe fluid problems.

B. Assessment.
1. Skin assessment.
   a. Color indicates the state of perfusion. Peripheral circulation decreases with decreasing extracellular volume.
   b. Warmth and color of the skin are indicators of perfusion.
   c. Skin turns from pink to pale to dusky to gray as perfusion decreases.
   d. Skin color should be even, not mottled.
   e. Skin becomes cool to the touch with increased capillary filling time.
      (1) Capillary refill is assessed by applying pressure to the nail bed, ear lobe, or fore-

head; observe the blanched area for
return of color.
(2) Normal capillary refill is less than 3 seconds.
2. Turgor.
a. Fluid loss causes the skin to become dry.
b. Decreased skin turgor results in "tenting"
of the skin.
(1) Pinch a fold of skin and subcutaneous
tissue.
(2) Normal turgor results in skin assuming
normal appearance.
(3) Pinched skin remaining raised in a "tenting" position indicates decreased fluid
state.
3. Mucous membranes.
a. Observe the amount of moisture in the mouth.
b. Observe for presence of wrinkled, dry,
cracked tongue.
c. Excessive mouth breathing can cause drying
of mouth.
d. Observe eyes for moist appearance.
(1) Eyes may appear dark and sunken.
(2) Tearing is generally present by 4 months
of age.
(3) Tears should be present if crying.
4. Fontanel.
a. The anterior fontanel remains open until the
age of 9 to 19 months.
b. The fontanel should be even with the contour
of the skull.
c. Depressed or sunken appearance is indicative
of a decreased fluid state.
5. Systemic perfusion.
a. Heart rate and blood pressure should be
within normal limits for age.
b. Extremities should be warm to the touch.
(1) Peripheral pulses should be palpable and
strong.
(2) Capillary refill should be brisk
(1–2 seconds).
6. Weight assessment.
a. Obtain current weight.
b. Compare pre-illness weight with current
weight.
c. If pre-illness weight is not available, other
indicators will need to be used.
7. Intake and output assessment.
a. Urine output.
(1) Observe urine output or diapers of infants
and toddlers.
(2) Note amount, color, and odor.
(a) Diapers can be weighed to estimate
urine volume (1 gm = 1 cc).
(b) Dark, concentrated, strong smelling
urine can indicate decreased fluid
volume.

(c) Specific gravity increases with fluid
deficit.
b. Stools.
(1) Observe the number, quantity, and characteristics of stool.
(2) Note presence of mucous or blood.
(3) If stools are watery, measure or estimate
volume and document as output.
c. Vomiting.
(1) Document the number and quantity of
vomitus.
(2) Document the appearance of vomitus.
d. Wound drainage.
(1) Wound losses can be excessive.
(2) Weigh dressings to estimate fluid loss.
e. Insensible fluid loss.
(1) Excessive perspiration may require
estimation of fluid loss by weighing
of clothing and linen.
(2) Use of warming lights and radiant
warmers increase fluid loss.
8. Behavioral assessment in dehydration.
a. Observe for decreased activity levels,
comfort-seeking behaviors, loss of interest
in the environment.
b. Anorexia may be present.
c. Note neurologic changes.
(1) Anxiety, restlessness, irritability, and
lethargy are significant changes.
(2) Infants may have a high-pitched cry.
(3) Lethargy or coma are late signs.
9. Diagnostic tests.
a. Serum sodium, (135–145 mEq/L).
(1) Primarily located in ECF.
(2) Hyponatremia (sodium < 135mEq/L)
occurs with fever, excessive sweating,
vomiting, diarrhea and renal disease.
(a) Signs and symptoms: abdominal cramps,
headache, apathy, confusion, muscle
weakness, nausea, restlessness, seizures.
(b) Water intoxication.
[1] Results from excessive oral intake,
overloading with hypo-tonic solutions, plain water enemas.
[2] Signs and symptoms: edema,
especially of eyelids and scrotum,
rales, decreased specific gravity,
hemodilution.
(3) Hypernatremia (sodium > 145 mEq/L).
(a) Occurs with high salt intake with feedings, renal disease, and increased fluid
loss without sodium loss.
(b) Signs and symptoms: flushed skin, dry
mucous membranes, elevated temperature, nausea, vomiting, and intense
thirst.

b. Serum potassium (3.5–5.0 mEq/L).
  (1) Largely contained in ICF.
  (2) Hypokalemia (potassium < 3.5 mEq/L).
    (a) Occurs with loss of gastric and/or intestinal secretions.
    (b) Occurs when IV fluid does not replace losses in urine and body fluids.
    (c) Lost from the ICF with dehydration or tissue injury.
    (d) Signs and symptoms: nausea, lethargy, dizziness, EKG changes (flattened T waves, ST depression), arrhythmias, diarrhea, confusion, decreased blood pressure.
  (3) Hyperkalemia (potassium > 5.0 mEq/L).
    (a) Occurs with hemolysis, tissue necrosis and with some diuretics.
    (b) Can occur with rapid administration of IV potassium or with renal failure.
    (c) Signs and symptoms: nausea, diarrhea, abdominal cramps, muscle weakness, EKG changes (tall peaked T waves, widened QRS progressing to sine waves), arrhythmias, cardiac arrest.
c. Serum chloride (98–108 mEq/L).
  (1) Found equally in ECF and ICF.
  (2) Levels generally parallel sodium levels.
  (3) Hypochloremia (chloride < 98 mEq/L).
    (a) Occurs with vomiting, diarrhea, gastric suction, sweating, and diuretic therapy.
    (b) Signs and symptoms: hypertonic muscles, decreased respirations, hyperirritability.
  (4) Hyperchloremia (chloride > 108 mEq/L).
    (a) Occurs with loss of body fluids, hyperventilation, head injury, and renal disease.
    (b) Signs and symptoms: tachypnea, weakness, lethargy.
d. Serum calcium (9.0–11.5 mEq/L).
  (1) Enters through the small intestine, deposited in bone.
  (2) Hypocalcemia (calcium < 9.0 mEq/L).
    (a) Pulled from ECF with burns or severe infection.
    (b) Calcium decreases with diarrhea, nephrosis, malabsorption, and ingestion of cow's milk in the newborn.
    (c) Signs and symptoms: neuromuscular irritability, seizures, tetany, abdominal cramps, EKG changes (prolonged Q-T interval), anxiety, twitching around the mouth.
  (3) Hypercalcemia (calcium < 11.5 mEq/L).
    (a) Occurs with hyperparathyroidism, prolonged immobilization, thyroid disease, and excessive use of diuretics.
    (b) Signs and symptoms: anorexia, constipation, dehydration, dry mouth, apathy, polyuria, hypotonic muscles, EKG changes (shortened Q-T interval).
e. Hemoglobin and hematocrit (see Table 2-1).
  (1) Hematocrit is the volume of cells and plasma in circulation.
  (2) Hemoglobin is found within the red cell and carries oxygen in the blood.
  (3) Hypervolemia decreases both hematocrit and hemoglobin due to dilution.
  (4) Hypovolemia raises both hematocrit and hemoglobin due to hemoconcentration.
  (5) Preexisting anemias may cause hematocrit and hemoglobin to stay within normal in decreased fluid volume states.
f. Serum blood urea nitrogen (5–20 mg/dl).
  (1) Cleared from the blood by the kidney.
  (2) Protein catabolism causes a rise in production of urea.
  (3) Dehydration causes decreased blood flow to the kidneys and decreased clearance of urea.
g. Serum creatinine (0.5–1.5 mg/dl).
  (1) Creatinine levels increase with renal dysfunction.
  (2) Levels increase with decreased blood flow to the kidney.
h. Serum osmolality (270–285 mOsm/kg).
  (1) Indicates the amount of solute in serum, general indication of hydration status.
  (2) Parallels sodium levels.
i. Urine specific gravity (1.002–1.030).
  (1) Measures the concentrating and diluting ability of the kidney.
  (2) General indicator of hydration in children.
  (3) Not reliable in infants due to immature renal function and an inability to concentrate urine.
  (4) Not reliable in children with underlying renal dysfunction.
j. Urine osmolality (0–4 months: 50–600 mOsm/kg H_2O; > 5 months: 50–1400 mOsm/kg H_2O).
  (1) Measures the number of solutes in solution.
  (2) More exact than specific gravity.
  (3) Best indicator of the kidneys' ability to concentrate urine.
k. Urine pH (5–8).
  (1) pH indicates acidity or alkalinity of urine.
  (2) A pH of < 5.0 occurs with diarrhea, dehydration, acidosis, nephritis, or uncontrolled diabetes.

Table 2-1
Hemoglobin (Hgb.) and Hematocrit (Hct.)

| Hemoglobin (Hgb.) and Hematocrit (Hct.) | | |
| Normal Values | | |
Age	Hgb. (gm/dl)	Hct. (%)
0–1 wk	18.0 (14.5–24.5)	54 (44–64)
1–3 wks	16.5 (12.5–20.5)	49 (39–59)
1–4 mo	14.0 (10.7–17.3)	42 (35–49)
4–7 mo	12.2 (9.9–14.5)	36 (29–43)
7–13 mo	11.8 (9.5–14.1)	35 (30–40)
13–25 mo	11.5 (9.2–13.8)	35 (30–40)
25 mo–3 yr	12.0 (10.2–14.8)	36 (31–41)
3–6 yr	12.6 (10.3–14.9)	37 (32–42)
6–9 yr	12.9 (10.6–15.2)	37 (32–42)
9–12 yr	13.4 (11.1–15.7)	39 (34–44)
12–16 yr	13.4 (11.1–15.7)	39 (34–44)

Reprinted with permission from O'Donnell, D., & Lathrop, J. (1993). *Pediatric fluids and electrolytes*. Milwaukee, WI: Maxishare, p. 31.

(3) A pH of > 7.0 occurs with urinary tract infections, vomiting, pyloric obstruction, alkalosis, and salicylate intoxication.
l. Urine ketones (negative).
  (1) Ketones are formed when fat is burned as fuel in the body.
  (2) Children are more susceptible to ketone production than adults.
  (3) Ketonuria accompanies dehydration, fevers, gastrointestinal disturbances, prolonged vomiting, and anorexia.
10. Fluid needs (see Table 2-2).
  a. Maintenance fluid needs are met by replacing fluids and electrolytes being lost through normal body processes.
  b. Deficit fluid needs are met by replacing fluids and electrolytes lost prior to the start of treatment.

C. Common outcomes and nursing interventions.
1. Outcomes: the child/adolescent and/or parent will:
  a. Verbalize knowledge of monitoring fluid status.
  b. Have serum electrolytes within normal limits for age.
  c. Weigh within normal limits for patient.
  d. Feel no excessive thirst.
2. Nursing interventions.
  a. Determine any active causes of fluid loss and use nursing actions to prevent further loss.
  b. Maintain IV for fluid replacement (if present).
  c. Encourage fluids by mouth if able to tolerate.
  d. Monitor intake and output.
  e. Monitor vital signs.
  f. Monitor urine specific gravity.
  g. Weigh daily.
  h. Monitor serum electrolytes.
  i. Repeat assessments to assess for fluid volume status.

D. Home care considerations.
1. Assess for fluid volume and electrolyte status.
2. Instruct family in signs and symptoms to observe and report.

Table 2-2
Daily Maintenance Fluid Needs

Scale: Daily Maintenance Fluid Needs	
Weight	**Fluid Needs per 24 Hours**
Newborn (0–72 hrs)	60–100 ml/kg
0–10 kg (0–22 lbs.)	100 ml/kg
11–20 kg (24–44 lbs)	1000 ml plus 50 ml/kg > 10 kg
> 20 kg (> 44 lbs.)	1500 ml plus 20 ml/kg > 20 kg

Reprinted with permission from O'Donnell, D., & Lathrop, J. (1993). *Pediatric fluid and electrolytes.* Milwaukee, WI: Maxishare, p. 38.

II. NUTRITION

◆ ◆ ◆ ◆ ◆ ◆ ◆ ◆ ◆ ◆ ◆ ◆ ◆ ◆ ◆ ◆ ◆ ◆ ◆

A. Overview.

Infants and children have high nutrient requirements relative to their body size due to the many growth processes occurring during this time. The body needs fuel to work properly. Nutrients are involved in all body processes, including repairing tissue, fighting infection, and thinking.

1. Definition: nutrition is the process by which an individual takes in and utilizes food.
2. Considerations across the life span.
   a. Nutrition during the first 12 months of life affects the future growth, health, and development of the infant. The infant grows faster during this time than during any other period. The infant's diet should supply nutrients for optimal growth and development, but should not exceed these requirements. The infant's organ systems are not fully developed; therefore, infants are not yet able to digest, metabolize, and excrete all nutrients.
   (1) Breast milk provides the essential nutrients needed and is ideal for absorption and utilization by the rapidly developing infant.
      (a) Colostrum provides enzymes that facilitate digestion, promote gut maturation, and assist in the passage of meconium.
      (b) Breast milk contains immunoglobulins and helps provide protection against infection and allergic diseases.
      (c) Breastfed infants need certain vitamin and mineral supplements.
         [1] Begin Vitamin D supplementation shortly after birth.
         [2] Do not start fluoride supplements until after 6 months of age to prevent dental fluorosis (brown discoloration).
         [3] Start iron supplementation after 6 months of age when fetal iron stores are diminished. Iron may be given in the format of iron-fortified cereal.
         [4] Breastfed infants of vegetarian mothers may need B-12 supplementation.
      (d) Contraindications to breastfeeding include mothers with HIV virus and those taking certain medications.
   (2) Commercially prepared formulas are nutritionally adequate alternatives to breastfeeding.
      (a) Infants fed commercial iron-fortified formula generally do not need vitamin or mineral supplementation.
      (b) Give fluoride supplements only if the community water contains less than 0.3 ppm of fluoride, and if the formula used is powdered or concentrated.
   (3) Solid foods may be introduced after 6 months of age.
      (a) Strained foods are best introduced one at a time to allow for detection of food allergies or intolerance.
      (b) Dry cereal may be mixed with formula but should not be added to a bottle unless specified for reflux.

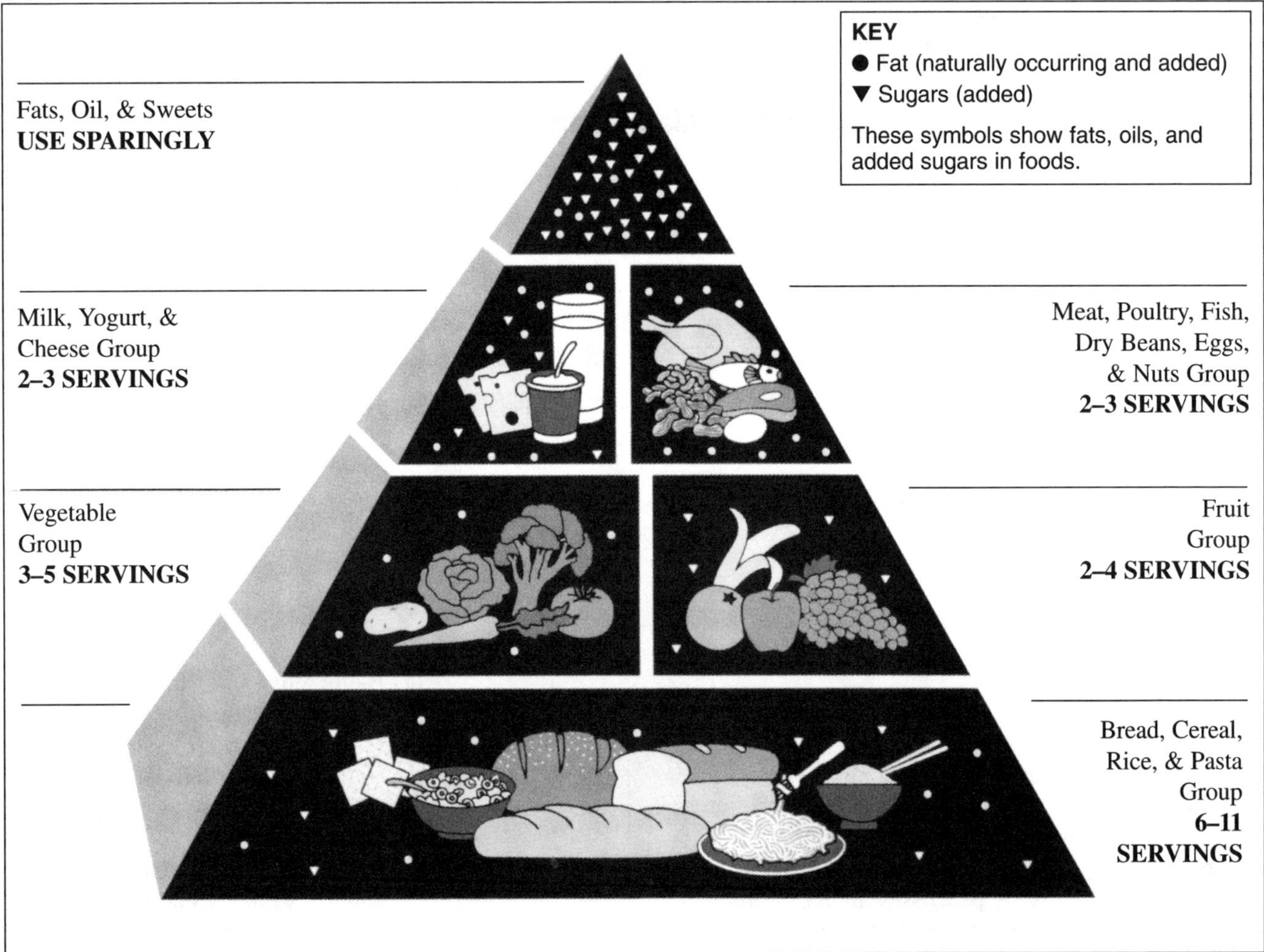

Figure 2-1
Food Guide Pyramid: A Guide to Daily Food Choices

Source: U.S. Department of Agriculture and the U.S. Department of Health and Human Services

b. A diet consisting of whole milk and soft cooked whole foods and ground meats may be used for children from 12 to 18 months of age. Do not use raw fruits (except bananas) or raw vegetables.

c. Children older than 1 year of age may be given a diet consisting of foods from the Food Pyramid Group (see Figure 2-1). The serving sizes are adjusted for age groups (see Table 2-3).

(1) Encourage children to try new foods, and to avoid excessive use of high fat, sugar, salt, and caffeinated beverages.

(2) Children less than 4 years of age are at risk for choking. Avoid raw carrots, nuts, grapes, and whole hot dogs in this age group.

B. Assessment. *Also see Chapter 4: Health, Psychosocial, and Developmental Screening and Assessment.*

1. History and physical exam.

a. An infant or child's general appearance will often give an initial impression of his/her nutritional status.

b. Use established growth charts to progressively follow height and weight changes.

c. Use weight to height ratio.

2. Diagnostic tests.

a. Blood samples may be used to assess for adequacy of protein, albumin, and triglyceride levels.

b. Anthropometric or skin caliper measurements may be used to assess fat percentage in the child and adolescent.

Table 2-3
Suggested Serving Sizes for Children

	1–3 Years	4–6 Years	7–10 Years
BREADS & GRAINS			
Bread	½ slice	1 slice	1 slice
Cooked cereal	¼–⅓ cup	⅓–½ cup	½–¾ cup
Dry cereal	¼–½ cup	⅓–¾ cup	¾–1 cup
Spaghetti	¼–⅓ cup	⅓–½ cup	½–¾ cup
Macaroni			
Noodles, Rice			
VEGETABLES			
Cooked or raw	2–3 tablespoons	⅓ cup	½ cup
Offer a dark green or yellow vegetable every day such as carrots, broccoli, greens, sweet potatoes.			
FRUITS			
Canned	2-3 tablespoons	⅓ cup	½ cup
Fresh	¼–½ small	½–1 small	1½ ounce
Juice	¼–⅓ cup	½ cup	1 cup
Offer a good source of vitamin C every day such as orange, grapefruit, strawberries, melon, kiwi, tomato.			
MILK PRODUCTS*			
Milk**	½ cup	¾ cup	1 cup
Cheese	½ ounce	1 ounce	1½ ounce
Yogurt	½ cup	¾ cup	1 cup*
*Offer 6 servings a day to 1–3 year olds and 4 servings to 4–6 year olds.			
**For children under 2 years of age, offer whole milk only.			
FISH, POULTRY, LEAN MEAT, DRY BEANS, NUTS & EGGS			
Fish, poultry, meat	½–1 ounce	½–1 ounce	2–3 ounces
Dry beans	⅓ cup cooked	⅓ cup cooked	½–1 cup cooked
Peanut Butter	1 tablespoon	1 tablespoon	2–3 tablespoons
Eggs	½–1	½–1	1–2
Nuts, peanuts & seeds are not suggested for children under 4 years of age as they may cause choking.			

Reprinted with permission from NCES, Inc. (1998). *Hot food facts for cool kids.* Olathe, KS: Author.

C. Common therapeutic modalities.
1. Medical interventions.
    a. A nasogastric (NG) or nasojejeunal (NJ) tube may be placed if the infant, child, or adolescent is unable to swallow foods.
    b. Intravenous parenteral nutrition may be necessary for some conditions.
2. Surgical interventions.
    a. A surgeon may place a gastrostomy tube (G-tube) when necessary to introduce nutrients directly into the stomach.
    b. A central venous line (CVL) may be necessary to provide long-term nutrition when enteral feeds are not an option.

D. Common outcomes and nursing interventions.
1. Outcomes.
    a. The infant or child will have a weight gain within his/her expected range on a growth chart.
    b. The infant, child, or adolescent will eat a diet consisting of appropriate foods and amounts for his/her age range.
    c. The infant, child, or adolescent will establish a pattern of rest/activity appropriate for his/her age range and ability.
2. Nursing interventions.
    a. Perform a nutritional assessment: general impression, height, weight, dietary intake, etc.

b. Repeat nutritional assessment on a regular basis.
c. Obtain a consult with a dietitian when necessary.
d. Teach child/adolescent and/or parent about age-appropriate diets.
e. Teach parents about appropriate feeding methods with infants and children.
f. Use a lactation consultant if necessary.

E. Home care considerations.
1. Do not force foods, or the infant or child may develop negative associations with eating.
2. Most children benefit from smaller meals in addition to planned nutritious snacks.
3. Adolescent girls going through puberty are often concerned about their weight and are at risk for developing poor dietary habits.

III. PHARMACODYNAMICS AND PHARMACOKINETICS

◆ ◆ ◆ ◆ ◆ ◆ ◆ ◆ ◆ ◆ ◆ ◆ ◆ ◆ ◆ ◆ ◆ ◆

A. Overview.
Children often respond to medications differently than adults. There are age-related differences that occur secondary to physiologic changes affecting the absorption, distribution, metabolism, and excretion of drugs. Ongoing growth and developmental changes will affect the dosage of medications in the pediatric patient. A knowledge of pharmacodynamics and pharmacokinetics will help to ensure safe and effective use of medication in children.
1. Definitions: pharmacodynamics studies how the drug molecule interacts with the receptor cell at the site of action to elicit the pharmacologic response. Pharmacokinetics studies how the drug is handled in the body, using mathematical concepts to describe the fate of the drug within the body.
2. Considerations across the life span.
   a. Drug absorption is affected by various physical and chemical properties of medications as well as various patient factors.
      (1) Oral absorption depends on a number of age-related patient variables.
         (a) The gastric pH is neutral at birth (probably due to amniotic fluid), decreases within a few hours of life until approximately day 10, when the pH then increases again to an alkaline level. Gastric pH reaches adult acidic levels at around 3 years of age. The difference in gastric pH affects the absorption of medications. Oral medications needing an acid medium for absorption are less effective in the neonate; whereas, some other drugs are absorbed more readily in the neonate's alkaline pH.
         (b) Neonates and infants less than 6 months old have prolonged gastric emptying time. This increases the absorption of medications needing an acid medium and causes delays in intestinal absorption.
         (c) Gastrointestinal transit time and peristaltic activity are variable in infants and children and depend on dietary intake. Breastfed infants typically have longer transit times than infants fed formula. Vomiting and diarrhea, which are often common in infants and children, will increase transit time, resulting in decreased absorption of medications in the intestine.
         (d) Infants have a proportionately greater surface area of small intestine. This results in greater absorption of some medications.
         (e) Pancreatic enzymes are decreased in infants. This results in decreased absorbency of medications that rely on a specific enzyme.
      (2) Percutaneous absorption of medications is increased in infants and children.
         (a) Infants and children have an immature, thinner layer of epidermis and increased skin hydration, which increases the absorption of topical medications. Less potent medications (i.e., steroid creams) are used.
         (b) Infants have an increased ratio of body surface area to weight, increasing the relative amount of medication being absorbed.
      (3) Intramuscular and subcutaneous absorption is variable and unpredictable in neonates and infants.
         (a) Neonates and infants have less muscle mass and subcutaneous fat, with a higher proportion of total body water.
         (b) Regional blood flow is variable in neonates and infants, depending on their perfusion.
      (4) Intravenous administration usually guarantees proper delivery of the medication dose. Slow infusion rates and restricted fluid in pediatrics influence when the medication actually reaches the vein. To

ensure that all of the medication reaches the child, use infusion pumps to deliver drugs to portals as close as possible to the child.

b. Drug distribution is affected by changes related to physical growth and development. The volume of distribution changes with each drug and with the age of the patient. The concentration of drug in the blood is equal to the dose of the drug divided by the volume of distribution of the drug (Vds).

(1) Neonates and infants have decreased levels of plasma protein, serum albumin, and altered plasma protein binding.

(a) Some drugs that bind with plasma proteins will not bind in the neonate and infant. This results in higher amounts of circulating unbound drugs that then can increase adverse effects.

(b) Drug binding reaches adult levels around 6 months of age.

(2) Neonates and infants have a greater proportion of body fluid for weight. Volume of distribution is greatest for neonates and decreases as one matures.

(a) At equal doses per body weight, the peak concentration of drugs in neonates and infants' bodies will be lower than adults, due to dilution of the drug.

(b) Adult levels of body fluid are reached at age 12.

(3) Neonates and infants have decreased muscle mass and fat tissue.

(a) Lipid soluble drugs have a decreased distribution volume due to the lower percentage of adipose tissue.

(b) Adult levels are reached at puberty.
  [1] Adolescent boys have an average of 12% body fat.
  [2] Adolescent girls have an average of 25% body fat.

c. Drug metabolism primarily occurs in the liver and has age-related differences.

(1) The newborn infant has an immature drug metabolic degradation system, resulting in a prolonged half-life of some drugs.

(2) Liver function does not reach adult levels until 1–2 years of age.

(3) Metabolism of many drugs may actually be enhanced from 2–3 months of age up until 12 years; pediatric patients may need more frequent dosage intervals.

(4) Drug metabolism reaches adult levels at puberty.

d. Drug excretion occurs mainly in the renal system and has associated age-related differences.

(1) Renal blood flow, glomerular filtration rate (GFR), and tubular function are decreased in neonates.

(a) Renal blood flow reaches adult levels at 5–12 months of age.

(b) GFR reaches adult levels at 3–5 months of age.

(c) Renal tubular function reaches adult levels at 7–8 months of age.

(2) Children 2–6 years old generally excrete drugs very rapidly and gradually slow down as they approach puberty.

B. Assessment.

1. Therapeutic drug monitoring is used for monitoring drug therapy in children.

a. There are some problems associated with drug monitoring in children.

(1) Most serum drug ranges were developed and tested in adults; reference values specific for pediatric age groups are not available.

(a) Neonates have increased potential for toxic effects of drugs due to their physiologic instabilities. Phenytoin, for example, is extensively bound to plasma proteins. Neonates have fewer proteins to bind drug; therefore, they have increased free phenytoin with increased side effects.

(b) Neonates require a higher serum concentration level of phenobarbital to stop seizures than in older children due to changes in the brain to blood concentration ratio.

(2) A single serum drug level is not generally representative of the average concentration. Do not make adjustments in dosage based on a single drug level without monitoring the clinical response.

b. Therapeutic drug monitoring can prevent serious toxic problems and is useful in symptomatic patients to determine nonadherence to treatment from treatment failure.

(1) Monitoring of aminoglycocides can prevent ototoxicity and nephrotoxicity in neonates and infants who often have impaired renal function.

(2) Drug monitoring is very important when the neonate, infant, or child presents with renal and/or hepatic failure.

c. Appropriate sampling methods will assist in obtaining diagnostic results. A free drug level (rather than serum concentration) is more diagnostic for highly protein bound drugs in neonates who have low albumin concentrations. Drug levels often require a relatively large volume of blood sample that could be detrimental in pediatric patients, especially to the neonate and infant.

  (1) Trough concentrations (blood drawn just before drug administration) are appropriate for most oral medications, antiseizure medications, and for medications such as digoxin, which takes considerable time to distribute to the tissue receptors.

  (2) Peak concentrations are used to monitor drugs with short half-lives and for determining toxicity.

  (3) Serial blood levels should be drawn if overdosing is suspected. Early blood levels may underestimate the severity of the problem since the drug may not be at a steady state, or the patient's clearance may change.

C. Common outcomes and nursing interventions.

  1. Outcomes: the child/adolescent and/or parent will:

    a. State why the medication is being used.

    b. State the correct dosage of the medication.

    c. Demonstrate how to administer the medication correctly.

    d. Recognize and report side-effects of the medication.

  2. Nursing interventions.

    a. Provide information about the medication: reason for medication, generic name, correct dosage, and possible side-effects.

    b. Allow the cooperative child to choose whether he or she would like to receive a medication in the liquid, chewable, or tablet form.

    c. Demonstrate how to draw up and administer the correct dosage.

    d. Explain need for drug level monitoring (if appropriate).

D. Home care considerations.

  1. Medications are usually ordered in mg/kg doses for neonates, infants, and children. Long-term medication dosages and intervals of administration need to be assessed at regular intervals and adjusted accordingly.

  2. Measure liquid medications accurately in syringes or cups with ml markings. Use a dropper only if it is included with a drug. Household teaspoons are inappropriate for use.

  3. Use the term "medication" rather than "drug" when dealing with school-age children, since

negative connotations surround the use of "drugs."

  4. Use alcohol-free and additive-free medications whenever possible. Do not crush or chew sustained-release products.

BIBLIOGRAPHY

Children's Hospital of Wisconsin Nutritional Services Department. (1995). *Children's Hospital of Wisconsin nutrition care manual.* Milwaukee, WI: Author.

Curley, M.A.Q., Bloedel Smith, J., & Moloney-Harmon, P. (1996). *Critical care nursing of infants and children.* Philadelphia: Saunders.

Hazinski, M.F. (1988). Understanding fluid balance in the seriously ill child. *Pediatric Nursing, 14*(3), 231–236.

Hazinski, M.F. (1990). Postoperative care of the critically ill child. *Critical Care Clinics of North America, 2*(4), 599–610.

Koren, G. (1997). Therapeutic drug monitoring principles in the neonate. *Clinical Chemistry, 43,* 222–227.

Milsap, R.L., & Jusko, W.J. (1994). Pharmacokinetics in the infant. *Environmental Health Perspectives, 102,* 107–110.

Niederhauser, V.P. (1997). Prescribing for children: Issues in pediatric pharmacology. *Nurse Practitioner, 22,* 16–18, 23, 26–29.

Nordeman, L., & Hamilton, R. (1996). Dehydration and gastroenteritis. *Topics in Emergency Medicine, 18*(3), 11–20.

O'Donnell, D., & Lathrop, J. (1993). *Pediatric fluids and electrolytes.* Milwaukee, WI: Maxishare.

Sagraves, R. (1995). Pediatric dosing information for health care providers. *Journal of Pediatric Health Care, 9,* 272–277.

Spencer, J.P. (1996). Practical nutrition for the healthy term infant. *American Family Physician, 54,* 138–144.

Acknowledgment

The authors wish to thank Pat Sowles, Rph, Children's Hospital of Wisconsin, for his assistance in editing the pharmacodynamics and pharmacokinetics section.

STUDY QUESTIONS

◆ ◆

1. The kidneys continue to mature and develop for:
   a. 6 months.
   b. 2 years.
   c. 5 years.
   d. 1 year.
   e. 2 months.

2. A child's metabolic rate is:
   a. slower than that of an adult.
   b. the same as an adult.
   c. 5 times faster than that of an adult.
   d. 2–3 times faster than that of an adult.

3. A prolonged capillary refill time can indicate decreased fluid volume in a child.
   a. True
   b. False

4. In a child with decreased fluid volume, the urine specific gravity is:
   a. higher than normal.
   b. lower than normal.
   c. remains the same.

5. Adult levels of body fluid are reached at age:
   a. 6 months.
   b. 9 months.
   c. 1 year.
   d. 6 years.
   e. 12 years.

6. Oral drug absorption in the neonate and infant is affected by:
   a. gastric pH.
   b. gastric emptying time.
   c. dietary intake.
   d. pancreatic enzymes.
   e. all of the above.

7. Billy is a 12-month-old with congenital heart disease who is on digoxin BID (0800 & 2000). He arrives at the clinic for a digoxin level at 9:00 a.m. His mother states that she has already given him his a.m. dose of digoxin at 8:00. Now is the best time to draw his digoxin level.
   a. True
   b. False

8. A suggested serving size of vegetables for a 2 year old is:
   a. 2–3 tablespoons.
   b. ⅓ cup.
   c ½ cup.
   d. 1 cup.
   e. none of the above.

9. Breast milk provides all of the essential nutrients except:
   a. Vitamin D.
   b. Fluoride.
   c. Vitamin C.
   d. Vitamin A.
   e. a and b.

10. Fluoride supplementation should be given to breast-fed infants:
   a. shortly after birth.
   b. at 6 months of age.
   c. only if there is < 0.3 ppm of fluoride in the community water.
   d. b & c

ANSWERS

◆ ◆ ◆ ◆ ◆ ◆ ◆ ◆ ◆ ◆ ◆ ◆ ◆ ◆ ◆ ◆ ◆ ◆ ◆

1.b 2.d 3.a 4 a 5.e 6.e 7.b 8.a 9.e 10.b

Chapter 3

Cognitive and Psychosocial Development

Mary A. Baroni, PhD, RN, CPNP

Concept

◆◆◆◆◆◆◆◆◆◆◆◆◆◆◆◆◆◆◆◆◆◆◆◆◆◆

◆ Anatomic structures and physiologic, psychologic, and spiritual processes in neonates, infants, children, and adolescents

Objectives

◆◆◆◆◆◆◆◆◆◆◆◆◆◆◆◆◆◆◆◆◆◆◆◆◆◆

At the completion of this chapter, the reader will be able to:

◆ Define growth and development in useable terms that include specification of associated domains.

◆ Identify classical developmental theories and theorists according to predominant focus on nature (heredity) or nurture (environment).

◆ Describe more recent interaction theories of development that focus on transactional effects of both nature (heredity) and nurture (environment).

◆ Identify key concepts and developmental challenges relevant to infants, toddlers, preschoolers, school-age children, and adolescents.

◆ Describe current systems of classifying child and adolescent behavioral disturbances, dysfunction, and/or disorders.

Key Points

◆◆◆◆◆◆◆◆◆◆◆◆◆◆◆◆◆◆◆◆◆◆◆◆◆◆

◆ Growth and development includes biologic, cognitive, and psychosocial domains.

◆ Classical developmental theories tend to focus on single domains of development.

◆ Newer theories focus on interactions across domains taking into account the impact of environmental context on growth and development.

◆ Nurses need to understand normal growth and developmental variations as well as behavioral disturbances that require early intervention.

◆ Interventions are needed for early recognition and treatment of common childhood behavioral problems before these problems become significant behavioral disorders.

3

Cognitive and Psychosocial Development

◆ ◆

I. OVERVIEW

A. Human growth and development: Underlying theory and science of child health.
1. Definition: How and why a person changes and/or stays the same over time (Berger, 1994).
2. There are three fundamental domains:
   a. Physical domain, which includes:
      (1) Genetic factors – genotype.
      (2) Physical stature and appearance – phenotype.
      (3) Temperament.
      (4) Nutritional status.
      (5) Physical health and well-being.
      (6) Fine and gross motor skills.
   b. Cognitive domain, which includes:
      (1) Communication.
      (2) Perception, thinking, and memory.
      (3) Receptive and expressive language.
   c. Psychosocial domain, which includes:
      (1) Emotional development.
      (2) Psychologic development and personality.
      (3) Social development and interpersonal relationships.
      (4) Home environment and other social contexts.

B. Behavioral development encompasses cognitive and psychosocial domains.
1. Domains are conceptual distinctions that are overlapping processes in reality.
2. Interaction and essential overlap between physical, cognitive, and psychosocial domains influence growth and developmental outcomes.

II. NATURE VS NURTURE CONTROVERSY

A. Controversy exists regarding the relative contribution of nature (heredity and genetic predisposition) or nurture (environmental influences) on behavioral development.

B. Developmental theories can be classified by nature vs. nurture perspectives.
1. Nature positions.
   a. Underlying assumptions.
      (1) Emphasize heredity and innate maturational processes.
      (2) Focus on active person and passive environment.
   b. Significant theorists and their focus.
      (1) Jacque Rousseau: child as an "untamed savage."
      (2) Charles Darwin: human evolution.
      (3) Arnold Gesell: maturational-organismic theory of infant development.
         (a) Focuses on "developmental milestones."
         (b) Provided the basis for items adapted for DDST/Denver II.
      (4) Sigmund Freud: psychosexual development.
      (5) Jean Piaget: cognitive development.
      (6) Noam Chomsky: language acquisition as innate process.
2. Nurture positions.
   a. Underlying assumptions.
      (1) Emphasize learning and environment.
      (2) Focus on passive person and active environment.
   b. Significant theorists and their focus.
      (1) John Locke: child as "tabula rasa" or "blank slate."
      (2) John Watson: behaviorism and classical conditioning.
      (3) B.F. Skinner: behaviorism and operant conditioning.
      (4) Albert Bandura, Walter Mischel, Robert Sears: social learning theory and modeling.
3. Dialectical-contextual perspective: nature and nurture position.
   a. Underlying assumptions.
      (1) Emphasize both nature and nurture with the notion that development of an individual cannot be understood in isolation or removed from environmental context.

(2) Focus on active person and active environment.

(3) View development as a result of imbalance and adaptations to disturbances in the person or environment.

b. Significant theorists and their focus.

(1) Georg Wilhelm Hegel: dialectic method.

(2) Lev Semanovich Vygotsky: zone of proximal development (ZPD) and language acquisition.

(3) Klaus Riegel: crisis and change as basis for development to occur; proposed life span perspective.

(4) Paul Baltes, Warner Schaie: life span model.

(5) Arnold Sameroff and Michael Chandler: transactional model.

(6) Urie Bronfenbrenner: ecological model.

(7) Michael Rutter, Emmie Werner: risk-resiliency model.

III. CLASSIC STAGE THEORIES OF BEHAVIORAL DEVELOPMENT

◆ ◆

A. Psychosexual development (Freud).

1. Human behavior is energized by psychodynamic forces divided among three components of personality.

a. Id: principle of pleasure.

b. Ego: principle of reality or self-interest.

c. Superego: principle of morality or conscience.

2. Personality development is viewed as the growth or unfolding of the general life force called sexual instinct.

3. Certain regions of the body assume prominent psychologic significance as the source of new sensual pleasures; new conflicts gradually shift from one part of the body to another at particular stages.

a. Oral stage (infancy).

b. Anal stage (toddler).

c. Phallic stage (preschool).

d. Latency stage (school-age).

e. Genital stage (adolescence).

B. Psychosocial development (Erikson).

1. This stage theory of life span psychosocial development, although built on Freudian theory, emphasizes the development of the healthy personality as opposed to Freud's pathologic approach.

2. Individuals strive to master key conflicts or core problems during critical stages in personality development.

a. Trust vs. mistrust (infancy).

b. Autonomy vs. shame and doubt (toddlers).

c. Initiative vs. guilt (preschool).

d. Industry vs. inferiority (school-age).

e. Identity vs. role confusion (adolescence).

f. Intimacy vs. isolation (young adulthood).

g. Generativity vs. stagnation (middle adulthood).

h. Integrity vs. despair (older adulthood).

C. Cognitive development (Piaget).

1. This interactionist-structuralist stage theory of cognitive development emphasizes knowledge as a process of acting physically or mentally on objects, images, and symbols.

2. Key concepts.

a. Schema: processes or ways of organizing experiences and coming to know the world, e.g., sucking and looking schema in the newborn; most schema in the newborn are inherited reaction patterns and reflexes.

b. Operations: mental or internalized equivalents of behavioral schemas; strategies, plans, or rules for problem-solving and classification.

c. Assimilation: "taking in" process of relating to a new experience and modifying it according to existing schema and/or operations available to the infant or child, e.g., pretend play is an example of assimilation.

d. Accommodation: adapting to new information;" complementary process to assimilation; adjustment of existing schemas to a new object or situation at hand, e.g., adjustment of sucking behavior necessary between breast and bottle feeding.

3. Age-related changes occur in mental activities in an orderly and sequential manner.

a. Sensorimotor thinking (birth–2 years).

(1) Stage of reflex activity (0–1 month): repetition of reflexive actions such as sucking, swallowing, and crying.

(2) Stage of primary circular reactions (1–4 months): functional repetition of simple body movements that may show beginning accommodation but no intention to actions; habitual behaviors, e.g., simple sucking, shaking a rattle.

(3) Stage of secondary circular reactions or "preserving interesting sights and sounds" (4–8 months): beginning of intentional, goal directed actions to get same result usually relating to external object; e.g., throwing a toy out of a crib, delight in making a particular noise.

(4) Stage of coordination of secondary schemas

(8–12 months): object permanence with awareness that people and objects continue to exist even when out of sight.
(5) Stage of tertiary circular reactions (12–18 months): active exploration with trial-and-error learning; e.g., putting a raisin in a small container and then exploring ways to get it out again (reaching in with fingers, shaking, turning upside down).
(6) Stage of mental combinations (18–24 months): ability to problem-solve simple situations without trial-and-error.
b. Preoperational thinking (2–7 years).
(1) Preconceptual (2–4 years).
(a) Major accomplishments relate to symbolic functions of language and imaginative play.
(b) Limitations include "egocentrism," the belief that the world is organized and centered on the child, and "animism," the belief that even inanimate objects have thoughts and feelings.
(2) Intuitive (4–7 years).
(a) Children begin to use mental processes and may get answers correct but cannot explain what principles were used to arrive at the answer.
(b) Thinking now encompasses "centration," which is focusing on one dimension of an object and believing that it characterizes the entire object.
(c) A major advance, the "5–7 shift," designates the period when a child may begin to appreciate conservation of number and mass.
c. Concrete operational thinking (7–12 years).
(1) Children gain increasing ability to understand logical processes when applied to concrete situations.
(2) Concepts.
(a) Reciprocity: notion that a change in one dimension of an object will result in a change in another dimension.
(b) Reversibility: notion that a process or action can be reversed, e.g., coming to understand that 2+3=5 and that 5–3=2.
(c) Classification: notion that objects can belong to particular categories, e.g., apples, oranges, and bananas are all fruit.
(d) Class inclusion: notion that a particular object or individual can belong to more than one category or class, e.g., bananas can fit into class of fruit as

well as class of yellow objects.
(e) Seriation: arrangement of objects in a particular logical order such as from smallest to largest.
(f) Conservation (number, mass, and volume): understanding that certain aspects or qualities of an object can change in appearance without changing the object itself.
d. Formal operational (abstract) thinking (12 years+).
(1) Children gain increasing ability to think in abstract terms.
(2) This ability to think abstractly allows them to speculate, form hypotheses, and think creatively about possibilities beyond the concrete and present realities.

D. Moral development (Kohlberg, 1958).
1. Kohlberg's theory developed from his original cross-sectional study of 84 school-aged boys recruited through two suburban Chicago schools, who were later followed up longitudinally (Colby et al., 1994; Kohlberg, 1958).
2. Children develop moral reasoning in an invariant developmental sequence.
3. Levels and stages of moral development are based on cognitive developmental theory.
a. Preconventional or premoral level.
(1) Stage 1: punishment-obedience – child behaves to avoid punishment.
(2) Stage 2: instrumental/exchange – child behaves well for some gain or reward.
b. Conventional level.
(1) Stage 3: good boy/good girl orientation – child behaves well to gain approval.
(2) Stage 4: law and order perspective – child behaves to avoid getting caught.
c. Postconventional level.
(1) Stage 5: social contract perspective – child or adolescent recognizes and respects generally accepted social mores.
(2) Stage 6: universal ethical principles – child or adolescent decides on moral standards of behavior through individual reflection and reasoning.
4. Gillian (1982; 1988) noted gender differences in moral development.
a. Male social development orients the child to ethic of principles with moral issues decided on the basis of fairness and justice.
b. Female social development orients the child to ethic of interpersonal relationships with moral issued decided on the basis of compassion and caring.

E. Spiritual development (James Fowler).
1. Spirituality extends beyond religion and affects the body, mind, and spirit.
2. Spiritual beliefs are related to the child's self-concept.
3. Stages in the development of faith are closely associated with cognitive and psychosocial development.
4. Fowler's stages of spiritual development (Fowler, 1981).
   a. Stage 0: undifferentiated (infancy) – infants have no concept of right or wrong, but spiritual groundwork is laid with the development of basic trust with primary caregivers.
   b. Stage 1: intuitive/projective faith (2–6 years) – children have magical, illogical faith with imitation of religious gestures and activities.
   c. Stage 2: mythical/literal (7–12 years) – spiritual development parallels cognitive gains as influenced by direct experiences and literal interpretation of religious teachings.
   d. Stage 3: synthetic/conventional (13–18 years) – adolescents generally accept religious beliefs and practices without significant questioning.
   e. Stage 4: individuating/reflexive (young adulthood) – there is increased skepticism and comparing of various spiritual beliefs to develop their own set of values and personal faith.
   f. Stage 5: conjunctive/faith (35–45 years) – Individuals integrate personal faith beliefs with respect for divergent perspectives.
   g. Stage 6: universalizing faith (45 years+) – individuals have unconditional regard for others, and a more detached perspective on life emerges.

F. Humanistic development (Maslow).
1. Maslow's theory of basic needs and human potential is derived from the study of healthy, creative adults.
2. Needs are ordered in a hierarchy, beginning with the most basic (Maslow, 1968).
   a. Physiologic.
   b. Safety, security, and stability.
   c. Affiliation, acceptance, and love.
   d. Ego, self-worth, confidence, competence, and success.
   e. Self-actualization.
3. Basic needs must be met to a certain degree before individuals can address those higher in the hierarchy.
4. Few individuals achieve self-actualization.

G. Touchpoints (Brazelton).
1. Touchpoints, which are universal, are those predictable times that occur just before a surge of rapid growth in motor, cognitive, or emotional development when, for a short time, the child's behavior falls apart (Brazelton, 1992).
2. The concept of touchpoints underlies a map of infancy and early child development with several dimensions:
   a. There are regressions as well as spurts.
   b. Psychologic growth takes place in many directions, not all at once.
   c. Each new achievement can temporarily disrupt the child's and even the whole family's progress.
3. These predictable periods of regression can become opportunities to understand the child more deeply and to support his or her growth.

IV. ETHOLOGICAL THEORIES
◆ ◆ ◆ ◆ ◆ ◆ ◆ ◆ ◆ ◆ ◆ ◆ ◆ ◆ ◆ ◆ ◆ ◆ ◆

A. Konrad Lorenz (1970; 1981).
1. Postulated sensitive periods as biologically programmed periods predisposed for particular learning similar to critical periods in animals.
2. Associated with the concept "imprinting," a rapid kind of learning of certain species-specific behavior patterns that occurs with exposure to the proper stimulus at a critical stage of early life.

B. Harry Harlow (1971; 1986).
1. Examined the effects of separation, isolation, and use of surrogate "terry cloth vs. wire" mothers on development of rhesus monkeys in his classic experiments at the Wisconsin Primate Laboratory.
2. Major study findings.
   a. Maternal separation and isolation resulted in dramatic impairment of social and emotional development.
   b. Physical contact and comfort are necessary components for normal social and emotional development.

C. John Bowlby (1969).
1. Defined attachment as "an affectional tie the infant forms to another specific person that binds the two together in space and endures over time."
2. Examined the importance of early mothering and the consequences of "maternal deprivation" as observed in orphanages and asylums.

D. Mary Ainsworth (1978).
1. Developed a laboratory paradigm (Strange Situation) to assess the quality of the attachment relationship in infants ranging from 12–24 months.
2. Key concepts.
    a. Early maternal responsiveness to infant cues and needs during the first 6 months of life promotes secure attachment at 12 months.
    b. Secure attachment provides a "safe base" from which the child can begin to actively explore the environment and continues to be a source of comfort when distressed.
    c. Infants who are securely attached and actively explore their environment show more optimal cognitive gains and later school performance illustrating the interconnectedness of psychosocial and cognitive development.

V. TRANSACTIONAL AND CONTEXTUAL THEORIES OF DEVELOPMENT
◆ ◆ ◆ ◆ ◆ ◆ ◆ ◆ ◆ ◆ ◆ ◆ ◆ ◆ ◆ ◆ ◆ ◆ ◆

A. Transactional Theory.
1. Development results from continual, dynamic, and reciprocal transactions between the individual and caretaking and/or social environment that occur over time (Sameroff & Chandler, 1975).
2. Key concepts.
    a. Genotype: genetic code that represents biological potential.
    b. Evirontype: family, social, economic, and cultural code that represents the type and range of environmental experiences available to a child.
    c. Phenotype: developmental status of the individual child at a particular point of assessment that results from ongoing genotype-evirontype transactions.
3. Examples of clinical problems with multifactorial etiology better understood through a transactional perspective.
    a. Failure-to-thrive.
    b. Child abuse and neglect.
    c. Attention-deficit-hyperactivity disorder.
    d. Conduct disorders.
    e. Anorexia nervosa and bulimia.

B. Ecological Theory.
1. A Person-Place-Process Model (Bronfenbrenner, 1979) proposes that understanding how and why a child (person) changes or stays the same over time requires examining the child's emerging capabilities plus:
    a. The quality of the settings (places and processes) where children spend time.
    b. Communication and linkages between settings.

c. The influence of policy decisions.
    d. Overall social, economic, cultural, and political context.
2. Key concepts.
    a. Microsystems: immediate settings within which a child may spend time during the course of development such as home, day care, school, hospital.
    b. Mesosystem: relationship or linkages between microsystems within which the child spends time such as communication between clinic staff and school; service coordination is essentially a mesosystem intervention.
    c. Exosystem: settings within which the developing child may not spend time but activities and decisions made within those settings may indirectly influence development, e.g., parent's workplace, school boards.
    d. Macrosystem: broad-based historical, cultural, political, and institutional context that influences development, e.g., introduction of managed care, welfare reform initiatives.
3. Examples of clinical interventions better understood through an ecological perspective.
    a. Early intervention programs, e.g., Birth-to-Three, Head Start.
    b. Home visiting programs.
    c. Case management or service coordination.

C. Risk-Resiliency Theory.
1. An individual's susceptibility or resistance to adverse developmental outcome is based in part by cumulative risk and protective factors innate to the child or within the social environment.
2. Certain factors are associated with vulnerability.
    a. Prematurity or other special health care needs.
    b. Difficult temperament.
    c. Male child.
    d. Maternal mental illness, particularly depression.
    e. Substance abuse in the family.
    f. Parent history of child abuse.
    g. Domestic or community violence.
    h. Poverty.
    i. Single-parent household.
3. Other factors promote resiliency.
    a. Maternal education.
    b. Easy temperament.
    c. Intelligence (child and/or caregiver).
    d. Adequate housing and income.
    e. Social support.
4. Classic studies.
    a. Werner (1982): Kauai Longitudinal Study from birth to adulthood on perinatal risk and

environmental factors in predicting developmental outcome.

b. Rutter (1979; 1987): epidemiologic studies of children of mentally ill parents on risk and protective factors predicting subsequent psychopathology as a developmental outcome.

VI. BEHAVIORAL CONCEPTS BY DEVELOPMENTAL AGE GROUPS

A. Infants and toddlers: social-emotional development.

1. Emotions represent an integration of affect as the "force" and cognition as the "structure" of mental life that includes the following components:
   a. Alteration in arousal (physiologic level).
   b. Subjective or experiential component that interprets arousal as pleasure or displeasure; precursors of emotional response in the newborn relates primarily to physiologic "comfort" or "discomfort."
   c. Behavioral or action component (response either toward or away from source of arousal).

2. Sequence of emotional development.
   a. Parent-infant synchrony.
      (1) Definition: sequencing of parent and infant behavioral signals and responses that may be highly coordinated and smooth or awkward and delayed as the acquaintance process unfolds.
      (2) This complex process of increasingly coordinated parent-infant interactions begins with parent's sensitivity and responsiveness to infant cues.
      (3) Highly synchronous parent-infant interactions in the first 6 months of life facilitate the development of a secure attachment relationship.
   b. Social smile.
      (1) Smiling in response to another person is seen at around 6 weeks.
      (2) Smiling and laughing in response to something that is amusing to infant is seen by 3–4 months.
   c. Stranger anxiety.
      (1) Definition: a tendency to inhibit approach or to avoid strangers; wariness of strangers.
      (2) This tendency:
         (a) May reflect curiosity as well as fearfulness.
         (b) Appears to be an innate response to

unfamiliar objects as well as people.
         (c) Is distinguished from fear, which includes a negative emotional response based on experience.
      (3) Stranger anxiety emerges between 6 and 8 months and peaks around 1 year.
   d. Separation anxiety.
      (1) Definition: fearfulness at being left alone by the mother or other primary caregiver.
      (2) Fearfulness.
         (a) Emerges between 8 and 9 months.
         (b) Peaks around 14 months.
         (c) Should begin to ease by 18 months.
      (3) Transition objects, such as a blanket as substitute for mother, are sometimes useful.

3. Attachment relationship.
   a. Definition: an emotional tie that develops between an infant and a specific person (usually the mother but may be another primary caregiver) that endures over time and that promotes a desire to be close.
   b. Attachment behaviors.
      (1) Proximity seeking: infant moves closer to parent when a stranger enters the room.
      (2) Contact seeking: infant who is distressed may crawl to caregiver and reach to be picked up.
      (3) Avoidance: infant may ignore or avoid proximity or interaction by turning away, hiding the face, or ignoring overtures by a caregiver.
      (4) Resistance: infant displays fussy, cranky, or angry behaviors in response to being picked up, held, or retrained, including squirming to be put down, becoming stiff, or other aggressive behavior in response to physical contact.
   c. Types of attachments.
      (1) Secure attachment with underlying emotion of love.
      (2) Insecure-anxious with underlying emotion of anxiety or ambivalence.
      (3) Insecure-avoidant with underlying emotion of anger.
      (4) Insecure-disorganized with underlying emotions being confused.
   d. Qualities of a secure attachment relationship.
      (1) The child, when distressed, is able to be comforted by attachment figure.
      (2) The child is free to be curious and explore the environment when the attachment figure is present.
   e. Secure attachment sets the stage of development whereby toddlers use their natural curiosity to explore the environment in active ways.

Table 3-1
Sequence of Language Acquisition

Age	Characteristics
Newborn	Cries as first means of oral communication
4–6 weeks	Coos
5 months	Makes monosyllabic sounds (e.g., "ba," "ga")
6–8 months	Babbles ("mamamama") Attends to own name
10 months	Uses first specific words with appropriate reference (e.g., "mama," "dada") Should comprehend word "no"
12 months	Uses 1–2 words other than "mama/dada" Increases vocabulary at an average of one word per week Comprehends simple commands
18–20 months	Uses an average of 20 words
24 months	Has a vocabulary of around 50 words Acquires one or more words per day Uses two word sentences ("want up") Should be able to follow simple two step commands (e.g., "sit down and drink your juice")
24–30 months	Uses telegraphic speech as 3–5 word sentences with subject, object and verb (e.g., "me want juice")
36 months	Has receptive language of about 800 words Understands simple prepositions (e.g., "put the ball under the table")
4 years	Uses intelligible speech most of the time

B. Preschool years: language acquisition, play, gender identity, impulse control, and delayed gratification.
1. Language acquisition.
   a. Elements of language. *Also see Chapter 30: Communication.*
      (1) Sound (phonology).
      (2) Meaning (semantics).
      (3) Order (syntax and grammar).
      (4) Use (pragmatics).
   b. The sequence of language acquisition begins with the cry of the newborn and progresses to intelligible speech most of the time at 4 years (see Table 3-1).
2. Play.
   a. Play is the major medium for early mastery of a variety of physical, cognitive, and psychosocial skills.
   b. Play has been appropriately described as the "work of children."
   c. Types of play.
      (1) Solitary play: earliest level of sensorimotor or skill mastery play by infants characterized by little awareness of other children.
      (2) Onlooker play: curious watching of other children playing, which is common among toddlers.
      (3) Parallel play: predominant style of toddler play with children engaged in similar play activity, often side-by-side, but with minimal interaction.
      (4) Associative play: some interaction and toy sharing, which occurs with older toddlers and young preschoolers, but the play is not organized enough to be considered a "game."
      (5) Cooperative play: turn-taking and active sharing when older preschool children (4–5 year olds) are actively playing together.
      (6) Dramatic or pretend play: highlight of preschool play during which children use "make-believe" play to create and act out familiar scenes like "dress up" or "playing house."
3. Gender identity.
   a. Gender identity includes the emerging self as a male or female person.

b. Toddlers can distinguish gender and will identify themselves as a boy or a girl (gender label).
c. Preschoolers tend to show sex-typed preferences; gender identity is usually firmly established and is unlikely to change.
d. Young school-agers (5–6 years) begin to express notions about how males and females should dress, behave, think, and feel.
4. Impulse control and delayed gratification.
   a. These are developmental challenges for older preschoolers and their parents in fostering school readiness.
   b. Difficulty in mastering these challenges may be related to difficult temperament, inconsistent parenting, and/or underlying attention-deficit-hyperactivity disorder.

C. School-age: adjustment to school, concrete thinking, self-esteem, and friends.
1. School entry is a major transition for children.
   a. School phobia: resistance to going to school because of dread of the school situation, concerns with leaving home, or both; usually relates to avoidance of school-related event or person such as a being picked on by a bully.
   b. School refusal: fear of school for a child under 13 years may more accurately be defined as a fear to leave love ones (separation anxiety); separation anxiety disorder may be masked as vague somatic complaints.
2. The issue of self-esteem (the competence to think, learn, and make decisions as well as the belief that one is worthy of love and respectful treatment from others) becomes a priority issue for school-agers.
3. Friends and peers take on increasing importance and influence; children who are unpopular and have few friends are frequently rejected because of excessive aggression or shyness and often have lower self-esteem.

D. Adolescence: independence, body image, sexuality, relationships, and identity.
1. Adolescence is divided into three psychosocial periods, each with distinct characteristics.
   a. Early adolescence.
      (1) Middle school period (11–14 years).
      (2) Priority issues.
          (a) Importance of peers/feeling "normal."
          (b) Moodiness with occasional withdrawal from family.
   b. Middle adolescence.
      (1) High school period (15–17 years).
      (2) Priority issues.

(a) Body image, dating, and sexuality.
(b) Asserting independence from the family.
   c. Late adolescence.
      (1) College or vocational training and career choices (18–21 years).
      (2) Priority issues.
          (a) Identity formation.
          (b) College, military, vocational training, and employment.
          (c) Intimacy in relationships.
2. Adolescent thinking may feature one or more of the following characteristics:
   a. Egocentrism: difficulty in thinking rationally about their personal experiences and interpreting them as particularly unique, e.g., "No one has ever felt so deeply as I do" about a particular issue.
   b. Invincibility fable: irrational belief that they are invincible and somehow protected from harm, which contributes to increased risk-taking behaviors among teens as well as the deeply experienced shock and disbelief when a peer is injured or dies.
   c. Personal fable: variation on egocentrism whereby adolescents view themselves as particularly gifted or special in some unusual way; this may contribute to a sense of "idealism" and belief that an individual can "change the world."
   d. Imaginary audience: an exaggerated self-consciousness and belief that "everyone" is watching them and taking note of every extra pound or facial flaw that emerges.
3. Identity formation as a key task of adolescence includes developing one's own sense of values and career/vocational goals, causing difficulty for many adolescents due to the following behaviors:
   a. Foreclosure: the adolescent simply accepts particular values or roles expected of him or her without exploring alternatives and making individualized choices; e.g., a teenage mother who drops out of school because that is what most of her peers are doing.
   b. Diffusion: the adolescent makes few commitments to any particular values or specific vocational or career path, remaining apathetic and undirected.
   c. Moratorium: the adolescent postpones clarifying values and making specific commitments while trying out alternatives; this is common among college students who may try out any number of majors before settling into an accepted path.

VII. BEHAVIORAL DEVIATIONS: MENTAL HEALTH ISSUES FOR CHILDREN

◆ ◆ ◆ ◆ ◆ ◆ ◆ ◆ ◆ ◆ ◆ ◆ ◆ ◆ ◆ ◆ ◆ ◆ ◆

A. Classification of early childhood behavioral deviations.
1. Behavioral deviations vary by degree and may be best expressed as a continuum from lesser to greater in terms of deviation from the norm.
2. Basic classifications.
    a. Perturbation: normal range of frustration and behavioral adjustments that occur in the course of normal growth and development, e.g., initial difficulties in establishing synchronous interactions in early breast feeding experience.
    b. Disturbance: behavioral difficulties that emerge when a child and family are not able to adapt to necessary changes in growth and development within a reasonable period of time, e.g., feeding experience becomes source of frustration and infant refuses to nurse.
    c. Disorder: behavioral difficulties adversely influence other domains, e.g., failure-to-thrive and subsequent delayed motor development.
3. Pitfalls of classification systems.
    a. Parent or child blaming can occur.
    b. Labeling may create an environment for self-perpetuation of expectations and maladaptation.
4. Potential advantages to using classification systems.
    a. They provide a common language for describing behavioral deviations.
    b. A continuum of perturbation, disturbance, and disorder may permit earlier identification of children at risk and appropriate interventions that avoid progression to disorder.
    c. Ongoing developmental surveillance of children and families at risk for behavioral deviations may detect earlier progression in severity and mobilization of resources.

B. *Diagnostic Classification of Mental Health and Developmental Disorders of Infancy and Early Childhood* (1995).
1. Regulatory disorders: difficulties in regulating behavior, physiologic functions including sensory, motor, attentional, or affective process.
    a. Hypersensitivity.
        (1) Fearful-cautious type.
        (2) Negative-defiant type.
    b. Underreactivity.
        (1) Withdrawn-difficult to engage.
        (2) Self-absorbed.
    c. Motor disorganization; impulsive, aggressive, fearless, and excitable.

    d. Sleep behavior disorder.
    e. Eating behavior disorder.
2. Affective disorders: relate to child's affective experience and/or distorted emotional expressiveness.
    a. Anxiety disorder.
        (1) Excessive stranger anxiety.
        (2) Separation anxiety.
    b. Mood disorders.
        (1) Prolonged bereavement-grief reaction.
        (2) Depression.
    c. Mixed disorder of emotional expressiveness.
    d. Gender identity disorder.
    e. Reactive attachment deprivation-maltreatment disorder.
3. Adjustment disorder: mild and transient behavioral disturbance associated with clearly identified event that resolves within 3–4 months.
4. Traumatic stress disorder: continuum of symptoms that emerge in response to a single or series of traumatic events and/or chronic stress. Common symptoms include:
    a. Reexperiencing trauma either through play or preoccupation.
    b. Numbed affect and/or social withdrawal.
    c. Sleep difficulties including night terrors.
    d. Increased fearfulness and/or aggression.
5. Multisystem developmental disorder: difficulty relating and communicating; autistic-like manifestations.
6. Relationship disorders: difficulties specific to particular caregiver-child relationship.
    a. Overinvolved.
    b. Underinvolved.
    c. Anxious-tense.
    d. Angry-hostile.
    e. Abusive.
        (1) Verbally-abusive.
        (2) Physically-abusive.
        (3) Sexually-abusive.

C. *DSM-IV* (1994) Classification of disorders usually first diagnosed in infancy, childhood, or adolescence.
1. Reactive attachment disorder of infancy or early childhood: a significant disturbance in social relationships that is associated with pathologic early caregiving including severe deprivation, neglect, or abuse.
2. Separation anxiety disorder: developmentally inappropriate and excessive anxiety related to separation from home or attachment figures, which is often related to school refusal.
3. Feeding/eating disorders: persistent disturbances in feeding and eating.

    a. Pica.
    b. Rumination.
    c. Failure-to-thrive.
    d. Anorexia nervosa.
    e. Bulimia.

4. Elimination disorders: disturbances in bowel and/or bladder control, voluntary or involuntary, in a child at least 4 years of age who would be expected to be toilet-trained.
    a. Encopresis.
    b. Enuresis.

5. Gender identity disorder: a persistent disturbance in a child's identification and/or comfort with their own gender that usually manifests itself during the preschool years and may cause anxiety and/or discomfort.

6. Attention-deficit-hyperactivity disorder: a persistent pattern of inattention, poor concentration, impulsivity, and overactivity that is beyond normal developmental variation.
    a. Inattentive type.
    b. Hyperactive-impulsive type.
    c. Combined type.

7. Oppositional-defiant disorder: a persistent dysfunctional pattern of negative, disobedient, defiant, and hostile behavior directed at authority figures.

8. Conduct disorder: a persistent dysfunctional pattern of aggressive behavior and/or disregard for rules or laws.

9. Pervasive developmental disorder (PDD): a spectrum of developmental disabilities that significantly affects a child's social interactions and communication, which is usually evident before 3 years of age and adversely affects learning and school performance.
    a. Autism.
    b. Rett's disorder.
    c. Childhood disintegrative disorder.
    d. Asperger's disorder.

10. Communication disorders: impairments in receptive or expressive language in terms of understanding and/or articulation.
    a. Expressive language.
    b. Mixed receptive-expressive language.
    c. Stuttering.

11. Learning disorders: significant learning problems that are usually diagnosed when a child's level of achievement is markedly below what would be expected for age, grade level, and intelligence.
    a. Reading.
    b. Mathematics.
    c. Writing.

BIBLIOGRAPHY

Ainsworth, M. (1978). *Patterns of attachment: A study of the strange situation.* Hillsdale, NJ: Lawrence Erlbaum Associates.

American Psychiatric Association. (1994). *Diagnostic and statistical manual of mental disorders* (4th ed.). Washington, DC: American Psychiatric Association.

Berger, K.S. (1994). *The developing person through the lifespan.* New York: Worth Publishers.

Bowlby, J. (1969). *Attachment and loss.* New York: Basic Books.

Brazelton, T.B. (1992). *Touchpoints.* Reading, MA: Addison-Wesley.

Bronfenbrenner, U. (1979). *The ecology of human development: Experiments by nature and design.* Cambridge, MA: Harvard University Press.

Colby, A., Kohlberg, L., Givvs, J., & Lieberman, M. (1994). A longitudinal study of moral judgement. In B. Puka (Ed.), *New research in moral development (pp. 1–96).* New York: Garland Publishing.

Coplon, J. (1995). Normal speech and language development: An overview. *Pediatrics in Review, 16*(3), 91–100.

Dixon, S.D., & Stein, M.T. (1992). *Encounters with children: Pediatric behavior and development* (2nd ed.). St. Louis: Mosby – Year Book, Inc.

Fowler, J.W. (1981). Stages of faith: *The psychology of human development and the quest for meaning.* New York: Harper and Row.

Garbarino, J. (1992). *Children and families in the social environment* (2nd ed.). New York: Aldine de Gruyter.

Gilligan, C. (1982). *In a different voice: Psychological theory and women's development.* Cambridge, MA: Harvard University Press.

Gilligan, C., & Attanucci, J. (1988). Two moral orientations: Gender differences and similarities. *Merrill-Palmer Quarterly, 34*(3), 223–237.

Harlow, C.M. (1986). *From learning to love: The selected papers of H.F. Harlow.* New York: Praeger Publishers.

Harlow, H.F. (1971). *Learning to love.* San Francisco: Albion Publishing Company.

Johnson, B.S. (1995). *Child, adolescent and family psychiatric nursing.* Philadelphia: Lippincott.

Kohlberg, L. (1958). *The development of modes of moral thinking and choice in the years 10–16.* Unpublished doctoral dissertation. University of Chicago.

Leiberman, A., Wieder, S., & Fenichel, E. (1997). *The DC casebook: A guide to the use of Zero to Three's diagnostic classification of mental health and developmental disorders of infancy and early childhood in assessment and treatment planning.* Washington, DC: Zero to Three.

Lorenz, K.Z. (1970). *Studies in animal and human behavior.* Cambridge, MA: Harvard University Press.

Lorenz, K.Z. (1986). *The foundations of ethology.* New York: Springer-Verlag.

Maslow, A. (1968). *Toward a psychology of being.* New York: Van Nostrand Reinhold.

Meisels, S.J., & Shonkoff, J.P. (1993). *Handbook of early*

childhood intervention. Cambridge, MA: Cambridge University Press.

Rutter, M. (1979). Protective factors in children's responses to stress and disadvantage. In M.W. Kent & J.E. Rolf (Eds.), *Primary prevention of psychopathology* (Vol. 3, pp. 49–74). Hanover, NH: University Press of New England.

Rutter, M. (1987). Psychosocial resilience and protective mechanisms. *American Journal of Orthopsychiatry, 57,* 316–331.

Sameroff, A., & Chandler, M. (1975). Reproductive risk and the continuum of caretaking casualty. In M. Horowitz, S. Hetherington, S. Scarr-Salapatek, & G. Siegal (Eds.), *Review of child development research* (Vol. 4, pp. 187–244). Chicago: University of Chicago Press.

Sameroff, A.J., & Emde, R.N. (1989). *Relationship disturbances in early childhood: A developmental approach.* New York: Basic Books.

Werner, E. (1982). *Vulnerable but invincible: A longitudinal study of resilient children and youth.* New York: McGraw-Hill.

Wong, D. (1995). *Whaley & Wong's nursing care of infants and children.* St. Louis: Mosby – Year Book, Inc.

Zero to Three. (1995). *Diagnostic classification: 0–3: Diagnostic classification of mental health and developmental disorders of infancy and early childhood.* Washington, DC: Zero to Three.

STUDY QUESTIONS

1. Which of the following developmental perspectives illustrates a passive person and active environment position?
   a. Maturational-organismic perspective
   b. Ecological perspective
   c. Behavioral perspective
   d. Dialectical perspective
   e. Risk-resiliency perspective

2. Clinical problems with multifactorial etiology such as failure-to-thrive is best explained by which theoretical perspective?
   a. Ethological theory
   b. Humanistic theory
   c. Transactional theory
   d. Social-learning theory
   e. Psychoanalytic theory

3. Home visiting as an intervention is an example of which ecological concept?
   a. Microsystems
   b. Mesosystem
   c. Exosystem
   d. Macrosystem
   e. Culturosystem

4. Development of synchronous parent-infant interaction during the first six months is related to what developmental task of infancy?
   a. Separation-individuation
   b. Circular reactions
   c. Initiative
   d. Autonomy
   e. Attachment

5. An infant who plays the "game" of repeatedly throwing a toy on the floor for someone's retrieval is illustrating:
   a. primary circular reactions.
   b. secondary circular reactions.
   c. tertiary circular reactions.
   d. object permanence.
   e. accommodation.

6. Egocentrism is a common characteristic of which two age groups?
   a. Toddlers and school-agers
   b. Infants and adolescents
   c. Preschoolers and school-agers
   d. Preschoolers and adolescents
   e. Preschoolers only

7. By what age should most of a child's expressive language be understandable?
   a. 30 months
   b. 36 months
   c. 48 months
   d. 5 years
   e. By school-entry

8. A major developmental stage associated with preschool development is:
   a. intuitive thinking of cognitive development.
   b. industry vs. inferiority stage of psychosocial development.
   c. "Good boy/good girl" perspective of moral development.
   d. mythical stage of spiritual development.
   e. anal stage of psychosexual development.

9. Which type of play is most characteristic of preschoolers?
   a. Solitary play
   b. Parallel play
   c. Associative play
   d. Pretend play
   e. Onlooker play

10. Which is a central developmental task of school-agers?
    a. Body image
    b. Identity
    c. Friendships
    d. Language acquisition
    e. Moratorium

11. Which of the following tasks or stages is not associated with school-age development?
    a. Industry vs. inferiority
    b. Conservation
    c. Concrete operations
    d. Latency
    e. Formal operations

12. A teenager who drops out of school, withdraws to his or her room, and shows little motivation to get a job would illustrate:
    a. identity moratorium.
    b. identity foreclosure.
    c. identity diffusion.
    d. separation-individuation.
    e. identity confusion.

13. Which characteristic of adolescent thinking would explain high risk-taking behaviors among this age group?
    a. Imaginary audience
    b. Personal fable
    c. Reversibility fable
    d. Invincibility fable
    e. Risk-resiliency rationale

ANSWERS

1.c 2.c 3.b 4.e 5.b 6.d 7.c 8.a 9.d 10.c
11.e 12.c 13.d

Chapter 4

Health, Psychosocial, and Developmental Screening and Assessment

Judith Schurr Salzer, MS, RN, CPNP

Concept

◆◆◆◆◆◆◆◆◆◆◆◆◆◆◆◆◆◆◆◆◆◆◆◆◆◆◆

◆ Anatomic structures and physiologic, psychologic, and spiritual processes in neonates, infants, children, and adolescents

Objectives

◆◆◆◆◆◆◆◆◆◆◆◆◆◆◆◆◆◆◆◆◆◆◆◆◆◆◆

At the completion of this chapter, the reader will be able to:

◆ Identify the components of a comprehensive health history on children from birth through adolescence.

◆ Develop age appropriate approaches to children from birth through adolescence.

◆ Identify the components of a comprehensive physical assessment.

◆ Differentiate between normal age appropriate physical findings and deviations from normal.

◆ Develop an age appropriate screening plan for children from birth through adolescence.

◆ Recognize age appropriate methods of developmental screening.

◆ Identify the components of anticipatory guidance.

Key Points

◆◆◆◆◆◆◆◆◆◆◆◆◆◆◆◆◆◆◆◆◆◆◆◆◆◆

◆ National guidelines provide age appropriate recommendations for preventive and health promotion services to children from birth through adolescence.

◆ A comprehensive health history and physical assessment provide the foundation for health supervision throughout childhood and adolescence.

◆ Developmental assessment is an integral part of health care services for children from birth through adolescence.

◆ Screening tests are conducted throughout childhood according to established guidelines.

◆ Age appropriate anticipatory guidance is provided to children and families at each health supervision contact.

Health, Psychosocial, and Developmental Screening and Assessment

I. NATIONAL RECOMMENDATIONS FOR HEALTH SUPERVISION

A. *Healthy People 2000: National Health Promotion and Disease Prevention Objectives for the Year 2000* (U.S. Department of Health and Human Services, 1990) provides specific goals for children's health status and risk reduction to be attained by the year 2000.

B. *Bright Futures: National Guidelines for Health Supervision of Infants, Children, and Adolescents* (U.S. Public Health Service, 1994) provides age-specific guidelines for preventive and health promotion services from birth through adolescence.

C. *AMA Guidelines for Adolescent Preventive Services* (GAPS) (Elster & Kuznets, 1994) provides specific guidelines for adolescent preventive health care.

D. *Guide to Clinical Preventive Services* (U.S. Preventive Services Task Force, 1989) provides preventive intervention recommendations for specific health problems across the life span.

E. The American Academy of Pediatrics' Committee on Practice and Ambulatory Medicine publishes *Recommendations for Preventive Pediatric Health Care* (1995) (see Figure 4-1).

II. HEALTH SUPERVISION

A. Obtain a comprehensive health history at initial contact and update during subsequent contacts.

B. Perform a complete physical assessment at each contact.

C. Conduct a developmental history and objective assessment at initial contact and update during subsequent contacts.

D. Conduct screening tests at each contact according to established guidelines.

E. Offer anticipatory guidance at each contact.

III. COMPREHENSIVE HEALTH HISTORY PREPARATION

A. Pause for a moment, clear the mind, and appear unhurried, professional, and calm.

B. Select an environment with privacy, comfortable seating arranged to encourage eye contact, and age-appropriate toys and/or activities.

C. Review the child's record to avoid unnecessary repetitive questioning and to identify information requiring clarification or confirmation.

D. Use an age-appropriate approach (see Table 4-1 and *Chapter 30: Communication*).

IV. COMPREHENSIVE HEALTH HISTORY COMPONENTS

A. Document identifying data including:
1. The child's full legal name.
2. Date of birth.
3. Parent or guardian's name.
4. Address.
5. Phone number.
6. The child's identifying number (hospital or clinic number/social security number).

B. Note information about the informant including:

Recommendations for Preventive Pediatric Health Care
Committee on Practice and Ambulatory Medicine

	INFANCY								EARLY CHILDHOOD					MIDDLE CHILDHOOD				ADOLESCENCE										
AGE	NEWBORN	2-4d	By 1mo	2mo	4mo	6mo	9mo	12mo	15mo	18mo	24mo	3y	4y	5y	6y	8y	10y	11y	12y	13y	14y	15y	16y	17y	18y	19y	20y	21y
HISTORY Initial/Interval	□	□	□	□	□	□	□	□	□	□	□	□	□	□	□	□	□	□	□	□	□	□	□	□	□	□	□	□
MEASUREMENTS Height and Weight	□	□	□	□	□	□	□	□	□	□	□	□	□	□	□	□	□	□	□	□	□	□	□	□	□	□	□	□
Head Circumference	□	□	□	□	□	□	□	□	□	□	□																	
Blood Pressure												□	□	□	□	□	□	□	□	□	□	□	□	□	□	□	□	□
SENSORY SCREENING Vision	S	S	S	S	S	S	S	S	S	S	S	O	O	O	S	S	O	S	O	S	S	O	S	S	O	S	S	S
Hearing	S	S	S	S	S	S	S	S	S	S	S	O	O	O	S	S	O	S	O	S	S	O	S	S	O	S	S	S
DEVELOPMENTAL/BEHAVIORAL ASSESSMENT	□	□	□	□	□	□	□	□	□	□	□	□	□	□	□	□	□	□	□	□	□	□	□	□	□	□	□	□
PHYSICAL EXAMINATION	□	□	□	□	□	□	□	□	□	□	□	□	□	□	□	□	□	□	□	□	□	□	□	□	□	□	□	□
PROCEDURES-GENERAL																												
Hereditary/Metabolic Screening	◄——	□																										
Immunization	□——		——►	□	□	□		◄——	□——	——►			◄-□-					□——					——►					
Lead Screening							□——	——►			□																	
Hematocrit or Hemoglobin			◄——					——□										◄——				□						——►
Urinalysis														□				◄——				□						——►
PROCEDURES-PATIENTS AT RISK Tuberculin Test								*	*	*	*	*	*	*	*	*	*	*	*	*	*	*	*	*	*	*	*	*
Cholesterol Screening											*	*	*	*	*	*	*	*	*	*	*	*	*	*	*	*	*	*
STD Screening																		*	*	*	*	*	*	*	*	*	*	*
Pelvic Exam																		*	*	*	*	*	*	*	*	*	*	*
ANTICIPATORY GUIDANCE	□	□	□	□	□	□	□	□	□	□	□	□	□	□	□	□	□	□	□	□	□	□	□	□	□	□	□	□
Injury Prevention	□	□	□	□	□	□	□	□	□	□	□	□	□	□	□	□	□	□	□	□	□	□	□	□	□	□	□	□
INITIAL DENTAL REFERRAL								◄——				——□																

Key:
□ to be performed
* to be performed for patients at risk
S subjective, by history
O objective, by a standard testing method
◄ - - - - - - - - - - the range during which a service may be provided

The recommendations in this publication do not indicate an exclusive course of treatment or serve as a standard of medical care. Variations, taking into account individual circumstances, may be appropriate.

Figure 4-1. Recommendations for Preventive Pediatric Health Care

From American Academy of Pediatrics Committee on Practice and Ambulatory Medicine. (1995). Recommendations for preventive pediatric health care. *Pediatrics, 92*(6), 751. Used with permission of the American Academy of Pediatrics.

1. His or her relationship to the child.
2. An assessment of the reliability of the information provided.

C. Record the stated reason for the visit including the presenting complaint or problem.

D. Obtain the child's birth history, which should be detailed for infants and young children, and include questions about the following topics:
1. Pregnancy.
   a. When was prenatal care initiated?
   b. How many pregnancies has the mother had and what were their outcomes?
   c. Was this pregnancy planned?
   d. How was the mother's health during the pregnancy?
   e. What medications (prescription or over-the-counter) did the mother take during the pregnancy, dosage, length of time taken, and during what month(s)?
   f. Was the mother hospitalized during the pregnancy?
      (1) Reason(s) and length of hospitalization.
      (2) Medications and treatments received.
      (3) The month(s) of pregnancy that hospitalization occurred.
   g. Did the mother use any tobacco, alcohol, or street drugs?
      (1) Name of the substance(s).
      (2) Amount.
      (3) How often.
      (4) During what month(s) of pregnancy.
   h. Did the mother's health care provider express concern about anything during the pregnancy?
2. Labor and delivery.
   a. What was the number of weeks of gestation?
   b. Was labor spontaneous or induced?
   c. Was delivery by cesarean or vaginal, and were forceps used?
   d. Were there any problems or complications?
   e. What was the baby's Apgar score?
   f. What was the baby's birth weight?
3. Neonatal period.
   a. Were there any problems with:
      (1) Breathing?
      (2) Jaundice?
      (3) Feeding?
   b. What was the baby's age at discharge?
   c. What was the baby's discharge weight?
   d. Were there any maternal complications?

E. Determine immunization status by:
1. Reviewing documentation of immunizations given and comparing it to current recommendations.

Table 4-1
Age-Appropriate Strategies for Conducting Interviews and Physical Assessments with Children and Youth

Age Group	Strategies
Infants	Have parent hold the infant.
	Comment on a positive aspect of the infant.
	Take advantage of times when infant or young child is quiet to auscultate.
Toddlers	Initially avoid direct eye contact.
	Approach slowly.
	Speak softly in a comforting tone.
	Distract with blocks or other age appropriate toys.
	Permit older toddlers to handle equipment.
Preschoolers and young school-agers	Greet the child directly.
	Provide age appropriate toys or activities.
	Ask the child a few simple questions during the interview.
	Demonstrate equipment and permit children to handle it.
Older school-agers and adolescents	Involve the child in the interview.
	Separate the child and family for part of the interview.
	Assure the child of confidentiality.
	Maintain a nonjudgmental attitude.
	Begin with nonthreatening topics.
	Respect privacy.
	Allow some choice in sequence of exam.
	Give child choice of having a parent present for exam.
	Discuss findings of exam with the child.

2. Asking the parent or guardian to bring records in for review if documentation is unavailable.

F. Obtain the child's medical history by asking questions about the following topics:
1. Allergies.
   a. What is the child allergic to?
   b. What type of reaction did the child have?
   c. Did a health care provider see the child?
   d. When did the reaction occur?
2. Illnesses.
   a. What illnesses has the child had?
   b. When did they occur?
   c. What treatments were used?
   d. Were there any complications?
3. Injuries or accidents.
   a. What types of injuries or accidents has the child experienced?
   b. What were the circumstances?

Table 4-2
Specific Health Problems

Tuberculosis
Diabetes
Heart disease
Hypertension
High cholesterol
Stroke
Kidney disease
Cancer
Allergies
Asthma
Seizures or epilepsy
Sickle cell disease or trait
Mental illness or retardation
Learning disabilities
Addictions or alcoholism
Sudden infant death
HIV, AIDS, or immune deficiency

    c. What treatments were used?
    d. What health care was obtained?
      (1) Was the child hospitalized or treated as an outpatient?
      (2) Where was treatment obtained?
    e. Were there any complications?
  4. Hospitalizations.
    a. Where and how long?
    b. What was the diagnosis?
    c. What was the treatment?
    d. Were there any complications?
  5. Surgeries.
    a. What type?
    b. As an inpatient or outpatient?
    c. Were there any complications?
  6. Medications.
    a. What medications does the child use regularly? (i.e., prescription, over-the-counter, vitamins, fluoride).
    b. What medications does the child use as needed?

G. Obtain family medical history by asking questions about the following topics:
  1. Health problems or deaths of immediate members of both parents' families.
    a. Type of condition.
    b. Age of diagnosis.
    c. Age of death.
    d. Relationship to child.

  2. Specific health problems (see Table 4-2)

H. Obtain a social history that includes questions about the following topics:
  1. Parents.
    a. Ages.
    b. Health status.
    c. Level of education.
    d. Marital status.
    e. Employment, including where, type of work, and hours.
  2. Siblings.
    a. Number, sex, and ages.
    b. Full or half siblings.
    c. Health status.
  3. Home. *Also see Chapter 7: Home and Family.*
    a. Occupants and their relationship to the child.
    b. House or apartment and its condition.
    c. Smoke detectors, fire extinguishers.
    d. Firearms, including location and presence of locks and safety mechanisms.
    e. Neighborhood safety.
  4. Support system, i.e., family, friends/neighbors, church.
  5. Financial resources, i.e., health insurance, Medicaid, contributions by noncustodial parent, food stamps.
  6. Child care.
    a. Type, location, and hours.
    b. Activities.

I. Review systems through questions about the following topics:
  1. Concerns or complaints.
    a. Has the child voiced any complaints?
    b. Does the parent/child have any concerns?
  2. Common complaints and problems.
    a. Skin rashes or lesions.
    b. Headaches.
    c. Chest pain.
    d. Wheezing or trouble breathing.
    e. Stomachaches.
    f. Urinary system.
      (1) Pain or frequency.
      (2) Number of wet diapers or voiding in 24 hours.
      (3) Day or night enuresis.
      (4) Age of toilet training or progress in training.
    h. Bowel habits.
    i. Extremity pain.
    j. Hearing.
      (1) Signs of deficit.
        (a) Lack of response to noise.
        (b) Delayed speech.
        (c) Regressed speech.
      (2) Date and results of last screening.

k. Vision.
  (1) Signs of deficit.
    (a) Trouble seeing the board in school.
    (b) Crossing of eyes.
  (2) Date and results of last screening.
l. Dental.
  (1) Brushing habits.
  (2) Fluorinated water supply or oral supplement.
  (3) Dental care.
    (a) Where and how often?
    (b) Dates of last and next screen.

J. Determine nutritional intake by asking questions about the following topics:
1. For infants under 6 months:
  a. Breastfed.
    (1) Frequency.
    (2) Length of feedings.
    (3) Total number of feedings in 24 hours.
  b. Formula fed.
    (1) Name and type of formula, i.e., ready-to-feed, concentrate, powder, and method of preparation.
    (2) Quantity per feeding.
    (3) Frequency of feedings.
    (4) Total number of feedings in 24 hours.
  c. Introduction of juice or baby foods.
    (1) Type.
    (2) Age at introduction.
    (3) Frequency and amount.
    (4) Adverse reactions.
  d. Problems.
2. For infants 6 to 12 months:
  a. Formula or breastfed assessment as for under 6 months.
  b. Cup or bottle.
  c. Solid foods, i.e., baby and/or table food, types of food introduced, frequency and amount.
  d. Problems.
3. For toddlers and preschoolers:
  a. Meal and snack schedule.
  b. Food preferences.
  c. Iron and calcium intake.
  d. Protein, carbohydrate, and fat intake.
  e. 24-hour recall.
  f. Problems.
4. For school-agers and adolescents, same as for toddler and preschoolers plus:
  a. Recent change in eating habits.
  b. Attitude toward eating and food.
  c. Recent gain or loss of weight.

K. Sleep history includes questions about the following topics:

Table 4-3
Major Early Developmental Milestones

Milestone	Usual Age of Attainment
Sits alone	6 ± 1 month
Drinks from cup	12 ± 3 months
Says first word	12 ± 3 months
Walks alone	12 ± 3 months
Scribbles	13 ± 2 months
Walks up steps	16 ± 3 months
Throws ball	18 ± 3 months
Combines words	20 ± 3 months
Pedals tricycle	36 ± 3 months
Dresses self	42 ± 6 months

1. Bedtime and bedtime routine, including sleep aids, such as bottle, pacifier, or special blanket or toy.
2. Nightmares or night terrors.
3. Bedwetting.
4. Own bed or with parent/sibling.
5. Own room or shared.
6. Time awakens.
7. Naps, including time and duration.

L. Obtain a developmental history by addressing the following issues:
1. Parents' evaluation of how this child's development compares with that of their other children at the same age.
2. Parents' expectations for what a child in this age group is capable of doing.
3. Parents' recollection regarding timing of major developmental milestones (see Table 4-3).
  a. How this compares with current development.
  b. The age of onset of any delay.
4. School progress.
  a. Current grade in school, grades skipped or repeated.
  b. Last report card.
    (1) Specific grades in specific subjects.
    (2) Comparison to previous report cards.
    (3) Teacher comments and conduct report.
  c. Parent contact with the teacher(s).
  d. Special classes or assistance child receives.
  e. Relationship with classmates.
  f. School attendance.
  g. Recent change in school performance.
  h. Concerns or problems.
5. Daily activities (see Table 4-4).

Table 4-4
Factors to Consider When Reviewing Daily Activities

Age Group	Activities
Infants	Frequency of holding
	Time in infant seat, bed, swing, and walker
	Frequency of talking and/or reading to infant
	Time prone and supine
	Frequency of moving from room to room
	Frequency of exposure to other people
Children	Time watching TV; type of programs
	Time alone playing video or computer games
	Participation in sports; level of exercise
	Frequency of playing board games
	Interaction with peers, including identification of best friend
	Participation in music, dance, or other lessons
	Maintenance of hobbies, collections
	Supervision before and after school
	Transportation to and from school
Adolescents	Relationship with parents
	Peer relationships
	Future plans for school or job
	Activities
	Drug, alcohol, tobacco use
	Sexual behavior
	Depression or suicidal thoughts
	Self-concept

6. Parents' philosophy and use of discipline for this child, including type, frequency, and reasons.

M. Ask parent(s) and child if they have additional concerns not previously expressed.

N. Observe parent-child interaction.
1. Begin observation on first sight, i.e., in the waiting room, walking down the hall, in the neighborhood or home.
2. Compare observations with parental reports.
3. Note interactions and individual actions/reactions of the parents and child.
   a. Is an infant being held or lying on an exam table?
   b. Does a toddler run to a parent for comfort or support?
   c. Is verbal communication supportive or harsh?

d. Is a child permitted to answer questions or does the parent answer for the child? *See Chapter 30: Communication.*
e. Does the child's behavior seem appropriate for age?
f. Are parents' expectations appropriate for the child's age?
g. Does the parent brag about the child or put the child down?

V. PHYSICAL ASSESSMENT

A. The purpose of physical assessment is to identify deviations from normal and determine the general state of health.

B. Physical assessment of children uses a systematic approach and considers the following characteristics:
1. Children of all ages need to be informed of what is going to be done next; other factors in the approach vary with the child's age and cooperation (see Table 4-1).
2. The scope is "head-to-toe" and comprehensive.
3. The sequence proceeds from the least threatening (heart, lungs) to the most threatening (abdomen, ears, mouth) components.
4. Use of assessment techniques varies with the child's age.
5. Range of normal findings varies with the child's age.

C. An appropriate environment for physical assessment is private, quiet, and well lighted.

D. Four basic techniques are used for physical assessment.
1. Inspection: observations made with the naked eye or aided by instruments.
   a. This is the most useful technique.
   b. Inspection requires concentration and attention to detail.
2. Palpation: using touch to obtain information
   a. Fingertips are used to assess fine tactile details such the distribution of a fine rash.
   b. The back of the fingers is most sensitive to variations in temperature.
   c. The ulnar side of the hand is used to assess vibrations such as a cardiac thrill.
   d. Light palpation is always used before deep palpation.
3. Percussion: tapping the skin and interpreting the sound produced; sounds tones include:
   a. Resonance: loud, low pitch, long, hollow (lung).

b. Hyperresonance: very loud, lower and longer than resonance, booming (lungs of a young child; not normally heard in adults).

c. Tympany: loud, high, musical, drum-like (gastric air bubbles).

d. Dullness: medium intensity, pitch and duration; thud-like (liver).

e. Flatness: soft, high pitch, short, flat (thigh).

4. Auscultation: listening to sounds produced by the body.

a. A stethoscope blocks out room noise and helps focus sound.

b. The stethoscope diaphragm held firmly against the skin hears high-pitched sounds such as normal breath, bowel, and heart sounds.

c. The stethoscope bell held lightly against the skin hears low-pitched sounds such as extra heart sounds and some murmurs.

E. Vital signs and growth parameters provide additional information for physical assessment.
See Chapter 1: Biologic Development.

VI. PHYSICAL ASSESSMENT COMPONENTS

A. General appearance.

1. Use inspection to assess the following characteristics:

a. Physical appearance.

b. Body structure.

c. Mobility.

d. Behavior.

2. Note:

a. Physical appearance (i.e., grooming, hygiene).

b. Body structure (i.e., tall, short, heavy, thin, husky, slight).

c. Mobility (i.e., coordination, symmetry, activity tolerance).

d. Behavior (i.e., age appropriate, fearful, passive, active, lethargic).

B. Integumentary system.

1. Inspect and palpate all skin surfaces, examining each body area as it is uncovered, and spreading skin folds to expose all surfaces of the neck, groin, and axillae. Note:

a. General condition.

(1) Texture and consistency.

(2) Turgor and mobility.

(3) Temperature.

(4) Moisture.

b. Color.

(1) Pigmentation.

(2) Cyanosis.

(3) Jaundice.

(4) Pallor.

(5) Erythema.

c. Birthmarks.

(1) Size.

(2) Color.

(3) Shape.

(4) Location.

d. Bruises.

(1) Size.

(2) Shape.

(3) Location.

e. Rashes and lesions.

(1) Type.

(2) Size.

(3) Color.

(4) Distribution.

(5) Configuration.

f. Nails.

(1) Color.

(2) Cleanliness and condition.

g. Hair and scalp.

(1) Hair.

(a) Condition.

(b) Consistency of color.

(c) Distribution on head and body.

(2) Scalp.

(a) Lesions.

(b) Excoriation.

(c) Bald spots.

2. Compare results with the following normal findings:

a. Circumoral cyanosis in young infants who are chilled or crying.

b. Slight peripheral cyanosis or mottling in young infants who are chilled or crying.

c. Generalized yellow skin due to carotenemia; sclera clear.

d. Mild pallor may be normal deviation.

e. Generalized erythema with fever.

f. Birthmarks.

(1) Café-au-lait spot: flat light brown patch; fewer than four is considered normal.

(2) Mongolian spot: flat bluish patch often on buttocks more often found in children with increased pigmentation; gradually fade and disappear.

(3) Simple hemangioma (stork bite): flat pink lesion present at birth, frequently on eyelids, midforehead, base of neck; fades over several years.

(4) Capillary hemangioma: flat pink lesion that appears soon after birth, becomes red and raised during the first year; gradually recedes over several years.

g. Bruises on the anterior lower legs of walking children.

3. Consider the following findings as deviations from normal:
   a. Poor hygiene.
   b. Rashes.
   c. Cyanosis.
      (1) Cyanotic heart disease.
      (2) Inadequate oxygenation.
      (3) Respiratory distress.
   d. Jaundice; yellow skin and sclera.
      (1) Physiologic: appears 24 hours after birth.
      (2) Breastfeeding: appears after the third day of life.
      (3) ABO incompatibility in newborns.
      (4) Sepsis in neonates.
      (5) Hepatitis.
      (6) Bile duct obstruction.
   e. Pallor.
      (1) Shock.
      (2) Chronic disease.
   f. Localized erythema.
      (1) Infection.
      (2) Sunburn.
   g. Bruises.
      (1) In infants who are not walking.
      (2) On face or trunk.
      (3) Linear or unusual shapes.
   h. Greater than four café-au-lait spots may indicate neurofibromatosis
   i. Areas of scalp baldness.
   j. Pubic or axillary hair before puberty.
   k. Hair tufts along spinal column.
   l. Presence of nits in hair.

C. Lymphatic system.
   1. Inspect visible nodes and erythema of nodes.
   2. Palpate nodes, using a circular motion, and note:
      a. Location.
      b. Size.
      c. Mobility.
      d. Consistency.
      e. Tenderness.
      f. Discrete or matted.
   2. Consider the following age variations:
      a. Cervical and inguinal nodes are common in children up to 12 years of age.
      b. Nodes are largest in 6- to 10-year-olds.
   3. Compare results with the following normal node characteristics:
      a. 1 cm or smaller in size.
      b. Discrete.
      c. Moveable.
      d. Not tender.
   4. Consider the following findings as deviations from normal:
      a. Palpable nodes in a young infant.
      b. Supraclavicular or axillary nodes without obvious cause.
      c. Response to infection.
         (1) Enlarged: 2 cm or less.
         (2) Discrete.
         (3) Slightly firm.
         (4) Mobile.
         (5) Tender.
      d. Associated with cancer.
         (1) Fixed.
         (2) Hard.
         (3) Matted.
         (4) Nontender.

D. Head, face, and neck.
   1. Measure and plot head circumference for children up to 2 years of age.
   2. Inspect head.
      a. Observe from the front, back, sides, and top.
      b. Note the shape, position, control, and movement.
      c. Note appearance of the anterior fontanelle in infants.
   3. Inspect face.
      a. Observe features for symmetric size and placement.
      b. Observe facial expressions for symmetric movement.
   4. Inspect neck.
      a. Note the appearance.
         (1) Symmetry.
         (2) Size.
         (3) Shape.
         (4) Pulsations.
         (5) Suprasternal retracting.
      b. Observe the degree of control.
   5. Palpate head in a systematic manner using both hands and focusing on the following:
      a. Suture lines in infants.
      b. Anterior and posterior fontanelles with the infant quiet and upright.
         (1) Size.
         (2) Shape.
         (3) Pulsations.
         (4) Degree of flatness.
   6. Palpate face focusing on the following:
      a. Irregularities.
      b. Consistency.
      c. Pain.
   7. Palpate the anterior, posterior, and lateral neck focusing on the following:
      a. Pulsations.
      b. Range of motion.
      c. Strength.
      d. Symmetry.
      e. Trachea.
      f. Thyroid.

8. Compare with normal findings, which vary with age.
   a. Head.
      (1) Growth in infants is rapid at a consistent rate and follows a percentile line.
      (2) Position is midline and held straight.
      (3) A closed posterior fontanelle is expected by 2 months of age.
      (4) An open anterior fontanel, slightly concave and perhaps with slight pulsations, is normal until 9–15 months of age.
      (5) A long thin shape is often seen in infants born prematurely.
      (6) Ridges along suture lines may be palpable in infants up to 6 months of age.
   b. Face.
      (1) Eyes are level and the same size.
      (2) Nostrils are the same size.
      (3) Lips are symmetric.
      (4) Ears are placed at the same level and are straight up and down.
      (5) Movement is symmetric with change of expression.
   c. Neck
      (1) Movement is smooth and symmetric.
      (2) Trachea is midline.
      (3) Thyroid may not be palpable in infants.
      (4) Thyroid in older children is a firm, smooth, symmetric mass that moves up with swallowing.
9. Consider the following findings as deviations from normal:
   a. Head.
      (1) Greater than expected growth may indicate hydrocephalus.
         (a) Serial measurements cross percentiles.
         (b) Suture lines are widely separated.
         (c) Fontanelles remain open past expected age.
      (2) Less than expected growth may indicate microcephaly.
      (3) Asymmetric shape may be the result of infant positioning or premature suture closure (craniosynostosis).
      (4) An edematous mass in a newborn may be the result of birth trauma.
         (a) Caput succedaneum crosses the suture line and resolves within a few days.
         (b) Cephalohematoma does not cross the suture line and requires several weeks or more to resolve.
      (5) A bulging anterior fontanelle indicates increased intracranial pressure.
      (6) A depressed anterior fontanelle is associated with dehydration and malnutrition.
      (7) An anterior fontanelle larger than 4–5 cm in diameter may indicate:
         (a) Chronically increased intracranial pressure.
         (b) Subdural hematoma.
         (c) Rickets.
         (d) Hypothyroidism.
         (e) Osteogenesis imperfecta.
      (8) Head tilting may result from muscular or sensory abnormalities such as torticollis, visual problems, or hearing problems.
   b. Face.
      (1) Asymmetric or dysmorphic features may be associated with various syndromes.
      (2) Asymmetry of movement may indicate paralysis.
      (3) Low set ears may be associated with mental retardation or kidney abnormalities.
   c. Neck.
      (1) A shift of the trachea from midline may indicate lung problems.
      (2) Resistance or pain with range of motion may indicate injury or meningitis.

E. Eyes.
   1. Observe eye shape, size, and placement.
   2. Inspect and palpate eyelids.
   3. Examine the sclera.
   4. Evaluate the pupils for size, shape, equality, and reaction to light.
   5. Inspect the conjunctiva.
   6. Assess ocular muscle movement.
      a. Have the child follow a toy or finger puppet through the six cardinal fields of gaze.
      b. Hold the child's chin to eliminate head movement.
   7. Evaluate for strabismus.
      a. Corneal light reflex test.
         (1) Note the placement of the reflection of a light shined into the eyes.
         (2) The reflection should be seen in the same place on each eye.
      b. Cover-uncover test.
         (1) Cover one eye and have the child focus on an object held at a distance of 12 inches.
         (2) Uncover the eye and observe it for movement.
         (3) Repeat the procedure with the other eye.
         (4) No movement should be seen as the eye is uncovered.
   8. Perform an ophthalmoscopic exam.
      a. Red reflex is evaluated on all infants and children.
      b. Full ophthalmoscopic exam is obtained on children who are able to cooperate by gazing straight ahead.
   9. Compare results with normal findings:

a. Eyes are symmetric and placed in a straight line.
b. Lids fully cover the eye when closed.
c. Sclera is clear white or slightly bluish in newborn infants.
d. Red reflex is clearly seen.

10. Consider the following findings abnormal:
a. Drooping eyelid (ptosis), which may be congenital or acquired.
b. Upward slanting eyes are present in Down syndrome.
c. Erythematous conjunctiva may indicate infection or allergy.
d. Continuous nystagmus often indicates neurologic disorder.
e. Unequal pupils may indicate central nervous system abnormality.
f. Lack of a red reflex is indicative of cataract.
g. Abnormal corneal light reflex or cover-uncover test indicates muscle imbalance.

F. Ears.
1. Note the structure of the outer ear.
2. Inspect for discharge from the canal, noting color, consistency, and odor.
3. Palpate the outer ear and mastoid.
4. Examine the canal and structures of the inner ear using an otoscope.
   a. Tympanic membrane.
   b. Bony landmarks.
   c. Light reflex.
5. Test the mobility of the tympanic membrane using a pneumatic bulb.
6. Compare results with normal findings:
   a. Firm cartilaginous outer ear.
   b. Patent canal often with a small amount of soft yellow-brown wax adhering to edges.
   c. Gray tympanic membrane.
   d. Clearly visualized bony landmarks.
   e. Sharp cone of light.
   f. Full mobility of tympanic membrane.
7. Consider the following findings as deviations from normal:
   a. Thin tissue-like outer ear may be found in premature infants.
   b. Pain on manipulation of the auricle is suspicious for an ear canal problem (e.g., infection, lesion, foreign body).
   c. Erythematous tympanic membrane may be normal or indicate pathology (e.g., infection).
   d. Immobility indicates infection or fluid behind the tympanic membrane.

G. Nose and sinuses.
1. Inspect the external area of the nose for lesions or discharge.

2. Palpate the nose for irregularities and tenderness.
3. Occlude each nostril to assure patency in infants.
4. Inspect the nasal interior using an otoscope with a short, broad speculum.
   a. Note color and condition of mucous membranes and turbinates.
   b. Observe for lesions.
   c. Inspect for foreign bodies.
   d. Note color and consistency of any discharge.
5. Consider child's age before assessing sinuses.
   a. Maxillary and ethmoid sinuses are present at birth.
   b. Frontal sinuses are fairly well developed by 8 years of age.
   c. Sphenoid sinus develops after puberty.
6. Evaluation of the sinuses in infancy is limited; evaluation in childhood includes inspection, palpation and percussion.
   a. Observe for swelling over sinus areas.
   b. Palpate below eyebrows for frontal sinuses.
   c. Palpate below cheekbones for maxillary sinuses.
   d. Use direct percussion over frontal and maxillary sinus areas.
7. Compare results with normal findings:
   a. Nasal turbinates are pink and moist.
   b. Sinus areas are nontender.
8. Consider the following as deviations from normal:
   a. Unilateral purulent nasal discharge is associated with foreign body.
   b. Clear nasal discharge may indicate upper respiratory infection or allergic rhinitis.
   c. Bilateral yellow or green nasal discharge in infants may indicate ethmoid sinusitis.
   d. Erythematous, edematous nasal turbinates are seen in infection.
   e. Pale, boggy, grayish turbinates are indicative of allergy.
   f. Swelling over a sinus area is associated with sinus infection.
   g. Pain on direct percussion of a sinus is indicative of sinus infection.

H. Mouth and throat.
1. Infants and young children are rarely cooperative for examination of the mouth and throat.
   a. Gently restrain if necessary.
   b. Supine position provides best visualization.
2. Inspection proceeds from the outside to the inside.
3. Note the color and condition of the lips.
4. Observe all mucous membrane surfaces using a tongue depressor to gently retract the lips and cheeks.

5. Inspect the tongue, noting color, size, movement, and surface characteristics.
6. Inspect the gums and teeth, noting color, condition, hygiene, and number of teeth.
7. Note the characteristics of the hard and soft palate.
8. Inspect the tonsils and pharynx.
9. Compare results with normal findings:
   a. Mucous membranes are pink and moist.
   b. Teeth are white without tartar accumulation.
   c. The tongue moves symmetrically.
   d. The hard palate is intact with a mild arch.
   e. The soft palate rises with crying.
10. Consider the following as deviations from normal:
   a. Red or white ulcerations may be related to trauma or viral infection.
   b. White patches on mucous membranes are indicative of thrush.
   c. Dry, tacky mucous membranes are associated with dehydration.
   d. A high arched hard palate may be associated with feeding problems.
   e. Erythematous tonsils with or without exudate are associated with viral or bacterial infection.
   f. A protruding tongue is found in children with Down syndrome or cerebral palsy.

I. Chest and lungs.
1. Inspect the chest, noting:
   a. Shape.
   b. Movement.
   c. Symmetry.
   d. Respiratory effort.
   e. Nipples, including shape, color, placement, and symmetry.
2. Palpate the chest, noting expansion, respiratory vibrations, lumps, irregularities, and nipple area.
3. Palpate the breasts, if present, and evaluate Tanner stage. *See Chapter 1: Biologic Development.*
4. Percuss the chest of older children.
   a. Compare one side with the other.
   b. Move symmetrically and systematically.
   c. Evaluate front, sides, and back.
5. Auscultate the chest, first listening with the ear for any audible sounds and then with the stethoscope diaphragm, alternating side to side and comparing sounds side to side.
6. Compare results with normal findings:
   a. Chest expansion is symmetric.
   b. Respiratory effort is unlabored.
   c. Breast tissue may be present in male and female young infants.
   d. Resonance is heard with percussion over lung surfaces.
   e. Dullness is heard with percussion over the heart and liver.
   f. Breath sounds are generally vesicular throughout the lungs.
   g. Supernumerary nipples may occur along the milk line.
   h. Breast tissue is soft, consistent and without masses or nodules.
7. Consider the following as abnormal findings:
   a. Retracting indicates increased respiratory effort.
   b. Increased respiratory rate is seen with fever and respiratory or systemic illness.
   c. Asymmetric chest expansion indicates a unilateral lung problem.
   d. Poor air exchange indicates severe obstruction.
   e. Grunting in an infant indicates respiratory distress.
   f. Stridor indicates compromise of the upper airway.
   g. Breast tissue in children less than 9 years may indicate precocious puberty.
   h. Breast tissue in a pubertal boy is most often associated with gynecomastia.
   i. Adventitious sounds are usually indicative of pathology.

J. Cardiovascular system.
1. Check pulse and blood pressure measurements.
2. Inspect the child's color and level of activity.
3. Observe the chest for visible pulsation.
4. Note any obvious bulge or heave.
5. Palpate and locate the apical impulse or point of maximum impulse (PMI), noting location and timing of any thrill.
6. Palpate and assess pulses for strength and equality.
7. Although not commonly used in infants and young children, indirect percussion may be used with older children to determine heart size.
8. Auscultate with the child in sitting and supine positions using the stethoscope diaphragm and bell at each listening area and focussing on the components of the cardiac cycle: systole, diastole, S1, and S2.
9. Note any splits or extra sounds (e.g., murmurs, clicks, snaps, S3, S4).
10. Listen to the back for any radiating murmurs.
11. Compare results with normal findings:
   a. Sinus arrhythmia may be heard in children of all ages.
   b. Splitting of S2 is heard in most young children at the second left intercostal space.
   c. A physiologic S3 may be heard at the apex in some children.

Table 4-5
Infant Automatisms (Reflexes)

Reflex	Age Present
Dazzle (blinking)	birth to 1 year
Babinski	birth to 2 years
Stepping	birth to 4–8 weeks
Extrusion	birth to 4 months
Galant's	birth to 4–8 weeks
Moro's	birth to 3–4 months
Palmar grasp	birth to 3–4 months
Rooting	birth to 3–4 months
Tonic neck	2–6 months

    d. A venous hum may be heard above or below the clavicles in some children.
    e. The PMI gradually changes location with growth.
      (1) Under 4 years: 4th intercostal space left of the midclavicular line.
      (2) At 4 to 6 years: 4th intercostal space at the midclavicular line.
      (3) By about 7 years: 5th intercostal space at the midclavicular line.
    f. The cardiac impulse may be visible in thin children.
    g. Innocent or functional systolic ejection murmurs (SEM) are commonly heard at the left lower sternal border; may be accentuated or only heard with fever, anemia, or pregnancy.
12. Consider the following as deviations from normal:
    a. Murmurs that are grade III/VI or louder, associated with a thrill, or heard during diastole.
    b. PMI at a location not expected for age.
    c. Absent, weak, or unequal pulses.
    d. An S4.
    e. Bounding visible cardiac impulse.

K. Abdomen.
  1. Inspect the abdomen noting symmetry, fullness, movement, and umbilicus.
  2. Inspect the anal area noting cleanliness and condition.
  3. Follow inspection with auscultation, listening for peristalsis in all four quadrants with stethoscope diaphragm.
  4. Using indirect percussion, percuss all areas systematically, noting areas of tympany and dullness.
  5. Palpate superficially then deeply in all quadrants and midline.
    a. Palpate during inspiration on a crying child.
    b. Note muscle tone, masses, or areas of tenderness.

6. Compare results with normal findings:
    a. Abdominal breathing is observed in young children.
    b. Bowel sounds are usually heard every 10 to 30 seconds.
    c. Tympany is heard over most of the abdomen.
    d. Dullness is heard over the liver margin, a full bladder, or a mass of feces.
    e. A reducible umbilical hernia may be found in young children.
    f. The anal area is clean and moist.
7. Consider the following as deviations from normal:
    a. Umbilical discharge may indicate infection.
    b. A palpable spleen is an indication of illness.
    c. Abdominal distention may be associated with organomegaly, tumor, or pregnancy.
    d. Visible peristaltic waves may indicate obstruction.
    e. Absent bowel sounds are associated with paralytic ileus.
    f. Frequent, high-pitched bowel sounds are heard with diarrhea or obstruction.
    g. Masses other than feces are indicative of malignancy.
    h. Anal fissures are indicative of constipation.
    i. An anal protrusion may be hemorrhoids or polyps.
    j. Venereal warts are indicative of sexual abuse.

L. Genitourinary system.
  1. Females.
    a. Inspect the external genitalia for presence and distribution of hair and deviations from normal.
    b. Spread the labia majora to observe the mucous membrane, clitoris, urethral orifice, and vaginal orifice.
    c. Determine Tanner developmental stage. *See Chapter 1: Biologic Development.*
    d. Perform a pelvic examination on sexually active females.
    e. Palpate the mons pubis and labia majora.
  2. Males.
    a. Inspect the penis, noting size, circumcision, and urethral meatus.
    b. Inspect the scrotum and visible testes.
    c. Note the presence and distribution of hair.
    d. Determine Tanner developmental stage. *See Chapter 1: Biologic Development.*
    e. Retract foreskin without force and palpate the testes, noting size, shape, consistency, mobility, and location.
  3. Compare results with normal findings.
    a. Females.
      (1) Structures are visible.

Table 4-6
Cranial Nerve Assessment

Cranial Nerve	Assessment
I. Olfactory	Not tested routinely
II. Optic	Direct and consensual light reflex
III. Oculomotor	Six cardinal fields of gaze
IV. Trochlear	Visual acuity
V. Trigeminal	Corneal reflex Jaw strength and symmetry as child bites down Light touch felt on cheeks
VI. Abducens	Full and symmetrical lid movement
VII. Facial	Symmetric grimace, eye squint, smile, frown Corneal reflex Taste not routinely tested
VIII. Acoustic	Hearing acuity
IX. Glossopharyngeal	Talking, swallowing; uvula & soft palate rise midline
X. Vagus	Gag reflex Taste not routinely tested
XI. Spinal	Symmetric strength of child's head turning against examiner's hand; symmetric strength of shoulder shrug against examiner's pressure
XII. Hypoglossal	Protruded tongue – midline

(2) Findings are consistent with age.
b. Males.
  (1) Urethral meatus is at the tip of the glans.
  (2) Foreskin is fully retractable after about 3 years of age in uncircumcised boys.
  (3) Testes are in the scrotum or can easily be "milked" down into the scrotum.
  (4) Penis and scrotum size are consistent with age.
3. Consider the following as deviations from normal:
a. Females.
  (1) Labial adhesions may obscure the view of the vaginal and urethral orifices.
  (2) Vaginal discharge is indicative of infection or foreign body.
b. Males.
  (1) Testes that are not in the scrotum of a child over 3 years of age may indicate undescended testes.
  (2) Fluid in the scrotum is most often a hydrocele.
  (3) Foreskin that is not easily retractable after the age of 3 years is phimosis.

M. Musculoskeletal system.
1. Inspect movement, noting:
a. Symmetry.
b. Use of all limbs.
c. Smoothness.
d. Gait.
2. Inspect structure, noting:
a. Symmetry.
b. Equality of limb length.
c. Equality of shoulder height.
d. Level of hips.
e. Straightness of spine when child is standing and when bending at the waist.
3. Palpate range of motion head to toe.
4. Palpate muscles down entire body, noting tone, strength, and symmetry.
5. Palpate bones from head to toe.
6. Palpate hips, performing for
a. All children: range of motion.
b. Infants: Ortolani maneuver and Barlow maneuver.
7. Compare results with normal findings.
a. Movement is symmetric and smooth.
b. Good muscle tone and strength are present.
c. Full range of motion is present throughout.
d. Some degree of in-toeing may be seen in toddlers.
e. Mild femoral anteversion may be seen in preschoolers.
8. Consider the following as deviations from normal:

a. Limp or asymmetry, which will require further evaluation.

b. Decreased muscle tone is noted in children with various syndromes including Down syndrome.

c. Hip click on Ortolani maneuver is associated with developmental dysplasia of the hip (formerly congenital dislocation of the hip).

d. Severe in-toeing or out-toeing may indicate a skeletal deformity.

e. Severe bowing of legs is associated with rickets.

f. Unequal shoulder or hip height may be associated with scoliosis.

g. Lateral curvature of the spine is indicative of scoliosis.

N. Nervous system.

1. Determine mental status for age by noting child's behavior, speech, response to questions, and school report.

2. Observe coordination as the child moves, plays, or responds during exam.

3. Observe gait when child is asked to "walk to the door."

4. Assess infant automatisms using Table 4-5 as a guide.

5. Perform cranial nerve assessment for age using methods listed in Table 4-6.

6. Assess deep tendon reflexes.

   a. In infants, obtain the patellar reflex and test for clonus.

   b. In children after infancy, obtain all deep tendon reflexes.

VII. ROUTINE SCREENING TESTS

A. Neonatal genetic screening is a legal requirement in all states.

1. Screening must be completed prior to hospital discharge and possibly repeated in cases of early discharge.

2. Although specific tests vary by state, tests commonly required include:

   a. PKU.

   b. Congenital hypothyroidism.

   c. Galactosemia.

   d. Hemoglobin type.

   e. Homocystinuria.

   f. Tyrosinemia.

   g. Maple syrup urine disease.

   h. Congenital adrenal hyperplasia.

B. Periodic screening should occur.

1. Timing is based on recommended intervals (see Figure 4-1) and according to risk factors, i.e., anemia, lead, urine, tuberculosis, cholesterol, STD.

2. At every health supervision visit:

   a. Plot growth parameters on growth chart.

      (1) Height.

      (2) Weight.

      (3) Head circumference for children up to 2 years of age.

   b. Check blood pressure beginning at 3 years of age.

   c. Assess vision.

      (1) Subjective to the age of 3 years of age; periodic objective testing beginning at 3 years of age using the Titmus or Snellen test.

      (2) Normal findings: 20/50 to 20/40 at 3 to 4 years of age; 20/20 by about 6 years of age.

   d. Test hearing.

      (1) Subjective to the age of 3 years of age; periodic objective testing beginning at 3 years of age using a screening audiogram.

      (2) Test at 20 decibels at frequencies of 500, 1000, 2000, and 4000 Hz.

   e. Assess speech by reviewing normal milestones of speech and using objective screening tools.

      (1) Clinical Linguistic Auditory Milestone Test (CLAMS) for 0–36 months of age.

      (2) Denver Articulation Screening Exam (DASE) for evaluation of articulation in 3–6 year olds.

      (3) Early Language Milestone scale (ELM) for 1–36 months of age.

      (4) Fluharty Preschool Speech and Language Screening Test for 2-6 year olds.

      (5) Receptive and Expressive Emergent Language scale (REEL) for 0–36 months of age.

   f. Assess development by obtaining an interval history and using objective screening tools.

      (1) Denver II.

         (a) Birth to 6 years of age.

         (b) Most frequently administered test.

         (c) Easily administered.

      (2) Bayley Infant Neurodevelopmental Screener (BINS).

         (a) 3– 24 months of age.

         (b) Newer developmental tool.

         (c) More difficult to score than Denver II.

VIII. ANTICIPATORY GUIDANCE

A. Provide anticipatory guidance during each contact.

B. Offer guidance that is developmentally appropriate.
1. Injury prevention. *See Chapter 10: Injury Control.*
2. Health behavior. *See Chapter 5: Health Behavior.*
3. Psychosocial issues. *See Chapter 3: Cognitive and Psychosocial Development* and *Chapter 7: Home and Family.*
4. Sexuality.

C. Provide anticipatory guidance appropriate to the child's environment.
1. Community. *See Chapter 8: Community Influences.*
    a. Urban.
    b. Rural.
    c. Affluent.
    d. Poor.
2. Season.
    a. Cold injury prevention.
    b. Danger of space heaters.
    c. Heat injury prevention.
    d. Sunburn prevention.
    e. Insect bite protection.

D. Provide anticipatory guidance that is culturally appropriate. *See Chapter 29: Cultural Influences.*

BIBLIOGRAPHY

◆ ◆ ◆ ◆ ◆ ◆ ◆ ◆ ◆ ◆ ◆ ◆ ◆ ◆ ◆ ◆ ◆ ◆

American Academy of Pediatrics Committee on Practice and Ambulatory Medicine. (1995). Recommendations for preventive pediatric health care. *Pediatrics, 92*(6), 751.

Burns, C.E., Barber, N., Brady, M.A., & Dunn, A.M. (1996). *Pediatric primary care: A handbook for nurse practitioners.* Philadelphia: Saunders.

Elster, A., & Kuznets, N. (1994). *AMA guidelines for adolescent preventive services* (GAPS). Baltimore: Williams & Wilkins.

Engel, J. (1997). *Pocket guide to pediatric assessment* (3rd ed.). St. Louis: Mosby.

U.S. Department of Health and Human Services (1990). *Healthy people 2000: National health promotion and disease prevention objectives for the year 2000.* (PHS) 91–50212. Washington, DC: U.S. Government Printing Office.

U.S. Preventive Services Task Force (1996). *Guide to clinical preventive services: Report of the U. S. Preventive Services Task Force.* Baltimore: Williams & Wilkins.

U.S. Public Health Service, Bureau of Maternal and Child Health (1994). *Bright futures: National guidelines for health supervision of infants, children, and adolescents.* Washington, DC: Author.

STUDY QUESTIONS

◆ ◆

1. Prior to obtaining a health history it is important for the interviewer to:
   a. discuss the case with the attending physician.
   b. call the family into the room and have the child undress.
   c. pause for a moment to prepare for the interview.
   d. request previous records.

2. What would be an appropriate approach to a toddler?
   a. Greet the child directly and ask a simple question.
   b. Initially avoid direct eye contact.
   c. Involve the child in the interview.
   d. Separate the child from the family for part of the interview.

3. In cases where immunization records are not available, it is advisable to:
   a. document what the parent recalls.
   b. document that records are not available.
   c. inform the parent that immunization records should always be carried.
   d. request that the parent bring records in for review.

4. When obtaining a nutritional history from school-agers and adolescents it is important to assess:
   a. attitude toward eating and food.
   b. the number of calories consumed daily.
   c. attitude toward school lunches.
   d. number of green vegetables eaten each day.

5. Questions about a child's school progress are part of:
   a. social history.
   b. family history.
   c. review of systems.
   d. developmental history.

6. A normal physical finding in a young infant who is crying is:
   a. erythematous lips.
   b. circumoral cyanosis.
   c. erythematous hands and feet.
   d. prominent abdominal veins.

7. Where are bruises commonly found?
   a. On the forehead of infants
   b. On the chest
   c. On the anterior legs of walking children
   d. On the anterior arms of school-aged children

8. Lymph nodes are commonly palpated in children. Normal palpable nodes in children under 12 years of age are:
   a. 2 cm. or smaller in size.
   b. firm or hard.
   c. tender.
   d. movable.

9. Normal findings of the anterior fontanelle of a 6-month-old infant include:
   a. slight pulsations.
   b. a feeling of fullness.
   c. a feeling of depression.
   d. no palpable fontanelle.

10. Evaluation of the sinuses of a young child requires:
    a. direct visualization of the sinuses.
    b. knowledge of sinus development.
    c. indirect visualization of the sinuses.
    d. assessment of the pharynx.

11. When assessing the abdomen, which technique follows inspection?
    a. Auscultation
    b. Palpation
    c. Direct percussion
    d. Indirect percussion

12. Which screening procedure is done based on risk factors?
    a. Blood pressure
    b. Vision
    c. Cholesterol
    d. Hearing

ANSWERS

◆ ◆

1.c 2.b 3.d 4.a 5.d 6.b 7.c 8.d 9.a 10.b 11.a 12.c

Chapter 5

Health Behavior

Ruth Bindler, MS, RN,C

Concept

◆◆◆◆◆◆◆◆◆◆◆◆◆◆◆◆◆◆◆◆◆◆◆◆◆◆◆◆

◆ Health behavior

Objectives

◆◆◆◆◆◆◆◆◆◆◆◆◆◆◆◆◆◆◆◆◆◆◆◆◆◆◆◆

At the completion of this chapter, the reader will be able to:

◆ Identify children's beliefs related to health and illness.

◆ State child health behaviors requiring assessment at health care encounters.

◆ Plan interventions to improve children's health behaviors.

◆ Use resources to consistently improve knowledge related to child health behaviors.

Key Points

◆◆◆◆◆◆◆◆◆◆◆◆◆◆◆◆◆◆◆◆◆◆◆◆◆◆◆◆

◆ Children's understanding of health and illness is influenced by cognitive level.

◆ Influences on health practices include children's knowledge, family patterns, cultural practices, social/economic factors, and the media.

◆ Early health behaviors influence health patterns later in life.

◆ Nurses should assess key points regarding health behaviors at all health care encounters with children.

◆ Interventions are needed to improve health behaviors of children.

5

Health Behavior

◆◆◆◆◆◆◆◆◆◆◆◆◆◆◆◆◆◆◆◆◆◆◆◆◆◆◆◆◆◆◆◆◆◆◆◆

I. CHILDREN'S VIEWS OF HEALTH AND ILLNESS

◆◆◆◆◆◆◆◆◆◆◆◆◆◆◆◆◆◆◆

A. Views of health and illness causality are based primarily on children's cognitive levels (see Table 5-1).
1. The cognitive theory of Jean Piaget forms the basis for the frameworks used to understand children's views of health and illness. *See Chapter 3: Cognitive and Psychosocial Development.*
2. Cognitive level determines the child's views of health and illness causation more than prior experiences with health care (Kury, 1995).

B. Health behaviors are learned progressively throughout life.
1. Explanations based on cognitive levels are needed by children during all encounters for health care.
2. Acquisition of knowledge at various ages is facilitated by:
   a. Increasing complexity of presentation.
   b. Different teaching methods.

C. All health supervision visits should include (Green, 1994):
   1. Assessment of the child's health status.
   2. Interventions to improve health.
   3. Teaching that anticipates the child and family needs for future information.

D. Both risk factor reduction and positive lifestyle changes (health promotion) are aims of health care teaching (Saucier, 1991).

E. Since many children receive limited health care, particularly for preventive services, each encounter with health professionals, for whatever reason, must be viewed as an opportunity to impart information and influence health behaviors.

II. FAMILY INFLUENCES ON CHILDREN'S HEALTH CARE BEHAVIORS

◆◆◆◆◆◆◆◆◆◆◆◆◆◆◆◆◆◆◆

A. Children's first experiences with health behaviors occur in their families.

B. Family structure plays an important part in health outcomes for children.
   1. Disrupted families more commonly have children with an accident, injury, or poisoning (Bloom & Dawson, 1991; Dawson, 1991).
   2. Asthma is more common in children from single parent families (Dawson, 1991).

C. Children's responsibility for self-care influences health behaviors and is related to the degree of parental supervision and management of these behaviors.

D. Health behavior changes are influenced by the support of family members.

E. Health behaviors learned in childhood are influential on adult patterns.

III. OTHER INFLUENCES ON CHILDREN'S HEALTH BEHAVIORS

◆◆◆◆◆◆◆◆◆◆◆◆◆◆◆◆◆

A. Cultural beliefs and practices (e.g., food habits, religious beliefs) influence health behaviors and may conflict with standard health practices and therapeutic interventions. *See Chapter 29: Cultural Influences.*

B. Nearly all children attend school, so this is a powerful medium for transmission of health related information.
   1. Despite this opportunity, less than half of the children in the United States receive school health education that spans multiple topics and occurs across all grade levels (U.S. Department of Health and Human Services, 1991).

Table 5-1
Children's Concepts of Health and Illness

Approximate Age	Cognitive Stage (Piaget)	Concept of Health	Concept of Illness	Strategies for Intervention
Under 7 years	Preoperational thought *Characteristics:* Egocentrism Transductive reasoning Present orientation	Health is seen as feeling good. Causation of loss of health poorly defined. Lacks understanding of relationship between present events and future health or illness.	Illness is caused by an event that occurs at the same time but is unrelated (phenomenism). People or objects in close proximity can cause illness (contagion).	Concentrate on teaching specific health practices (e.g., hand-washing) and their direct effects (e.g., hands feel clean, you stay healthy). Tell child that he/she did not cause illness. Clarify causes.
7–10 years	Concrete thought *Characteristics:* Logical thought based on concrete experiences Conservation Reversibility	Health is ability to perform desired activities. The effect of behaviors on health and illness is understood.	People or objects that are harmful and in direct contact cause illness (contamination). Although contact with someone or something harmful causes illness, the illness is viewed as inside one's body (internalization).	Teach the relationship between concrete health behaviors and health or illness (e.g., hand-washing and illness, exercise, and healthy heart, bicycle helmet and safety). A high level of interest in health in this age group makes it an ideal time for targeting children in various settings for health care teaching.
11 years and over	Formal thought *Characteristics:* Abstract reasoning Future orientation	Health is ability to perform desired activity. Importance of mental health is noted. One's future health is of interest and concern.	External events trigger illness, which then occurs with physiologic changes in the body (physiologic). Psychologic events are also seen as a cause of illness. Thoughts and feelings can relate to state of health or illness (psychophysiologic).	Add more information about illness causation and psycho/physiologic functioning on the body. Emphasize the relationship between present health practices and future ability to perform desired activities.

Adapted from Natapoff, J.N. (1988). A developmental analysis of children's ideas of health. *Health Education Quarterly, 9*(2,3), 130-141; and Bibace, R., & Walsh, M.E. (1981). *Children's conceptions of health, illness, and bodily functions.* San Francisco: Jossey Bass.

2. Curricula from kindergarten through 12th grade should include health related knowledge, attitudes, and skills regarding multiple topics such as:
   a. Nutrition.
   b. Physical activity.
   c. Family life.
   d. Injury prevention.
   e. Substance abuse.

3. Nurses can help plan health curricula for children and facilitate their integration into school programs.

C. Media plays an important role in the lives of all children and therefore has potential to influence their health behaviors.
1. The number of hours the average child views

Table 5-2
Lipid Recommendations for Children

	Total Cholesterol (mg/dl)	Triglycerides (mg/dl)	LDL Cholesterol (mg/dl)	HDL Cholesterol (mg/dl)
Recommended	<170	<100	<110	>35
Borderline	170–199	100–129	110–129	
High	≥200	≥130	≥130	

Adapted from National Cholesterol Education Program. (1991). *Report of the Expert Panel on Blood Cholesterol Levels in Children and Adolescents.* Washington, DC: U.S. Department of Health & Human Services.

television is significant and related to the child's health.
   a. Most children watch more television hours than the hours they attend school.
   b. Incidence of obesity and overweight are significantly correlated with number of hours of television viewed daily.
2. Computers, video games, movies, and other media are influential in the lives of children.
   a. Most media does not focus on concepts of health promotion.
   b. Violence and related concepts are frequently viewed.
   c. Characters who engage in risk-taking behaviors seldom experience realistic consequences.
3. More programs are needed that use the familiar media format to teach health concepts to children.

D. Communities play a part in fostering health behaviors in children.
1. Proximity of public health and other services to needed areas influences health patterns and practices.
2. Integration of community services can be influential (e.g., a local health district providing hepatitis B immunization and health-related information in a local public school).
3. Recreation departments and sports complexes provide a vehicle for health practices and dissemination of information regarding activities.
4. Synagogues, mosques, and churches can offer classes and services to foster mental health and other supports and resources.
5. Day care services can teach health practices to young children.
6. Violence in communities is a growing threat to the health of children (Garbarino, 1995).
   a. Homicide and personal crimes (rape, assault, robbery) are increasingly common among teens and occur at a high rate compared to other age groups (Lewit & Baker, 1996).
   b. Exposure to violence can influence a child's mental as well as physical health.
7. Individuals, communities, and government are responsible for providing interventions that reduce children's exposure to violence, which include:
   a. Control of and education about firearms.
   b. Provision of safe after-school and summer programs.
   c. Decrease in substance abuse.
   d. Provision of safe and affordable housing.
   e. Provision of safe schools.

E. A Lifestyle Questionnaire is available to assess health behaviors in children (VanAntwerp, 1995).

IV. HEALTH BEHAVIORS OF CHILDREN

◆ ◆ ◆ ◆ ◆ ◆ ◆ ◆ ◆ ◆ ◆ ◆ ◆ ◆ ◆ ◆ ◆ ◆

A. Nutrition.
1. The average American child:
   a. Obtains 35% of calories from fat, with 14% from saturated fat.
   b. Consumes from 193 mg (1–5 years) to 255 mg (6–11 years) to 296 mg (12–19 years) of cholesterol daily (National Cholesterol Education Program, 1991).
2. The National Cholesterol Education Program (1991) recommends that a diet for children over 2 years be balanced by approximately 55% of calories from carbohydrate and 15–20% from protein and include:
   a. No more than 30% of total calories from fat.
   b. Less than 10% of total calories from saturated fat.
   c. Dietary cholesterol of less than 300 mg daily.

Table 5-3
Nutritional Measurements

Measurement	Age To Be Performed
Height and weight	By 1 month, at 2, 4, 6, 9, 12, 15, 18, 24 months; at 3, 4, 5, 6, 8, 20, 23, 24, 26, 28 years
Hematocrit or hemoglobin	9, 24 months; 8, 18 years

Adapted from Committee on Psychosocial Aspects of Child and Family Health. (1997). *Guidelines for health supervision* (3rd ed.). Elk Grove Village, IL: American Academy of Pediatrics.

3. Healthy dietary and exercise habits are reflected in lipid profiles (see Table 5-2 for recommendations).
4. Healthy school lunches and day care nutrition programs should follow nutrition principles in Dietary Guidelines for Americans (1985).
5. Height, weight, and hematocrit should be checked at regular intervals and used as basis for additional assessment and intervention (see Table 5-3).
6. Identification of nutritional disorders such as obesity, anorexia, bulimia, and inadequate intake is needed at each health care visit; about 11% of children are overweight, double the percentage of one decade ago (Troiano, 1995).
   a. Height and weight should generally be within the 5th to 95th percentiles, and should track in similar percentiles over time.
   b. Height and weight should be roughly the same percentile.
   c. Physical examination may reveal signs of inadequate intake (e.g., pallor, lethargy, dry skin, listless eyes).
   d. Signs of anorexia and bulimia commonly occur in adolescence and may include:
      (1) Low weight.
      (2) Signs of malnutrition.
      (3) Calluses on knuckles.
      (4) Eroded tooth enamel.
      (5) Cessation of menses in the female.
      (6) History of excessive exercise.

B. Physical activity.
1. Youth in the United States get increasingly less physical activity.
   a. Only 66% of youths engage in vigorous activity three or more times weekly for at least 20 minutes (U.S. Department of Health and Human Services, 1991).
   b. While all children exercise less the older they become, girls' activity decreases with age even more than boys.'
2. Recommendations to increase children's physical activity include the following:
   a. Parents and children can exercise together to facilitate physical activity for all in the family.
   b. Children should have aerobic activity at least 3–5 times weekly for a minimum of 20–30 minutes each time; additional strength and stretching exercise is also recommended.
3. School physical education programs are underused resources.
   a. Less than half of all children participate in a daily physical education program at school.
   b. Increasing physical education at school can influence health and teach positive health behaviors.
4. Children engage in the passive activity of watching television, which limits time spent in more active pursuits.
   a. Children watch an average of 4.8 hours of television daily (Gortmaker et al., 1996).
   b. Strategies to increase physical activity should suggest postponing television until exercise is completed each day and limiting total television viewing time.

C. Blood pressure.
1. Blood pressure is an important health parameter that can be influenced by an individual's health behaviors.
2. Blood pressure should be measured routinely in children, beginning in infancy and toddlerhood, to establish baseline measures for each child.
3. The child should be sitting and relaxed with the right arm (the arm preferable for measurement) at heart level.
4. The mercury sphygmomanometer is the preferred instrument for measuring blood pressure.
5. Average blood pressure levels are available for children of various ages (Hohn, 1997) (see Table 5-4).
6. New nomograms have been developed that consider the age, gender, and height of the child when evaluating blood pressures (Sinaiko, 1996) (see Table 5-5).

Table 5-4
Diagnosis of Hypertension by Age (Modified from Task Force Report)

Age	Systolic BP (mm Hg) Signif†	Serious‡	Diastolic BP (mm Hg) Signif	Serious
Newborn (8 to 30 days)	104	110		
Infant (<2 years)	112	118	74	82
Child (2 to 5 years)	116	124	76	84
Child (6 to 9 years)	122	130	78	86
Child (10 to 12 years)	126	134	82	90
Adolescent (13 to 15 years)	136	144	86	92
Adolescent (16 to 18 years)	142	150	92	98

† > 95% for age and gender ‡ >99% for age and gender

Used with permission from Hohn, A.R. (1997). Diagnosis and management of hypertension in childhood. *Pediatric Annals, 26*(2), 105–110.

Table 5-5
Blood Pressure According to Age, Gender, and Height

*95th Percentile of Blood Pressure in Boys and Girls 3 to 16 Years of Age, According to Height**

Blood Pressure	Age	Height Percentile For Boys 5th	25th	75th	95th	Height Percentile For Girls 5th	25th	75th	95th
	yr	mm Hg				mm Hg			
Systolic	3	104	107	111	113	104	105	108	110
	6	109	112	115	117	108	110	112	114
	10	114	117	121	123	116	117	120	122
	13	121	124	128	130	121	123	126	128
	16	129	132	136	138	125	127	130	132
Diastolic	3	63	64	66	67	65	65	67	68
	6	72	73	75	76	71	72	73	75
	10	77	79	80	82	77	77	79	80
	13	79	81	83	84	80	81	82	84
	16	83	84	86	87	83	83	85	86

* The height percentiles were determined with standard growth curves. Data are adapted from those of the Task Force on High Blood Pressure in Children and Adolescents.

Used with permission from Sinaiko, A.R. (1996). Hypertension in children. *The New England Journal of Medicine, 335*(26), 1968–1973.

7. Blood pressure is evaluated as:
  a. normal: systolic and diastolic <90th percentile for age and gender.
  b. high normal: systolic and/or diastolic blood pressure consistently between 90th and 95th percentile for age and gender.
  c. significant hypertension: three separate systolic and/or diastolic measures are >95th percentile for age and gender.
  d. serious hypertension: three separate systolic and/or diastolic measures are >99th percentile for age and gender.
8. Prevention of hypertension is important since blood pressure tracks into adulthood.
  a. Blood pressure is a strong cardiovascular risk factor.
  b. A familial influence on blood pressure is evident early in life.
9. Various measures are used to decrease blood pressure in children.

Vaccines[1] are listed under the routinely recommended ages. Bars indicate range of acceptable ages for immunization. Catch-up immunization should be done during any visit when feasible. Shaded ovals indicate vaccines to be assessed and given if necessary during the early adolescent visit.

Age ▶ Vaccine ▼	Birth	1 mo	2 mos	4 mos	6 mos	12 mos	15 mos	18 mos	4-6 yrs	11-12 yrs	14-16 yrs
Hepatitis B[2,3]	Hep B-1										
		Hep B-2			Hep B-3					Hep B[3]	
Diphtheria, Tetanus, Pertussis[4]		DTaP or DTP	DTaP or DTP	DTaP or DTP		DTaP or DTP[4]			DTaP or DTP	Td	
H influenzae type b[5]		Hib	Hib	Hib		Hib					
Polio[6]		Polio[6]	Polio		Polio[6]				Polio		
Measles, Mumps, Rubella[7]						MMR			MMR[7]	MMR[7]	
Varicella[8]						Var				Var[8]	

Approved by the Advisory Committee on Immunization Practices (ACIP), the American Academy of Pediatrics (AAP), and the American Academy of Family Physicians (AAFP).

1 This schedule indicates the recommended age for routine administration of currently licensed childhood vaccines. Some combination vaccines are available and may be used whenever administration of all components of all vaccine is indicated. Providers should consult the manufacturers' package inserts for detailed recommendations.

2 Infants born to HBsAg-negative mothers should receive 2.5 mcg of Merck vaccine (Recombivax HB) or 10 mcg of SmithKline Beecham (SB) vaccine (Energix-B). The second dose should be administered at least 1 month after the 1st dose. The third dose should be given at least 2 months after the second, but not before 6 months of age.

Infants born to HBsAg-positive mothers should receive 0.5 mL of hepatitis B immune globulin (HBIG) within 12 hrs of birth, and either 5 mcg of Merck vaccine (Recombivax HB) or 10 mcg of SB vaccine (Energix-B) at a separate site. The second dose is recommended at 1-2 months of age and the third dose at 6 months of age.

Infants born to mothers whose HBsAg status is unknown should receive either 5 mcg of Merck vaccine (Recombivax HB) or 10 mcg of SD vaccine (Energix-B) within 12 hours of birth. The second dose of vaccine is recommended at 1 month of age and the third dose at 6 months of age. Blood should be drawn at the time of delivery to determine the mother's HBsAg status; if it is positive, the infant should receive HBIG as soon as possible (no later than 1 week of age). The dosage and timing of subsequent vaccine doses should be based upon the mother's HBsAg status.

3 Children and adolescents who have not been vaccinated against hepatitis B in infancy may begin the series during any visit. Those who have not previously received 3 doses of hepatitis B vaccine should initiate or complete the series during the 11- to 12-year-old visit, and unvaccinated older adolescents should be vaccinated whenever possible. The second dose should be administered at least 1 month after the first dose, and the third dose should be administered at least 4 months after the first dose and at least 2 months after the second dose.

4 DTaP (diphtheria and tetanus toxoids and acellular pertussis vaccine) is the preferred vaccine for all doses in the vaccination series, including completion of the series in children who have received 1 or more doses of whole-cell DTP vaccine. Whole-cell DTP is an acceptable alternative to DTaP. The fourth dose (DTP or DTaP) may be administered as early as 12 months of age, provided 6 months have elapsed since the third dose, and if the child is unlikely to return at 15-18 months. Td (tetanus and diphtheria toxoids) is recommended at 11-12 years of age if at least 5 years have elapsed since the last dose of DTP, DTaP, or DT. Subsequent routine Td boosters are recommended every 10 years.

5 Three H influenza type b (Hib) conjugate vaccines are licensed for infant use. If PRP-OMP (PedvaxHIB [Merck]) is administered at 2 and 4 months of age, a dose at 6 months is not required.

6 Two poliovirus vaccines are currently licensed in the U.S.: inactivated poliovirus vaccine (IPV) and oral poliovirus (OPV). The following schedules are all acceptable to the ACIP, the AAP, and the AAFP. Parents and providers may choose among these options:
a. Two doses of IPV followed by 2 doses of OPV.
b. Four doses of IPV.
c. Four doses of OPV.

The ACIP recommends 2 doses of IPV at 2 and 4 months of age followed by 2 doses of OPV at 12-18 months and 4-6 years of age. IPV is the only poliovirus vaccine recommended for immunocompromised persons and their household contacts.

7 The 2nd dose of MMR is recommended routinely at 4-6 years of age but may be administered during any visit, provided at least 1 month has elapsed since receipt of the first dose and that both doses are administered beginning at or after 12 months of age. Those who have not previously received the second dose should complete the schedule no later than the 11- to 12-year visit.

8 Susceptible children may receive varicella vaccine (Var) at any visit after the first birthday, and those who lack a reliable history of chickenpox should be immunized during the 11- to 12-year visit. Susceptible children 13 years of age or older should receive 2 doses, at least 1 month apart.

Figure 5-1
Recommended childhood immunization schedule* – United States, January–December 1998

Used with permission from Selekman, J. (1998). Infectious diseases and the immunizations of today and tomorrow. *Pediatric Nursing, 24*(4). Originally from the Advisory Committee on Immunization Practices (ACIP), the American Academy of Pediatrics (AAP), and the American Academy of Family Physicians (AAFP).

a. Elimination of obesity and overweight.
b. A low sodium and high potassium diet.
c. Adequate calcium and fiber intake.
d. Low intake of saturated fats.
e. Regular exercise.
f. Avoidance of smoking.
g. Avoidance of alcohol, street drugs, and other substances of abuse.
h. Behavior modification and biofeedback.
10. Drug therapy is used for those with persistent significant hypertension.
a. Single dose therapy is initiated with a calcium entry blocker, ACE inhibitor, beta blocker, or diuretic.
b. Multiple dose therapy is tried if one drug is not effective.
11. The goal for blood pressure is to maintain systolic and diastolic levels below the 95th percentile for age and gender.

D. Immunizations.
1. A large number of immunizations is needed during infancy, childhood, and adolescence (see Figure 5-1).
2. Immunization schedules should be reviewed at every health care encounter and the greatest possible number of needed immunizations administered.
3. Health professionals should use only true contraindications (see Table 5-6) as reason for not administering an immunization during a health care visit to minimize missed opportunities for immunization.
4. All health care providers should review and be knowledgeable about annually updated immunization schedules from the American Academy of Pediatrics and the Centers for Disease Control and Prevention (see "Resources" in Table 5-7).
5. Immunization recommendations are available in the American Academy of Pediatrics Committee on Infectious Diseases most current Redbook and in the Centers for Communicable Disease publication *Morbidity and Mortality Weekly Report*.

E. Safety factors.
1. Health teaching for the major safety hazards at each age should be incorporated into health care visits, school curricula, and community programs. *See Chapter 10: Injury Control.*
2. Both parents and children should be adequately informed about common hazards such as bicycle accidents, car crashes, firearm use, drowning, and fires.

F. Substance abuse.
1. Substance abuse among children and adolescents is a growing problem.
a. Marijuana use among youth doubled from 1992 to 1994 (Children's Defense Fund, 1996).
b. Twenty-two percent of youths use alcohol regularly (Children's Defense Fund, 1996).
c. Smoking occurs at increasingly younger ages (American Medical Association, 1990).
(1) Thirty-five percent of 9th–12th graders smoke.
(2) Every day 3,000 young people begin smoking (American Heart Association, 1993).
(3) Children often begin smoking in grades 5 or 6.
2. Children are also exposed to secondhand smoke (environmental tobacco smoke or ETS).
a. Nine million children under 5 years old live with a smoker (American Heart Association, 1993).
b. Secondhand smoke is known to have many of the same health risks as direct smoking.
3. Children may grow up in homes where substance abuse is a problem and need strategies to deal with this issue.
4. Prevention and intervention strategies are needed.
a. Both the physical examination and mental status examination reveal symptoms of substance abuse. *See Chapter 18: Acute Illness: Injuries.*
b. Educational programs are needed in schools and communities to prevent substance abuse.
c. Families should address substance abuse issues and be alert for signs of use.

V. HEALTH PROGRAMS FOR CHILDREN
◆ ◆ ◆ ◆ ◆ ◆ ◆ ◆ ◆ ◆ ◆ ◆ ◆ ◆ ◆ ◆ ◆ ◆ ◆ ◆

A. Health screening should occur on a regularly scheduled basis during childhood.

B. Interventions based on the child's cognitive level and other assessment data should be offered at each health care encounter to enhance the health behaviors that support positive lifestyles.

C. Model curricula have been developed to implement teaching on health behaviors with children (see Table 5-7).

D. Information should be presented and later reinforced and built upon to encourage maintenance of new health behaviors.

Table 5-6. Summary of Rules for Childhood Immunization

Adapted from ACIP, AAP and AAFP by the Immunization Action Coalition, March 1997

Vaccine	Ages usually given, route of administration, and other guidelines	If children fall behind - minimum intervals	Contraindications (Remember, mild illness is not a contraindication.)
DTaP (contains acellular pertussis vaccine) **DTP/ or DTwP** (contains whole cell pertussis vaccine)	• DTaP is preferred for all doses in the series but DTwP is acceptable. • Give at 2m, 4m, 6m, 15-18m, 4-6yrs of age. • May give #1 as early as 6wks of age. • May give #4 as early as 12m of age if 6m has elapsed since #3 and you think the child is unlikely to return by 18m of age. • If started with DTwP, may complete series with DTaP. • Do not give DTaP or DTwP to children ≥7yrs of age (give Td). • DTaP/DTwP may be given with all other vaccines but at a separate site. • DTaP/DTwP are given IM.	• #2 & #3 may be given 4wks after previous dose. • #4 may be given 6m after #3. • If #4 is given before 4th birthday, wait at least 6m for #5. • If #4 is given after 4th birthday, #5 is not needed. • Don't restart series, no matter how long since previous dose.	(DTaP and DTwP have the same contraindications and precautions.) • Anaphylactic reaction to a prior dose or to any vaccine component. • Moderate or severe acute illness. Don't postpone for minor illness. • Previous encephalopathy within 7 days after DTwP/DTaP. • Undiagnosed progressive neurologic problem. **Precautions:** The following are precautions not contraindications. Generally when these conditions are present, the vaccine shouldn't be given. But, there are situations when the benefit outweighs risk so vaccination should be considered (e.g., pertussis outbreak). • Previous rxn of T≥105°F (40.5°C) within 48 hrs after dose. • Previous continuous crying lasting 3 or more hours within 48 hrs after dose. • Previous convulsion within 3 days after immunization. • Previous pale or limp episode, or collapse within 48 hrs after dose.
DT	• Give to children < 7yrs of age if the child has had a serious reaction to the "P" in DTaP/DTwP, or if the parents refuse the pertussis component. • DT can be given with all other vaccines but at a separate site. • Give IM.	For children who have fallen behind, use information in box directly above.	• Anaphylactic reaction to a prior dose or to any vaccine component. • Moderate or severe acute illness. Don't postpone for minor illness.
Td	• Use for persons ≥7yrs of age. • A booster dose is now recommended for children 11-12yrs of age if 5yrs have elapsed since previous dose. Then boost every 10 years. • Td may be given with all other vaccines but at a separate site. • Give IM.	For those never vaccinated or behind give dose #1 now; dose #2 1m later; dose #3 6m after #2, and then boost every 10 years.	• Anaphylactic reaction to a prior dose or to any vaccine component. • Moderate or severe acute illness. Don't postpone for minor illness.
Polio IPV and OPV	• Give at 2m, 4m, 12-18m, 4-6yrs of age. • ACIP recommends "Sequential Schedule": IPV for #1 and #2, and OPV for #3 and #4. ACIP also says all-OPV or all-IPV schedule is acceptable. • AAFP/AAP recommend that clinicians/parents discuss the 3 schedules (sequential [IPV/OPV], all-OPV, and all-IPV) and choose among them. • If all OPV is given, #3 may be given as early as 6m. • Not routinely given to anyone ≥18yrs of age (except certain travelers). • OPV/IPV may be given with all other vaccines but at a separate site. • OPV is given PO. • IPV is given SC.	• #1 & #2 (IPV or OPV) should be separated by at least 4wks. • If #3 (IPV or OPV) is given at ≥4yrs of age, a 4th dose is not needed. • All IPV: In children under 4yrs of age, #3 may be given as early as 4wks after #2 but a 6m interval is preferred for best response. • All OPV: minimum of 4wks between #1, #2, & #3 and a supplemental dose between 4-6yrs of age. • Don't restart series, no matter how long since previous dose.	• Anaphylactic reaction to a prior dose or to any vaccine component. • Moderate or severe acute illness. Don't postpone for minor illness. • Use IPV when an adult in the household or other close contact has never been vaccinated against polio. • In pregnancy, neither OPV nor IPV is recommended, but if immediate protection is needed, use OPV. **The following are contraindications for OPV so use IPV in these situations:** • Cancer, leukemia, lymphoma, immunodeficiency or HIV/AIDS. • Taking a drug that lowers resistance to infection, e.g., anti-cancer, high-dose steroids. • Someone in the household has any of the above medical problems.
Varicella Var	• Routinely give at 12-18m. • Vaccinate all children ≥12m of age including adolescents who have not had prior infection with chickenpox. • If Var and MMR are not given on the same day, space them ≥30d apart. • Var may be given with all other vaccines but at a separate site. • Give SC.	• Do not give to children <12m of age. • Susceptible children ≤12 yrs of age receive 1 dose. • Susceptible persons ≥13 yrs of age receive 2 doses 4-8wks apart. • Don't restart series, no matter how long since previous dose.	• Anaphylactic reaction to a prior dose or to any vaccine component. • Moderate or severe acute illness. Don't postpone for minor illness. • Pregnancy, or possibility of pregnancy within 1 month. • If blood products or immunoglobulin have been administered during the past 11 months, consult ACIP recommendations before vaccinating. • Immunocompromised persons due to malignancies and primary or acquired immunodeficiency including HIV/AIDS. Note: For patients on high-dose immunosuppressive therapy, consult ACIP recommendations regarding delay time. Note: Manufacturer recommends "no salicylates" for 6wks following this vaccine.

* Hepatitis A, influenza, and pneumococcal vaccines are indicated for many children, so make sure you provide these vaccines to at-risk children. The newer combination vaccines are not listed on this table. They may be used whenever administration of all components of the vaccine is indicated. Read the package inserts.

For full immunization information, see recent ACIP statements as published in the *MMWR* or the *AAP's Red Book–Report of the Committee on Infectious Diseases.*

Table 5-6 continues on opposite page

Table 5-6. Summary of Rules for Childhood Immunization (continued)

Vaccine	Ages usually given, route of administration, and other guidelines	For children fallen behind (minimum intervals)	Contraindications (Remember, mild illness is not a contraindication.)
MMR	• Give #1 at 12-15m. Give #2 at 4-6yrs or by 11-12yrs of age. • Can give as early as 6m of age in an outbreak, but two routine doses will still need to be given at ≥12m of age. • If a dose was given before 12m of age, give #1 at 12-15m of age with a minimum interval of 1m between these doses. • If MMR and Var are not given on the same day, space them ≥30d apart. • May give with all other vaccines but at a separate site. • Give SC.	• Give whenever behind. There should be a minimum interval of 1m between MMR #1 and MMR #2. • Dose #2 can be given at any time if at least 1m has elapsed since dose #1, and both doses are administered after 1 year of age. • Don't restart series, no matter how long since previous dose.	• Anaphylactic reaction to a prior dose or to any vaccine component or to eggs. • Pregnancy or possible pregnancy within next 3m (use contraception). • Moderate or severe acute illness. Don't postpone for minor illness. • HIV positivity is NOT a contraindication to MMR except for those who are severely immunocompromised. • Immunosuppressed patients due to cancer, leukemia, lymphoma, immunosuppressive drug therapy (including high-dose steroids). • If blood products or immunoglobulin have been administered during the past 11 months consult ACIP recommendations regarding time to wait before vaccinating. Note: MMR is NOT contraindicated if a PPD test was done recently, but PPD should be delayed if MMR was given 1-30 days before the PPD.
Hib	• HibTITER (HbOC) & ActHib (PRP-T): give at 2m, 4m, 6m, 12-15m. • PedvaxHiB (PRP-OMP): give at 2m, 4m, 12-15m. • Dose #1 of all Hib vaccines may be given as early as 6wks of age but do NOT give it any earlier than than 6 wks of age. • May give with all other vaccines but at a separate site. • Give IM.	**Rules for all Hib vaccines:** • If the child is ≥15m of age, only 1 dose is given. • Not routinely given to children ≥5yrs of age. • Give booster dose a minimum of 2m after previous dose. • Don't restart series, no matter how long since previous dose. **Rules for HbOC (HibTITER) & PRP-T (ActHib) only:** • If #1 is given up to 7m, give #2 & #3 spaced 1-2m after previous dose and boost at 12-15m. • If #1 is given at 7-11m only 3 doses are needed: #2 given 1-2m after #1, then boost at 12-15m. • If #1 is given at 12-14m, give a booster dose in 2 m. **Rules for PRP-OMP (PedvaxHiB) only:** • If #1 is given at 3-11m of age, give #2 1-2m later and boost at 12-15m. • If #1 is given at 12-14m, boost 2m later.	• Anaphylactic reaction to a prior dose or to any vaccine component. • Moderate or severe acute illness. Don't postpone for minor illness.
Hep-B	• For infants, give at 0-2m, 1-4m, 6-18m of age. • **If mother is HBsAg positive**: give HBIG and Hep-B #1 within 12 hrs of birth, #2 at 1-2m, and #3 at 6m of age. • **If mother is not a carrier but from an endemic area:** complete series by 12m of age. • ACIP says to vaccinate 1) all children born after 11/21/91; 2) all 11-12yr olds if not previously vaccinated; 3) all children ≤12yrs of age who are or whose parents are from endemic areas; and 4) all children and teens in high risk groups. • AAP recommends vaccination of 1) all infants; 2) all adolescents; 3) all children in populations of high HBV endemicity; and 4) all children in other high-risk groups. • May give with all other vaccines but at a separate site. • Give IM. Note: Your state health department may recommend broader coverage for the use of hepatitis B vaccine. Give them a call to find out.	• Series can be started at any age. • Commonly used spacing options for older children and teens: • **0m, 1m, 6m** or • **0m, 2m, 4m** or • **0m, 1m, 4m.** • Minimum spacing for children and teens: 1m between #1 & #2, and 2m between #2 & #3. Overall there must be 4m between #1 and #3. • Don't restart series, no matter how long since previous dose. ***Dosing of Hepatitis B vaccine:** Engerix-B: 1) 10 µg=dose for 0-19 yr olds (including infants of HBsAg positive mothers). 2) 20 µg=dose for those ≥20 yrs. old. Recombivax-HB: 1) 2.5 µg=dose for infants born to HBsAg negative mothers and children up to age 11; 2) 5 µg=dose for infants of HBsAg positive mothers and for children ages 11-19; 3) 10µg=dose for ages ≥20 yrs. **NOTE: Engerix-B and Recombivax-HB have different packaging and concentrations. Read the package insert carefully to determine the proper volume of vaccine to administer.**	• Anaphylactic reaction to a prior dose or to any vaccine component. • Moderate or severe acute illness. Don't postpone for minor illness.

This two-sided table was developed to combine the "rules for childhood immunization" onto one page. It was devised especially to assist health care workers in immunization clinics to determine the appropriate use and scheduling of vaccines. It can be posted in immunization clinics or clinicians' offices. The table will be revised yearly due to the changing nature of national immunization recommendations.

Thank you to the following individuals for their review and comments regarding this document: William Atkinson, MD, Karl Chun, MD, Jacqueline Gindler, MD, Caroline Breese Hall, MD, John Hollister, Muriel Hoyt, PHN, Sam Katz, MD, Sanford Kaufman, Anne Kuettel, PHN, Lucinda Long, Frank Mahoney, MD, Edgar Marcuse, MD, Harold Margolis, MD, James McCord, MD, Linda Moyer, PHN, Paul Offit, MD, Diane Peterson, Tom Saari, MD, Jane Seward, MD, Linda Thompson, MD, and Tom Vernon, MD. Final responsibility for errors or omissions lies with the editors.

Your comments are welcome. Please send them to Lynn Bahta, PHN, or Deborah Wexler, MD, Immunization Action Coalition, 1573 Selby Ave., Suite 229, St. Paul, MN 55104 or call 612-647-9009, fax 612-647-9131, or e-mail: editor@immunize.org.

Item #P2010 (3/97)

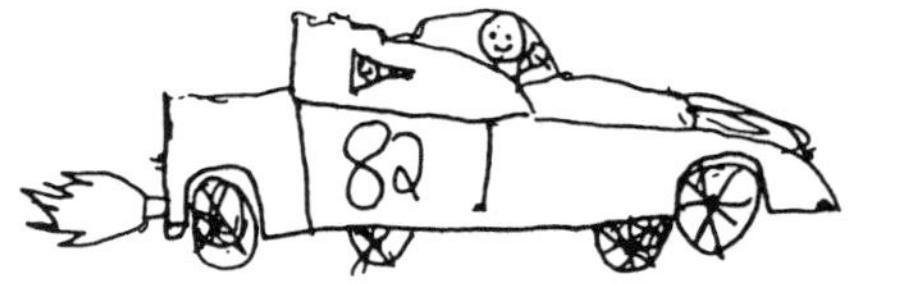

Adapted from the Advisory Committee on Immunization Practices (ACIP), the American Academy of Pediatrics (AAP), and the American Academy of Family Physicians (AAFP) by the Immunization Action Coalition, February 1997.

Table 5-7
Programs and Resources for Promotion of Health Behaviors in Children

PROGRAMS	RESOURCES
Heart Smart Family Health Promotion Program A school based program for cardiovascular risk reduction among high risk children and their families; adaptable to clinical practice 　Department of Medicine 　Louisiana State University Medical Center 　New Orleans, LA 70112 　504-568-4808 **Minnesota Heart Health Program** An educational program for 6th grade students 　Division of Epidemiology, School of Public Health 　University of Minnesota at Minneapolis 　Minneapolis, MN 55454-1015 　612-624-1818 **San Diego Family Health Project** A family based cardiovascular disease risk reduction intervention taking place in schools 　San Diego State University and 　Division of Pediatrics at 　University of California, San Diego 　La Jolla, CA 92093 　619-534-4161	**American Academy of Pediatrics** P.O. Box 927 141 Northwest Point Blvd. Elk Grove Village, IL 60009-0927 847-228-5005 **American Heart Association** 7320 Greenville Avenue Dallas, TX 75231 214-373-6300 Each state chapter of the American Heart Association has various materials available. **Centers for Disease Control and Prevention** 1600 Clifton Road, NE Atlanta, GA 30333 404-639-3291 **National Institutes of Health** National Heart, Lung, and Blood Institute 9000 Rockville Pike Bethesda, MD 20892 301-496-2411 The State Dairy Council of each state has educational materials related to nutrition.

E. All agencies and programs serving children should obtain and/or develop materials to address important health behaviors.

BIBLIOGRAPHY

American Heart Association. (1993). *Fact sheet.* Southfield, MI: Author.

American Medical Association. (1990). *Healthy youth 2000.* Chicago, IL: Author.

Bloom, B., & Dawson, D. (1991). Family structure and child health. *American Journal of Public Health, 81*(11), 1526–1528.

Children's Defense Fund. (1996). *The state of America's children.* Washington, DC: Author.

Committee on Infectious Diseases. (1997). *Redbook* (24th ed.). Elk Grove Village, IL: American Academy of Pediatrics.

Dawson, D.A. (1991). Family structure and children's health and well-being: Data from the 1988 national health interview survey on child health. *Journal of Marriage and the Family, 53,* 573–584.

Garbarino, J. (1995). The American war zone: What children tell us about living with violence. *Journal of Developmental Behavioral Pediatrics, 16*(6), 431–435.

Gortmaker, S.L., Must, A., Sobol, A.M., Peterson, K., Colditz, G.A., & Dietz, W.H. (1996). Television viewing as a cause of increasing obesity among children in the United States, 1986-1990. *Archives of Pediatric and Adolescent Medicine, 150,* 356–362.

Green, M. (Ed.) (1994). *Bright futures: Guidelines for health supervision of infants, children, and adolescents.* Arlington, VA: National Center for Education in Maternal and Child Health.

Hohn, A.R. (1997). Diagnosis and management of hypertension in childhood. *Pediatric Annals, 26*(2), 105–110.

Kury, S.P., & Rodrigue, J.R. (1995). Concepts of illness causality in a pediatric sample: Relationship to illness duration, frequency of hospitalization, and degree of life-threat. *Clinical Pediatrics, 34,* 178–182.

Lewit, E.M., & Baker, L.S. (1996). Children as victims of violence. [Monograph]. In R.E. Behrman (Ed.), *The future of children: The juvenile court, 6*(3), 147–156.

Milsum, J.H. (1991). Health, risk factor reduction, and lifestyle change. In K.A. Saucier (Ed.), *Perspective in fam-*

ily and community health (pp. 176–184). St. Louis: Mosby Year Book.

National Cholesterol Education Program (1991). *Report of the expert panel on blood cholesterol levels in children and adolescents.* Washington, DC: U.S. Department of Health and Human Services.

Sinaiko, A.R. (1996). Hypertension in children. *The New England Journal of Medicine, 335*(26), 1968–1973.

Troiano, R.P., Flegal, K.M., Kuczmarski, R.J., Campbell, S.M., & Johnson, C.L. (1995). Overweight prevalence and trends for children and adolescents. *Archives of Pediatrics and Adolescent Medicine, 149,* 1085–1091.

U.S. Department of Health and Human Services. (1991). *Healthy children 2000.* Washington, DC: Author.

VanAntwerp, C.A. (1995). The lifestyle questionnaire for school-aged children: A tool for primary care. *Journal of Pediatric Health Care, 9*(6), 251–255.

STUDY QUESTIONS

1. Which health condition is known to be more common in children from single parent families?
   a. Depression
   b. Glomerulonephritis
   c. Asthma
   d. Leukemia

2. What percentage of children in the United States receive health teaching about numerous health topics across all grade levels?
   a. < 50%
   b. 50%
   c. 75%
   d. Nearly 100%

3. Homicide and personal crimes are highest in which age group?
   a. < 3 years
   b. 5–9 years
   c. 9–12 years
   d. Teens

4. The recommendation for the amount of daily calories to be supplied by dietary fat in children's diets is:
   a. 15%
   b. <30%
   c. 50%
   d. >45%

5. Which is a true statement about overweight in children?
   a. About 5% of children are overweight.
   b. The percentage of children who are overweight has remained fairly constant over the past several years.
   c. Most children outgrow overweight as they grow older.
   d. About twice as many children are overweight now as were a decade ago.

6. The minimum number of times weekly that a child should have an aerobic activity is:
   a. 7
   b. 5
   c. 3
   d. 1

7. Eroded tooth enamel and knuckle calluses are a sign of which disorder?
   a. Vitamin deficiency
   b. Poor dental hygiene
   c. Obesity
   d. Bulimia

8. For a diagnosis of significant hypertension to be made, which condition must be present?
   a. Three separate systolic and/or diastolic blood pressure measures above the 95th percentile for age and gender.
   b. Systolic and/or diastolic blood pressure consistently between the 90th and 95th percentile for age and gender.
   c. Three separate systolic and diastolic blood pressure measures above the 75th percentile for age and gender.
   d. Systolic and/or diastolic blood pressure consistently above the 50th percentile for age, gender, and weight.

9. Which of the following has been shown to be ineffective in lowering blood pressure in children?
   a. Low sodium diet
   b. Adequate fiber intake
   c. Low potassium diet
   d. Low saturated fat intake

10. Recommended total cholesterol level for children is:
    a. <170 mg/dL
    b. <190 mg/dL
    c. <200 mg/dL
    d. <240 mg/dL

11. Recommended immunizations for teens include:
    a. hepatitis A and pertussis.
    b. hepatitis B and varicella.
    c. haemophilus influenzae type b and pneumococcal.
    d. typhoid and polio.

12. Which characteristic of cognitive ability at 9 years is important to remember when planning health teaching for this age?
    a. Egocentrism; inability to understand the views and experiences of others.
    b. Ability to focus on the future results of present activities.
    c. A need for concrete experiences to learn information.
    d. An emphasis on mental health concepts.

ANSWERS

1.c 2.a 3.d 4.b 5.d 6.c 7.d 8.a 9.c 10.a 11.b 12.c

Chapter 6

Separation, Loss, and Bereavement

Lois J. Pearson, MEd, CCLS

Concept

◆◆◆◆◆◆◆◆◆◆◆◆◆◆◆◆◆◆◆◆◆◆◆◆◆◆

◆ Separation, loss, and bereavement

Objectives

◆◆◆◆◆◆◆◆◆◆◆◆◆◆◆◆◆◆◆◆◆◆◆◆◆

At the completion of this chapter, the reader will be able to:

◆ Recognize the components of separation, loss, and bereavement.

◆ Describe the impact of death of a child upon parents and surviving siblings.

◆ Demonstrate knowledge of children's understanding of death by age.

◆ Identify interventions that are most supportive to grieving families.

◆ Assess the needs of the dying child and family.

Key Points

◆◆◆◆◆◆◆◆◆◆◆◆◆◆◆◆◆◆◆◆◆◆◆◆◆

◆ Knowledge of the developmental characteristics of each age group is fundamental to providing family-centered care when a child is dying.

◆ Participation by parents is essential to coping with the death of a child.

◆ Interventions with families at the bedside of a dying child must be focused on preparation and support.

◆ Children's grief is unique and needs careful attention to what is felt rather than to what is understood.

Separation, Loss, and Bereavement

I. OVERVIEW OF SEPARATION, LOSS, AND GRIEF

A. Definitions (Wolfelt, 1996).
1. Grief: the thoughts and feelings that are experienced when someone loved dies; the internal meaning given to the experience of bereavement.
2. Mourning: taking the external experience of grief and expressing it outside oneself, i.e., "grief gone public."
3. Bereavement: the state of having suffered a loss; to be bereaved means to have the experience of loss.

B. Historical perspective.
1. Up until the 20th century, death experiences were an integral part of living from day to day.
2. A number of factors have recently changed the way death is experienced (DeSpelder, 1987).
   a. Life expectancies have increased, and mortality rates have decreased so that death is not encountered as frequently.
   b. Geographic mobility isolates families so that the death of a member may occur away from the extended family.
   c. Causes of death have changed; in the past, people died quickly and suddenly because medical treatments were so limited.
   d. Generations live apart from one another due to changing demands of the work force.
   e. Death most often occurs in an institutional setting rather than at home.
   f. Advances in medical technology enable people to live much longer in varying states of health or ill health.
   g. Advanced Directives allow people some autonomy in how they experience death. *See Chapter 31: Legal, Moral, and Ethical Issues of Care.*

C. Classic studies of separation.
1. Spitz (1945) studied effects of separation on hospitalized children.
   a. Noted that infants and young children stopped eating, became marasmic, and often died after suffering an overwhelming sense of loss.
   b. Identified term "hospitalism" to describe the intense sense of loss experienced by infants and preschool age children.
2. Robertson (1958) described three stages of response to separation.
   a. Protest: acute distress characterized by screaming, crying with expectation of parent's return.
   b. Despair: increasing hopelessness about return of parent accompanied by withdrawing behaviors.
   c. Detachment or denial: child appears to be recovered but then greets parent's return with apathy.
3. Bowlby (1969) used the same stages as Robertson, but detailed the effect of separation as related to repeated losses of the young child, and an eventual inability of the child to attach to anyone.
   a. Described attachment behaviors derived from need for security and safety.
   b. Identified that attachment behaviors have survival value for children and adults.
4. Piaget (1960) identified a child's understanding of death as related to his or her stage of cognitive development.
   a. Preoperational: death is reversible.
   b. Concrete operational: what lives also dies.
   c. Formal operations: death has physiologic explanation and everyone will eventually die.

D. Research specific to grief as separation.
1. Lindemann (1944) described grief as a definite syndrome with somatic and psychologic components.
   a. Stated three goals of grief work to be:
      (1) Emancipation from the bondage of the deceased.
      (2) Readjustment to the environment.
      (3) Ability to form new relationships.
   b. Documented that the most severe reactions

seemed to occur in mothers who lost young children.

2. Nagy (1948) studied 378 Hungarian children ages 3–10 years and described stages of children's grief:
   a. Children under 5 years of age did not see death as irreversible, but rather as living under changed circumstances.
   b. Children 5–9 years old personified death.
   c. Children 9 years old and older saw death as final.

3. Speece and Brent (1995) reviewed more than 100 research studies conducted between 1934 and 1990 to discover children's understanding of deaths and identified five principal subconcepts applicable across age groups.
   a. Universality: all living things must eventually die.
   b. Irreversibility: the physical body cannot be restored to life.
   c. Nonfunctionality: death means the end of all physiologic functions.
   d. Causality: attempts to understand what causes death to occur.
   e. Some type of continued life form: a belief in what happens after death, i.e., the soul or spirit.

II. PARENTAL GRIEF

◆ ◆ ◆ ◆ ◆ ◆ ◆ ◆ ◆ ◆ ◆ ◆ ◆ ◆ ◆ ◆ ◆ ◆ ◆ ◆

"Physiologically, psychologically and socially, the relationship that exists between parents and their children may well be the most intense that life can generate. Obviously then, vulnerability to loss through death is most acute when one child dies. Not only is the death of a child inappropriate in the context of living, but its tragic and untimely nature is a basic threat to the function of parenthood to preserve some dimension to the self, the family, and the social group" (Jackson, 1977, p. 187).

A. Review of research.
1. Bowlby (1969) described four phases of parental grief.
   a. Numbness.
      (1) Feelings of shock and denial.
      (2) Motions devoid of emotion.
      (3) Self-preservation response to allow time.
   b. Yearning and searching.
      (1) Preoccupation with dying or deceased person.
      (2) Strong urge to recover what has been lost.
      (3) Crying, anger, hostility.
   c. Disorganization and despair.
      (1) Inability to concentrate.

      (2) Bleak state of mind.
      (3) Feelings of depression.
   d. Reorganization.
      (1) Formation of new attachments.
      (2) Working through of attachments to the deceased.

2. Kalish (1969) identified difficulty of society to support parents who lose children as compared to children who lose a parent.
   a. Reported that the death of a child causes more stress than any other loss.
   b. Related this to the exceptional social value of a child in today's society.

3. Sanders (1979) identified intensity of grief reaction for three losses — spouse, child, or parent — and noted significant increase in intensity of grief for parents who survive the death of their child.

4. Furman (1978) combined research on parent child relationships and bereavement and mourning.
   a. Stated that our culture does not contain social supports for parents who have lost a child.
   b. Noted that grief must be shared with other grieving parents (thus an advantage of support groups), and that the pain must be tolerated.

5. Worden (1982) developed a four-step model toward successful recovery, which is more effective with adult loss than loss of a child:
   a. Accepting reality of the loss.
   b. Experiencing the pain of grief.
   c. Adjusting to an environment in which the deceased is missing.
   d. Withdrawing emotional energy and reinvesting in another relationship.

B. Parental reactions to loss of a child (Rando, 1986).
1. Compared to other losses, the death of a child is severe, complicated, and long lasting.
2. The death of a child has an impact on four areas.
   a. Individual parent.
      (1) Child represents future hopes and dreams.
      (2) Loss of child = loss of part of parent.
   b. Marital relationship.
      (1) Emotional relationship affected.
      (2) Severe grieving affects partnership.
      (3) Dissimilar grief responses found between spouses.
      (4) Reaction to losses based on roles in marriage.
   c. Family system.
      (1) Roles of family members change after loss.
      (2) Surviving children experience many difficulties.

d. Society.
  (1) Inappropriate social expectations about grief exist that do not fit the intensity of feelings over the loss of a child, i.e., that grief reactions will follow the pattern of other losses, which is often not the case.
  (2) Anxiety of would-be supporters of grieving parents felt when contemplating the potential loss of their own child.
  (3) Stigma of loss of child experienced; no term for grieving parent, wherein child without parent is called "orphan" and person without spouse is termed "widow" or "widower."
3. Phases of parental grief (Rando, 1986).
  a. Avoidance phase.
    (1) Feels overwhelmed, numb, bewildered.
    (2) Experiences disbelief; needs to know exactly what happened.
    (3) Intellectualizes response to loss.
  b. Confrontation phase.
    (1) Shock wears off; most intense period of grief.
    (2) Rando describes phase as "angry sadness."
    (3) Experiences feelings of extreme emotions.
  c. Fear and anxiety.
    (1) Extreme emotional reactions trigger fear of loss of sanity.
    (2) Chronic or intermittent feelings of panic occur.
    (3) Feels complete vulnerability and loss of control over life.
  d. Anger and guilt.
    (1) Vented at God, physicians, or others.
    (2) Angry at deceased for abandonment.
    (3) Guilt is the single most pervasive parental response to loss (Miles & Demi, 1986):
      (a) Guilt over cause of death.
      (b) Illness-related guilt.
      (c) Parental role guilt.
      (d) Moral guilt.
      (e) Survival guilt.
      (f) Grief guilt.
  e. Separation and longing.
    (1) Experiences acute physical feelings of emptiness.
    (2) Has vivid visual or auditory dreams and recollections.
    (3) Experiences unparalleled feelings of yearning for the lost child.
  f. Depression.
    (1) Feels utter despair.
    (2) Disregards personal matters of care due to preoccupation with thoughts of child.
    (3) Is irritable and unable to concentrate.
  g. Obsession.
    (1) Constantly reviews death event with attempts to gain control.
    (2) Behavior magnified in this phase if sudden death.
  h. Search for meaning to death.
    (1) Important part of grief process because loss of child is so unnatural.
    (2) Creates facts that give reasons, even if information is incomplete.
  i. Grief attacks.
    (1) Sudden acute upsurges of grief occur.
    (2) Grief is accompanied by physical sensations.
    (3) Becomes confused over these renewed acute feelings.
  j. Identification.
    (1) Engages in activities to keep ties to dead child at forefront.
    (2) Acts positively to support association with importance of child's life.
  k. Social manifestations.
    (1) Socially withdraws.
    (2) Is unable to maintain patterns of interaction with others; friends appear to abandon parent.
    (3) Refuses to accept support offered by friends.
  l. Common physiologic manifestations.
    (1) Anorexia.
    (2) Insomnia.
    (3) Loss of interest in sex.
    (4) Weight loss.
    (5) Crying.
  m. Reestablishment phase.
    (1) Grief feelings gradually decrease.
    (2) Can reengage in everyday activities.
    (3) Has feeling of beginning to grow up with the loss, recognizing that there will be a normal reactivation of grief and sadness at certain times, i.e., graduation of classmates, anniversary of death, birthday, child's friend's wedding.

C. Anticipatory coping and its effect on parental grief.
1. Positive effects resulting from supporting parents during child's illness include (Rando, 1986):
  a. Fewer incidences of abnormal grief responses following an anticipated death.
  b. Parental reports of more positive responses to loss.
2. Illnesses of longer than 18 months do not seem to enhance the value of anticipatory grief (Rando, 1986).
3. Parents who have high level of previous losses

Table 6-1. Children's Understanding of Death by Age

AGE	UNDERSTANDING OF DEATH	CHARACTERISTIC BEHAVIORS	LANGUAGE	INTERVENTIONS
Newborn to 3 Years A 2½ year old has begun having temper tantrums each morning 2 weeks after the death of her 1-week-old sister. Her mother admits that she cries each morning upon awakening to another day of grieving. When questioning the 2-year-old child about why she is acting that way, she replies that she "wants Mommy not to be sad anymore!"	• Does not comprehend death • Aware of constant buzz of activity in the house • Aware of Mom and Dad looking sad and teary-eyed • Aware that someone in the home is missing	• Has altered eating and sleeping patterns • Is irritable • Clings	• Use the 'D' words: dying, death, dead. • Avoid euphemisms like "lost, passed away, gone to sleep," which confuse young children. • Explain in physiologic terms, i.e., person who is dead does not eat or drink, or feel feelings, like being cold after burial in the ground. • Expect questions to change. • Expect repeated questioning & testing to confirm information.	• Maintain routines but allow for flexibility. • Choose familiar and supportive caregivers. • Assign a support person for each child during funeral, burial, and other rituals. • Acknowledge all feelings of child and adult by naming feelings and giving permission to express anger and sadness in developmentally appropriate ways. • Give extra hugs when needed to help child feel secure.
3 to 5 Year Olds A 4-year-old girl was thought to not know anything about the anticipated death of her soon-to-be-born baby brother, until she was observed playing "dead baby" with her dolls. It was only then that the family realized how perceptive this 4 year old was to the surrounding grief.	• Sees death as temporary and reversible; child continually asks if person will return • May feel ambivalent • Through magical thinking, may assume responsibility for the death	• Is concerned about own well-being • Feels confused and guilty • May use imaginative play, reenacting scene of CPR, etc. • Withdraws • Is irritable • Regresses	• Explain cause of death factually; that which is mentionable is manageable. • Answer questions honestly, e.g., clarify wellness of sibling, unlike that of dying child. • Avoid abstracts. • Diffuse magical thinking. • Be consistent and persistent.	• Reinforce that when people are sad, they cry; crying is natural. • Read stories (see bibliography of children's books). • Provide materials for child to draw pictures. • Encourage dialogue/family meetings. • Expect misbehavior as child struggles with confusing feelings and issues. • Offer play with themes of death while providing supportive guidance.
6 to 9 Year Olds A 6-year-old boy, who has just returned from the bedside of his dying newborn sister, explains in a matter-of-fact style to his 5-year-old sister, "We cannot go to heaven after Mindy goes there, because you would have to have a spaceship. Heaven is way father away. You have to go past Mars." Another 6-year-old whose 12-year-old brother had just been struck by a car and was declared brain dead, tried to relate what was happening to herself and her family but was completely unable to organize the experience in a cognitive way. In her sadness and confusion at the bedside, she said "Ah Buddy...We had some great times together, but he never died before."	• Begins to understand concept of death • Feels it happens to others • May be superstitious about death • May be uncomfortable in expressing feelings • Worries that other important people will die	• May seem outwardly uncaring, inwardly upset • May use denial to cope • May attempt to "parent" parent • May act out in school or home • May play death games	• Look for questions within questions. • Expect a more global view. • Encourage child to answer own questions. • Explore feelings by questions such as "What do you think?"	• Listen to determine what kind of information the child is seeking. • Increase physical activity while role modeling stress-reducing behaviors. • Work on identifying feelings, which are becoming more sophisticated, i.e., frustration, confusion. • Encourage creative outlets for feelings, i.e., drawing, painting clay, blank books.

continued on next page

Table 6-1. Children's Understanding of Death by Age (continued)

AGE	UNDERSTANDING OF DEATH	CHARACTERISTIC BEHAVIORS	LANGUAGE	INTERVENTIONS
9 to 12 Year Olds A 10-year-old girl describing her feelings following the unexpected death of her father... "Sure I thought he would die before me. He was older than I am. But I certainly didn't expect him to die when I was only 10 years old!" A 9 year old, in explaining why his baby sister did not look like herself at the open casket visitation, stated that "Her soul is gone, and that's what gives people their light."	• Accepts death as final • Has personal fear of death • May be morbidly interested in skeletons, gruesome details of violent deaths • Concerned with practical matters about child's lifestyle	• May appear tough or funny • May express and demonstrate anger or sadness • May act like adult, but regress to earlier stage of emotional response	• Provide more detail as needed, especially to explain cause of death in physiologic context. • Probe for thoughts and feelings. • Allow for spiritual development. • May answer questions about an afterlife by stating, "We don't really know but we believe that..."	• Encourage creative expressions of feelings. • Explore support group/peer-to-peer connection (see Box 6-2 describing grief support group session). • Establish family traditions and memorials. • Incorporate children into rituals not just at time of death, but at important anniversaries (e.g., taking balloons to the cemetery; creating a special ornament for the Christmas tree, which is always hung first; having birthday dinners and memory nights).
Adolescents An adolescent girl wrote these words after her father died and her mother was diagnosed with cancer: "While I was tending to my mom, all I felt was anguish and despair. I tried to kill myself in an adverse way by driving my Firebird at 100mph on a winding road. It was stupid, but it was the only way to rid myself of my anger. I had bad feelings that my mom was going to leave me alone and I would be without the two people I loved the most, my mom and dad" (Snoddy, 1992, p. 13).	• Has adult concept of death, but ability to deal with loss is based on experience and developmental factors • Experiences thrill of recklessness • Focuses on present • Is developing strong philosophical view • Questions existence of an afterlife	• Increased reliance on peers instead of family • Moodiness and irritability • May engage in risk-taking behaviors • Appears rebellious and tests limits • May act impulsively or without common sense	• Treat as adult with information, respect, and responsibility. • Role model adult behaviors. • Allow to make informed choices.	• Allow for informed participation. • Encourage peer support. • Suggest individualized and group expressions of grief, e.g., school memorials. • Support group advocacy for causes, e.g., Students Against Drunk Driving (SADD). • Recommend creative outlets, e.g., writing, art, and music.

may not demonstrate positive effects of anticipatory grief work.

4. Anticipatory coping builds on the trust level of the family and the health care professionals working together over time prior to the death.

5. Stages of parental anticipatory mourning (Futterman & Hoffman, 1983).
   a. Acknowledgement: a growing awareness of approach of inevitable death accompanied by alternating feelings of hope and despair.
   b. Grieving: emotional reactions to the loss that start as intense undifferentiated responses and mellow in quantity and intensity.
   c. Reconciliation: attempts to find meaning for life and death.
   d. Detachment: process whereby parents gradually withdraw their emotional investment from child.
   e. Memorialization: idealization of child results in parents developing mental image of child that will live beyond the death.

D. Behaviors by health care professionals that support positive grief work (Worden, 1982).
   1. Present information carefully.
   2. Intervene with sensitivity.
   3. Help parents to actualize the loss by providing an opportunity for them to view the dead body.
   4. Clarify the cause of death.
   5. Provide information about subsequent emotional reactions.

E. Supportive interventions at the time of death.
   1. Allow parents to make choices whenever possible, but limit those choices that are not helpful, i.e., what time to discontinue life support.
   2. Determine the significant support persons among family and staff, and encourage their presence at the bedside.
   3. Provide privacy for family.
   4. Voice empathy by acknowledging feelings to family.
   5. Access available resources within the health care setting:
      a. Social Work for crises intervention and support.
      b. Chaplaincy to offer spiritual support.
      c. Child Life to address issues of surviving siblings and other children involved in the death.
      d. Bereavement counselors for additional support.
      e. Hospice or palliative care, if appropriate.
   6. Describe process at time of death, including preparation of the body.
   7. Allow adequate time for good-byes at the bed-

side, but be sensitive to helping family leave when necessary.

8. Offer concrete memorials:
   a. Lock of hair.
   b. Ink prints of hand and/or foot.
   c. Plaster casts of hand or foot.
   d. Photographs of family with dying child or after death.
   e. Comfort objects used at time of death, i.e., infant dress and hat, baby quilt used for last holding.
   f. Certificates, plaque, seashell used for bedside rituals like baptism.
9. Allow parents to participate in cares at time of death, e.g., holding, bathing, dressing.
10. Assure parents and other family members that all rituals, requests, or plans at the time of death are acceptable and based solely on parents needs and wishes (see "Culture, Grief, and Mourning," in this chapter and *Chapter 29: Cultural Influences.*
11. Offer for nurse to accompany the body from the unit to the morgue, if appropriate.
12. Accompany and support parents and other family members as they leave the hospital.
13. Provide bereavement resources as available.
14. Follow up with bereavement services and support through funeral, anniversaries, birthdays, and first year.

III. CHILDREN'S GRIEF
◆ ◆ ◆ ◆ ◆ ◆ ◆ ◆ ◆ ◆ ◆ ◆ ◆ ◆ ◆ ◆ ◆

A. Unique characteristics of children's grief.
   1. Children of any age focus on their ability to feel, rather than their ability to understand. (Rando, 1986; Wolfelt, 1996).
   2. The grief responses of children are affected by the following factors:
      a. Anticipated versus unanticipated death.
         (1) The more sudden a death, the more likely a child is to mourn in doses and intermittently.
         (2) Response to sudden death may appear to be without feeling.
         (3) Less outward mourning may be characteristic of sudden death.
      b. Age of the person who died.
         (1) Deaths that are "out of the natural order" are more difficult for children to reconcile.
         (2) The death of a child is especially frightening for other children who believe that only old people die.
      c. Child's sense of culpability.
         (1) Magical thinking may cause children to believe that what they wished or thought

could hurt someone or make someone die.
  (2) Magical thinking is characteristic of young children.
  d. Stigma surrounding death.
    (1) Certain causes of death are less acceptable within society, i.e., suicide, violent death.
    (2) Deaths accompanied by stigma are more difficult for children.
3. A child's world is based on play, and play is an important tool to assist bereaved children in the work of mourning (see Table 6-1 for age-appropriate interventions).
4. There are three primary questions the child needs to have answered:
  a. Did I cause this to happen?
  b. Could I die too?
  c. Who will take care of me now?
5. How a child grieves is dependent on developmental level, family communication, and coping style.

B. Children's perceptions of death by developmental age (see Table 6-1 and Box 6-1. "What Does 'Dead' Mean?").

C. The unique grief of siblings.
1. Siblings cannot relate to past or future as adults do.
2. Grief is complicated by the unavailability of grieving parents to surviving children.
3. Siblings spend more time together than any other family members.
4. The bond between siblings begins before birth as one prepares to become "big brother or sister."
5. Common characteristics of sibling grief include:
  a. Guilt that they caused the illness and death.
  b. Fear that they could also die.
  c. Confusion over their role in changed family structure.
  d. Inability to compete with dead sibling.
  e. Sense of responsibility that all parental expectations are now placed upon them.
6. Siblings need additional information over time as their developmental and cognitive abilities expand.
7. Factors associated with favorable adjustment include:
  a. Children who are involved in illness experience and prepared for death may have fewer abnormal responses than those who face sudden death.
  b. Children who are involved in the rituals of sibling's death have fewer behavioral problems up to 3 years later (Grollman, 1995).

WHAT DOES "DEAD" MEAN?

The following responses to the question "What does 'dead' mean?" are from children who have had first hand experience with the death of a family member.

Angie, age 6…
"I think dead means that the person who is dead, their heart's not beating and their brain's not thinking, their lungs not breathing and then their spirit goes up to heaven and then I don't know what else."

Matthew, age 7…
"I think dead means that people's skin go away from their bodies and the bones are left."

Tyler, age 8….
"Dead means to me that when you're dead, you can't come back to life and you live a new life up in heaven."

Robert, age 9…
"I think dead means that people don't live no more and you can do whatever with the body. You can either cremate them or just bury them in the casket."

Melissa, age 10…
"I think dead means that when someone dies, your heart stops beating and you're just dead. And the body starts to disintegrate. Also, they just don't come back."

Antonio, age 18…
"I think death is when your time is up. You're ready to leave and you've lived your life. Maybe you didn't live it to its fullest, but when you're dead I look at it from a religious point of view and it depends on your deeds. If you were good or you were bad. If you were good, you will get your reward in heaven. If you were bad, maybe you can have another chance on judgment day and see if you can be forgiven. But death is really just another part of life. I believe there's two parts, one living and one dead. And we shouldn't really say that death is bad because when you're dead, you'll finally have peace of mind and you'll have peace within yourself and maybe the people that knew you will also have peace. That's what I think death is."

Box 6-1

c. Siblings who are emotionally close demonstrate more favorable adjustment following a loss than siblings who are not close (Davies, 1988).
d. Higher levels of extended family and friends support enhances family adaptation.

A GLIMPSE INTO A CHILDREN'S SUPPORT GROUP SESSION...

The two brothers share the auspicious moment. Circle rounds have been completed and the time for sharing has arrived. Together the boys present a large, brown, worn looking case with tattered leather straps and buckles, which are lovingly handled by the young boys. An awesome silence settles over the giggly, rambunctious circle of children as the lid is slowly lifted to reveal the precious contents. It is a much-loved guitar.

To an adult, the scene touches one's heart, realizing that the instrument's music has been silenced by the sudden death of the boys' father. To the children, who all share the common experience of having had a parent die, the moment isn't perceived as a sad one, but rather as a means to get to know the boys' father through sharing a special memory.

With respect and tenderness, the boys pass the guitar from child to child in the circle, allowing each to tug gently at a string, or touch the highly polished wood of its face. Circle is completed when all others have shared a memento, cherished photo, or favorite memory of their dead parent — a fishing trip, a shell they collected along the beach. The sharing and expression of feelings is the common tie.

Unlike adults, the children make an almost spontaneous transition from the quiet rather serious sharing within the circle, to the more typical activity at the art table. Animated conversation mingles with laughter and continued sharing as the children begin work on their memory mobiles. Each construction paper creation symbolizes a special time or favorite activity of the parent who died.

The scene is complete with the realization that accompanying the busy sounds of the children at work, a tape recorder in the center of the table is filling the room with the rich warmth of Jacob's and David's father singing the country folk music he loved so much.

Box 6-2

D. Interventions for siblings.
1. Provide medical play, if appropriate, during critical illness.
2. Encourage creative expression of feelings:
   a. Art work (family drawings, collages).
   b. Writing diaries, blank books, simple poetry, letters to dying sibling.
   c. Dramatic play, audiotapes, videotapes.
3. Identify support persons.

4. Provide information for teachers and students on ways to support the surviving sibling.
5. Prepare for procedures, treatments, and visits to bedside.
6. Include in family sessions with support of family if appropriate.
7. Provide ongoing interventions by trusted health care professional.

E. Reconciliation of children's grief (Wolfelt, 1989).
1. Reconciliation: a changed reality of moving forward in life without the physical presence of the person who has died (Wolfelt, 1996).
   a. It is accompanied by a renewed sense of energy and an ability to become reinvolved in activities of living.
   b. It does not indicate a total return to normalcy as the experience of grief changes the bereaved.
2. Determinants of successful grief reconciliation for children include:
   a. Previously healthy relationship with deceased person.
   b. Prompt and accurate information.
   c. Encouragement to ask questions and receive responses.
   d. Participation in family mourning process.
   e. Supportive presence of continued trusting relationships (see Box 6-2. "A Glimpse Into a Children's Support Group Session").
3. Indicators of reconciliation.
   a. Return to stable eating and sleeping behavior patterns.
   b. Renewed sense of energy.
   c. Capacity to enjoy life.
   d. Recognition of the reality and finality of death.
   e. Establishment of new, healthy relationships.

IV. THE DYING CHILD AND FAMILY

◆ ◆ ◆ ◆ ◆ ◆ ◆ ◆ ◆ ◆ ◆ ◆ ◆ ◆ ◆ ◆ ◆ ◆ ◆ ◆

A. Overview of terminal illness.
1. How a child faces death depends upon the:
   a. Child's developmental capacity to understand its meaning.
   b. Environmental climate provided by child's caretakers.
2. The grief of the dying child is similar to those feelings other bereaved children experience.
3. *The Private Worlds of Dying Children* by Myra Bluebond-Langner (1978) describes a socialization study of children on a leukemia ward of the hospital (see Box 6-3. "Life and Death on the Oncology Unit").

LIFE AND DEATH ON THE ONCOLOGY UNIT

The Private Worlds of Dying Children by Myra Bluebond-Langner (1978) details by observation and interview how children come to know they are dying and the mutual pretense they create between parent and child and children and medical personnel.

How children acquired the knowledge of their disease process, treatment and prognosis was accomplished in stages, each marked by the acquisition of important information.

1. Realization that "It" is a serious illness.
2. Understanding names of drugs, uses, and side effects.
3. Knowledge of procedures and treatments, relationships between symptoms and procedures, each viewed as unique and isolated events.
4. Realization that the disease is a series of remissions and relapses
5. Understanding that the disease would cause death when drugs were no longer effective

Experience provided the necessary movement from one stage to the next. At the same time, as children passed through the stages of information acquisition, they also passed through five stages of differing self-concepts (see Figure 6-1).

1. Well at diagnosis
2. Seriously ill and will get better (evidenced by responses of family and friends and physical changes in themselves)
3. Always ill and will get better
4. Always ill and will never get better (relapses and drug complications threatened the child's sense of well-being)
5. Dying (only realized when child heard of the death of a peer)

The behaviors of dying children provided clues to the child's knowledge of impending death despite adults' refusal to prepare the children. Children who were dying avoided the name and belongings of a child who had died on the unit; lacked interest in nondisease-related conversation and play; became preoccupied with death and disease imagery in play, art, and literature; engaged selected individuals in either disclosure conversations or disclosure speeches; appeared anxious about increased debilitation and about going home, but for different reasons than earlier on in the disease process; avoided talking about the future; displayed concern that things be done immediately; refused to cooperate with relatively simple, painless procedures; and established distance from others through displays of anger or silence.

According to Bluebond-Langner (1978, p. 235): "The answer lies in devising a policy that allows children to maintain open awareness with those who can handle it, and at the same time to maintain mutual pretense with those who want to practice it. The children know both what their parents know and what they want to hear. They are more concerned with having their parents near than with them telling them the prognosis."

Box 6-3

B. Guidelines for intervention with the dying child (Wolfelt, 1996).

1. Do not underestimate the child's capacity to understand.
2. Create open communication but do not force it.
   a. Listen first, then offer support.
   b. Provide honest information.
   c. Remember that it is okay to say, "I don't know."
   d. Answer only what child wants to know.
3. Provide creative outlets for anger, such as art therapy.
4. Follow the child's lead.
5. Be honest with the child about impending death.
6. Allow the child time to say good-byes.
7. Permit the child to decide when he or she wants to share the pain of grief.
8. Remember that the child may choose to protect the parent (mutual pretense).
9. Help the dying child to live.
   a. Make the child comfortable.
      (1) Arrange physical setting for the child to be with family.
         (a) Create space for the child in family living area.
         (b) Plan family activities for the child to participate in or observe.
         (c) Arrange for medical equipment, i.e., hospital bed, only as needed.
      (2) Address pain control measures and methods.
      (3) Focus on keeping environment and routine child-focused as much as possible.
   b. Create special, memorable moments.
   c. Continue some routine.
   d. Surround the child with people who mean the most to the child.
   e. Help the child maintain peer friendships.

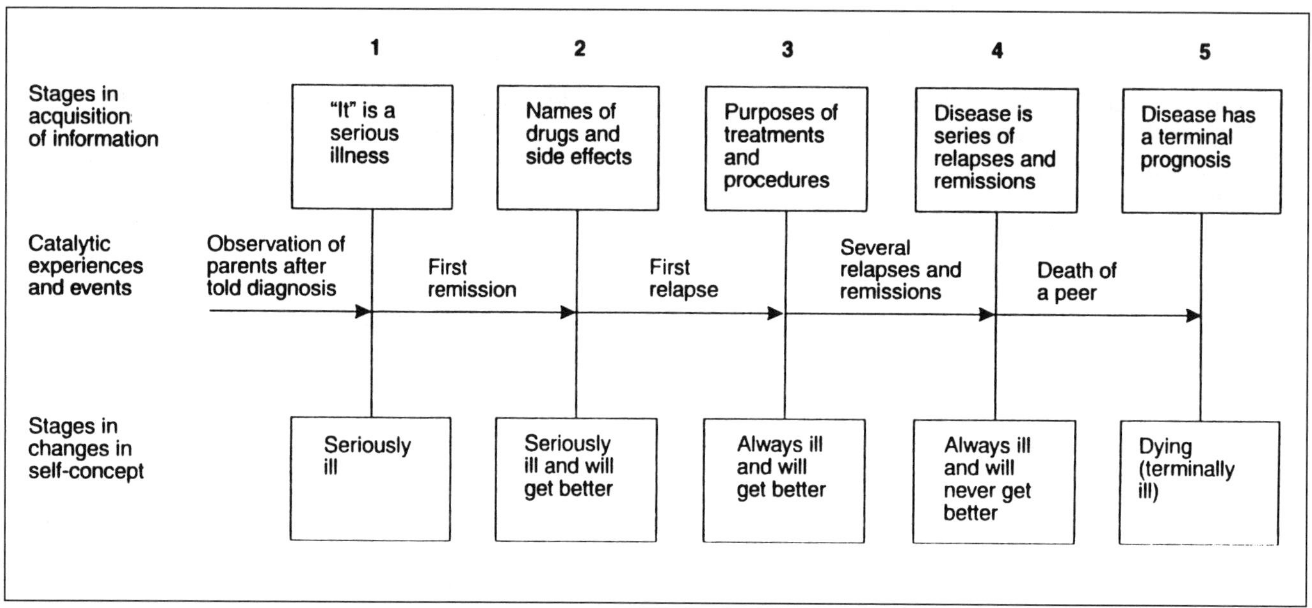

Figure 6-1
Children acquire knowledge of their disease process, treatment, and prognosis in stages.
Reprinted with permission from Doka, K.J. (1995). *Children mourning: Mourning children.* Bristol, PA: Hospice Foundation of America, p. 117.

C. Particular issues for the dying adolescent.
1. Response to terminal illness is similar to that of an adult.
2. Tolerance of physical ravages of terminal illness is poor.
3. Tends to feel that time spent growing up was wasted.
4. Fears increased dependency, bodily deterioration.
5. Is comforted by religious beliefs.

D. Guidelines for communicating with the dying adolescent (Pazola & Gerberg, 1990).
1. Tell the adolescent he/she is dying.
   a. When disease is progressing and treatment is not working, the adolescent needs to be given permission to talk about death.
   b. Plan for supportive presence of parents, physician, nurse, and significant others.
   c. Answer questions of "Why?" and "What will happen next?" with honesty, sensitivity, and directness.
   d. Adolescents will confide in caregivers who are able to tolerate the overwhelming sadness of impending death.
2. Acknowledge sadness of this news on patient, parents, and caregivers.
3. Allow adolescent time to make plans, bring closure.
4. Intervene if denial occurs.
   a. The adolescent who states she's going to be an Olympic swimmer may be expressing wishes of what she had hoped would be her future.
   b. Redirect communication, "You wish that you could be well enough to do that."
   c. Reframe the situation with reassurance that the adolescent will not be alone.
5. Respond to indirect pleas for support.
   a. Adolescent may need confirmation from caregivers that death is imminent or treatment is no longer working.
   b. Last wishes may be made of caregivers to protect family members; teens are often especially protective of their parents' feelings.
6. Enable expression of needs and wishes to pursue unfinished business, i.e., make accommodations for teen to travel to say goodbye to close friends.
7. Advocate for the adolescent in ethical dilemmas of treatment and end of treatment choices.
8. Support decisions on how and where the adolescent wants to die.

E. The hospice movement in the United States.
1. Hospice: a concept of care started in England that provides physical, psychologic, social, and spiritual support to children and families with life-threatening conditions, their families, and health care professionals.
2. The National Hospice Organization's 1992

survey indicated that 1% of 240,000 hospice patients were children (Grollman, 1995).

3. Hospice care includes:
   a. Palliative care and symptom management.
   b. Respite care.
   c. Anticipatory grief.
   d. Bereavement care.
4. Death occurs in the home, hospital, or other facility.
5. Preparation and coordination of services are essential to support parents caring for child in the home.
6. Hospice care provides attention to the whole family, support of parents, the child who is ill, and surviving siblings.

V. Culture, Grief, and Mourning

A. Overview of the effects of culture.
   Also see Chapter 29: Cultural Influences.
   1. "What people who have experienced a loss believe, feel and do, varies enormously from culture to culture" (Irish, Lundquist, & Nelsen, 1993, p. 14).
   2. Cross cultural variations in behaviors of bereaved people are not random, but arise out of societal ways of understanding the world.
   3. Cultural differences include:
      a. What people believe and understand about death.
      b. What people feel about death.
      c. What elicits these feelings.
      d. Perceived implications of these feelings.
      e. Ways to express these feelings.
      f. Appropriateness of certain feelings.
      g. Techniques for dealing with feelings that cannot be expressed.

B. Implications for health care professionals (Grollman, 1995).
   1. Identify the individual or family's cultural beliefs.
   2. Understand and respect the values reflected in all cultures.
   3. Enhance communication effectiveness by providing medical interpreters.
   4. Remember that in some cultures the age of a child is not an accurate predictor of experience with death.
   5. Avoid conclusions based on limited information about another culture.
   6. Ask questions about the beliefs and bereavement rituals of both adults and children.
   7. Avoid broad generalizations as there is much diversity within common ethnic groups.
   8. Make allowances for partial assimilation into the dominant culture, especially for children.
   9. Ask family what cultural values are most important to them.
   10. Acknowledge the significance of collective losses for some cultures, i.e., loss of homeland, traditions.
   11. Be aware of the implications of one's own beliefs as they may affect the role of caregivers in life and death experiences.

VI. Summary

A. The experience of the death of a child has an impact that forever changes the bereaved family.

B. To provide sensitive care for bereaved families requires knowledge of:
   1. Children's understanding of death by developmental age.
   2. The unique grief reactions and responses of the bereaved adolescent.
   3. The characteristics of parental grief.
   4. The needs of the dying child and surviving family members.
   5. The role of cultural diversity in grief and mourning.

C. The provision of sensitive and supportive care of the family through the experience of the death of a child will have significant effect upon the bereaved family's ability to reconcile the loss in a meaningful way and move toward a changed future.

D. Being able to identify the interventions that have a significant impact upon a family's adjustment to loss will enable the health care professional to respond effectively when facing the difficult issues of the death of a child.

Bibliography

Bluebond-Langner, M. (1978). *The private worlds of dying children.* Princeton, NJ: Princeton University Press.

Bowlby, J. (1969). In *Attachment and loss: Vol. 1. Attachment.* New York: Basic Books.

Bowlby, J. (1980). In *Attachment and loss: Vol. 3. Loss, sadness and depression.* New York: Basic Books.

Davies, B. (1988). The family environment in bereaved families and its relationship to surviving sibling behavior. *Children's Health Care, 17*(1), 22–30.

DeSpelder, L., & Strickland, A. (1987). *The last dance: Encountering death and dying.* Palo Alto, CA: Mayfield Publishing Company.

Doka, K. (Ed.). (1995). *Children mourning: Mourning children*. Bristol, PA: Hospice Foundation of America.

Furman, E. (1978). The death of a newborn: Care of the parents. *Birth and the Family Journal 5*(4), 214–218.

Futterman, E.H., & Hoffman, I. (1983). Mourning the fatally ill child. In J. Schowalter, P. Patterson, M. Tallmer, A. Kutscher, S. Gullo, & D. Peretz (Eds.), *The child and death* (pp. 366–381). New York: Columbia University Press.

Grollman, E. (1995). *Bereaved children and teens: A support guide for parents and professionals*. Boston: Beacon Press.

Irish, D.P., Lundquist, K.F., & Nelsen, V.J. (1993). *Ethnic variations in dying, death and grief: Diversity in universality*. Washington, DC: Taylor and Francis.

Jackson, E. (1977). Comments in section on "The Parents." In N. Linzer (Ed.), *Understanding bereavement and grief*. New York: Yeshiva University Press.

Kalish, R.A. (1969). The effects of death upon the family. In L. Pearson (Ed.), *Death and dying: Current issues in the treatment of the dying person* (pp. 79–107). Cleveland: The Press of Case Western Reserve University.

Lindemann, E. (1944). Symptomatology and management of acute grief. *American Journal of Psychiatry, 101,* 141–148.

Miles, M.S., & Demi, A.S. (1986). Guilt in bereaved parents. In T. Rando (Ed.), *Parental loss of a child (pp*. 97–118). Champaign, IL: Research Press Company.

Nagy, M. (1948). The child's theories concerning death. *Journal of Genetic Psychology, 73,* 3–27.

Pazola, K.J, & Gerberg, A.K. (1990). Privileged communication — Talking with a dying adolescent. *Maternal Child Nursing, 15,* 16–21.

Piaget, J. (1960). *The child's conception of the world*. Patterson, NJ: Littlefield, Adams & Company.

Rando, T. (1986). *Parental loss of a child*. Champaign, IL: Research Press Company.

Robertson, J. (1958). *Young children in hospitals*. New York: Basic Books, Inc.

Sanders, C.M. (1979-80). A comparison of adult bereavement in the death of a spouse, child, and parent. *Omega, 10,* 303–322.

Snoddy, A. (1992). A teenager's personal account of tragedy. *Thanatos, 17*(2), 13–15.

Speece, M.W., & Brent, S.B. (1985). The development of children's understanding of death. In C.A. Corr, & D.M. Corr (Eds.), *Helping children cope with death and bereavement*. New York: Springer Publishing Company.

Spitz, R. (1945). Hospitalism: An enquiry into the genesis of psychiatric conditions in early childhood. *Psycho-analytical Study of the Child, 1,* 53–74.

Wolfelt, A. D. (1996). *Healing the bereaved child*. Fort Collins, CO: Companion Press.

Worden, J.W. (1982). *Grief counseling and grief therapy*. New York: Springer.

STUDY QUESTIONS

◆ ◆

The 14-day-old infant daughter of Mr. and Mrs. Sullivan was admitted to the hospital late yesterday afternoon after she stopped breathing at home. Her neurologic condition has deteriorated throughout the day. Medical staff have told the parents that her prognosis is grim and will order brain flow studies in the morning. As you begin your shift, Mrs. Sullivan tells you that she does not know what to do about her three other children, ages 2, 4, and 10 years, who were all at home at the time of the incident.

1. Identify the age appropriate intervention that would be of most importance for the 2-year-old sibling.
   a. Have her brought to the hospital to be close to her parents.
   b. Be careful that she does not see the baby after the death.
   c. Keep her in the care of familiar and loving caretakers.
   d. Explain exactly what happened so she does not feel that the death is her fault.
   e. Do not say anything about what happened until the parents return home.

2. Identify the age-appropriate interventions that are most important for the 4-year-old sibling.
   a. Provide accurate and honest information about the cause of the baby's illness and probable death.
   b. Assure the 4-year-old that nothing she did or thought caused this to happen.
   c. Insist that the sibling hold the baby before she dies.
   d. Encourage her to draw pictures about what happened at home.
   e. All except c

3. Identify the age-appropriate interventions that are most important for the 10-year-old sibling.
   a. Explain the physiologic reasons for what is happening to the baby.
   b. Provide opportunities to express feelings through artwork.
   c. Encourage sibling to attend school to keep him from worrying about the baby.
   d. Reassure him that the baby has been baptized and will go to heaven to be with great-grandma.
   e. a and b

4. Mr. and Mrs. Sullivan are struggling with the impact of their infant daughter's sudden illness and impending death. Much medical information has been presented and now the plan is simply to wait for the results of the brain flow studies. What role should the health care professional have in addressing the needs of the other children?
   a. The nurse should simply tell the parents that a visit to the bedside at this time would be too overwhelming for the other siblings.
   b. Information focused on the value of preparing siblings to visit the baby to say goodbye should be given to Mr. and Mrs. Sullivan so that they can decide what is best for their family.
   c. Ask parents to wait until after the tests results are known before telling the other children what has happened.
   d. Suggest that the parents try to get some sleep and not worry about the other children who are being well taken care of by the grandparents.
   e. Ask the attending physician to talk with the parents about their questions.

5. Hospital practices and policies related to family participation at the bedside of a dying child are being challenged and changes are occurring. Why?
   a. Parents have increased knowledge of their rights and responsibilities within the health care system.
   b. Health care professionals are receiving more advanced training in addressing the sensitive issues of death and dying.
   c. Extended family and friends are more easily accessible to offer support during crises.
   d. Current research demonstrates that participation by the family at the bedside of a dying child offers potential for more favorable adjustment following the death.
   e. Sophisticated medical technology makes the realities of death more difficult for families to accept.

6. A hospitalized child who refuses to eat, interact or play when the family is absent from the bedside, may be in which of the following stages as described by Robertson?
   a. Protest
   b. Denial
   c. Despair

7. A child's apparent lack of response to the news of the sudden death of a sibling:
   a. reassures the parent that the sibling will not be too upset by the loss.
   b. demonstrates a developmentally appropriate response of a child to an overwhelming experience.
   c. indicates that the child feels angry and guilty about the death.
   d. requires immediate intervention to force the child to accept the reality of the situation.
   e. demonstrates need for the child to view the body in order to be able to believe the loss.

continued on next page

STUDY QUESTIONS (CONTINUED)

8. A 6-year-old girl was admitted to the hospital with minor effects of smoke inhalation. However, her mother and younger brother died in the fire, and her father is hospitalized in another hospital. The nursing staff is concerned that the girl is asking to go to the playroom and has not cried since her admission last night. What might be the best intervention at this time?
   a. Wait until the father is discharged before talking to the girl about what happened.
   b. Ask the child to draw a picture of what happened and have a conversation together about what she draws.
   c. Distract her with activities so she does not think about the fire or ask any questions until other family members get to the hospital.
   d. Obtain a psychiatry consult as soon as possible.
   e. Transfer the child to the adult hospital where her father is a patient.

9. Accepting the death of a newborn may be described as complicated mourning due to:
   a. guilt feelings of the parent.
   b. inability to clearly identify the cause of death.
   c. society's influence and discomfort to address feelings over loss of an infant.
   d. well-meaning friends who suggest that the loss of an infant is easier than that of an older child with whom more time has been spent.
   e. all of the above.

10. Physical mementos provided to parents at the time of a child's death:
   a. have no particular value for grief work.
   b. may become painful reminders of the accident or illness.
   c. should be kept out of sight of young siblings who may ask questions.
   d. help fill the physical needs of acute grief of parents.
   e. should only be offered in situations of sudden and unexpected death.

11. A Native American adolescent is dying in the Intensive Care Unit. A large group of family and friends is gathered at the bedside. They are insistent that a ritualistic ceremony involving burning and the creation of smoke must be performed to ensure passage of the teen's soul beyond death. The hospital should:
   a. suggest that the family return home to conduct the ceremony and return to the hospital when it is finished.
   b. explain sensitively that fire laws prohibit burning of anything within the hospital building.
   c. ask a hospital chaplain to suggest a more suitable blessing for the dying.
   d. meet with administration and facilities engineers to determine a place where this ritual might safely be conducted.
   e. remind the family that rules prohibit more than two visitors at the bedside at one time.

ANSWERS

1.c 2.e 3.e 4.b 5.d 6.c 7.b 8.b 9.e 10.d 11.d

Chapter 7

Home and Family

Martha J. Bradshaw, PhD, RN

Concept

◆◆◆◆◆◆◆◆◆◆◆◆◆◆◆◆◆◆◆◆◆◆◆◆◆◆

◆ Economic, social, and political influences

Objectives

◆◆◆◆◆◆◆◆◆◆◆◆◆◆◆◆◆◆◆◆◆◆◆◆◆◆

At the completion of this chapter, the reader will be able to:

◆ Use a theoretical framework as a basis for family assessment.

◆ Recognize key factors influential on family health and unity.

◆ Select appropriate assessment tools pertinent for use with a specified family.

◆ Determine the impact of life-changing events on the family and the child.

◆ Apply family perspectives to child health issues.

Key Points

◆◆◆◆◆◆◆◆◆◆◆◆◆◆◆◆◆◆◆◆◆◆◆◆◆◆

◆ Home and family connote security and acceptance to the child.

◆ A child's view of the world is governed by the values, attitudes, and lifestyle patterns of the family.

◆ Family structure, function, and interaction are universal attributes, yet are characterized in ways unique to each family.

◆ Family coping, in the face of life-changing events, is directly related to the cohesiveness of the family and will influence the child into adulthood.

◆ A thorough nursing assessment of home and family may uncover critical areas of concern that affect the health of the child.

7

Home and Family

I. THE HOME

A. The physical setting of the home has a major impact on the child's health and development.

1. Sleeping arrangements.
   a. Availability of consistent, designated bed for each family member.
   b. Amount of sharing of bedrooms and beds.
   c. Placement of infants in room or bed with parent(s).
2. Eating rituals.
   a. Meal preparation.
   b. Food selection and storage.
   c. Eating patterns.
      (1) Family/common meal.
      (2) Adults first.
   d. Use of alcohol.
      (1) Daily.
      (2) Special occasions.
      (3) Introduction of alcohol to minors.
3. Hygiene, clothing, and cleanliness.
   a. Access to running water.
   b. Adequacy of ventilation.
   c. Hygienic practices.
   d. Adequacy and practicality of clothing and shoes.
   e. Health beliefs.
   f. Pets and pet care.
4. Safety factors.
   a. Childproofing.
   b. Antitheft.
   c. Fire safety.
   d. Repair needs.
   e. Weapons control.
   f. Secondhand smoke.
   g. External hazards: yard, traffic.
5. Social interaction.
   a. Common rooms.
   b. Privacy.
   c. Communications.
      (1) Access to telephone and door.
      (2) Freedom and control, e.g., Does the mother of an adolescent:
         (a) Listen in on telephone conversations?
         (b) Turn friends away at the door?
      (3) Amount and types of conversations.
         (a) Domination by family member (e.g, Does the male head of household control the conversation at the table?).
         (b) Types of conversations.
            [1] Discussing family business.
            [2] Giving instructions.
            [3] Discussing ideas.
            [4] Describing interesting or significant events in member's daily life.
         (c) Persons involved.
   d. Cultural or religious practices.
      (1) Commemorating holidays, anniversaries, or significant historical events to transmit family traditions through generations (e.g., the American holiday of Thanksgiving).
      (2) Culturally-oriented foods and rituals associated with event are included in family gathering (e.g., Seder for Passover).
   e. Neighborhood activities (e.g., block parties, community clean-up events).
6. Comfort and entertainment.
   a. Sources of warmth and cooling.
   b. Areas for relaxation.
   c. Types of entertainment.
   d. Age-appropriate sources of play or entertainment.

B. The home environment has direct and indirect impact on the child.

1. Family circumstances.
   a. Traditional or alternative family pattern.
   b. Source(s) and stability of income and other resources.
   c. Transient members.
   d. Cultural or religious practices.
   e. Supervision of children.
2. Household members.
   a. Nuclear or extended family in home.
   b. Health and well-being of household members.
   c. Caregiver responsibilities.
   d. Effects of crowding.
3. Education and development.

a. Access to schools or home schooling practices.
b. Support for learning in the home.
 (1) Books.
 (2) Newspaper.
 (3) Computer.
c. Interferences with learning.
 (1) Television or video games instead of homework.
 (2) Disruptive home life, e.g., violence, family crisis.
 (3) Schedule problems, largely due to outside activities.

II. THE FAMILY

◆ ◆ ◆ ◆ ◆ ◆ ◆ ◆ ◆ ◆ ◆ ◆ ◆ ◆ ◆ ◆ ◆ ◆

A. Several theoretical frameworks are used to describe families.
1. Developmental tasks (Duval, 1977).
 a. The family must accomplish specific, critical tasks to insure its survival.
 b. The basic tasks for American families.
 (1) Provide shelter, food, clothing, and health care.
 (2) Allocate resources such as finances, space, and time.
 (3) Assign roles for support, management, and caretaking.
 (4) Promote socialization and maturation both within the family and in society.
 (5) Establish forms of communication, interaction, and self-expression that are acceptable table both within the family and in society.
 (6) Bear and/or adopt children and rear them.
 (7) Relate to the extended family, friends, school, church, and relevant society.
 (8) Provide motivation, values, rewards.
 (a) Motivation example: encouraging a new mother by letting her know she is doing a good job with her baby.
 (b) Values example: explaining to a child why she or he should be courteous and respectful of others.
 (c) Rewards example: treating a child to ice cream for completing a good school year.
 (9) Develop goals and set priorities.
 (10) Cope with crises.
2. Family Life Cycle and Developmental Tasks (Duval, 1977) (see Table 7-1).
 a. Addresses period of time in the family, as a unit, progresses through certain stages of life, from inception to dissolution.
 b. Includes eight stages that are based upon growth and developmental experiences of oldest child.

c. Assumes repetition of family experiences with successive children.
d. Emphasizes that stage-critical family developmental tasks must be achieved.
3. Systems perspective (Allmond, Buckman, & Gofman, 1979).
 a. The family is an open, self-regulating system, interacting with external environments that include:
 (1) The mesosystem, the immediate larger environment, such as neighborhood or community.
 (2) The macrosystem, the broad environment, such as culture or social setting.
 b. There are multiple related microsystems or subsystems (e.g., dyads, siblings).
 c. Families can create balance between stability and change.
 d. Families have selective boundaries: residences, traditions, shared experiences.
 e. Family patterns reflect other institutions and society (e.g., economics, values).
 f. Change in one family member affects all family members.
 g. The family as a whole is greater than the sum of its parts.
4. Interactional theory (Wong, 1995).
 a. The family is a unit of interacting personalities, each with assigned roles, purposes, and expectations.
 b. Reactions by members and family as a unit are based upon the meaning the event has for member(s).
 c. The family is a closed unit that addresses conflicts and makes decisions internally.
 d. The family is affected more by interfamilial factors than by social norms.

B. Family structure provides organization by which family functions can be accomplished.
1. Type of family structure is based on characteristics of individual members.
 a. Nuclear family: husband, wife, children.
 b. Extended family: nuclear family plus individuals related by blood or marriage.
 c. Blended or reconstituted family: creation of a new family from two previously separate families, most often by the marriage of the two adult family members.
 d. Cohabiting family: adult partners are not joined legally but live together and share commitment and responsibilities.
 e. Single parent family: household consists of one adult and children, who usually are the offspring of the adult.
 f. Gay or lesbian family: two same-sex adult

Table 7-1
Stage-Critical Family Developmental Tasks Through the Family Life Cycle

Stage of the Family Life Cycle	Positions in the Family	Stage-Critical Family Developmental Tasks
Married couple	Wife Husband	Establishing a mutually satisfying marriage Adjusting to pregnancy and the promise of parenthood Fitting into the kin network
Childbearing	Wife-mother Husband-father Infant daughter or son or both	Having, adjusting to, and encouraging the development of infants Establishing a satisfying home for both parents and infant(s)
Preschool-age	Wife-mother Husband-father Daughter-sister Son-brother	Adapting to the critical needs and interests of preschool children in stimulating, growth-promoting ways Coping with energy depletion and lack of privacy as parents
School-age	Wife-mother Husband-father Daughter-sister Son-brother	Fitting into the community of school-age families in constructive ways Encouraging children's educational achievement
Teenage	Wife-mother Husband-father Daughter-sister Son-brother	Balancing freedom with responsibility as teenagers mature and emancipate themselves Establishing postparental interests and careers as growing parents
Launching center	Wife-mother-grandmother Husband-father-grandfather Daughter-sister-aunt Son-brother-uncle	Releasing young adults into work, military service, college, marriage, etc., with appropriate rituals and assistance Maintaining a supportive home base
Middle-aged parents	Wife-mother-grandmother Husband-father-grandfather	Rebuilding the marriage relationship Maintaining kin ties with older and younger generations
Aging family members	Widow/widower Wife-mother-grandmother Husband-father-grandfather	Coping with bereavement and living alone Closing the family home or adapting it to aging Adjusting to retirement

Used with permission from Duval, E.M. (1977). *Marriage and family development.* Philadelphia: Lippincott.

partners establishing a household; often one of the adult members brings children into the household from a previous heterosexual relationship.

2. Power structure characteristics.
   a. Position or status: placement in family, by virtue of age, experience, or other forms of authority gives power.
   b. Roles: each family individually defines which roles are of higher value, and thus carry more influence or power.

C. Family function is the outcome or consequence of family structure, and is defined as the reason the family exists or purpose that it serves.

1. Affective function: to meet psychologic or emotional needs of members.
2. Economic function: provide sufficient economic resources and allocate them effectively.
3. Health maintenance function: provision of physical needs that maintain well being.
4. Reproductive function: to insure survival of species and family continuity.
5. Socialization function: primarily to socialize younger members, to make them productive, contributing members of the society.

D. Family composition, size and configuration considers roles, number of family members, and birth order.
1. Composition.
   a. Paired roles.
      (1) Husband-father.
      (2) Wife-mother.
      (3) Child-sibling.
   b. Individual roles.
      (1) Wage earner/provider.
      (2) Keeper of the home.
      (3) Childrearing.
      (4) Recreation and companionship.
      (5) Affective.
      (6) Sexual.
2. Size and configuration.
   a. The number of family members governs structure, power, and role assumption.
   b. Birth order influences developmental patterns of each child (Murray & Zentner, 1993).
      (1) First or only child: responsible, independent, good intellectual potential, less opportunity for peer interactions.
      (2) Middle child(ren): learns multiple roles, adaptability to multiple persons, may experience jealousy or envy with other siblings, less individuality.
      (3) Last-born child: emotionally secure due to acceptance and attention by other family members, more dependent on others, matures at a slower rate.
      (4) Multiple births: multiple-birth siblings are usually closer than other children, sharing a unique understanding, way of communicating, and intuition about each other. Expectations from them by parents may be different than for singleton children.

E. Family assessment.
1. Environment.
   a. Physical characteristics and condition of family dwelling.
   b. Family's view of adequacy of dwelling.
   c. Environment external to home.
2. Family structure, role, and function.
   a. Overt and covert patterns of structure.
   b. Role assumption and task assignment.
   c. Unfulfilled roles/role strain.
3. Communication patterns.
   a. Adult-to-adult patterns.
   b. Adult-to-child patterns.
   c. Child-to-child or adult patterns.
   d. Decision-making patterns.
   e. Affective or emotional expression.
   f. Extent of openness, clarity, and suitability.
   g. Methods of conflict management.

4. Resources and problem-solving skills.
   a. Key individuals in problem recognition.
   b. Perceived needs and threats.
   c. Awareness of resources.
   d. Conflicting problems or priorities.
   e. Business skills.
   f. Previous coping experiences.
   g. Family cohesiveness in problem resolution.
5. Health beliefs and behaviors.
   a. Health rituals.
      (1) Nutrition and nutritional supplements.
      (2) Personal hygiene.
      (3) Dental care.
      (4) Rest and exercise.
   b. Family values related to health and health practices.
      (1) Physical examinations.
      (2) Immunizations.
      (3) Contraception.
      (4) Emergency care.
      (5) Health promotion.
      (6) Alternative and/or complementary therapies.
      (7) Financial aspects of health care.
   c. Unhealthy behaviors/situations.
      (1) Substance usage.
      (2) Reckless endangerment.
      (3) Stress.
6. Social, cultural, and religious values.
   a. Incorporation into and acceptance of family by society.
   b. Agreement among family members about social, religious, and cultural mores adopted by family.
   c. Socioeconomic status (SES).
      (1) Direction of SES mobility.
      (2) Family's feelings about status.
7. Lifestyle.
   a. Recreational patterns.
   b. Safety measures.
   c. Amount of and use of free time.
8. Coping mechanisms.
   a. Resources.
   b. Problem-solving skills.
   c. Support from significant others.
   d. Family cohesion.
9. Risk factors or potential stressors.
   a. Conflicts in parenting.
   b. Alterations in health.
   c. Family goals conflicts.
10. Assessment tools.
   a. Calgary Family Assessment Model (Wright & Leahey, 1994).
      (1) Multidimensional scale consisting of three categories: structural, functional, and developmental.

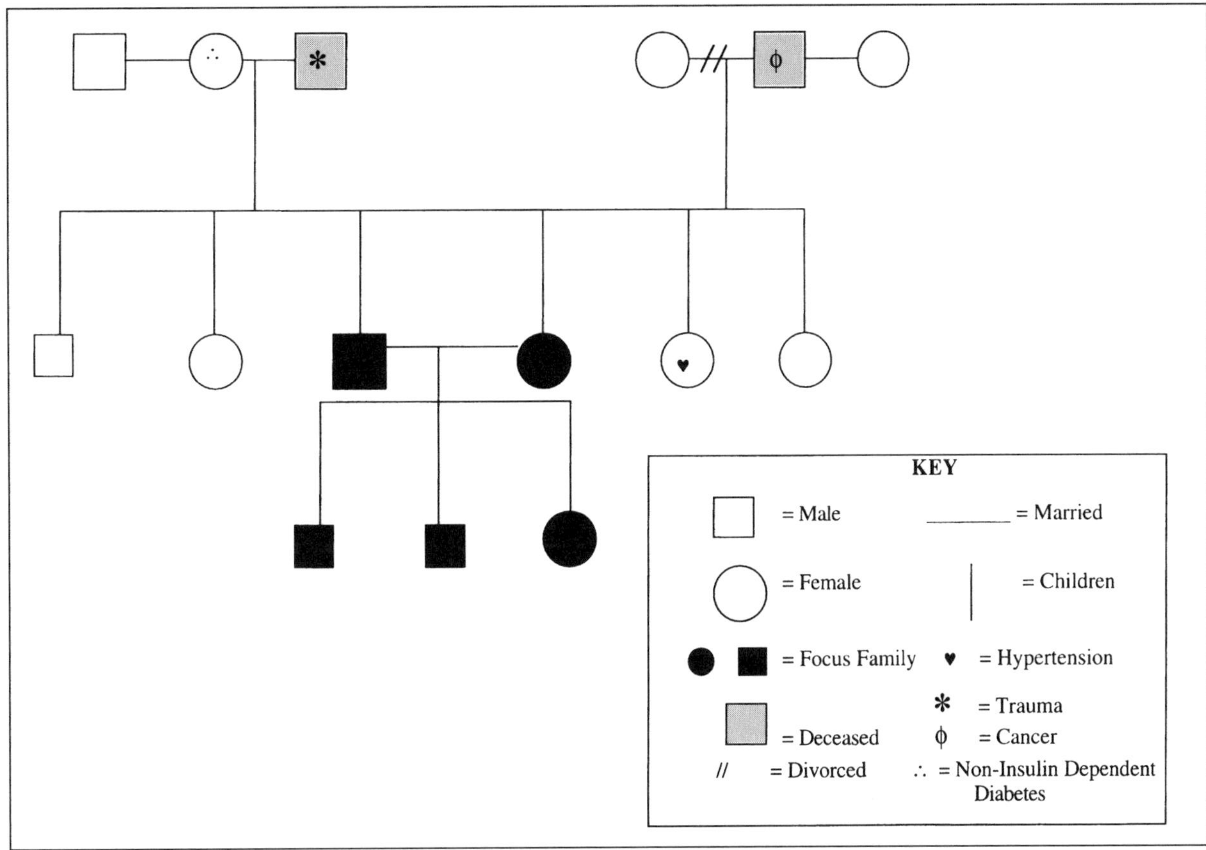

Figure 7-1
Sample Genogram

(2) Model is used to assess and draw conclusions about family strengths and problems.
(3) Problem areas can undergo more in-depth assessment or interventions.
(4) Areas of strength can be used as family resources.
b. Feetham Family Functioning Survey (Feetham, 1982).
  (1) A 25-question survey assessing family functioning, along a seven-point scale.
  (2) Assesses parents' views of relationships among family members and between family and other social systems.
  (3) Respondents are asked to indicate own perception of:
    (a) Degree (amount) of function that currently exists.
    (b) How much there should be.
    (c) How important it is to that family member.
c. Friedman Family Assessment Model and Form (Friedman, 1992).
  (1) A 29-item instrument (with subcategories), based upon structural-functional view of family.

(2) Consists of four assumptions.
  (a) The family is a social system with functional requirements.
  (b) These functions serve the individual family member as well as society.
  (c) A family is a small group that possesses features that are generic to other small groups.
  (d) Family members act according to internalized values and norms that are perpetuated by the family.
(3) Subcategory structure enables nurse to individualize assessment according to family functioning and needs.
d. Family Apgar test (Smilkstein, 1982).
  (1) Five-item scale, scored in same manner as neonatal Apgar (2,1,0 per item).
  (2) Respondent indicates level of satisfaction with home and family life.
  (3) Assesses family functioning in areas of adaptability, partnership, growth, affection, and resolve.
e. The HOME (Home Observation for Measurement of the Environment Inventory) instrument (Lotas et al., 1992).

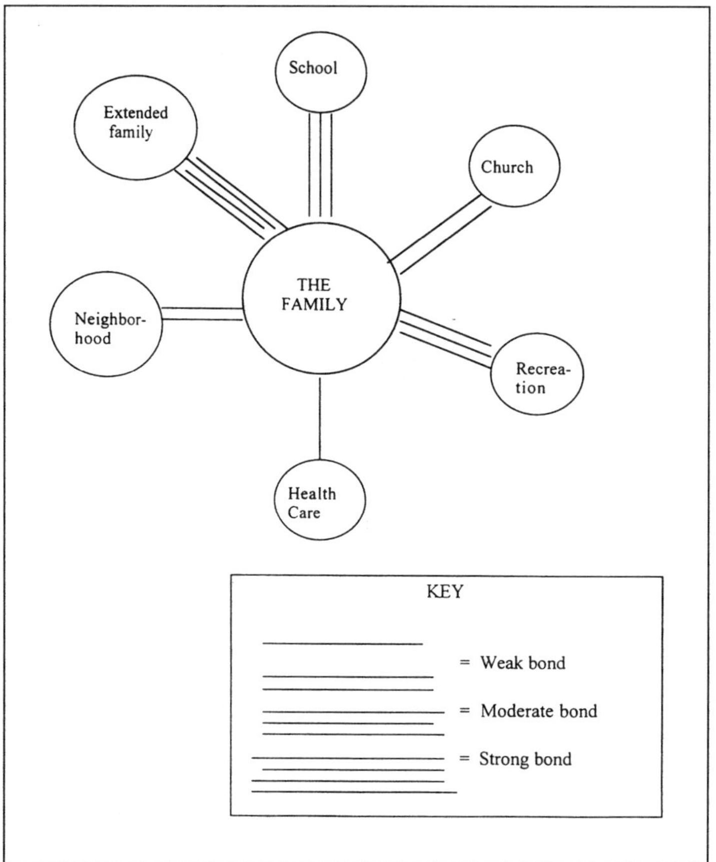

Figure 7-2
Sample Ecomap

(1) Instrument consisting of two subscales: 45 items target children ages birth to 3 years of age; 55 items focus on children 3 to 6 years of age.
(2) Subscales address:
   (a) Emotional and verbal responses from mother/caregiver.
   (b) Amount of vocal and developmental stimulation.
   (c) Maternal involvement in basic need gratification.
   (d) Physical and temporal environment.
   (e) Avoidance of restriction on exploratory behavior.
   (f) Availability of play materials indicative of parental concern for learning in the child.
(3) Instrument designed to provide information about the home as a stimulus for learning and development of the children in the family.

f. Genogram (see Figure 7-1).
   (1) Diagrammatic representation of connections between family members through birth and marriage.
   (2) Assesses family structure.
   (3) Enables health care providers to identify family patterns, determine significant family relationships.
g. Ecomap (see Figure 7-2).
   (1) Diagrammatic representation of contacts and relationships between family and outside units with whom the family interacts.
   (2) Enables health care providers to identify strengths of relationships and valuable resources that are external to the family.

III. PARENTING

◆ ◆ ◆ ◆ ◆ ◆ ◆ ◆ ◆ ◆ ◆ ◆ ◆ ◆ ◆ ◆ ◆ ◆ ◆ ◆

A. Parental development occurs over time and

considers factors such as:
1. Adaptation to parenthood.
   a. Recognition and acceptance of multitudinous new, interwoven, and demanding roles and way of living.
   b. Relinquishment or modification of old roles or lifestyle.
   c. Amount of adaptation and rate of needed changes.
      (1) Directly influences success of acceptance of parenting roles.
      (2) Consciously or subconsciously governed by how adult was parented as a child.
   d. Use of a parental leave plan.
      (1) In many organizations, is available for both father and mother.
      (2) Allows time for recovery from birth and adaptation to new family member and way of living.
2. Parenting classes, which provide:
   a. Formal instruction in selected aspects of parenting, e.g., feeding, caregiving, discipline, detecting and managing illness.
   b. Opportunity for new parents to interact, share concerns and experiences.
   c. Means by which new parents can develop a sense of competence and independence in role.
3. Anticipatory guidance.
   a. Definition: conscious, planned awareness of the child's development and changing needs, and appropriate responses to these changes.
   b. For each child, anticipatory guidance should address specific areas.
      (1) Physical.
      (2) Cognitive.
      (3) Emotional.
      (4) Social.
   c. Also addresses incorporation of additional members into the family.
4. Parenting goals.
   a. Establishing goals, priorities, and values; changing as family changes.
   b. Balancing conflicts between goals as a parent versus goals as an individual.
   c. Promoting survival and continued reproduction of family generations.

B. Styles of parenting incorporate behaviors, traditions, and cultural influences. *See Chapter 29: Cultural Influences.*
1. Parenting behaviors.
   a. Behaviors are usually determined by parent's own role model(s), most often their own parents.
   b. Parental control styles.
      (1) Authoritarian/dictatorial.
      (2) Permissive.
      (3) Democratic.
   c. Discipline and limit-setting.
      (1) Positive and necessary aspect of childrearing.
      (2) Protects child and teaches acceptable behavior.
      (3) Enables child to redirect inappropriate feelings or behaviors.
      (4) Consistency from parents provides sense of security in child.
2. Typical maternal styles.
   a. Initial attachment.
   b. Nurturing.
   c. Internally focused: more directed at issues within the family.
3. Typical paternal styles.
   a. Engrossment or interaction.
   b. Protective and responsible: directed to influence of external environment on family.
   c. Accessible.
4. Influence of ethnicity or culture on parenting style.
   a. Male or female dominated cultures.
   b. Forms of punishment and discipline.
   c. Primary (home/family) and secondary (external environment) interactions and conflicts.

C. Factors that influence parenting
1. Economic status.
   a. Affects amount of time each parent is able to spend with child(ren).
   b. Creates unsupervised setting for child(ren) if parents are absent.
   c. Families living in poverty.
      (1) May have frequently absent wage-earner or single, working head of household.
      (2) Often consist of multigenerational families, which provide for child care.
      (3) May be dependent upon subsidized programs for health care and food.
   d. Families of affluence.
      (1) May consist of strong career commitments from one or both parents.
      (2) May provide substitutes for parents, such as nannies, governesses, or boarding school.
2. Level of education.
   a. Has direct influence on wage-earning potential, health beliefs and behaviors, and problem-solving abilities of parents.
   b. Contributes to extent to which parents are involved in child's school work.
      (1) Low literacy level in parent hinders verbal development in child.

(2) Level of education related to extent to which parent role models problem solving, business skills, and use of technology.
3. Occupation.
   a. Work hours may be opposite to hours of other family members, such as school hours.
   b. Exposure to contaminants endangers health of wage earner; may endanger other family members.
   c. Job stress may disrupt harmonious family life.
4. Resources.
   a. Personal.
     (1) Previous experience that results in learned strategies and coping skills.
     (2) Support that provides encouragement and additional resources.
     (3) Skills, especially intellectual, communications, enable parents to make decisions and reach goals effectively.
   b. Social/environmental.
     (1) Network external to home valuable for problem-solving.
     (2) Community resources provide services that can not be met in the home.
5. Family and individual goals.
   a. Family goals change as families change (see Table 7-1).
   b. Family goals should be negotiated among family members.
   c. Individual goals or needs may supersede family goals.
   d. Decisions about family goals and priorities should be made by parent(s).
6. Role strain/role conflict.
   a. Strain: difficulty parent has enacting role; may be a result of:
     (1) Caregiver burden, especially if combined with caregiving for another adult.
     (2) Unwillingness or unpreparedness to assume parenting role.
   b. Conflict: difficulty individual has effectively enacting parenting role in combination with other roles, such as:
     (1) Spouse.
     (2) Wage earner.
     (3) Student.
     (4) Community leader.
     (5) Extended family member.

IV. SPECIAL ISSUES

◆ ◆ ◆ ◆ ◆ ◆ ◆ ◆ ◆ ◆ ◆ ◆ ◆ ◆ ◆ ◆ ◆ ◆ ◆ ◆

A. Transient families have challenges or opportunities unique to their circumstances.
1. Migrant.

   a. Economic and social instability.
   b. Interruption of education.
   c. Lack of access to and continuity of health care.
   d. Language and cultural barriers.
   e. Child labor.
   f. Lack of resources and social support.
2. Military or business-related.
   a. Interruption of education and social support.
   b. Experiences with different cultures.
   c. Resources from the work organization.
   d. Absent parent.
3. Homelessness.
   a. Incidence.
     (1) The number of homeless children is on the rise.
     (2) Most homeless children are preschoolers, between infancy and 5 years of age.
   b. Types.
     (1) Sharing living space with family or friends.
     (2) Living outside; may or may not have access to temporary shelter.
   c. Impact on family.
     (1) May become single-parent family.
     (2) Exposed to consequences of loss of income and other resources.
     (3) Experiences profound changes in home life and lifestyle.
   d. Priority problems for children who are homeless.
     (1) Physical needs.
     (2) Health care.
     (3) Education.
     (4) Play.
     (5) Emotional security.

B. Single-parent households are increasingly commonplace and may be led by either the mother or the father.
1. Divorce is the primary reason for single parent households.
   a. Results in change of lifestyle, adaptation of home life, sometimes for the better.
   b. Child may become involved in anger or resentment between parents.
   c. Parental coping and decision-making often compromised during divorce process.
   d. Custody often becomes a major issue that can lead to:
     (1) Manipulation of children.
     (2) Guilt on part of child.
   e. Common responses in the child.
     (1) Disturbed patterns of eating or sleeping.
     (2) Fears, irritability, anxiety, or tantrums.
     (3) Regression to previous developmental level.

(4) Desire for reconciliation in parents.
  f. Amount of family or social support influences adjustment and recovery from divorce.
2. Death of a parent creates a single parent household with similar and additional issues.
  a. Grief by survivors.
  b. Psychologic ramifications, depending on the circumstances of death, such as:
    (1) Prolonged illness.
    (2) Accident.
    (3) Homicide or suicide.
  c. Adaptation of home life without the parent.
  d. Interpretation of death by child.
  e. Family or social support

C. Gay or lesbian families.
1. May evolve from "blended" families or from adoption by a gay/lesbian couple or individual.
2. Legal decision regarding child custody or adoption tend to not favor a homosexual couple family (Patterson & Redding, 1996).
3. Gay couples have more equitable and satisfying division of labor and roles within the family than do heterosexual couples (McPherson, 1995).
4. Research suggests that gay/lesbian families are as capable of providing as nurturing and supportive of a home environment as may a heterosexual family (Patterson & Redding, 1996).

D. Abuse can take various forms within the home and family.
1. Physical abuse.
  a. Arises from a culture that sanctions physical measures for discipline or control and often used as an outlet for anger or frustration.
  b. Is usually a repetitive pattern. Adults or parents who are abusers likely were abused as children.
  c. Likely involves a victim who is dependent, has low self-worth, and who internalizes reasons for abuse.
  d. Is typically precipitated by a stressful episode such as job pressures or an argument.
  e. May include subtle forms of mistreatment such as animal abuse, child neglect, verbal or emotional abuse.
  f. Physical findings in the victim.
    (1) Bruises, welts, or cuts.
    (2) Fractures of skull, facial bones, limbs, or digits; findings of old fractures on x-ray.
    (3) Burns or scald.
    (4) Lacerations or abrasions.
    (5) Sprains, torsion of extremity (wringing), "shaken baby syndrome."
    (6) Internal bleeding.
  g. Behavioral findings in the victim.

    (1) Somatizing, e.g., vomiting, shock.
    (2) Extreme aggressiveness.
    (3) Unusual fears.
    (4) No eye contact, flat affect.
    (5) Uninterested in parents.
    (6) Strong positive responses to attention.
2. Sexual abuse.
  a. Defined as use of a child for sexual purposes, which includes incest, rape, molestation, or pornography.
  b. Causes and patterns similar to that of physical abuse and may occur simultaneously.
  c. May be known to other family members who may themselves be victims.
3. Substance abuse.
  a. Defined as the regular use of drugs for purposes other than medically recommended reasons.
    (1) Abuse results in physical and/or psychologic injury.
    (2) Abuser may become involved in acts detrimental to society.
  b. Causative factors.
    (1) Boredom.
    (2) Escape.
    (3) Pressure from others.
    (4) Desire to prove independence/maturity.
  c. More common among adolescents than younger children.
    (1) Alcohol is most commonly abused drug.
    (2) Drug use/abuse is highly correlated to adolescent's need for acceptance by peers.
  d. Family involvement: strategies for avoiding substance abuse also are effective in treatment plan.
    (1) Value of role modeling by parent(s).
    (2) Open communication patterns.
    (3) Measures to relieve stress or pressure.

E. Life-changing events can have short-term and long-term implications for the child and family.
1. Catastrophic illness or trauma.
  a. Impact on family members.
    (1) Guilt, grief, fears.
    (2) Simultaneous hospitalization of other members.
    (3) Physical demands as caregivers.
    (4) Demands on family resources.
  b. Possible long-term implications.
    (1) Change in individual abilities or function.
    (2) Change in family roles and functions.
    (3) Adjustments in lifestyle.
2. Adolescent pregnancy.
  a. Physiologic and physical demands of pregnancy and adolescence.
    (1) Nutrition.

(2) Development of reproductive structures.
(3) Cardiovascular demands and anemia.
(4) Sexually transmitted diseases.
  b. Psychosocial aspects to consider.
    (1) Initial reactions.
    (2) Revealing pregnancy to family.
    (3) The conflicting developmental tasks of adolescence and pregnancy.
      (a) Tasks of adolescence.
        [1] Becoming comfortable with own body and how to use it effectively.
        [2] Developing a satisfying and socially acceptable identity.
        [3] Building relationships with both sexes.
        [4] Gaining emotional independence from nuclear family.
        [5] Selecting goals and preparing for economic independence.
        [6] Developing mature intellectual skills, concepts, and a value system.
      (b) Tasks of pregnancy.
        [1] Pregnancy confirmation.
        [2] Incorporating fetus into body image.
        [3] Viewing fetus as separate entity.
        [4] Acceptance and preparation for birth.
    (4) Interruption of education and goals.
  c. Preparation for childbirth and parenting.
    (1) Acceptance of pregnancy and mothering role.
    (2) Prenatal health care.
  d. Issues for the adolescent father.
    (1) Acceptance by his own family and family of his pregnant partner.
    (2) Role assumption and involvement in childbearing.
  e. Family issues.
    (1) Acceptance of and incorporation of new family member.
    (2) Primary caregiver role assumption.
    (3) Acceptance of pregnancy outside of family.
    (4) Recidivism.
3. Suicide/attempted suicide.
  a. Along with accidents and homicide, suicide is among the top three causes of death in children and adolescents.
  b. These acts are usually related to depression and helplessness.
  c. Suicide attempts are a call for help or attention.
  d. Impact on family may include guilt, grief, and/or rage.

4. Natural disaster (flood, fire, tornado).
  a. Impact on family.
    (1) Resources and social support.
    (2) Posttraumatic stress.
    (3) Disaster recovery.
    (4) Personal injury.
  b. Meaning of disaster to family members.
    (1) Loss of loved one(s).
    (2) Loss of home and possessions.

BIBLIOGRAPHY

Allmond, B.W., Buckman, W., & Gofman, H.F. (1979). *The family is the patient*. St. Louis: Mosby.

Duval, E. (1977). *Marriage and the family*. Philadelphia: Lippincott.

Feetham, S. (1982) The Feetham Family Functioning Scale. In S. Humenick (Ed.). *Analysis of current assessment strategies in the health care of young children and childbearing families* (pp. 259–268). New York: Appleton-Century-Crofts.

Friedman, M.M. (1992). *Family nursing: Theory and practice* (3rd ed.). Norwalk, CT: Appleton-Lange.

Lotas, M., Penticuff, J., Medoff-Cooper, B., Brooten, D, & Brown, L. (1992). The HOME Scale: The influence of socioeconomic status on the evaluation of the home environment. *Nursing Research, 41*, 338–341.

McPherson, D. (1995). Perfect partners (gay families). *Psychology Today, 28*, 14.

Murray, R.B., & Zentner, J.P. (1993). *Nursing assessment and health promotion: Strategies through the life span* (5th ed.). Norwalk, CT: Appleton & Lange.

Patterson, C.J., & Redding, R.E. (1996). Lesbian and gay families with children: Implications of social science research or policy. *The Journal of Social Issues, 52*, 29–50.

Smilkstein, G., (1982). Validity and reliability of the family by APGAR as a test of family function. *Journal of Family Practice, 15*, 303–311.

Wong, D. (1995). *Whaley & Wong's nursing care of infants and children* (5th ed.). St. Louis: Mosby.

Wright, L., & Leahey, M. (1994). *Nurses and families: A guide to family assessment and intervention* (2nd ed.). Philadelphia: Davis

STUDY QUESTIONS

1. Which of the following home situations would alert the nurse to unhealthy health beliefs or behaviors?
   a. Adolescent family members are permitted to have a glass of wine at holiday meals.
   b. A 13-year-old girl shares a bed with her 11-year-old brother.
   c. The household has indoor toilets but uses well water for drinking and bathing.
   d. The home has no locking windows and no smoke detector.

2. According to Duval, a stage in the Family Life Cycle is determined by:
   a. age of the parents.
   b. number of years parents have been married.
   c. number of children in the family.
   d. age of oldest child.
   e. age of youngest child.

3. The relationship between family structure and family function is that:
   a. functions mandate family structure.
   b. structure provides organization by which family functions can be accomplished.
   c. family structure is determined by individuals, whereas family function is determined by the entire unit.
   d. both are affected by family developmental tasks.

4. The Family Life Cycle of families in poverty differs from typical families because:
   a. there are fewer available resources.
   b. health problems often interfere with family development.
   c. events and stressors are predictable.
   d. the extended family is absent.
   e. there are a larger number of children in families of poverty.

5. In conducting a family assessment, nurses must recognize and respect ethnicity because it:
   a. produces a barrier to societal interaction.
   b. predicts family behaviors.
   c. provides traditions that enrich family life.
   d. has a strong impact on economic mobility.
   e. influences family resources.

6. The Calgary Assessment Model, Family APGAR, and the Feetham Assessment Scale all focus on which aspect of the family?
   a. Function
   b. Parenting
   c. Roles
   d. Economics
   e. Structure

7. For new parents, formal classes in parenting would be helpful for all of the following EXCEPT:
   a. learning how to safely bathe and child and detect illness.
   b. developing a better sense of competence.
   c. sharing concerns or questions about parenting.
   d. anticipating developmental changes in the child.
   e. determining which form of discipline works best.

8. As a family nurse practitioner, you are talking with a mother about her concerns that she may become physically abusive with her three young children. Which statement would be most indicative of the potential for abuse?
   a. "No one in my family ever hit or shoved anyone."
   b. "I usually discipline them with time out or restriction."
   c. "My children seem to want a lot of attention right now."
   d. "Being a single mother, I sometimes wonder how I'm managing to make ends meet."

9. Natural disasters and/or homelessness can create anxieties or fears in children predominantly because of:
   a. change in lifestyle.
   b. loss of possessions.
   c. withdrawal from school.
   d. separation from loved ones.
   e. change in sleeping and eating patterns.

10. Adolescent pregnancy is a complex family issue. What is the most significant psychologic issue for the pregnant adolescent and her family?
    a. Learning to love the baby
    b. Conflict between tasks of adolescence and tasks of pregnancy and parenting
    c. Acceptance of the father of the baby
    d. Confronting the adolescent's sexuality
    e. Acceptance of adolescent and family by society

ANSWERS

1.b   2.d   3.b   4.a   5.c   6.a   7.e   8.d   9.d   10.b

Chapter 8

Community Influences

Marion L. Donohoe, MSN, RN, PNP

◆◆◆◆◆◆◆◆◆◆◆◆◆◆◆◆◆◆◆◆◆◆◆◆

◆◆◆◆◆◆◆◆◆◆◆◆◆◆◆◆◆◆◆◆◆◆◆◆

Concept

◆◆◆◆◆◆◆◆◆◆◆◆◆◆◆◆◆◆◆◆◆◆◆◆◆◆◆◆◆

◆ Economic, social, and political influences

Objectives

◆◆◆◆◆◆◆◆◆◆◆◆◆◆◆◆◆◆◆◆◆◆◆◆◆◆◆◆◆

At the completion of this chapter, the reader will be able to:

◆ Identify community influences on the health of children and their families.

◆ Assess, plan strategies, and implement therapeutic approaches to children's health care that are community-based, coordinated, comprehensive, culturally sensitive, and in accord with the family's economic and social situation and available resources.

◆ Identify community strengths and needs to enable families to implement the health care needs of their child(ren).

◆ Develop strategies to network with public and private community agencies that provide health services and resources for children and their families.

Key Points

◆◆◆◆◆◆◆◆◆◆◆◆◆◆◆◆◆◆◆◆◆◆◆◆◆◆◆◆◆

◆ The child's well being is linked to the community in which he or she lives and grows.

◆ Identifying the risks and strengths of a child's community promotes understanding that drives the collaborative efforts of parents and health care providers to insure a safe, nurturing environment. Defining a community is the first strategy to understanding the strengths and needs of children and their families.

◆ The nurse's understanding of how children and their families function in their community is the foundation for promoting health and preventing illness.

◆ Understanding the impact of community on the growth and development of a child is multifaceted and requires ongoing assessment.

8

Community Influences

I. OVERVIEW

A. Community is the base setting in which a child lives, grows, and works.
1. The first community a child enters is the family. *See Chapter 7: Home and Family.*
2. As the child grows and explores the communal environment, there are community resources consisting of extended family members, health care providers, day care providers, friends, teachers, coaches, and others.
   a. These community allies form a web of interaction and learning.
   b. Each encounter within this web has an impact on the development of the child.

B. Every aspect of the community surrounding the child influences the physical and mental health of the child (see Figure 8-1).
1. If the community is safe and nurturing, the web of learning can build a strong, self-assured, productive member of society (Green, 1994).
2. If the web is unsafe with hazards and risks, the child's ability to grow and learn is challenged, but more important, the physical, emotional, and mental health of the child are at risk.

C. The immediate family is the child's first community.
1. This family is embedded within other social systems that define the child's community.
2. The challenge of the community is to provide resources and services that meet a child's strengths and needs.
   a. To adequately assess a child's growth and development, attention must be focused on assessing the community where the child lives, plays, and learns.
   b. Typical social systems that surround and support the family can be:
      (1) Kinship groups, grandparents, aunts, uncles, cousins.
      (2) Neighborhoods with parent support groups including PTAs, neighborhood

friends, playmates' families, Girl Scouts/Boy Scouts.
      (3) Religious affiliations including minister/priest/rabbi, church members.
      (4) Culture (language, customs).
      (5) Professionals and organizations (doctor, public health clinic, day care, teachers, schools).
      (6) Larger influences in society such as media, advertising, local and state government, school board, inflation/poverty, employment trends, and legislation.

D. Socioeconomic factors influence how a family functions in its community.
1. Children only may be taken for health care at times of acute illness when parents have employers who do not offer health insurance benefits.
2. Early Periodic Screening Diagnosis and Treatment (EPSDT) has been mandated by federal legislation, but the child only experiences it during well-child visits.
3. Without well-child visits, the child and family miss important health surveillance, anticipatory guidance, and immunizations that are crucial to good growth and development.

E. The nurse must be aware of and able to assess the economic, social, and political environment influencing the child's health and the family caring for the child.

F. Defining a child's community helps the pediatric nurse partner with the child, family, and community, which is the key to providing comprehensive, culturally sensitive interventions to meet the physical and mental health needs for a child (Grason & Guyer, 1995).
1. Community can be defined in several ways.
   a. Natural boundaries of a community are geographic regions, social planning areas, socioeconomic status, demographic characteristics, cultural, and ethnic groups.
   b. Business planners define communities by

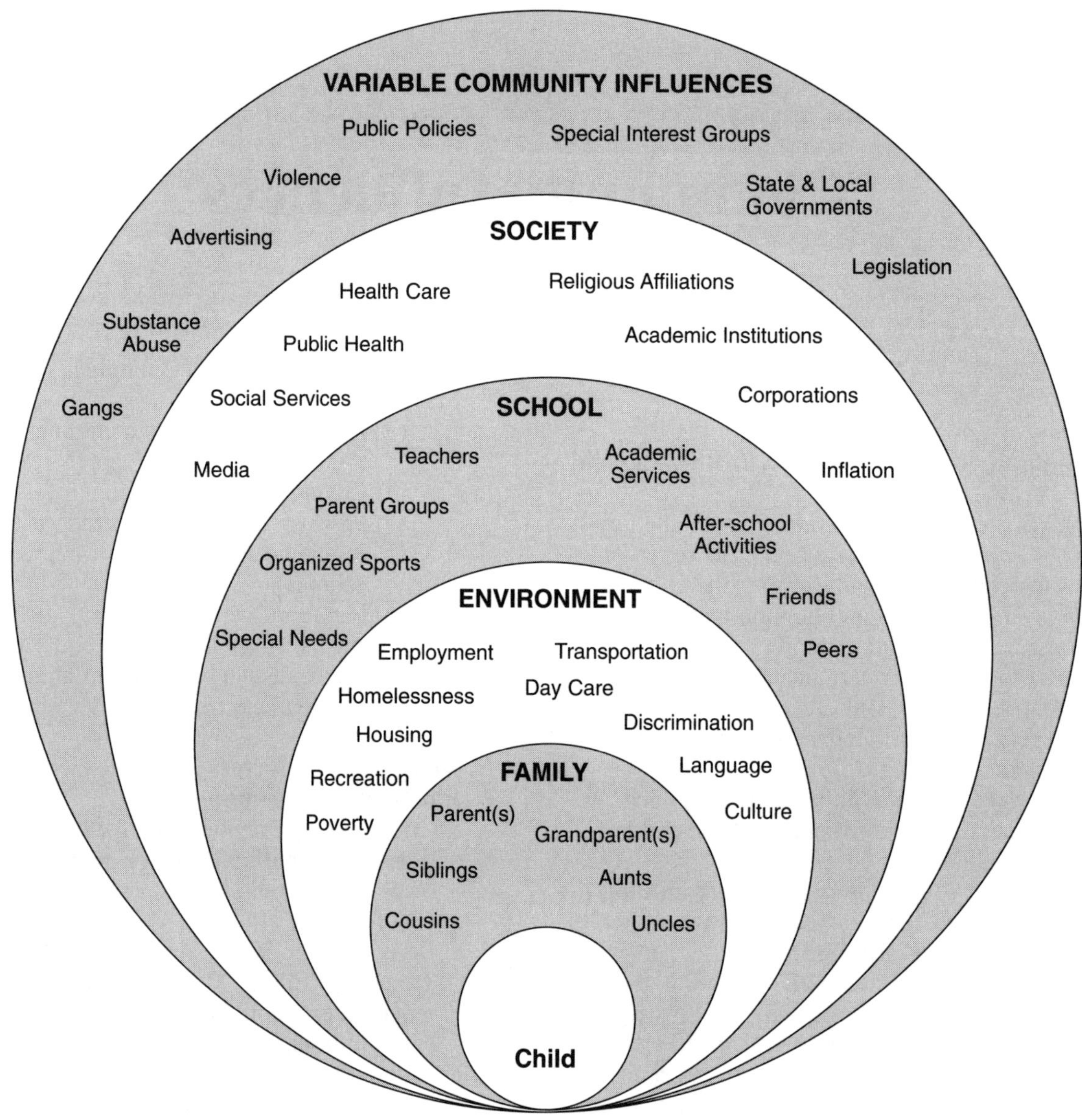

Figure 8-1
Dynamic Variables of Child's Community

Adapted from Dunst, C., Trivette, C., & Deal, A. (1988). *Enabling and empowering families: Principles and guidelines for practice.* Cambridge, MA: Brookline Books; and Leininger, M. (1996). Cultural care theory, research, and practice. *Nursing Science Quarterly, 9*(2), 71–78.

specific business opportunities, professional groupings, consumer supply, and demand for services.

c. Health care professionals define communities by health status and health needs and access to care including gender (male and female), age (pediatric, adolescent, adult, geriatric), medical specialties (pulmonary, cardiac, special needs), and disease-specific diagnoses (asthma, HIV/AIDS, cancer).

2. Legislation, political boundaries, and public policy may also define a community. For example:

a. Policy makers would not provide a communi-ty of senior citizens with parks and recreational facilities geared to children.

b. Similarly, a senior citizen community without children may not vote for higher school taxes.

c. Accordingly, organizations that offer services for children would best be located in geographic areas populated by children and their families.

3. The key to understanding and knowing a community is a coordinated approach to defining a community.

a. Quantitative data can be found in governmental services such as vital statistics, public health departments, and social services.

  b. Qualitative community data comes from networking with organizations and agencies that provide resources and services to the community. These organizations and agencies can be:

    (1) Governmental.

    (2) Public or private.

    (3) Formal or informal.

    (4) Religious groups.

    (5) Academic institutions.

    (6) Special interest groups that have addressed specific needs of the community.

4. Identification of subgroups provides a frame of reference to assist in understanding how a community functions.

  a. Focus groups, ethnic, and cultural groups are examples of subgroups within the framework of community.

  b. Organizations with a specific objective such as colleges or universities, or professional or social organizations, also form subgroups of community.

5. The definition of community and understanding of the social networks of the community have an impact on how the nurse, child, and family will function in the community.

  a. The child's growth and development is affected both positively and negatively by the various community issues.

  b. The child and family recognize the commitment of the nurse who knows their community.

G. Assessing the child's living situation involves knowing the home conditions including cultural and ethnic patterns.

1. Expectations of a child differ among cultures. *See Chapter 29: Cultural Influences.*

2. These expectations or values define the role the child plays in the home, family, and neighborhood. For example:

  a. In the Hispanic community, extended family members can have equally responsible roles for parenting and care of the child.

  b. In the subculture of poverty, a 5-year-old child may be trusted with "minding the baby" while the mother goes to the store for milk.

3. Close attention to the parent(s)' social, economic, and cultural resources is necessary for making assessments, planning strategies, and implementing approaches that are appropriately sensitive to the child's family and community (Gross, 1996).

4. The child's growth and development is the first social expectation and is molded and shaped by influences in the home, school, neighborhood,

Table 8-1
Examples of Broad-Based Community Projects

State	WIC Office: Women, Infants, Children is a supplemental food program for women and their children who meet financial and medical requirements.
Local	Teen Clinic: Teen Clinic is part of the School-Based Health Care Clinic developed to address the special health care needs of adolescents in the community.
National	Title V: Block grant funding for children with special health care needs and their families.
Private	Sickle Cell Clinic: Clinic and staff provide education and referral services supported by private funding and benefactors.
Academic	Pediatric Mobile Van: Mobile clinic that provides comprehensive pediatric services to children living in public housing.
Special Interest Group	Children's Advocacy Centers: Centers funded by private interest foundations, citizens, and corporations to provide shelter, support, and services needed by children who are abused, neglected, or victims of sexual assault.

and community as a whole.

5. Poverty, transportation, homelessness, and violence are barriers to health care (U.S. Public Health Service, 1990).

  a. Recognizing environmental factors and preventable injury as priorities can promote health, prevent illness, and improve the status of child health.

  b. Comprehensive community assessment highlights the importance of these issues, even though many are deeply embedded in communities and may appear insurmountable.

6. Reviewing nursing and interdisciplinary child health journals can provide insight about the impact that community can have on a child's health, and strategies necessary to make positive changes.

  a. Based on existing literature, the following are community factors that influence a child's health:

    (1) Family.

    (2) Hazard-free environment.

    (3) Safe neighborhood.

    (4) Social support.

(5) Access to health care.

(6) Schools that provide appropriate education.

b. Research that demonstrates what other communities and health care providers have effectively implemented can serve as the planning framework that follows assessment. For example, the state of Arizona uses a community development model to approach the needs of the individual communities.

c. Nurses and nurse practitioners can facilitate collaborative action in the community where decisions and accountability for effective outcomes are planned around the needs of children and their families.

d. Professional literature documents and supports the premise that community characteristics and influences have a decisive impact on a child's growth, development, and overall health.

H. For a summary of broad-based community projects, see Table 8-1.

II. COMMUNITY OF FAMILY

◆ ◆

A. The parent's role in the community influences the expectations of the child, the child's performance, and personal autonomy.

1. Employment, access to transportation, health care, food, housing, police and fire protection, child care, and recreation affect the parental status and directly translates to the child's well-being.

a. Abrupt changes from employment to unemployment will dramatically change the family structure and expectations of the child.

b. A growing shortage of safe, affordable low-income housing, declining incomes, and lack of family supports contributes to the financial, mental, and emotional stress of families.

2. Domestic violence, discrimination against families with children or those on public assistance, lack of community supports, mental health issues, substance abuse, and family tension contribute to the lack of parenting.

3. Adequate parenting gives structure to a child's life that is needed for health promotion and health surveillance.

B. Eliciting health beliefs that are ethnically and culturally based provides the health care provider with insight to the child's immediate community, its values, strengths, and differences. *Also see Chapter 29: Cultural Influences.*

1. When the child's parents are immigrants, language can also be the determining factors for the absence or presence of access to health care.

2. Target goals of Healthy People 2000, such as immunizations and well child health surveillance, are at risk when challenged by language, culture, and affordable accessible health care among some populations.

3. An understanding of cultural diversity enables the provider to sensitively negotiate with the family to implement needed health care strategies to improve health and education.

C. In 1995, 20.8% of children under the age of 18 were poor, making them the largest age component of the poverty population (Census Bureau, 1997). *See Chapter 9: Influences of Regulatory Mechanisms and Policies of Health Care.*

1. Although children represent 25% of the total population, they make up 40% of all poor people.

2. The trends recently identified in the United States include (National Center for Children in Poverty [NCCP], 1997):

a. Young child poverty rate grew faster in the suburbs (59%) than it did in cities(39%).

b. Poverty rate among white children grew twice as fast (38%) as black children(19%).

c. Close to 45% of young children were living in near poverty.

3. For young children living with married parents one of who was working, the poverty rate grew 6% in 1975 to 15% in 1995.

D. The scope of homelessness is difficult to assess in the health care delivery equation given the lack of a concrete definition of homelessness and the variety of ways state and federal agencies track homelessness. *See Chapter 9: Influences of Regulatory Mechanisms and Policies of Health Care.*

1. The evolving term "homelessness" is now being used to describe a continuum extending from those individuals who may be subjected to multiple unplanned moves in a single year to others who live on the streets or in abandoned buildings and cars.

2. The number of families with children who are homeless has increased from 27% of the population in 1985 to 38% of the population in 1996 (Children's Defense Fund, 1997).

3. The major cause of homelessness is poverty.

a. In 1995, 14.7 million children (21% of America's children) were living in poverty (Children's Defense Fund, 1997).

b. Of these children, 24% were under the age of 6 (Children's Defense Fund, 1997).

4. Homelessness compounds the risks and stresses

of poverty on children's physical growth and development and mental health.

   a. Infants and toddlers of parents who are homeless are at greater risk for developmental delays and unidentified disabilities (Carnegie, 1994).

   b. Young children who experience developmental delays without intervention may demonstrate further developmental delay and disorders later in life affecting school performance if they remain without access to early intervention services.

5. Homelessness also places children at risk for physical health disorders such as chicken pox, ringworm, hepatitis, and upper respiratory disorders (National Center for Children in Poverty, 1997).

6. Networking with state and federal agencies is imperative for linking these families with children who are homeless to appropriate services that are legally mandated by the McKinney Act of 1994 and can be provided locally if community agencies are tasked to provide services.

E. Another component of community that touches a child's growth and development is child care, which is a necessity for millions of families.

1. Approximately 7.7 million children under 5 years of age are being cared for by someone other than their parents while their mothers work; 59% are in daycare centers and family daycare homes (Children's Defense Fund, 1997).

2. Young children who are cared for in day care centers are at risk for a variety of infections.

   a. Variables that contribute to this health environment include (Kendall & Moukaddem, 1992):

      (1) A large number of children are in diapers.

      (2) Gathering large numbers of children and adults together increases exposure to infection.

      (3) Children's frequent exploration of their mouths spread respiratory secretions.

      (4) Young children have immature immune systems.

   b. The impact these variables have on a child's health has positively influenced policies that have been developed through the collaboration of American Public Health Association and American Academy of Pediatrics to minimize risks and maximize health.

3. Well-child surveillance visits should include questions regarding the developmentally appropriate activities and expectations of the children in their day care setting.

   a. Nurses can advocate for children by teaching parents and teachers to incorporate handwashing in play activities and acting as consultants for daycare centers.

   b. Surveillance, assessment, anticipatory guidance, and advocacy for the growing child spending the daytime hours out of the home are specific, positive ways to collaborate with parents to improve the child's environment.

III. Environment of the Community

◆◆◆◆◆◆◆◆◆◆◆◆◆◆◆◆◆◆◆◆◆

A. Environmental community components that have an impact on a child's health. *See Chapter 9: Influences of Regulatory Mechanisms and Policies of Health Care.*

1. The American Public Health Association (1992) identified the following health indicators for a building a healthy community:

   a. Access to medical care.

   b. Healthy environment.

   c. Healthy neighborhoods.

   d. Community services.

2. Barriers to accessing community services.

   a. Knowledge deficit.

   b. Language

   c. Transportation.

   d. Health care access.

   e. Cultural diversity and respect.

B. Access to medical care is related to children's health, for access to health care is not available to all children if health insurance or funding is not available. According to the Census Bureau (1997):

1. In 1995, 9.8 million children (13.1%) under the age of 18 had no health insurance.

2. Hispanic children are less likely to have health insurance (26.8%) than are White or Black children, and Black children are less likely to have health insurance (15.3%) than White children are (13.4%).

3. In 1995, Medicaid covered 45% of all Black children, 37.4% of all Hispanic children, and 18.3% of all White children.

C. Recreational and play opportunities for children and families should be identified in the community.

1. As a child develops from the hand-holding toddler to the playground-bound first grader, new assessments must be made regarding the community environment.

2. The safety of playgrounds located in relation to the child's home depends on the housing avail-

able to the family.

3. Safety issues where children play and grow are often addressed by school nurses because of the number of injuries that occur on school playgrounds.

D. The physical environment where a child lives and grows can influence the child's health status.

1. Research studies, as well as anecdotal evidence, suggest that health damaging environmental pollutants are more prevalent in low-income communities and are found disproportionately in neighborhoods of people of color.

   a. Inadequate housing, nutrition, and access to care exacerbate the health-related consequences of these environmental risk factors.

   b. Adolescents need an environment that provides opportunities for healthy recreation, constructive activities, and access to the educational and health services they need (Blyth, 1990).

   c. Neighborhoods need to build a sense of community that motivates young people to help each other and help the community provide positive support for mental and physical health.

2. Children remain exposed to environmental hazards despite a decrease in the overall number of hazards in the environment.

   a. Once these hazards are identified, they are calculated as "risks" in the assessment of a child's environment.

   b. Children are at higher risk than adults due to physiologic, behavioral, and dietary factors related to the accumulation of pesticides from food, and exposure to the outside environment such as yards and playgrounds.

   c. Advocacy and education about these risks influence federal agencies such as the Environmental Protection Agency (EPA).

      (1) The 1996 Safe Drinking Water and Food Quality Protection Acts underscore the link between environment and children's health.

      (2) New EPA proposals provide protection to 40 million children from environment risks.

      (3) The EPA acknowledges that children could benefit from research that addresses their unique characteristics, but to date has not conducted such research.

IV. SCHOOL COMMUNITY
◆ ◆ ◆ ◆ ◆ ◆ ◆ ◆ ◆ ◆ ◆ ◆ ◆ ◆ ◆ ◆ ◆ ◆ ◆

A. A relationship exists between economic

prosperity and an educated work force.

1. Schools provide the education that fosters the child's productivity and eventual autonomy.

   a. America's schools provide the single most comprehensive, coordinated, child-centered developmentally appropriate environment for children.

   b. Schools provide the opportunity for continued growth and development outside the family.

2. Former Surgeon General Novello is attributed with identifying the relationship between health and the readiness of a child to learn.

3. Given this relationship, it is important to remember that public school budgets are financed by local and state sources with supplementary resources from the federal government.

4. Nurses need to know the funding factors, the curriculum, and the safety of the school environment that affect school objectives and outcomes. Considerations include:

   a. Values.

   b. Transportation.

   c. Educational goals.

   d. Education resources.

   e. Building safety.

   f. Playground safety.

   g. Personal safety.

B. School-based health clinics are promoting and implementing children's education and health while collaborating with communities groups and organizations to address their individual needs (Walker et al., 1996).

1. School-based health clinics offer an opportunity to remove the greatest barrier of access to health care by placing the services where they are needed and can be delivered effectively.

2. The opportunity to research children's health within their immediate community can lead to a better grounded health practice research and guidelines that are based on quality outcome studies (Primas et al., 1994).

V. SOCIAL SUPPORT IN THE COMMUNITY
◆ ◆ ◆ ◆ ◆ ◆ ◆ ◆ ◆ ◆ ◆ ◆ ◆ ◆ ◆ ◆ ◆ ◆ ◆

A. Foster care caseloads rose to 468,000 in 1994, a 16% increase since 1990 (Children's Defense Fund, 1997).

1. On a single day in 1993, 445,000 children were in foster family homes, groups homes, or residential treatment centers, an increase of about two-thirds over the 1-day count of 10 years earlier (Children's Defense Fund, 1997).

2. Dubowitz (1990, cited in Halfon & Klee, 1991) found the following:

a. One-third of the children in foster care have potentially serious health and problems:
   (1) 20% had growth failure
   (2) 19% had cardiovascular problems
   (3) 14% had dental problems
   (4) 38% of children under 5 years of age showed developmental delay
   (5) 87% of children under 4 years had abnormal behavioral assessments.
   b. Children in foster home placement were 3 to 6 times more likely to have depression, conduct disorders, difficulties in school, impaired social relationships, and need appropriate school placements than child in nonfoster home.
3. Length of out-of-home stay has also dramatically increased in recent years.

B. The number of children in kinship care is growing (Children's Defense Fund, 1997).
1. In 1995, more than 1.4 million children lived with grandparents with no parents present in the household, up 66% since 1989.
2. Many grandparents and other relatives providing kinship care do not receive foster care payments as policy varies by state.

C. Child Welfare advocates warn that welfare reform initiatives that affect family income are significant parental stressors, affect a family's access to services, and affect the health and development of their children.
1. Creation and implementation of comprehensive plans should consider all vulnerable families.
2. National Center for Children in Poverty (NCCP) publishes recurring themes that emphasize the need for plans that monitor and track children's services, especially child welfare and protective services.
3. Welfare reform requires collaboration and mutual understanding among communities and state and federal government agencies.

D. Communities are sometimes defined by their functional capacity and patterns rather than in terms of demographics.
1. When community coalitions form, they become the cornerstone of activity and leadership.
2. For example, Healthy Foundations in Iowa demonstrated the "plan-do-study-act" cycle that identifies, analyzes, and promotes improvement in local systems of care and keeps the systems "individualized" for the community they serve rather than using the same system across the state (DeWitt & Roberts, 1996).

VI. SIGNIFICANT VARIABLES IN THE COMMUNITY

◆ ◆ ◆ ◆ ◆ ◆ ◆ ◆ ◆ ◆ ◆ ◆ ◆ ◆ ◆ ◆ ◆ ◆ ◆ ◆

A. Substance abuse is a serious and growing problem that has an impact on the health and well-being of childbearing women and their infants.
1. Many pregnant women who abuse drugs do not seek treatment and either receive no prenatal care or come for care late in the pregnancy (Haauk & Budetti, 1993).
   a. The impact of this phenomenon on the urban maternity units has been observed and felt in many communities.
   b. While the incidence of substance abuse among pregnant women has been documented at 10% (Farkus & Parran, 1993), few programs have been established to meet these women's health care needs. Reasons include (Farkus & Parran, 1993; Haauk & Budetti, 1993):
      (1) Limited funding.
      (2) Inadequate models of intervention.
      (3) Few opportunities for comprehensive, coordinated services for women and children.
2. Researchers have found that many effects of in-utero substance exposure on the growth and development of infants are transitory (Robbins & Mills, 1993).
3. Many of the previously described drug-related disabilities of infants are actually the effects of poverty, violence, abuse, neglect, prostitution, mental illness, and psychologic and physical abandonment, which are identifiable community issues that have an impact on a child of any age (Haack & Burdetti, 1993).

B. Children witness violence in the electronic media and in their communities.
1. The average child in America spends more time watching television than in any other activity except sleeping (American Academy of Pediatrics, 1990); the quality of programming has been debated for many decades, but it is documented that much of what a child views on TV is violent.
2. Studies document that in communities such as the District of Columbia and Detroit, Michigan, 30–60% of school age children are witnessing violent crimes in their neighborhoods, compared to 6–13% percent in suburban or rural areas (Fry-Bower, 1997).

C. Health providers identify the availability of firearms as contributing to the alarming number of deaths among children under 19 years of age.

D. Exposure to community violence affects children in several ways.

1. Children exposed to violence show signs of depression including low self-esteem, excessive crying, and worries about death or being injured.
2. Many inner city children who are regularly exposed to violence develop physiologic defense mechanisms that inhibit their abilities to learn, leading to aggressive and atypical social behavior.
3. Children who are exposed to violence as witnesses and victims demonstrate the negative impact of violence through behavior that affects their cognitive, moral, and social development.
4. Children may decide to align with a group or gang for a sense of belonging, protection, or power.

E. A significant number of children are victims of child abuse and neglect.

1. Between 1985 and 1995, the number of children in the United States reported abused or neglected rose 61%, to 3.1 million (Children's Defense Fund, 1997).
2. The 1994 data released in Children's Defense Fund Yearbook 1997 indicate an increasing prevalence of child abuse and neglect, domestic violence, and children in foster care.
3. Children who have disabilities experience abuse and neglect at a higher rate than children without disabilities.

F. State and local laws, policies, and resources provide the framework for the educational, health care, and social welfare systems available to the child and family.

1. Many low-income children with severe disabilities qualified for cash assistance though the children's SSI program.
2. The Maternal and Child Health Bureau (MCHB) provides support and resources for parents and communities that offer information, education, multidisciplinary care, and services including respite care for the families who care for children with special needs (Austin & Donohoe, 1996).
3. MCHB endorses and promotes care that is family centered, coordinated, comprehensive, culturally sensitive, and developed through collaboration with the child and family (Grayson & Guyer, 1994).

Table 8-2
Interdisciplinary Team Community Members

Medical health professionals
Social workers
Nurses
Physical therapists
Speech therapists
Occupational therapists
Psychologists
Child advocates
Educational specialists
Family

VII. INTEGRATING STRATEGIES

A. Identifying and understanding the risks and strengths of a child's community supports the collaborative efforts that can insure a safe, nurturing environment for all children.

1. Recognizing that communities consist of a significant number of external influences that affect health care delivery enables the provider to integrate strategies that can improve the influences on a child's growth and development.
2. Communities can plan and support programs offering respite care and other resources needed by families with children with special needs (Tannen, 1996).
3. An important outcome of reforming health care service systems is the service model that includes the concept of case management and care coordination (Austin & Donohoe, 1996).
4. Principles of community assessment for a specific population should include:
   a. Defining what constitutes the community (e.g., demographics, social, economic indicators).
   b. Deciding what data needs to be known and what needs to be measured.
   c. Knowing the source of the data and its validity.
   d. Identifying the health status and health risks.
   e. Determining the importance of the data in relation to the health status and health risks for the child and family.
   f. Identifying health care access, available services, and the costs involved.
   g. Presenting the data in a meaningful way that ensures a common understanding to the family, provider, and collaborative community members.

B. Health service models that include the concept of case management and care coordination should incorporate the following principles (Austin & Donohoe, 1996)**:**
1. Assessment.
2. Primary care provided with ongoing health coordination.
3. Linkage with resources.
4. Collaboration with families.
5. Provision and access to counseling and social supports as needed.
6. Collaboration with health care providers of an interdisciplinary team providing services to identify the strengths and needs of the child and family (see Table 8-2).
7. Advocacy and care coordination facilitated by a case manager.
8. Inclusion of the child and family in appropriate educational services.
9. Crisis intervention and monitoring.

C. Assimilating community assessment and care coordination principles in health care delivery enables the nurse and the family to design a community that provides the child with a safe, nurturing environment that facilitates growth and development.

BIBLIOGRAPHY

American Academy of Pediatrics. (1990). Children, adolescents and television. *Pediatrics, 85*(6), 1119–1120.

American Public Health Association. (1991). *Healthy communities 2000: Model standards. Guidelines for community attainment of the Year 2000 National Health Objectives.* Washington, DC: APHA.

American Public Health Association & American Academy of Pediatrics. (1992). *Caring for our children. National health and safety performance standards: Guidelines for out-of-home child care programs.* Washington, DC: APHA.

Austin, J.R.D., & Donohoe, M. (1996). *Continuing education needs for nurses caring for children with special health care needs.* Washington, DC: Georgetown University and National Center for Education in Maternal and Child Health.

Blyth, D. (1990). *Six steps toward improving adolescent health.* Washington, DC: National Center for Education in Maternal and Child Health.

Carnegie Corporation of New York. (1994). *Starting points: Meeting the needs of our youngest children.* New York: Carnegie Task Force on Meeting the Needs of Young Children.

Census Bureau. (1997). *Children's health insurance.* (On-line). Housing and household economic statistics division. Available: hhes-info@census.gov

Children's Defense Fund. (1997). *The state of America's children yearbook.* Washington, DC: CDF.

DeWitt, T., & Roberts, K. (Eds.). (1996). *Pediatric education in community settings: A manual.* Arlington, VA: National Center for Education in Maternal and Child Health.

Farkas, K.J., & Parran, T.V. (1993). Treatment of cocaine addition during pregnancy. *Clinics on Perinatology, 20,* 29–45.

Fry-Bower. E.K. (1997). Community violence: Its impact on the development of children and implications for nursing practice. *Pediatric Nursing, 23*(2), 117–127.

Grason, H.A., & Guyer, B. (1995). *Assessing and developing primary care for children: Reforms in health systems.* Arlington, VA: National Center for Education in Maternal and Child Health.

Green, M. (Ed.). (1994). *Bright futures: Guidelines for health supervision of infants, children, and adolescents.* Arlington, VA: National Center for Education in Maternal and Child Health.

Gross, D. (1996). What is a "good parent?" *Maternal and Child Nursing, 21,* 178–182.

Haack, M.R., & Budetti, P.P. (1993). An analysis of resources to aid drug exposed infants and their families. *Addictions Nursing Network (Pt. 1),* 5, 107–114.

Halfen, N., & Klee, L. (1991). Health and development services for children with multiple needs: The child in foster care. *Yale Law and Policy Review, 9*(46), 71–96.

Kendall, E., & Moukaddem, V. (1992). Who's vulnerable in infant child care centers? *Issues in Contemporary Pediatric Nursing, 16*(2), 99–108.

Leininger, M. (1996). Cultural care theory, research, and practice. *Nursing Science Quarterly, 9*(2), 71–78.

National Center for Children in Poverty. (1997). *One in four: America's youngest poor.* Columbia School of Public Health: NY.

Primas, P.J., Mileham, T., Torono, C., & McCoy, B.J. (1994). A nursing system of health care: Breaking the cycle of disadvantage. *Nursing and Health Care, 15*(1), 10–17.

Public Health Service. (1990). *Healthy people 2000: National health promotion and disease prevention objectives.* Washington, DC: U.S. Department of Health and Human Services.

Robbins, L.N., & Mills, J.L. (Eds.). (1993). Effects of in utero exposure to street drugs. *American Journal of Public Health, 83(Suppl.),* 1–32.

Tannen, N. (1996). *Families at the center of the development of a system of care.* Washington, DC: Maternal and Child Health Bureau of the Health Resources and Services Administration.

Walker, P.H., Bowllan, N., Chevalier, N., Gullo, S., & Lawrence, L. (1996). School-based care: Clinical challenges and research opportunities. *Journal of the Society of Pediatric Nursing, 1*(2), 64–74.

STUDY QUESTIONS

◆◆

1. The child's first community is:
   a. the immediate family.
   b. the extended family.
   c. the church.
   d. the daycare center.

2. Which of the following topic areas form the foundation for community issues that influence a child's health?
   a. Family and a hazard-free environment
   b. Social support and a safe neighborhood
   c. Access to health care and schools that provide appropriate education
   d. a and b
   e. a, b, and c

3. Which of the following statements about homelessness is true?
   a. The scope of homelessness is difficult to assess because a concrete definition of the term does not exist.
   b. All state and federal agencies use the same methods to track homelessness.
   c. The term *homelessness* is used only to describe persons who live on the streets, in abandoned buildings, cars, or homeless shelters.
   d. a and b
   e. a and c

4. Young children who are cared for in daycare centers are at risk for:
   a. developmental delays.
   b. injuries.
   c. malnutrition.
   d. infections.
   e. none of the above.

5. What percentage of children in foster care experience growth failure?
   a. 4%
   b. 10%
   c. 16%
   d. 20%
   e. 25%

6. Which population of children in the United States is least likely to have health insurance?
   a. Hispanic
   b. Black
   c. White
   d. Asian

7. Which of the following provides the single most comprehensive, coordinated, child-centered developmentally appropriate environment for children?
   a. Immediate family
   b. Extended family
   c. School
   d. Church

8. Many of the effects of in-utero substance exposure on the growth and development of infants are transitory.
   a. True
   b. False

9. On a clinic visit for immunizations for her 5-year-old daughter Rosa, Mrs. Rodriquez reports to the nurse that Rosa was once a very happy child, but now seems sad much of the time. "Rosa asks me question after question about people and animals dying," she adds. These signs would alert the nurse to explore which of the following issues with Rosa and her mother?
   a. The amount of television and types of programming Rosa watches each day
   b. The nutritional value of Rosa's diet
   c. Any recent deaths or life-threatening illnesses or injuries of a family member, friend, or neighbor
   d. Exposure to violence in the home or neighborhood
   e. a, b, and c
   f. a, c, and d

10. Principles of community assessment include:
    a. identifying the health status and health risks of the community.
    b. determining what data needs to be known and what needs to be measured.
    c. identifying health care access, available services, and the costs involved.
    d. presenting the data in a meaningful way that ensures a common understanding to the family, provider, and collaborative community members.
    e. all of the above.

ANSWERS

◆◆◆◆◆◆◆◆◆◆◆◆◆◆◆◆◆◆◆◆◆◆◆◆◆

1.a 2.e 3.a 4.d 5.d 6.a 7.c 8.a 9.f 10.e

Chapter 9

Influences of Regulatory Mechanisms and Policies of Health Care

Barbara Velsor-Friedrich, PhD, RN

Concept

◆◆◆◆◆◆◆◆◆◆◆◆◆◆◆◆◆◆◆◆◆◆◆◆◆◆◆◆

◆ Economic, social, and political influences

Objectives

◆◆◆◆◆◆◆◆◆◆◆◆◆◆◆◆◆◆◆◆◆◆◆◆◆◆◆◆

At the completion of this chapter, the reader will be able to:

◆ Identify the role that the federal government has played in the development and regulation of child health and welfare policies/programs.

◆ Describe the current status of selected critical issues affecting children, i.e., poverty, lack of health insurance, homelessness.

◆ Discuss federal and state programs that address these critical issues.

◆ Identify the nurse's role in supporting and empowering vulnerable children and their families to access child health and welfare programs.

Key Points

◆◆◆◆◆◆◆◆◆◆◆◆◆◆◆◆◆◆◆◆◆◆◆◆◆◆◆◆

◆ Children occupy a small but important segment of society.

◆ The federal government has had a significant impact on the development and regulation of child health and welfare programs.

◆ Proposed reductions in federal funding of child and family programs threaten to significantly alter or completely remove the "safety net" from many children and their families.

◆ All child health/welfare programs must be structured within the context of the family.

◆ Nurses have a strategic role in planning, implementing, coordinating, and evaluating health care delivery models and safeguarding the current federal/state programs.

Influences of Regulatory Mechanisms and Policies of Health Care

I. OVERVIEW

Child health care remained completely under the control and concern of individual families without any government regulation or support until the early 1900s. Although great strides have been made in developing and implementing government supported child health and welfare programs, there are major gaps in coverage. Millions of children in America are without food, shelter, or routine health care.

A. Although the federal government has been instrumental in helping to set important policies related to child health and welfare, a recent shift in values and priorities threatens to dramatically change programs for vulnerable children and their families.

B. Nurses are positioned to serve as a strong advocates for children and their families by supporting existing and proposed child health and welfare programs.

II. DEFINITIONS

A. Regulation.
1. A rule or order prescribed by an authority.
2. A governing direction or law (Webster, 1996).

B. Policy.
1. The principles that govern action toward given ends (Titmus, 1974).
2. The result of decisions on resource allocation (Natapoff & Wieczorek, 1990).
3. The choices that a society or segment of society makes regarding its goals and priorities and how it will allocate its resources (Mason, Talbott, & Leavitt, 1993).

C. Health policy: directives and goals for promoting the health of a country's citizens (Mason, Talbott, & Leavitt, 1993).

III. FEDERAL GOVERNMENT'S INVOLVEMENT IN CHILD HEALTH CARE DELIVERY (See Table 9-1)

A. The issue of problems affecting the health and welfare of children first received national attention when President Theodore Roosevelt called the first White House Conference on Children in 1910.

B. As an outcome of the White House Conference, the Children's Bureau was created in 1912 to investigate problems such as infant mortality, dangerous occupations, and diseases of children.

C. The Sheppard-Towner Act was passed in 1921, authorizing $1.2 million to improve health services for all classes of children.
1. Passage of this act marked the first direct federal grant-in-aid program for health services.
2. This act was responsible for the registration of all births and the establishment of well baby clinics.

D. In 1935, Title V of the Social Security Act was passed.
1. Programs under this title were directed to address the integration of health services for poor children and their mothers and for crippled children.
2. Services provided included prenatal care, well child care, school health, immunizations, public health nursing, day care, and some nutritional assistance.

E. Medicaid is the largest public medical care program for children in the United States.
1. Federal and state governments jointly administer this program on a cost-sharing basis, with each state agency administering its own Medicaid program using federal guidelines.
2. Medicaid eligibility is based on financial need.
   a. Medicaid has substantially improved access

Table 9-1
Federal Involvement in Maternal Child Health Welfare Programs

Date	Program/Legislation
1910	First White House Conference called by President Teddy Roosevelt
1912	Children's Bureau established
1921	Sheppard-Towner Act enacted (1st Maternity/ Infant Act)
1935	Title V of Social Security Act enacted (established many MCH services)
1943	Federal Emergency Maternal and Infant Program enacted, providing medical and hospital care for servicemen's wives and children
1965	Title XIX of Social Security Act enacted; Project Headstart initiated
1967	Early Periodic Screening and Diagnostic Testing (EPSDT) initiated
1972	Women Infant and Children (WIC) food assistance program started
1975	P.L. 94-142 Education for all Handicapped Children Act (covers children ages 5-21 years)
1981	Block Grants initiated
1986	P.L. 99-457 Education of the Handicapped Amendment extends PL 94-142 to infants and toddlers
1996	Personal Responsibility and Work Opportunity Reconciliation Act

to health care for economically disadvantaged children in poor health.
  b. Children in low-income families make up 50% of the beneficiaries although they account for only 15% of Medicaid expenditures (The Kasier Common Future of Medicaid, 1995).
  3. In the 1980s, Congress passed a series of amendments that expanded women and children's Medicaid coverage.

F. Supplemental Program for Women, Infants, and Children (WIC) provides assistance and nutritional screening to low-income pregnant women and postpartum women, infants, and children up to the age 5 years.
  1. Congress established the program in 1972.
  2. The WIC program is designed to provide eligible women and children with nutritious supplemental food, nutrition education, and to promote the optimal use of existing health services, i.e.,

preventive and therapeutic infant and child care (Natapoff & Wieczorek, 1990).

G. PL 94-142 Education for All Handicapped Children assures that anyone with disabilities is entitled to a free public education in the least restrictive environment with services appropriate to meet the child's unique needs, including the administration of medicines and tube feedings.

H. PL 99- 457 extends PL 94-142 to children with disabilities between the ages of 3 and 5 years.

I. Early Periodic Screening and Diagnostic Testing (EPSDT) was established through the Social Security Amendments in 1967.
  1. The program provides comprehensive and periodic assessment of children's health, including screening for development, nutrition, vision, dentition, and hearing.
  2. States provide EPSDT services to all children under 21 years who are Medicaid beneficiaries.

J. Aid to Families with Dependent Children (AFDC), established by the Social Security Act of 1935, targets children living in a single-parent family and in some two-parent families with incomes below state-established eligibility levels to assure that some minimum amount of funding is available to help meet poor families' daily needs.

IV. FINANCING AND MANAGEMENT OF CURRENT CHILD HEALTH AND WELFARE PROGRAMS
◆ ◆ ◆ ◆ ◆ ◆ ◆ ◆ ◆ ◆ ◆ ◆ ◆ ◆ ◆ ◆ ◆ ◆ ◆

A. Health and welfare programs for children have experienced many changes in the methods of payment and reimbursement.

B. Maternal Child Health (MCH) Block Grants: the consolidation of all MCH funds into primary health care grants funded directly to the states brought about through the passage of the Omnibus Budget Reconciliation Act, 1981 (OBRA P.L. 97-35).
  1. Programs were combined into four blocks.
    a. MCH.
    b. ETOH (alcohol and drugs).
    c. Preventive Health.
    d. Primary Care.
  2. Although this new "federalism" gives states greater authority and control over health and

welfare programs, they receive 20% less federal support.

3. If this deficit is not met through state and local taxes, health and welfare programs for children and their families could be drastically reduced (Videka-Sherman & Viggiani, 1996).

C. Adequate funding continues to plague federally sponsored health programs.

1. Costs associated with the Medicaid program have grown in excess of 10% per year in recent years.
2. The budget resolution for FY 1997-2002 recommends reducing Medicaid spending by $72 billion (Ford, 1996).

D. Managed Care: a system of health care delivery that combines clinical decision making with resource use by shifting the locus of clinical control from solely the health care provider to an organization that manages the care; encompasses any measure that favorably affects the price of services, the site at which services are received, or their utilization (Ferguson, 1996).

1. This system is rapidly becoming a major source of health care delivery for beneficiaries of both employer-funded care and of publicly funded programs, Medicaid, and Medicare (U.S. Department of Heath and Human Services [USDHHS], 1996).
2. Managed Care requires that Medicaid programs be responsible for both the organization and delivery of care (Ferguson, 1996).
   a. The primary aim is to cap Medicaid increases.
   b. Many states have implemented Managed Care Medicaid Programs to improve access and continuity of care and to decrease inappropriate and unnecessary utilization.
3. Nurses' involvement with managed care has focused on a concern for quality and access as well as reducing costs.

E. Case management: a model of care delivery that has been identified as a process for achieving optimal patient outcomes in expected time frames while containing costs.

1. Some overlap exists regarding the terms nurse managed care and case management.
2. Case management programs for special pediatric populations, i.e., children with chronic illnesses, have been developed, and demonstrate an effective way to balance expected outcomes, the process of care delivery, and cost (Schryer, 1993; Smith, 1994).
3. Case management has been incorporated into the process of implementing and evaluating procedures such as preadmission services, and

found effective in moving the child/family through the hospital experience in a caring, efficient, and cost-effective manner (Lauffer, 1992).

4. The nurse as case manager coordinates multidisciplinary care and acts as a liaison for patients and families through a continuum of care across settings while maintaining a cost-conscious focus (Newell, 1995).

V. CRITICAL CHILD HEALTH AND WELFARE ISSUES

◆ ◆ ◆ ◆ ◆ ◆ ◆ ◆ ◆ ◆ ◆ ◆ ◆ ◆ ◆ ◆ ◆ ◆ ◆

A. Poverty.

1. The official 1997 federal government's poverty guideline for a family of four is $16,050 (Federal Register, 1997).
2. Children continue to make up the largest portion of the population living in poverty.
   a. The percent of children living in poverty is at its highest rate in 30 years, from 16.8% in 1975 to 22% in 1993 (Annie E. Casey Foundation, 1995).
   b. There are 7.1 million children growing up in poor communities (Annie E. Casey Foundation, 1997).
   c. Children from ethnically diverse populations are more likely to live in poor families, with 44% of African-American children, 36% of Hispanic children, and 15% of white children living in poverty (Allen, 1994).
   d. Children living in poverty are at greater risk of:
      (1) Being sick and having inadequate health care.
      (2) Being parents before they complete high school.
      (3) Being exposed to violence.
      (4) Being incarcerated before they are old enough to vote (Annie E. Casey Foundation, 1997).
3. Current federal programs available to poor children and their families include Aid to Families of Dependent Children (AFDC), Medicaid, WIC, and Food Stamps.
   a. Drastic reductions in funding of these programs have occurred.
   b. Changes in eligibility criteria have led to the elimination of many of the "working poor" from these programs.
4. The Welfare System underwent major changes with the passage of P.L. 104-193, The Personal Responsibility and Work Opportunity Reconciliation Act of 1996 (Buckley, 1996), also known as the Welfare Reform Act, which ended the federal government's 61-year-old guarantee of providing welfare checks to

eligible low-income mothers and their children.
  a. Funds now are distributed using the following criteria:
    (1) There is a 2-year time limit with a lifetime cap of 5 years.
    (2) The recipient must actively seek a job.
    (3) Unmarried teenage mothers are required to live at home and stay in school to get benefits.
    (4) Food stamps are limited to a 3-month period for adults between the ages of 18 and 50 years.
    (5) Legal immigrants are denied benefits; however, states may provide Medicaid for legal immigrants already in the U.S. (Church, 1996).
  b. Concerns regarding the act.
    (1) Finding and paying for child care to get and keep a job.
    (2) Availability of jobs for welfare recipients.
    (3) Whether states can find effective means to take care of its low-income mothers and children.
5. Improving the odds for children in low-income communities will require:
  a. Employment opportunities for parents.
  b. Quality health care.
  c. Formal and informal support networks.
  d. Organized recreation.
  e. Safe streets.
  f. High quality schools (Annie E. Casey Foundation, 1997).

B. Uninsured children and their families.
1. More than 10 million children (14.4%) in this country are without health insurance (USDHHS, 1996).
2. Of children whose families live in poverty, 62% are publicly insured primarily through Medicaid; 15% have private coverage; and 22% have no health coverage (USDHHS, 1996).
3. The number of uninsured children is expected to increase due to welfare reform and changes in employer-based insurance plans.
  a. In 1993, over 18 million people worked for companies that did not sponsor any health insurance; 5 million companies sponsored coverage only for employees.
  b. If current trends continue, it is estimated that by the year 2002, 13 million children will be uninsured (Hosansky, 1997).
4. Several state and federal proposals/programs are aimed at decreasing the number of uninsured children.
  a. Some states have implemented programs to insure children whose parents earn too much

to qualify for Medicaid, or have passed plans to expand Medicaid programs to cover more children.
  b. State programs may have a minimal impact and may reach only a small percentage of the 10 million uninsured children.

C. Homeless children and their families.
1. Homelessness has become one of this country's most significant social problems affecting a growing number of men, women, and children.
2. The nation's homeless population is estimated to be anywhere from 350,000 to 3,000,000 people (Bassuk & Rosenberg, 1990).
3. The increase in the homeless rate is thought to be associated with:
  a. An increase in the number of people who live in poverty.
  b. A decrease in the number of affordable housing units.
  c. Loss of employment.
  d. Emergency demand on income.
  e. Gentrification of neighborhoods.
  f. Alcohol or other drug abuse problems.
  g. A decrease in the number of alternative housing facilities.
4. Children and their families (single mothers and their children) are the largest growing segment of the homeless population (Interagency Council on the Homeless, 1991).
5. Children who are homeless are at risk for developing a variety of acute and chronic medical problems as well as psychologic and emotional problems.
6. Health care services for the homeless tend to be fragmented and limited in scope.
7. The Stewart B. McKinney Assistance Act of 1987 created the Interagency Council of the Homeless to coordinate and direct federal homeless efforts.
  a. The act allocated 1 billion dollars ($355 million was authorized) for housing demonstration projects, job training, and health care for homeless elderly persons, individuals with handicaps, families with children, Native Americans, and veterans.
  b. Additional funding from this act has supported emergency shelter grants, emergency nutrition assistance, grants for delivery of primary health care, and substance abuse services that include outreach, mental health, and assistance in obtaining entitlements.
8. Nutritional assistance, i.e., WIC, food stamps, school meals, is available to most homeless individuals.
9. Health care needs of homeless children and

their families should be addressed through the establishment of statewide comprehensive services that are coordinated and accessible to the population.

  a. Health screening, diagnosis, treatment, and referrals should be available in shelters.

  b. Services should include on-site services and day care services (Alperstein & Arnstein 1988).

10. Nurses can play a significant role in meeting the needs of homeless children and families.

  a. Nurses have helped to establish clinics and outreach services for the homeless.

  b. Nurses must educate themselves and the public about homelessness as a broad and complex social issue facing American society today (Natapoff & Wieczorek, 1990).

  c. Nurses can support legislation to prevent homelessness and increase legislation to provide services to individuals who are homeless, i.e., affordable housing and accessible health services.

D. Family violence.

1. The incidence of family violence is widespread and complex.

  a. Women and children are the primary victims.

  b. In 1991, 2–4 million children were abused or neglected, and 2 million women were battered by their partners (Kroll, 1993).

2. The Centers for Disease Control and Prevention has identified interpersonal or family violence as a major public health problem (Kroll, 1993).

3. Psychologic and physical abuse has been linked to deficiencies in a child's social and psychologic development, i.e., short attention span, impulsive behavior, heightened physical activity, and impairment of intellectual and language development (Craig, 1992).

4. Youths ages 12–17 years make up 38% of the child population but make up 47% of the victims of all forms of child violence (American Medical Association, 1992).

5. Violence is the second leading cause of injuries in women ages 14–44 years, with falls reported to be the leading cause of death overall (Novello, 1992).

6. Pregnant women are also affected by violence; one study reported between 4% and 8% of women attending prenatal clinics were abused during their pregnancy (Novello, 1992).

7. Child welfare systems have been advocating programs that seek to preserve families with services that include:

  a. Parent education and skills training.

  b. Family therapy.

  c. Psychologic support and counseling.

8. Title XX Social Services Block Grant is the largest source of funds directed to the states for child protective services, but appropriations have decrease since 1981 (Natapoff & Wieczorel, 1990).

9. Health care institutions are taking steps to address the issue of violence.

  a. In 1990, the Joint Commission on the Accreditation of Health Care Organizations (JCAHCO) added requirements for emergency and ambulatory care services to develop and use protocols to identify violence among patients.

  b. Some hospitals have developed hospital-based domestic violence programs (Sheridan & Taylor, 1993).

10. In 1993, 83 professional organizations, including the American Nurses Association (ANA) and the American Medical Association (AMA), set priorities in the area of family violence and recommended:

  a. Support for community-based efforts.

  b. Protection and empowerment of persons who experience violence.

  c. A national coalition to work in partnership with the media to promote safe, nonviolent families and home life (Stanley, 1994).

11. Nursing organizations have developed position statements that address the issue of violence.

  a. Recommendations from the ANA's Position Statement on Physical Violence (1991).

  (1) Routine education of all nurses and health care providers in the skills necessary to prevent violence against women.

  (2) Routine assessment and documentation for physical abuse of all women in any health care setting.

  (3) Research on violence against women, including the development and evaluation of nursing models for preventive assessment, intervention, and treatment of abused women, their children, and perpetrators.

  (4) Education of school-age children and adolescents in public schools about relationships without violence and community resources for help.

  b. Recommendations from the Society of Pediatric Nurses Position Statement on Pediatric Firearm Injuries (1995).

  (1) The focus of health care providers must shift to primary prevention through education.

  (2) Pediatric nurses, employed in a variety of settings, have the opportunity to educate

parents and children about gun violence and the prevention of firearm injuries.
- (3) Firearm safety should be included as part of safety assessment on hospital admission, homecare intake, and outpatient assessment forms.
- (4) Nurses should support programs for children and teens that limit violence, including conflict management workshops, after-school programs, recreational activities, and parent education programs.
12. Pediatric nurses will encounter victims of physical, sexual, and psychologic violence in every health care setting and therefore must assess all pediatric patients for the potential of abuse and recommend treatment.

VI. THE NURSE'S ROLE IN SUPPORTING AND EMPOWERING VULNERABLE FAMILIES

A. Nurses can assume the role of child advocate.
1. Child Advocacy has been defined as operating on three levels (Margolis, Cole & Kotch, 1997).
   a. On the individual or case level, the advocate is an individual acting on the behalf of a child, and serves as a defender, protector, mediator, supporter, investigator, or negotiator.
   b. On the organizational level, the advocate attempts to alter and monitor legislative, budgetary, and administrative processes and at times, monitors professionals and professionalism.
   c. On the systems or class level, the advocate helps to reform an organization or a system to benefit a group of people or the users of the organization.
2. Strategies that a child advocate may pursue include educating policy makers and citizens, lobbying for legislation and/or regulation, and adjudicating when rights or interests cannot be satisfied.
3. Advocates need to be active at each of the three levels of regulatory authority for public health:
   a. Federal.
   b. State.
   c. Local.

B. Nurses can participate in the public policy process.
1. Because interest groups compete for a limited number of resources, nurses must be familiar with and participate in the public policy process to ensure that the needs of women and children are better served.

2. Nurses must be able to identify the stakeholders (i.e., elected officials, interest groups, representatives, individuals) who are directly involved in shaping a particular policy and may be directly affected by its outcome (Mason, Talbott, & Leavitt, 1993).
3. Because a policy may be affected at any point in the process, nurses need to be aware of the stages of policy development (Anderson, 1990).
   a. Policy agenda setting.
   b. Policy formation.
   c. Policy adoption.
   d. Policy implementation, and
   e. Policy evaluation.
4. Policy decisions should be designed to safeguard the health and welfare of children and their families.

VII. CONCLUSION

A. Although the government has played an important role in the advancement of child health and welfare issues, much progress is needed to strengthen vulnerable families and protect children at risk.

B. Healthy intact families are the fundamental resource for the development of healthy children.

C. By strengthening and preserving families, children will have a better chance to grow up in safety and security (Chicago Child Care Society, 1994).

D. Due to their clinical knowledge base, the nurse is in a favorable position to influence policy decision making.
1. Nurses must serve on policy-making boards.
2. Nurses should always be consulted when child health and welfare policies are being made.

BIBLIOGRAPHY

Allen, C.E. (1994). Families in poverty. *Nursing Clinics in North America, 29*(3), 377–392.

Alperstein, G., & Arnstein, E. (1988). Homeless children — A challenge for pediatricians. *Pediatric Clinics of North America. 35,*1413–1425.

American Medical Association. (1992). Medical news & perspectives. ACOG renew domestic violence campaign, calls for changes in medical school curricula. *Journal of the American Medical Association, 267*(23), 3131.

American Nurses Association. (1991). *Position statement on physical violence against women.* Washington DC: ANA.

Anderson, J.E. (1990). *Public policymaking.* Boston, MA: Houghton Mifflin.

Annie E. Casey Foundation. (1995). *Kids count data book.* St. Paul, MN: Annie E. Casey Foundation.

Annie E. Casey Foundation. (1997). *Kids count data book.* St. Paul, MN: Annie E. Casey Foundation.

Bassuk, E., & Rosenberg, L. (1990). Psychological characteristics of homeless children and children with homes. *Pediatrics, 85*(3), 257-261.

Buckley, W. (1996, August 2). Understanding the welfare-reform bill. *National Review, 48*(174), 2.

Chicago Child Care Society. (1994). *Annual report.* Chicago: Author.

Church, G. (1996). Ripping up welfare. *Time, 148*(8), 18–22.

Craig, S. (1992, September). The education needs of children living with violence. *Phi Delta Kappa,* 67–71.

Federal Register. (1997, March 10). *Annual update of the HHS poverty guidelines, 62*(46), 10856–10859.

Ferguson, S. (1996). The use of Medicaid managed care: A case study of two states. *Journal of Pediatric Nursing, 11*(3), 189–191.

Ford, M. (1996, July 19). *Medicaid reform, Congressional research services.* Washington, DC: Library of Congress.

Hosansky, D. (1997, April 12). Concern for uninsured children has not led to agreement. *Congressional Quarterly Weekly Report, 55*(15), 850–852.

Interagency Council on the Homeless. (1991). *The 1990 annual report of the Interagency Council on the Homeless.* Washington, DC: Author.

Kroll, L. (1993). The American Medical Association's Family Violence Campaign. *Journal of the American Medical Association, 269*(14), 1875.

Lauffer, D. (1992). Integrated preadmission services and case management: The foundation for achievable patient outcomes in a hospital-based ambulatory surgery setting. *Seminars in Perioperative Nursing, 1*(3), 136–141.

Margolis, L., Cole, G., & Kotch, J. (1997). Children's rights, social justice, and advocacy in maternal and child health. In J. Kotch (Ed.), *Maternal and child health: Programs, problems, and policy in public health (pp. 19–43).* Gaithersburg, MD: Aspen.

Mason, D., Talbott, S., & Leavitt, J. (1993). *Policy and politics for nurses.* Philadelphia: Saunders.

Natapoff, J., & Wieczorek, R. (1990). *Maternal-child health policy: A nursing perspective.* New York, NY: Springer.

Newell, M. (1995). *Using nursing case management to improve health outcomes: Recasting theory, tools and care delivery.* Gaithersburg, MD: Aspen.

Novello, A. (1992). From the Surgeon General, U.S. Public Health Service. *Journal of the American Medical Association, 267*(23), 3132.

Schryer, N.M. (1993). Nursing case management for children undergoing craniofacial reconstruction. *Plastic Surgery Nursing, 12*(1), 17–26.

Sheridan, D.J., & Taylor, W.K. (1993). Developing hospital-based domestic violence programs, protocols, policies and procedures. *Clinical Issues in Perinatal and Women's Health Nursing, 4*(3), 471–482.

Smith, L.D. (1994). Continuity of care through nursing case management of the chronically ill child. *Clinical Nurse Specialists, 8*(2), 65–68.

Society of Pediatric Nurses. (1995). *Position statement on pediatric firearm injuries.* Denver: Author.

Stanley, S. (1994, May). Heath care groups discuss family violence. *The American Nurse,* 17.

The Kasier Family Foundation. (1995). *Medicaid facts.* Washington, DC: The Kasier Commission on the Future of Medicaid.

Titmus, R.M. (1974). *Social policy: An introduction.* New York: Pantheon Books.

U.S. Department of Health and Human Services. (1996). *Child health USA.* Washington DC: Government Printing Office.

Uzark, K., LeRoy, S., Callow, L., Cameron, J., & Rosenthal, A. (1994). The pediatric nurse practitioner as a case manager in the delivery of services to children with heart disease. *Journal of Pediatric Health Care, 8*(2), 74–78.

Videka-Sherman, L., & Viggiani, P. (1996). The impact of federal policy changes on children: Research needs for the future. *Social Work, 41*(7), 594.

Webster, M. (1996). *The collegiate dictionary* (10th ed.). Springfield, MA: Merriam-Webster.

Study Questions

1. Which of the following pieces of legislation marked the first direct federal grant-in-aid program for health services?
   a. The Sheppard-Towner Act of 1921
   b. Title V of the Social Security Act 1935
   c. Medicaid Act
   d. Education for All Handicapped
   e. Amendment to the Education for All Handicapped

2. The Block Grant form of health care financing and management has resulted in which of the following outcomes?
   a. Primary health care grants were consolidated into six major areas.
   b. The federal government maintained the authority and control of all funds.
   c. States received 20% more federal support for their programs.
   d. States determined how a portion of the block grant was allocated.
   e. None of the above

3. Children who live in poverty are at greater risk for:
   a. having inadequate health care.
   b. becoming parents before completing high school.
   c. being exposed to violence.
   d. being incarcerated before they are 21 years of age.
   e. all of the above.

4. Improving the outcomes for low-income children should include which of the following?
   a. High quality schools
   b. Organized recreation
   c. Employment opportunities for parents
   d. Quality health care
   e. All of the above

5. Which of the following statements is false regarding nurses' involvement in the public policy process?
   a. It is important to identify the stakeholders.
   b. A policy may be influenced until the stage of policy formation.
   c. Interest groups may be competing for the same limited number of resources.
   d. Child health policies should be formulated within the context of the family.
   e. All of the above

6. Managed care is:
   a. a system of health care delivery that shifts the locus of clinical control from solely the health care provider to an organization that manages care.
   b. a model of care delivery that has been identified as a process for achieving optimal patient outcomes in expected time frames while containing costs.
   c. any measure that favorably affects the price of services, the site at which services are received, or their utilization.
   d. a and b.
   e. a and c.

7. Children make up the largest portion of the population living in poverty.
   a. True
   b. False

8. Which age group makes up nearly half of the victims of all forms of child violence?
   a. Infants
   b. Toddlers
   c. Preschoolers
   d. School-agers
   e. Adolescents

9. The Welfare Reform Act limits receipt of welfare funding to:
   a. 1 year with a lifetime cap of 3 years.
   b. 2 years with a lifetime cap of 5 years.
   c. 2 years with a lifetime cap of 7 years.
   d. 3 years with a lifetime cap of 5 years.
   e. 5 years.

10. Due to their clinical knowledge base, nurses should always be consulted when child health and welfare policies are being made.
    a. True
    b. False

Answers

1.a 2.d 3.e 4.e 5.b 6.e 7.a 8.e 9.b 10.a

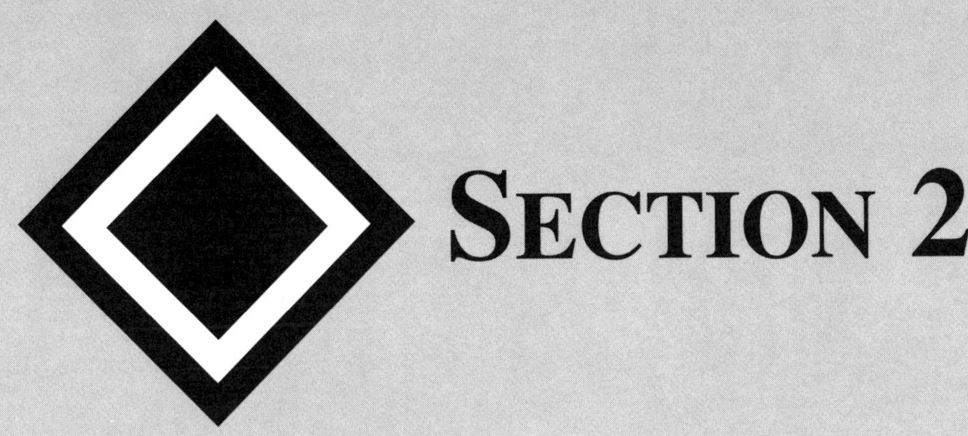

SECTION 2

Clinical Problems or Areas

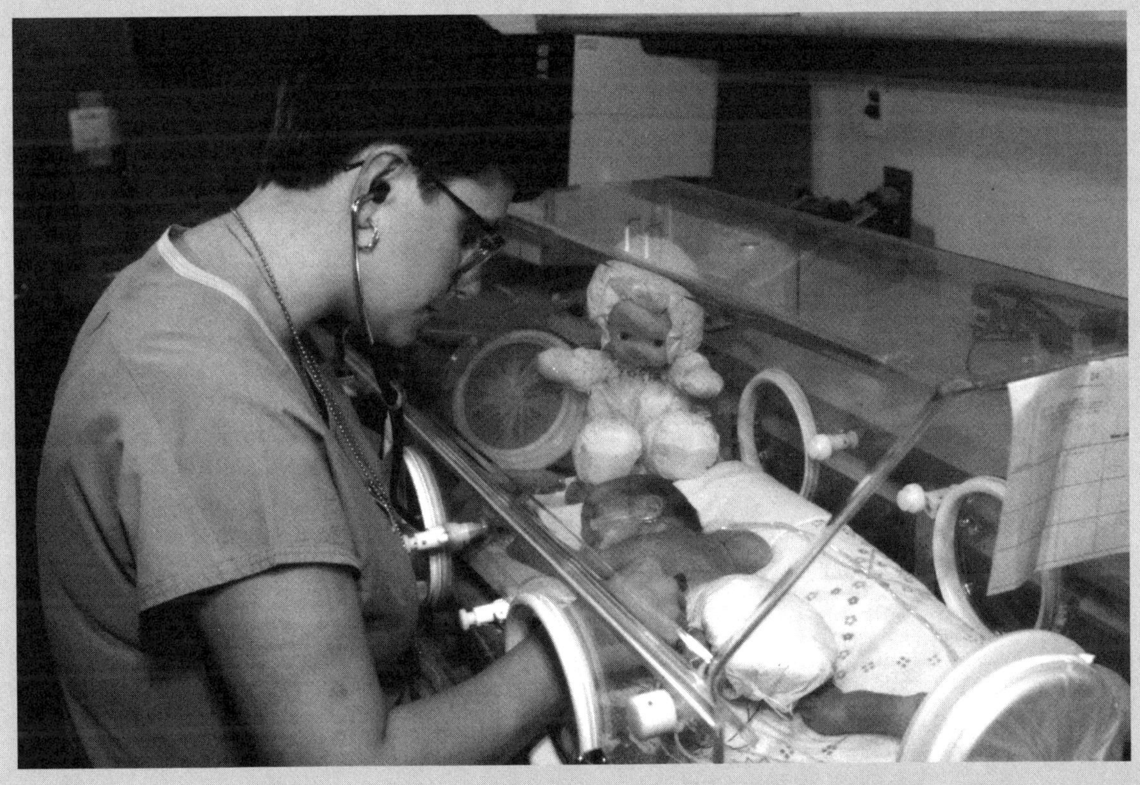

Chapter 10

Injury Control

Jenifer M. Wincek, MSN, RN, CPNP

Concept

◆◆◆◆◆◆◆◆◆◆◆◆◆◆◆◆◆◆◆◆◆◆◆◆◆◆◆

◆ Safety and injury prevention

Objectives

◆◆◆◆◆◆◆◆◆◆◆◆◆◆◆◆◆◆◆◆◆◆◆◆◆◆◆

At the completion of this chapter, the reader will be able to:

◆ Define and discuss the interaction of host, agent, and environment in an injury event.

◆ Conduct an injury event analysis and identify at least nine opportunities to modify the injury risk.

◆ For a given injury risk, identify at least six specific countermeasures to reduce the injury risk.

◆ Identify the most common approaches used for successful injury prevention.

◆ For a given age group, identify developmental factors that contribute to injury risk and discuss the most common injury patterns for that age group.

◆ For a given injury mechanism, identify at least three multifaceted strategies to reduce the risk of injury.

Key Points

◆◆◆◆◆◆◆◆◆◆◆◆◆◆◆◆◆◆◆◆◆◆◆◆◆◆◆

◆ Injuries result from an interaction between a force, the environment, and humans; manipulating any one of these factors will reduce injury morbidity and mortality.

◆ Approaches to injury control that focus on human factors must be developmentally appropriate; strategies that are most effective for infants may not be as effective with adolescents.

◆ Changes in the environment or product will have more of an impact on injury control versus attempting to change human behavior.

◆ The most effective injury control approach is one that combines educational, technologic, and legislative strategies.

10

Injury Control

◆◆◆◆◆◆◆◆◆◆◆◆◆◆◆◆◆◆◆◆◆◆◆◆◆◆◆◆◆◆◆◆◆◆◆◆◆◆

I. OVERVIEW

Each year, one out of every four children ages 14 and under sustain injuries that are serious enough to require medical attention, resulting in 246,000 hospitalizations, nearly 8,700,000 emergency department visits, and more than 11,000,000 visits to physicians' offices (National Safe Kids Campaign, 1996). In 1995, more than 6,600 children in this age group died from unintentional injuries and nearly 120,000 were permanently disabled. Injuries kill more children than all other causes of childhood death combined.

A. Most injuries occur as a result of predictable and preventable events that can be described using public health principles.

B. Applying an epidemiologic triad, injuries result from an interaction between an energy source or force (see Table 10-1), human factors, and environmental factors.

C. In some instances a "vehicle" is required to transmit the energy force to the human (see Figure 10-1). Example: A gun (vehicle) found under the bed (environment) is shot and transmits a bullet (physical energy force) to the host (child) resulting in an injury.

II. UNDERSTANDING INJURY EVENTS

◆◆◆◆◆◆◆◆◆◆◆◆◆◆◆◆◆◆◆◆◆◆◆◆◆

Effective prevention depends upon adequate understanding of the conditions that contribute to injury risk, or injury morbidity and mortality.

A. Conditions to consider.
1. Agents: What are the possible causes?
2. Host: Who is most likely to be effected?
3. Environment: Where is it most likely to happen?
4. Primary prevention: What can be done to reduce the risk?
5. Secondary prevention: What is the best intervention once an injury occurs?

Table 1
Factors Contributing to Injury Risk or Morbidity

Energy (agent)*	Human (host)	Environment
Gravity	Age	Physical
Mechanical	Developmental capabilities	Socioeconomic
Radiation	Supervision (parenting)	
Thermal		
Chemical		
Electrical		

A **vehicle** may be used to transmit the energy source to the host.

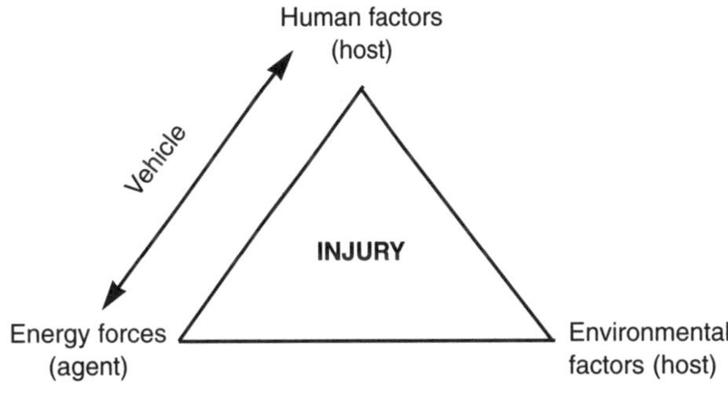

Figure 10-1
A vehicle is required to transmit the energy force to the human.

◆◆◆◆◆◆◆◆◆◆◆◆◆◆◆◆◆◆◆◆◆◆◆◆◆

B. William F. Haddon (1980) described a continuum of time for the injury event.
1. Pre-event phase: point in time prior to the interaction of energy and the host.
2. Event: point in time when the energy is being transmitted to the host
3. Postevent: point in time after the energy transfer has occurred

C. The Haddon Matrix.
1. Serves as a framework to analyze epidemiologic factors (agent, host, and environment) over an

entire continuum of time for an injury event (see Table 10-2).
2. Illustrates prevention strategies that can be used to reduce the risk or severity of injury by modifying one or more of the variables within the nine areas of the matrix.

D. The most common forces of injury in children.
1. Gravity.
   a. The force of gravity is one of the most common injury agents.
   b. It is most commonly transmitted through a falling event.
   c. Falls are the most commonly occurring injury in children.
      (1) Falls from heights greater than 10 feet are associated with more severe injuries.
      (2) Falls in combination with acceleration/deceleration events such as bike falls, automobile ejection, or mechanism that throw the victim often lead to more serious injuries.
      (3) Since the head is larger and proportionately heavier in young children, it often leads the body in a fall and sustains a forceful injury during falls from great heights or speed.
      (4) Falls on playgrounds, during sports and active play, or while climbing occur most often in the school-age child and adolescent.
      (5) Falls in the home from changing tables, beds, down stairs, out of windows or off balconies occur most often in infants and children under 5 years.
2. Mechanical.
   a. Mechanical forces typically result in crushing tissue and bone injury.
   b. Examples of injury mechanisms producing mechanical forces.
      (1) Motor vehicle crash.
         (a) The greater the speed and mass of the car the greater the mechanical force generated.
         (b) Vehicles of greater mass will also absorb a greater degree of mechanical force without transmitting to the host within the vehicle.
         (c) Example: The proliferation of larger utility and 4-wheel drive vehicles has resulted in a greater frequency of large vehicle to small vehicle traffic fatalities, particularly to victims in the smaller vehicle.
      (2) Motor vehicle versus pedestrian.
         (a) Large mechanical forces are transmitted directly to the unprotected child, resulting in devastating head, trunk, or orthopedic injuries.
         (b) Often a combination of mechanical and gravitational forces occur as the child is propelled into the air.
      (3) Bike falls.
         (a) Bike speed is a determinant of the degree of mechanical force that is transmitted.
         (b) Direct mechanical force, often in combination with gravitational forces can lead to serious head, chest, abdomen, or orthopedic injuries.
      (4) Cutting or penetrating devices.
         (a) Cutting or penetrating devices localize the delivery of mechanical energy, causing less diffuse tissue destruction.
         (b) Localized injury can be severe, particularly when vital organs are penetrated.
         (c) The type of injury resulting from a firearm varies with the type of gun and velocity of projectile.
         (d) High velocity weapons cause direct mechanical injury as well as collateral tissue injury.
      (5) Sports.
         (a) Mechanical forces during sports vary greatly depending on the sport type.
         (b) Sports with high-speed objects (balls) or with a large amount of contact will generate more mechanical force than other types.
      (6) Child abuse and assault.
         (a) Hitting or kicking, with or without an object leads to direct transmission of mechanical energy to the child.
         (b) The size of the striking object and strength of blow will have an impact on the degree of tissue injury.
         (c) Diffuse cerebral injury in Shaken Baby Syndrome is caused by the shifting of brain tissue within the skull resulting in a tearing and crushing injury.
3. Thermal.
   a. Thermal forces cause direct and diffuse tissue destruction.
   b. Examples of injury mechanisms producing thermal forces.
      (1) Flame.
         (a) Fire causes direct tissue destruction.
         (b) Ambient heat forces and smoke may also lead to inhalation injuries.
      (2) Hot liquid.

Table 10-2
The Haddon Matrix
Example: Motor vehicle crash

	Agent/Vehicle	Host	Environment
Pre-event phase	*Examples of prevention strategies*		
Period of time prior to the injury event where action may be taken to reduce injury risk.	• Reduced speed of vehicle • Testing of brakes • Lower center of gravity	• Avoidance of alcohol intoxication • Reduced fatigue • Driver's training • Polarized sunglasses to improve driver's vision	• Divided highways • Improved lighting • Road free of ice • Designated driver programs
Event phase	*Examples of prevention strategies*		
Period of time while the injury event is taking place where factors can be modified to reduce injury.	• Increased vehicle size • Release of automatic restraint devices	• Passive restraint device properly secured • Maturity of skeletal system	• Occupant restraint laws • Automotive production safety standards • Guard rails
Post-event phase	*Examples of prevention strategies*		
Period of time following injury where action can be taken to improve outcome or prevent secondary problems related to the primary injury.	• Fuel system integrity • Use of "Jaws of Life" to speed vehicle extrication	• Age • Intact cardiorespiratory system	• Availability of trained EMS providers • Proximity to Trauma Center • Access to Rehabilitation Center

(a) The heat generated by hot liquids can cause massive tissue destruction until the liquid in contact with the skin has cooled below burning temperatures.

(b) Less dense fluids (water) cool faster than higher density liquids (oil, hot cereal).

(3) Hot objects.

(a) As long as the hot object is in contact with host, the transmission of energy will continue.

(b) A less mobile infant is not likely to move away from a hot, burning object and will sustain greater tissue injury.

(4) Temperature extremes.

(a) Either cold exposure or heat exposure can result in thermal injury.

(b) Temperature extremes cause tissue damage at the cellular level.

4. Radiation.

a. Radiation forces cause tissue damage at the cellular level.

b. Higher doses can lead to burn-type tissue injury.

c. Examples of injury mechanisms producing radiation forces.

(1) Sunburn.

(2) Overexposure to radiation waves.

5. Chemical.

a. The type of chemical injury produced depends on the injury mechanism.

b. Examples of injury mechanisms producing chemical forces.

(1) Poison ingestion cause cellular destruction or cellular level dysfunction.

(2) Anoxia, an absence of oxygen, leads to cellular level dysfunction or destruction.

(3) Contact with caustic agents causes burn-type tissue destruction.

6. Electrical.

a. Contact with electrical current leads to tissue destruction.

b. This destruction occurs along the path of electrical flow.

E. Host factors.

1. Patterns of injury are greatly affected by a child's age and developmental capabilities.

a. Infants less than 1 year old.

(1) Developmental considerations contributing to risk.

(a) Is completely dependent on others to provide a safe environment.

(b) Learns by exploring, touching, and putting things into mouth.
(c) Motor skills rapidly advancing.
(d) Cannot recognize and avoid unsafe situations.
(e) Lacks object permanence; will not remember previous injury events.
(2) The most common injury mechanisms.
(a) Homicide from child abuse or shaking is the leading cause of injury-related death in infants.
(b) Suffocation is the leading cause of unintentional injury deaths in infants.
[1] Strangulation from draperies, cords, and cribs with slats spaced more than 2½ inches apart.
[2] Choking on small pieces of toys and food.
(c) Motor vehicle crashes when the infant is not properly restrained are one of the leading causes of injury-related deaths in infants.
(d) Other common causes of injury.
[1] Burns and smoke inhalation from home fires.
[2] Scalds from hot drinks, hot water, bath water.
[3] Drowning in bathtubs, buckets.
[4] Falls from beds, changing tables, baby walkers.
[5] Ingestion of poisons.
[6] Electrocution from uncovered sockets, frayed cords, chewing cords.
[7] Bike injuries when riding as passenger without helmet.
b. Toddlers and preschoolers.
(1) Developmental considerations contributing to risk.
(a) Motor skills rapidly advancing.
(b) May not remember or recognize dangerous situations.
(c) Is egocentric with a high degree of autonomy.
(d) Does not always understand difference between right and wrong, safe and unsafe.
(e) Very curious and will explore without recognizing consequences.
(f) Can follow simple directions but will not remember them.
(g) Has magical thinking, which may lead to misperceptions of risks.
(h) Does not fully understand cause and effect.
(2) The most common injury mechanisms.

(a) Burns from fire and hot liquid are the leading cause of injury-related deaths in children 1–4 years; fires are most often caused by young children playing with matches and lighters.
(b) Drowning in backyard pools, buckets, toilets, and bathtubs is one of the top causes of toddler mortality.
(c) Pedestrian injuries when playing in or near the street rank in the top causes of injury related deaths in children 1–4 years.
(d) Motor vehicle crashes when child is not properly restrained or positioned in the car also rank as one of the top causes of injury-related death in young children.
(e) Other common causes of injury.
[1] Child abuse.
[2] Falls from playground structures, windows, balconies, steps, and other high places.
[3] Ingestion of poisonous or caustic agents.
[4] Unintentional firearms discharge.
[5] Choking on small pieces of toys and food, particularly while active.
[6] Strangulation from draperies and cords.
[7] Electrocution from uncovered sockets, frayed cords, chewing cords.
[8] Bike injuries when riding as passenger without helmet.
c. School-age child.
(1) Developmental considerations contributing to risk.
(a) Is testing independence.
(b) Is beginning to conduct experiments with motor skills, physical and chemical agents.
(c) Does not fully understand causal relationships.
(d) Has rudimentary problem-solving skills; "good" ideas might have unrecognized dangers.
(e) Is beginning to apply rules, challenge rules, and understand consequences of breaking rules.
(f) Social acceptance and peer pressure may have a negative or positive effect on safety practices.
(g) Is learning how to deal with frustration; good role models and problem-solving skills will reduce aggression

and rage as child moves toward adolescence.
(h) Use and abuse of chemical substances increases the risk of injury significantly.
(2) The most common injury mechanisms.
(a) Motor vehicle occupant injuries when the child is not properly restrained or positioned in the car are the leading cause of injury related death in children 5–10 years.
(b) Pedestrian versus motor vehicle injuries when playing near the street is the second most common cause of injury-related deaths.
(c) Other common injury mechanisms.
[1] Burns from playing with gasoline or fire.
[2] Drowning in pools, drainage reservoirs, large bodies of water.
[3] Child abuse and interpersonal violence.
[4] Bike injuries, particularly when riding without helmet.
[5] Fireworks and explosive devices.
[6] Firearm injuries.
[7] Falls from roofs, playground equipment, trees.
[8] Sports and playground injuries.
[9] Intentional ingestion or inhalation of chemical agents.
d. Adolescent.
(1) Developmental considerations contributing to risk.
(a) Substance use and abuse is associated with 70% of adolescent injuries.
(b) Peer pressure is strong; teens may undertake risky activities to impress peers.
(c) Feels infallible and omnipotent.
(d) Wants to establish independence.
(e) Rebellious activities are common.
(f) Does not consider future consequences of risky behavior.
(g) Poor self-esteem may lead to greater substance use or greater risk-taking behaviors; unconcerned about the consequences.
(h) Good safety habits started earlier in life will usually remain.
(i) Violent reactions may result from inadequate problem-solving skills or role modeling.
(2) The most common injury mechanisms.
(a) Motor vehicle crashes when the adolescent is not properly restrained, with inattentive or inexperience drivers,

with substance use or risk-taking behaviors are the leading cause of unintentional injury-related deaths in youth ages 11–18 years.
(b) In some regions, interpersonal violence including assault with firearms, blunt, or cutting objects is the leading cause of adolescent injury-related deaths.
(c) Suicide, often repeated attempts, is one of the top three causes of adolescent injury-related deaths.
(d) Other common injury mechanisms.
[1] Bike, motorcycle, and off-road vehicle accidents particularly when riding without helmet.
[2] Drowning in pools after climbing fences or diving in unknown waters.
[3] Drowning or diving injuries in unknown water.
[4] Pedestrian hit by automobile.
[5] Firearms.
[6] Intentional ingestion or inhalation of chemical agents.
[7] Sports injuries.

F. Environmental factors include both social and physical elements.
1. Factors in the social environment associated with injury risk.
a. Family.
(1) Family member safety practices greatly affect children; safe and unsafe practices are modeled by adult family members.
(2) Attentiveness and supervision patterns may increase or decrease injury risk.
(a) Children with more unstructured time are more at risk for injuries.
(b) Young and inexperienced parents, daycare providers, and sitters may not be prepared to assess or reduce injury risks.
(c) Single-parent households have greater injury rates.
(3) Children may be influenced by television or music, acting out what they see or hear.
(4) Substance use in the home, while driving, or during recreational activities increases injury risk.
(5) Undue stressors at home or work may distract families, leading to decreased attention and supervision of children.
b. Peers.
(1) Beginning in the school-age child, peers

greatly influence a child's safety practices, risk-taking behaviors, and decisions.
(2) In adolescence, peers are often the single most influential force in a youth's decisions about substance use, experimentation, and risk-taking practices.
(3) Youth left in unsupervised or unstructured settings are more likely to engage in higher risk activities.

c. School.
(1) School playground injuries are commonplace during unstructured play.
(2) Properly conditioned youth, knowledgeable coaches, and use of protective gear greatly reduce sports injury risk.
(3) Fights in school or schoolyards may result from competition, peer pressure, gang activities, or inadequate levels of adult supervision.

d. Community.
(1) The community as a whole sets the standards for safety practices.
(a) Unsafe practices may be difficult to change if the practice has been a longstanding community norm.
(b) Community members can be powerful forces in monitoring and enhancing youth safety practices.
(2) Laws to enhance or reduce safe practices are generated from community members and their elected leadership.
(3) As school-age children and adolescents spend more and more time away from the home, the community becomes a greater influence in monitoring and enforcing safe behaviors.
(4) Media (television, movies, and music) have a great influence over youth behavior, including safety practices.

e. Economic variables.
(1) Children from low socioeconomic families have significantly higher injury and injury-related death rates.
(2) Injury rates in non-Whites are 2–3 times greater than those of White children
(3) Safety devices may be too expensive or not valued as being as important as other household necessities.
(4) Hopelessness about the future may reduce the likelihood that individuals will undertake life-saving practices.
(5) Higher percentage of rental housing or houses in poor condition may lead to greater injury risks.
(6) In impoverished communities there are fewer safe places for youth to play due to poorly maintained playgrounds, and increased sale and use of drugs and violent behaviors.
(7) Secondhand clothes, toys, safety devices, and furniture may not meet current safety standards.

2. Factors in the physical environment associated with injury risk.
a. Infants and young children spend the majority of time in the home where environmental hazards are the greatest.
b. The physical structure of the home presents a variety of serious risks to children.
(1) Fire and carbon monoxide poisoning risks, which vary depending on heating sources, modernization of electrical system, accessibility of matches and lighters, and proper installation and maintenance of fire and smoke detectors.
(2) Lead exposure from lead-based painted surfaces.
(3) Fall hazards presented by stairways, balconies, and windows, particularly in older, poorly maintained homes.
c. Specific rooms in the home have common risks and injury patterns.
(1) Kitchens.
(a) The kitchen is the most hazardous room in the house.
(b) Cooking with children underfoot leads to scald burns from hot food and liquid spills.
(c) Cleaning substances, often stored under sink cabinets, pose a substantial risk to young children.
(d) Knives and sharp objects stored in accessible drawers or on countertops pose a cutting and stabbing hazard.
(e) Accessible appliances such as stoves, toasters, and refrigerators pose safety hazards to young and independent children.
(f) Routinely taken medications such as vitamins or pain relievers are often stored in easy to reach places.
(2) Bathrooms.
(a) Bathrooms are particularly dangerous for young children.
(b) Bathtubs present scald burn and drowning risk.
(c) Toilets are a drowning hazard to infants and toddlers.
(d) Medications, hygiene products, cosmetics, and cleansers are often readily accessible in sink cabinets.
(3) Basements and garages.

(a) These areas are often filled with dangerous chemicals and mechanical hazards.
(b) Stored paint, cleaners, and combustible products may be ingested by younger children and used as recreational substances in school-age and adolescent youth.
(c) Automatic garage doors pose a strangulation risk if not properly installed.
(d) Gas-powered engines such as lawn mowers may lead to mechanical injuries if children are near them when operated.
(4) Bedrooms.
  (a) Furniture such as cribs, changing tables, and toy chests may pose strangulation or fall hazards.
  (b) Toys that are not age-appropriate may pose a choking risk.
  (c) Drapery, blind, and toy pull cords may strangulate children, particularly if located near the bed.
  (d) Second-story windows with or without screens may be pushed out and pose a falling hazard, particularly when furniture that the child can climb upon is located near windows.
(5) Yards.
  (a) Play sets or play surfaces may contribute to fall-related injuries.
  (b) Poisonous plants may present a hazard to young children.
  (c) Play areas near streets or driveways may pose risk of pedestrian versus motor vehicle injuries.
(6) School.
  (a) Most schools are designed to meet environmental standards for childhood safety.
  (b) The most common school injuries occur on the playground or in the gym during unstructured play.
  (c) Injuries related to school-based interpersonal violence are increasing in incidence.
(7) Community.
  (a) Building codes regulate many environmental conditions such as home construction, playgrounds, bike paths, and sidewalks.
  (b) Transportation crash data are used to develop standards for street and highway construction and traffic control.
  (c) Crime and injury data help to design safe and effective lighting products and other security measures.

III. APPROACHES TO PREVENTION

Using the epidemiologic model for injury analysis, it becomes evident that there are multiple opportunities for prevention along the entire continuum of the injury event.

A. Effective prevention reduces the economic burden caused by injuries
1. Products for prevention are far less costly than treatment costs provided by hospitals or primary care settings following injury.
2. Serious injuries may require parents to expend resources for long-term care.

B. The three E's of prevention include Education, Enforcement, and Engineering approaches to injury control. Although each of the approaches may be effective independently, the most effective prevention strategy is to combine the three approaches.
1. Education or persuasion.
  a. From early childhood, safety practices are taught and modeled. Consistent, repeated messages over time, particularly by parents, teachers, and local community members, are critical.
  b. Health care providers play a key role in reinforcing, recommending, and teaching family safety practices. During each health care encounter, safety practices should be evaluated and reinforced.
  (1) Parents need to understand their child's cognitive and physical capabilities.
    (a) They should also be able to anticipate the next developmental steps so that they can alter their environment accordingly.
    (b) Example: It is not necessary to keep poisons out of reach of a 3-month-old infant since the infant does not possess the developmental skills to independently obtain and ingest the poison. The parent does need to be concerned about the infant rolling over and falling from changing surfaces. By the time the infant is 6 to 8 months, all poisons should be securely stored out of reach.
  (2) Parents and older children need to understand the most common injury patterns in children.

(3) Parents and older children should understand the possible strategies to reduce injury risk, which ones are likely to be most effective, and the local resources to obtain certain safety devices.

c. The best learning takes place when the learner:
   (1) Plays an active role in his or her education.
   (2) Is exposed to a multitude of learning modalities.
   (3) Is provided with ample reinforcement.

d. One-time educational programs have not been found to change safety practices.

e. Educational programs and materials available at low or no cost to community members and health care professionals.
   (1) Tipp: The Injury Prevention Program by the American Academy of Pediatrics.
   (2) The National Safe Kids Campaign's educational materials.
   (3) National Safety Town curriculum.
   (4) Department of Transportation educational materials.
   (5) Police and Fire Department safety programs.
   (6) American Red Cross safety and first aid programs.
   (7) American Trauma Society educational materials.
   (8) National Safety Council educational materials.
   (9) National Crime Prevention Council safety and educational materials.

f. Knowledge of appropriate safety practices does not always result in action. Once the best safety practices are understood, other persuasive strategies may be necessary to gain compliance (e.g., rewards, incentives, feedback, role modeling).

g. Effective safety education programs consider:
   (1) The developmental level of the child.
   (2) The educational level of the parent.
   (3) Socioeconomic or cultural variations.

2. Engineering.
   a. Modifying the environment or products associated with injuries can be the most effective strategy for injury control since this strategy does not rely on the "human element" for success.
   b. Health care providers, particularly emergency department and trauma care providers, play a critical role in identifying patterns of injury, reporting product-related injuries, and recommending designs that would reduce traumatic injury.
   c. Examples of safety engineering.
      (1) Redesign of cars and restraint devices.
      (2) Design of interstate highways, streets, or sidewalks.
      (3) Maximum temperature regulation on hot water heaters.
      (4) Fire and carbon monoxide detectors.
      (5) Protective sports equipment such as bike helmets and kneepads.
   d. The Consumer Product Safety Commission helps to monitor product-related injuries and promote improved safety designs.
   e. The Department of Transportation and Highway Safety monitors traffic injuries and develops the standards for road construction and vehicle safety.
   f. Economic barriers may limit those who can benefit from environmental or product redesign. Often, products with the safest design are the most costly.
   g. Many technical or design improvements result from legislative actions such as building code regulations.

3. Enforcement.
   a. A key role of government is to protect its citizens. Safety legislation plays a major role in all of our lives.
   b. Examples of common safety legislation.
      (1) Traffic regulations.
      (2) Occupant restraint laws.
      (3) Toy, clothing, and product manufacturing regulations.
      (4) Allocation of safety education and training funds.
      (5) Environmental cleanup legislation.
      (6) Teen curfews.
      (7) Drug and alcohol prohibition for youth.
   c. Organizations that are actively involved in child safety legislation include the National Safe Kids Campaign, the American Academy of Pediatrics, the American Trauma Society, and the regional Centers for Injury Control.
   d. Health care providers are effective advocates and should work with community members and legislators in enhancing safety legislation. They provide a unique perspective as providers of care following traumatic injuries.

C. Certain educational, enforcement, and engineering approaches are more successful than others.

1. Haddon (1980) defined several strategies called "Injury Countermeasures" that can be used to mediate the forces causing injury. When the chosen strategy involves human action or

behavior change, many variables will contribute to the success of that strategy.

a. One or more of these strategies can be used to design the most effective approach to reducing injury risk, morbidity, and mortality.

(1) Prevent the hazard from being made. With comprehensive injury-tracking measures, products or devices that are most hazardous are often removed from production lines in lieu of more safely designed products.

(a) Three-wheel all-terrain vehicles.

(b) Accordion-type infant gates.

(c) Lead-based paints.

(2) Reduce the amount of the hazard present.

(a) Smaller drug packages with reduced available total dose.

(b) Lower speed limits.

(c) Point-of-delivery hot water controls.

(3) Prevent the release of the hazard.

(a) Child-resistant containers.

(b) Window guards.

(c) Childproof lighters.

(4) Disperse the forces to reduce the effect.

(a) Cushioned landing surfaces.

(b) Airbags.

(c) Protective athletic gear such as pads and helmets.

(5) Separate the hazard from that which is to be protected.

(a) Time (e.g., reduced speed during school beginning and end times).

(b) Space (e.g., sidewalks and bike paths, poisons stored in higher cabinets).

(c) Barrier (e.g., pool gates, cabinets locks, road barricades, bunk bed rails).

(6) Modify the hazard so that risks are reduced.

(a) Reduced water heater temperatures.

(b) Narrowed spaces between crib slats.

(c) Larger, stronger automobiles.

(7) Make potential victim more resistant to damage.

(a) Improved general health.

(b) Use of protective gear.

(c) Improved conditioning.

(8) Begin to counter the damage already done by hazard.

(a) First aid and CPR training.

(b) Effective emergency medical responses.

(9) Stabilize, repair, or rehabilitate person who has been damaged.

(a) Trauma centers.

(b) Burn and rehabilitation centers.

2. Changing individual safety behaviors depends upon several variables.

a. Frequency that the action must be taken.

(1) Behaviors that must be done often or every time are less likely to be done consistently.

(2) Example: testing the hot water each time is less effective than turning the water heater down once.

b. Degree of effort required.

(1) If a considerable amount of effort is required, the behavior is less likely to be done.

(2) Example: transferring infant seats from one vehicle to another is less effective than two sets of seats or built in seats.

(3) Passive strategies are more effective than active strategies.

(a) Passive strategies.

[1] Are designed so safety happens automatically with little or no effort required.

[2] Does not depend on person taking action.

[3] Examples: automatic airbags, 10-year smoke detector batteries.

(b) Active strategies.

[1] Requires a person to change behavior.

[2] Requires action to be taken.

[3] Examples: manual passenger restraint devices, trigger locks, infant gates.

c. Degree of comfort or discomfort created by the action.

(1) A more comfortable safety device is more likely to be used versus one that causes discomfort.

(2) Example: a well-fitting, stylish bike helmet is more likely to be worn by school-age children.

d. Perceived consequences of taking or not taking action.

(1) If an individual believes that there will be personal costs of not taking action, they are more likely change their safety practices (e.g., consistently enforced laws with costly penalties are more effective than inconsistently enforced laws or laws with little personal cost).

(2) If individuals believe that there will be benefits to safety behaviors, they will be more likely to continue those actions (e.g., if an adolescent believes that his or her risk of serious head injury is reduced by wearing a bike helmet, he or she is most likely to consistently wear the helmet).

e. Perceived relative risk or susceptibility to sustaining injury.
  (1) If individuals believe that they are at greater risk for injury, they will be more likely to protect themselves.
  (2) Examples.
    (a) If parents have never worn a bike helmet and have never sustained a bike-related head injury, they may have difficulty understanding the value of a bike helmet for themselves or their child.
    (b) If parents feel they are at risk of intruders, they are more likely to have a loaded and accessible fire-arm available for protection.
f. Barriers to taking action.
  (1) The most common barriers are economic and educational barriers.
  (2) If there are considerable barriers to taking action, an individual is less likely to carry out those behaviors.
  (3) Examples.
    (a) If a tenant does not know how to turn down a water heater, he or she will not complete the action.
    (b) If a safety product is too costly, parents with no or low income may not purchase it.
    (c) If a tenant does not own a ladder, he or she may not be able to reach the smoke detector to change batteries.

IV. PREVENTION STRATEGIES FOR SPECIFIC INJURY MECHANISMS

◆ ◆ ◆ ◆ ◆ ◆ ◆ ◆ ◆ ◆ ◆ ◆ ◆ ◆ ◆ ◆ ◆ ◆ ◆

The most successful prevention strategies are multi-faceted and customized to the agent, host, and environment. Intervention across the injury event continuum (pre-event, event, and post-event) will have a positive impact on both incidence and severity of injury.

A. Motor vehicle occupant injuries are addressed through the following prevention strategies:
1. Education.
  a. Driver's education programs.
  b. Child passenger restraint device training.
  c. Prevention programs on drinking and driving.
    (1) Mothers Against Drunk Driving (MADD).
    (2) Students Against Drunk Driving (SADD).
    (3) Emergency Nurses CARE (ENCARE).
    (4) Pre-prom night demonstration rescues.
  d. Child passenger restraint education programs.
    (1) Department of Transportation.
    (2) National Safe Kids Campaign.
    (3) National Safety Towns.
2. Enforcement.
  a. Seat belt and child passenger restraint laws.
  b. Driver's license testing.
  c. Speed limits.
  d. Zero tolerance blood alcohol legislation.
  e. Driver imposed rules ("Car does not start until everyone is buckled-up").
3. Engineering.
  a. Improved automotive safety design standards.
  b. Children correctly placed in appropriately sized restraint devices.
  c. Interstate highway construction codes.
  d. Traffic lights.

B. Motor vehicle vs. pedestrian injuries are addressed through the following prevention strategies:
1. Education.
  a. Pedestrian crossing skill training and practice.
  b. Trained crossing guards.
  c. Safety public service announcements (PSAs) warning drivers about school zones.
2. Enforcement.
  a. School crossing guards.
  b. Parent rules ("Never cross without an adult").
  c. Police patrol of school crossing zones.
  d. Drivers stop for school buses.
3. Engineering.
  a. No parallel parking on neighborhood streets.
  b. Sidewalks.
  c. Pedestrian crossing zones.
  d. Speed zones in school zones and neighborhoods.
  e. Improved lighting on neighborhood streets.

C. Bike injuries are addressed through the following prevention strategies:
1. Education.
  a. Bike rodeos that enforce safe riding practices.
  b. Bike helmet awareness campaigns.
  c. Purchasing a helmet with the first bike.
  d. Parents wearing helmets when riding with youth.
  e. TV commercial showing youth riding with helmets.
  f. Health care providers discussing bike safety practices.
2. Enforcement.
  a. Helmet laws.
  b. Police officer reward patrols for youth wearing helmets.
  c. Parent rules ("Wear helmets when riding, or walk").
  d. Peer pressure to own and wear a designer helmet.

3. Engineering.
   a. Bike paths.
   b. Helmet distribution campaigns.
   c. Well-fit bike.
   d. Bright clothes.
   e. Properly maintained bike and accessories (working brakes, reflectors).

D. Falls are addressed through the following prevention strategies:
1. Education.
   a. Window fall awareness campaigns.
   b. New mother classes teaching about walker and other fall hazards.
   c. Seminars on safe playground construction.
2. Enforcement
   a. Infant safety gate production standards.
   b. Parent rules ("No climbing on top of hazardous surfaces").
   c. School rules ("No running in the halls").
   d. Laws to ban production of infant walkers.
3. Engineering.
   a. Installation of window guards in second and third story windows.
   b. Locked balcony doors.
   c. Railings on stairways.
   d. Changing infants on floor versus changing table.
   e. More impact-absorbing playground surfaces.
   f. Removal of wheels from infant walkers or production or alternative devices for infant mobility.

E. Poisoning is addressed through the following prevention strategies:
1. Education.
   a. Poison Control Centers.
   b. Hazardous product sticker (Mr. Yuk) or labels.
   c. Campaigns to raise awareness about household poisonings.
   d. Poison prevention classes for preschool children.
   e. Education on medication storage and use of syrup of ipecac.
   f. Skull and bones symbol.
2. Enforcement.
   a. Medication packaging regulations.
   b. Lead paint abatement regulations.
   c. Waste disposal requirements.
3. Engineering.
   a. Child-resistant containers.
   b. Medicine cabinet locks.
   c. Storage of hazardous products high and out of reach.
   d. Locked garages.

F. Drowning is addressed through the following prevention strategies:
1. Education
   a. Swimming lessons.
   b. Boater's safety courses.
   c. Diver precaution signs.
   d. Educational campaigns about the hazards of water sports while using alcohol.
   e. Cardiopulmonary resuscitation training.
2. Enforcement.
   a. Pool rules
   b. Lifeguards.
   c. Prohibition of alcohol consumption with boat drivers.
   d. Parent rules ("Buddy swimming" or "No pool use without an adult present").
   e. Personal flotation device regulations for boat passengers.
3. Engineering.
   a. Four-sided, locked fences surrounding pools.
   b. Antislip surfaces around inground pools.
   c. Improved flotation systems in boats.
   d. Toilet lid covers in the down position.
   e. Door handle covers on exterior bathroom doors; doors closed.

G. Sports injuries are addressed through the following prevention strategies:
1. Education.
   a. Training and proper conditioning.
   b. First aid training for coaches.
   c. Instructions on proper use of safety gear.
2. Enforcement.
   a. League sport rules to enhance safety.
   b. Adults setting standards and expectation on the use of protective gear.
   c. Umpires' enforcement of safety breach penalties.
3. Engineering.
   a. Impact absorbing and dispersing protective gear and play surfaces.
   b. Running lanes on a race track.
   c. Padded goal posts.

H. Playground injuries are addressed through the following strategies:
1. Education.
   a. Parent education on safe yard playground design.
   b. Classroom programs on playground safety.
   c. Playground safety inspections.
   d. Parent education on age limits on playground devices based on developmental skills.
2. Enforcement.
   a. Playground monitors, adult supervision.
   b. Play area rules ("No contact activities").

3. Engineering.
   a. Rounded edges on playground equipment.
   b. Soft landing surfaces.
   c. Height limitations on play equipment.
   d. Narrowed slats between rails.

I. Motorized equipment injuries (e.g., lawnmowers, farm machinery, boats) are addressed through the following prevention strategies:
   1. Education.
      a. Farm safety programs.
      b. Warning information in product literature.
      c. Public service announcement on lawnmower hazards.
      d. Motorcyclist safety programs.
   2. Enforcement.
      a. Age restrictions on all terrain vehicles (ATVs).
      b. Helmet legislation.
      c. Boating speed regulations.
      d. Parent rules ("No children around operating equipment or lawnmowers").
   3. Engineering.
      a. Motor "kill" switches.
      b. Farm equipment shields.
      c. Approved riding tracks.
      d. Lawnmower blade guards.

J. Animal bites are addressed through the following prevention strategies:
   1. Education.
      a. Instruction to children to never to approach an unfamiliar animal or take food from an animal.
      b. Public service announcement regarding potential hazards of small children left near unsupervised animal.
   2. Enforcement.
      a. Animal control, leash, and vaccine laws.
      b. Prohibition of keeping wild or notoriously vicious animals.
   3. Engineering.
      a. Kennels of sufficient height to prevent escape.
      b. Locked gates to prohibit children from entering animal quarters.
      c. Muzzles on animal that may potentially bite.
      d. Feeding of animals away from children.

K. Choking is addressed through the following prevention strategies:
   1. Education.
      a. Hospital display of objects that have choked children.
      b. Rescue classes demonstrating techniques to help a choking child.
      c. Parent classes on choking hazards.

   2. Enforcement.
      a. Parent rules ("Pick up toy parts so that younger child does not find" and "Always sit down when eating").
      b. Toy safety standards and laws.
   3. Engineering.
      a. Cutting up food into small pieces or never feeding small, round food pieces to young children.
      b. Lifesaver® hard candy with a hole in the center and sides less than ¼″ so that air can pass in the event that the candy is aspirated into the trachea.
      c. Age-appropriate toy construction.
      d. Stuffed toys with nonremovable eyes.

L. Flame burns are addressed through the following strategies:
   1. Education.
      a. Child safety programs teaching stop, drop, and roll.
      b. Family fire escape plan.
   2. Enforcement.
      a. Laws requiring smoke and fire detectors installed in all rental units.
      b. Laws requiring fire alarms in public building.
   3. Engineering.
      a. Fire and smoke detectors installed, checked monthly, and new batteries installed semiannually.
      b. Fire retardant fabrics.
      c. Fire resistant building materials.
      d. Child resistant lighters.
      e. Store matches out of reach of children.
      f. No storage of food over stove.

M. Scald burns are addressed through the following prevention strategies:
   1. Education.
      a. Public awareness campaign depicting common mechanism for scald burns (hot coffee, boiling liquid on stove, hot tap water for baths).
      b. Teach children to stay out of kitchen while cooking.
   2. Enforcement.
      a. Laws regulating maximum water heater temperatures.
      b. Parent rules ("Never run bath water by self" or "No children in kitchen while cooking").
   3. Engineering.
      a. Water heater temperature adjusted to low setting.
      b. Point of delivery temperature regulators.
      c. Pan handles turned to inside of stove.
      d. Bath thermometer.

N. Interpersonal violence (child abuse) is addressed through the following prevention strategies:
1. Education.
   a. Public awareness campaign about the hazards of shaking babies.
   b. Teaching parents anger management.
   c. Infant-parent nurturing classes, and fostering infant-parent attachment.
   d. Positive adult role models.
2. Enforcement.
   a. Child protection agencies.
   b. Child abuse and neglect laws.
3. Engineering.
   a. "Timeouts" versus spanking.
   b. Alternative physical outlets for anger and frustration.

O. Interpersonal violence (Older children/adolescents).
1. Education.
   a. Anger management and mediation classes.
   b. SafeNight America activities and message ("No arguments, No drugs or alcohol, No weapons").
   c. Gang awareness and prevention campaigns.
   d. Monitoring media exposure.
   e. Parent and adult modeling of alternative anger management practices.
2. Enforcement.
   a. Childhood curfew laws.
   b. Firearm ownership restrictions.
   c. Juvenile delinquency centers.
   d. Parent boundaries on activities and behavior.
3. Engineering.
   a. Trigger locks and proper firearm storage (locked, trigger lock secure, ammunition in a separate place).
   b. Alternative settings for safe youth activities (recreation centers, jobs, school).
   c. Well-lighted neighborhoods.

P. Intrapersonal violence (suicide) is addressed through the following prevention strategies:
1. Education.
   a. Parent and teacher training on suicide risk factors.
   b. Youth self development classes.
   c. Peer training on suicide prevention.
   d. Parent and school-based education on alternatives.
2. Enforcement.
   a. Laws mandating 24-hour detention following suicidal gesture.
   b. Dispensing regulations for controlled prescriptive medication.

   c. Firearm sale waiting periods.
3. Engineering.
   a. Trigger locks for guns.
   b. Proper firearm storage.
   c. Suicide crisis phone lines.

BIBLIOGRAPHY

American Academy of Pediatrics. (1987). *TIPP: The injury prevention program.* Elk Grove Village, IL: Author.

Centers for Disease Control. (1990). Childhood injuries in the United States. *American Journal of Diseases in Children, 144,* 627–646.

Haddon, W. (1980). Advances in the epidemiology of injuries as a basis for public policy. *Public Health Reports, 95,* 411–421.

Jones, N.E. (1992). Childhood injuries: An epidemiologic approach. *Pediatric Nursing, 18,* 235–239.

Jones, N.E. (1993). Childhood residential injuries. *American Journal of Maternal Child Nursing, 18,* 168–172.

National Committee for Injury Prevention and Control (1989). *Injury prevention: Meeting the challenge.* New York: Oxford University Press.

National Safe Kids Campaign. (1996). *Fact sheet.* Washington, DC: Author.

Rivera, F.P. (1994). Unintentional Injuries. In I.B. Pless (Ed.), *The epidemiology of childhood disorders* (pp. 369–391). New York: Oxford University Press.

Wilson, M.H., Baker, S.P., Teret, S.P., Shock, S., & Garbarino, J. (1991). *Saving children: A guide to injury prevention.* New York: Oxford University Press.

STUDY QUESTIONS

◆ ◆

1. Jessica Williams will be discharged from the hospital tomorrow after delivering Colin, a healthy 8-pound boy. She is enrolled in an infant care class. In teaching Jessica about scald burn prevention, what strategy is most likely going to be effective for Jessica?
    a. Test the water with her elbow each time prior to giving Colin a bath.
    b. Use a wash tub versus the bathtub or sink.
    c. Obtain a thermometer and dip it into the bath water prior to putting Colin in.
    d. Have the water heater turned down to 110 degrees.
    e. Write to encourage her legislator to promote a law for installation of water heaters pre-set on low setting.

2. Which of the following is least effective in reducing bike related head injuries?
    a. Constructing bike paths parallel to well-traveled roads
    b. Insisting that 15-year-old son wear sister's helmet
    c. Passing helmet usage regulation in community
    d. Conducting bike rodeos at school
    e. Offering affordable helmets for sale

3. Several teen mothers of 18–24-month-olds are participating in a parenting class. The topic today is poison prevention. Which of the following strategies is most effective?
    a. Install under the sink cabinet latches
    b. Brightly colored "Mr. Yuk" avoidance stickers on all poisonous products
    c. Medicines stored out of sight in bedside stand drawer.
    d. Watch child carefully "all the time"
    e. Poisonous products stored in container on top shelf in closet

4. Emergency department nurses have witnessed several serious injuries resulting from dog bites. They have decided that they need to do something to combat the problem. The nurses have developed three strategies. Which set of strategies is most likely to have a greater impact?
    a. Develop brochures that could be given out at safety fairs and in the emergency department, warning of the hazards of dogs and listing several safety actions.
    b. Work with city legislators to strengthen city ordinances related to animal control and ownership of attack-dog breeds.
    c. Work with law enforcement and judges to strengthen enforcement practices.
    d. Conduct a multimedia public awareness campaign with short public service announcements.

5. Which of the following is NOT a developmental trait affecting injury risk in the infant?
    a. Rapidly advancing motor skills
    b. Remembers and avoids painful events
    c. Learns by exploring, touching and putting objects in mouth
    d. Does not recognize hazardous situations
    e. Is completely dependent on others for safety

6. Which of the following is NOT a developmental trait affecting injury risk in the toddler?
    a. Rapidly advancing motor skills
    b. Magical thinking
    c. High desire to assert autonomy
    d. Does not recognize unsafe situations
    e. Will consistently follow safety rules that have been taught

7. Which of the following is NOT a developmental trait affecting injury risk in the school-age child?
    a. Has difficulty resisting peer pressure
    b. Understands rules and consequences of not following rules
    c. Can fully analyze risk situations
    d. Chemical substance use increases injury risk
    e. Uses the experimental approach to problem solving

8. Which of the following is NOT a developmental trait effecting injury risk in the adolescent?
    a. Usually retain safety habits that have been performed from early childhood
    b. Poor self-esteem may contribute to greater risk taking
    c. Understands future consequences of risk taking behaviors
    d. Undertakes great risks to impress peers
    e. Substance use greatly increases injury risk

9. Which of the following prevention strategies will be most successful?
    a. Teaching clients about safety hazards and actions to take to reduce risk
    b. Passing laws that require individuals to take proper precautions
    c. Redesigning the hazards so that risk will be reduced
    d. a and c
    e. a, b, and c

10. The pediatric clinic nurse notices that Justin's mother does not restrain Justin when they travel in the taxicab to the clinic. The nurse explicitly remembers counseling Justin's mother on this issue on prior visits. What steps should be taken to produce a more positive safety behavior in Justin's mother?
    a. Determine if Justin's mother knows how to properly restrain him.
    b. Ascertain if Justin's mother is concerned about motor vehicle injuries.
    c. Counsel Justin's mother about the child passenger restraint laws.
    d. Report the fact that Justin is not consistently restrained to the pediatrician.
    e a, b, and c

ANSWERS

◆ ◆

1.d   2.b   3.e   4.b   5.b   6.e   7.c   8.c   9.e   10.e

Chapter 11

Acute Illness, Injury, and Hospitalization: Effects on the Child

Virginia E. Maikler, PhD, RN

Concept

◆◆◆◆◆◆◆◆◆◆◆◆◆◆◆◆◆◆◆◆◆◆◆◆◆◆

◆ Children with acute illness or injuries and their families

Objectives

◆◆◆◆◆◆◆◆◆◆◆◆◆◆◆◆◆◆◆◆◆◆◆◆◆◆

At the completion of this chapter, the reader will be able to:

◆ Describe the influence of cognitive development on a child's understanding of illness.

◆ Describe common stressors confronting hospitalized children and their families.

◆ Identify modifiers that alter the stress associated with hospitalization.

◆ Recognize coping strategies commonly used by ill children.

◆ Discuss stressors associated with hospitalization in an intensive care environment.

Key Points

◆◆◆◆◆◆◆◆◆◆◆◆◆◆◆◆◆◆◆◆◆◆◆◆◆◆

◆ A child's understanding of illness is influenced by his/her cognitive maturity level.

◆ Hospitals, especially emergent and intensive care environments, are all stressors for the child.

◆ Common responses to hospitalization, such as fear, anxiety, and coping, are influenced by the child's cognitive level.

◆ Children vary in the type of coping strategies they use to manage the stressors of hospitalization.

Acute Illness, Injury, and Hospitalization: Effects on the Child

I. CHILDREN'S UNDERSTANDING OF ILLNESS

A. Children's understanding of illness proceeds in progressive developmental patterns, rather than distinct, predictable stages.

B. Children's understanding, as they grow older, moves from global and undifferentiated to concrete and abstract patterns.

C. Influences associated with understanding of illness concepts.
1. Cognitive maturity.
2. Information.
3. Experience with altered health patterns.
4. Cultural differences.
   a. Some cultures view illness as something to be resisted.
   b. Other cultures view illness as natural and to be accepted.

D. Meaning of illness according to age.
1. Infant: no understanding.
2. Toddler: no understanding.
3. Preschool child.
   a. Phenomenistic.
      (1) Understands connection exists between illness and the body.
      (2) Believes illness causes external, remote.
      (3) Explanations may be magical or circular.
   b. Beliefs about contagion.
      (1) Cause is related to proximity of source.
      (2) Illness is punishment for past "bad" deeds.
      (3) Things can be done to prevent illness.
4. School-age child.
   a. Beliefs about cause of illness.
      (1) Links illness to direct contact with some source such as germs.
      (2) Believes cause can be external, but located in the body.
      (3) Sometimes confuses cause and effect.

     (4) Distinguishes between a number of symptoms related to illness.
   b. Children older than 8 years show greater understanding about the location and function of internal organs.
5. Adolescent.
   a. Has a more mature understanding of illness.
   b. More aware of own role in health and illness and the importance of avoidance of illness to maintain health.
   c. Illness is the result of internalizing some contaminant.
   d. Understands a person can be somewhat sick, somewhat healthy.
   e. Differentiates between internal and external factors involved in health and illness.
   f. Aware that feelings and thoughts can contribute to health and illness.

II. ILLNESS AND HOSPITALIZATION AS STRESSORS

A. Majority of children are unprepared for hospitalization.

B. For some children (e.g., low-income, inner city, and/or multiproblem families), hospitalization may be a positive experience.
1. Structured environment.
2. Safe from violence.
3. Emotional support.

C. Common stressors confronting children in hospitals.
1. Separation from family and loved ones.
2. Strange people.
   a. Multiple caregivers.
   b. Caregivers are sources of information and may provide:
      (1) Too little information.
      (2) Too much information.
      (3) Upsetting, distressful information.
   c. Can be a source of pain.

3. Strange environment.
   a. Group living.
      (1) Loss of privacy.
      (2) Unmet needs.
      (3) Witnessing the care/treatment of other children.
   b. Disrupted routines.
      (1) Interrupted sleep.
      (2) Food.
         (a) Quality.
         (b) Quantity.
         (c) Timing of meals, snacks.
   c. Excessive noise, light.
   d. Unfamiliar, unpleasant smells.
   e. Uncertainty about limits, expectations.
   f. Loss of control.
4. Communication barriers.
   (1) Unfamiliar medical terminology.
   (2) Language barriers (e.g., non-English-speaking/comprehension).
5. Strange sensations.
   a. Pain.
      (1) Disease-related.
      (2) Treatment-related.
   b. Prolonged physical restraint.
   c. Loss of control.
      (1) Emotional, such as crying.
      (2) Physical, such as throwing up, bleeding, personal care by others.
6. Strange experiences.
   a. Intrusive procedures.
   b. Stress points during hospitalization for surgery.
      (1) Admission.
      (2) Blood sampling.
      (3) Prior to surgery.
      (4) Premedication injection.
      (5) Transport to operating room.
      (6) Return from recovery room.

D. Modifiers that can decrease or increase stress.
1. Stress point modifiers.
   a. Trend toward same-day, short-stay, and ambulatory surgery.
   b. Prehospital blood sampling.
   c. Trend toward oral, rectal, or no premedication.
   d. Discharge to home from recovery room.
2. Stress point enhancers.
   a. Play deprivation.
   b. Prolonged illness and/or hospitalization.
   c. Increased parental anxiety and distress behavior.
   d. Temperament of child if a poor fit with a specific environment.

III. RESPONSES TO STRESS OF ILLNESS AND HOSPITALIZATION

◆ ◆ ◆ ◆ ◆ ◆ ◆ ◆ ◆ ◆ ◆ ◆ ◆ ◆ ◆ ◆ ◆ ◆

A. Child's perception of the stressors determines whether a situation will result in a stress response.
1. Threat.
2. Challenge.
3. Benefit to well-being.

B. Responses will be influenced by cognitive maturity.
1. Children ages 6 months to 4 years usually most vulnerable.
2. School-age child has been studied more than any other age group; adolescents least.
3. School-age child may be less susceptible to the effects of hospitalization.

C. Lower family income is associated with greater fear of hospitalization.

D. Common responses to hospitalization.
1. Fear.
2. Anxiety.
   a. Separation anxiety.
   b. Stages of separation anxiety peaking in toddlerhood.
      (1) Protest.
         (a) Crying loudly, angrily with parental departure.
         (b) Refuses to eat.
         (c) Escape behavior.
      (2) Despair.
         (a) Depression deepens.
         (b) Sad, withdrawn, less angry.
      (3) Detachment.
         (a) Loss of trust in parents.
         (b) Superficially relates to others.
         (c) Compliant with care.
         (d) Also called "settling in."
   c. May decrease or increase during the course of a hospitalization.
3. Attitudinal and affective changes.
   a. Sense of mastery.
   b. Adopting the sick role.
   c. Adapting to the sick role.
4. Anger.
5. Coping. See Section IV on next page.

E. Age-related responses.
1. Infant.
   a. Separation anxiety.
   b. Distress.
      (1) Irritability.

(2) Extreme restlessness.
(3) Inconsolable crying.
(4) Poor feeding.
2. Toddler.
  a. Separation anxiety: highest in this age group.
  b. Distress.
    (1) Sleep disturbance.
    (2) Aggression.
  c. Fear of unfamiliar.
3. Preschooler.
  a. Eating, sleeping, speech disturbances.
  b. Fears.
    (1) Pain.
    (2) Bodily harm, castration, mutilation.
    (3) Loss of control.
    (4) Intrusive experience.
  c. Regressive behavior.
4. School-age.
  a. Separation anxiety: less, but still most common response.
  b. Physical and verbal aggression.
  c. Attitudinal and affective changes.
    (1) Fear and anxiety.
      (a) Mutilation.
      (b) Pain.
      (c) Death.
      (d) Loss of control.
      (e) Unknown.
    (2) Anger.
5. Adolescent.
  a. Fear related to:
    (1) Loss of control.
    (2) Loss of independence.
    (3) Loss of privacy.
    (4) Loss of identity.
    (5) Pain.
    (6) Disfigurement.
  b. Separation anxiety: from peers; family.

F. Modifiers of appropriate responses.
1. Past experiences.
2. Developmental needs.
3. Knowledge/information.

G. Responses associated with timing of hospitalization.
1. Prehospitalization.
  a. Planned admission/preparation.
  b. Unplanned/emergency admission.
2. Postdischarge reactions more severe in younger child.
  a. Increased separation anxiety.
  b. Sleep anxiety.
  c. Eating disturbances.
  d. Regression.
  e. Aggression.

f. Withdrawal.
g. Depression.
h. Increased bodily concerns.

IV. COPING WITH THE STRESS

◆ ◆ ◆ ◆ ◆ ◆ ◆ ◆ ◆ ◆ ◆ ◆ ◆ ◆ ◆ ◆ ◆ ◆

A. Child appraises the illness and hospitalization.
1. Primary appraisal: determines the relevance of the event for personal well-being.
2. Secondary appraisal: focuses on the resources available for coping.

B. Coping styles are different from coping strategies.
1. Coping styles.
  a. Are partly learned, partly innate behavior patterns that are characteristic of the way the child adapts to the environment.
  b. Become personality traits that are relatively stable over time.
2. Coping strategies.
  a. Specific cognitive and behavioral methods of dealing with stressors.
  b. Influenced by:
    (1) Age and maturation.
    (2) Cognitive development.
      (a) Increasing attention span.
      (b) Problem-solving ability.
      (c) Understanding of cause and effect.
    (3) Increasing impulse control.
    (4) Experience.
  c. Are amenable to intervention by health care professionals.
  d. Young children primarily use behavioral strategies.
  e. Cognitive strategies increase with age.

C. Ryan-Wenger's (1989) healthy children coping strategies taxonomy.
1. Aggressive behavior: verbal or motor activities that may be hurtful to people, animals, or objects.
2. Behavioral avoidance: behavior other than isolating that is a deliberate attempt to keep oneself away from a stressor.
3. Behavioral distraction: behavior other than isolating or avoidant that delays the need to deal with the stressor.
4. Cognitive avoidance: deliberate cognitive attempts to avoid acknowledging the existence of a stressor.
5. Cognitive distraction: deliberate cognitive attempts to keep thoughts away from a stressor.
6. Cognitive problem-solving: thoughts focused on ways to modify, prevent, or eliminate the stressor.

7. Cognitive restructuring: thoughts that alter one's perception of the characteristics of the stressor.
8. Emotional expression: behavior other than aggressive motor and verbal activities that expresses feelings or emotions.
9. Endurance: behavior that causes one to face the stressor and accept its consequences.
10. Information-seeking: behavior that involves obtaining information about the stressor.
11. Isolating activities: behavior that serves to separate the individual from the presence of others.
12. Self-controlling activities: behavior or cognition that serve to reduce tensions or control one's behavior or emotions.
13. Social support: nonaggressive behavior that involves seeking the presence of an individual.
14. Spiritual support: behavior that suggests an appeal to a higher being.
15. Stressor modification: noncognitive behavior that eliminates the stressor or modifies the characteristics of the stressor.

D. Coping strategies more commonly used by hospitalized children.
1. Social support.
2. Stressor modification.
3. "Hospital veterans" use following strategies:
   a. Information-seeking.
   b. Information-limiting.
   c. Avoidant.
   d. Active.
   e. Avoidant-active.

E. Age-related coping.
1. Infant.
   a. Inaction.
   b. Behavior avoidance.
2. Toddler and preschool.
   a. Limited cognitive ability.
   b. Social support.
   c. Aggressive behavior.
   d. Behavior avoidance.
3. School-age.
   a. Countermeasure.
   b. Control.
   c. Social support.
   d. Cognitive restructuring.
   e. Cooperation.
   f. Cognitive processing.
4. Adolescent.
   a. Emotion-focused.
      (1) Cognitive distraction.
      (2) Inaction.
      (3) Self-controlling activity.
      (4) Social support.
   b. Problem-focused.

(1) Stressor modification.
(2) Situational control.

V. INTENSIVE CARE ENVIRONMENTS – ADDITIONAL CONSIDERATIONS
◆ ◆ ◆ ◆ ◆ ◆ ◆ ◆ ◆ ◆ ◆ ◆ ◆ ◆ ◆ ◆ ◆ ◆ ◆ ◆
A. Stressors.
1. Family-related.
   a. Restricted visitation.
   b. Interrupted visitation.
   c. Parental anxiety high and distress behaviors common.
   d. Interrupted bonding with neonates.
2. Environmental.
   a. Sleep interruption.
   b. Continuous light/sound.
   c. Time distortion.
   d. Unfamiliar, high-tech equipment.
   e. Urgency of care.
3. Strange sensations.
   a. Intubation.
   b. Inability to communicate.
   c. Inability to eat or drink.
   d. Frequency of painful, irritating procedures.

B. Response to trauma, emergent, intensive care.
1. Influenced by length and severity of situation.
2. Progressive, rather than distinct phases.
   a. Impact phase: shock both physical and emotional.
   b. Denial phase: avoidance and withdrawal.
   c. Panic: interrupts and breaks through the denial.
   d. Protest and regression.
   e. Oppositionalism: positive sign of mobilizing defenses.
   f. Mourning: reaction to loss of threatened loss.
   g. Readjustment.

BIBLIOGRAPHY
◆ ◆ ◆ ◆ ◆ ◆ ◆ ◆ ◆ ◆ ◆ ◆ ◆ ◆ ◆ ◆ ◆ ◆ ◆ ◆

Bibace, R., & Walsh, M. (1980). Development of children's concepts of illness. *Pediatrics, 66,* 912–917.

Carson, D., Gravley, J., & Council, J. (1992). Children's prehospitalization conceptions of illness, cognitive development, and personal adjustment. *Children's Health Care, 21*(2), 103–110.

Inagaki, K., & Hatano, G. (1993). Young children's understanding of the mind–body distinction. *Child Development, 64*(5), 1534–49.

Jansen, M., DeWitt, P., Meshul, R., Krasnoff, J., Lau, A., & Kerns, T. (1989). Meeting psychosocial and developmental needs of children during prolonged intensive care unit hospitalization. *Children's Health Care, 18*(2), 91–95.

Kalish, C. (1996). Causes and symptoms in preschoolers' conceptions of illness. *Child Development, 67*(4), 1647–1670.

Mabe, P., Treiber, F., & Riley, W. (1991). Examining emotional distress during pediatric hospitalization for school-age children. *Children's Health Care, 20*(3), 162–169.

Rudolph, K., Dennig, M., & Weisz, J. (1995). Determinants and consequences of children's coping in the medical setting: Conceptualization, review and critique. *Psychological Bulletin, 118*(3), 328–357.

Ryan-Wenger, N. (1989) Stress-coping strategies identified from school-age children's perspective. *Research in Nursing and Health, 12,* 111–122.

Stevens, M. (1989). Coping strategies of hospitalized adolescents. *Children's Health Care, 18*(3), 163–169.

Thompson, M. (1994). Information-seeking coping and anxiety in school-age children anticipating surgery. *Children's Health Care, 23*(2), 87–97.

STUDY QUESTIONS

1. At what developmental stage does the child understand only that a connection exists between illness and the body?
   a. Infant
   b. Toddler
   c. Preschooler
   d. School-age child
   e. Adolescent

2. Which practice may increase the stress of hospitalization?
   a. Primary nursing
   b. Private rooms
   c. Early discharge
   d. Visiting hours
   e. Detailed information

3. Which of these children would have the most difficulty with hospitalization?
   a. Alice, whose parents cannot visit
   b. Lucy, who is having ambulatory surgery
   c. Jerry, who lives in the inner city
   d. Jonny, who doesn't like his roommate
   e. Tom, who had his appendix removed

4. To facilitate a 4-year-old child's coping with admission to the hospital, which statement by the nurse is most helpful?
   a. "I'll be your mother while you're here."
   b. "Would you like Dad to check your temperature?"
   c. "This won't hurt."
   d. "Dad, children this age are the least affected by hospitalization."
   e. "Mom and Dad need to go home now."

5. Children with multiple hospitalizations are less stressed by hospitalization than first-time admissions.
   a. True
   b. False

6 Which phrase best describes separation distress?
   a. Begins in toddler, peaks in preschooler, and declines in school-age child
   b. For a given child, all losses are viewed the same
   c. Involves protest, despair, and detachment
   d. Resolves with discharge

7. Which age group may be least susceptible to the effects of hospitalization?
   a. Infant
   b. Toddler
   c. Preschooler
   d. School-age child
   e. Adolescent

8. Which is the most commonly used coping strategy by hospitalized children?
   a. Aggressive behavior
   b. Cognitive avoidance
   c. Emotional expression
   d. Information-seeking
   e. Social support

9. Inaction and behavior avoidance are most commonly observed in which age group?
   a. Infant
   b. Toddler
   c. Preschooler
   d. School-age child
   e. Adolescent

10. The intensive care environment is less stressful to children because a nurse is always nearby to meet all their needs.
    a. True
    b. False

ANSWERS

1.c 2.d 3.a 4.b 5.b 6.c 7.d 8.e 9.a 10.b

Chapter 12

Acute Illness: Effects on the Child's Family

Elizabeth A. Bossert, DNS, RN
Dynnette E. Hart, DrPH, RN

Concept

◆◆◆◆◆◆◆◆◆◆◆◆◆◆◆◆◆◆◆◆◆◆◆◆◆◆◆◆◆

◆ Children with acute illness or injuries and their families

Objectives

◆◆◆◆◆◆◆◆◆◆◆◆◆◆◆◆◆◆◆◆◆◆◆◆◆◆◆◆

At the completion of this chapter, the reader will be able to:

◆ Identify sources of stress for parents and siblings during the acute illness and hospitalization of a child.

◆ Describe common parental and sibling reactions, needs, and coping behaviors during the acute illness and hospitalization of a child.

◆ Describe cultural influences on a family experiencing hospitalization of a child with an acute illness.

◆ Appropriately assess cultural factors and respond to assessment information with culturally congruent planning and nursing interventions.

◆ Identify strengths and resources that will enable the family to successfully negotiate the acute illness and hospitalization of a child.

Key Points

◆◆◆◆◆◆◆◆◆◆◆◆◆◆◆◆◆◆◆◆◆◆◆◆◆◆◆◆

◆ Hospitalization of a child with an acute illness is a great source of stress for families.

◆ Reactions to stressors and coping behaviors vary with each family – parents and siblings.

◆ A basic cultural assessment should be a standard component of every hospital admission process.

◆ Parents and siblings need information and involvement in caregiving to assist them in coping.

◆ Every family brings strengths into the nurse-ill child-family relationship, which need to be identified and nurtured as resources for positive coping.

12

Acute Illness: Effects on the Child's Family

I. PARENTAL RESPONSES TO ACUTE ILLNESS AND HOSPITALIZATION OF A CHILD

A. Illness and hospitalization of a child usually produce some level of stress for a family, although the perception of the event differs from family to family. The evaluation of stress includes:

1. A person (the parent) and the environment (having a sick child) mutually act on each other, resulting in an event (seeking health care).
2. The event (seeking health care) is appraised by the person (parent) who asks:
   a. Does the event effect my well-being?
   b. What can I do in response to the event?
3. Possible responses to appraisal of event (seeking health care).
   a. Event is appraised as irrelevant so does not cause stress; an unlikely response from most parents.
   b. Event is appraised as benign so does not cause stress; unlikely response from most parents.
   c. Event is appraised as causing stress; common response from most parents.

B. Sources of stress for parents during acute illness of child.

1. Child's illness.
   a. Diagnosis as a source of stress.
      (1) Waiting for diagnosis.
      (2) If diagnosis is unknown, uncertainty exists re: meaning of illness for child's well-being.
      (3) If diagnosis is known, concerns will vary based on parent's perception of meaning of illness for child.
   b. Decisions about management of illness as a source of stress.
      (1) Possible knowledge deficit about pathophysiology of illness and subsequent recommended treatment.
      (2) Unfamiliar medical jargon.
      (3) Not sure if health care personnel are qualified to provide appropriate care for child.
      (4) Unclear about what role to take in determining child's treatment.
      (5) Consent for invasive and/or painful treatments.
      (6) Consent for treatment with outcomes that will affect child throughout life.
   c. Appraisal of severity of illness as a source of stress.
      (1) Perception of illness may be influenced by several factors.
         (a) Past experience with same or similar diagnosis.
         (b) Degree of familiarity with hospital environment.
         (c) Cues from health care personnel.
      (2) Perception of greater severity increases stress.
2. Hospital environment as a source of stress.
   a. Unfamiliar environment and equipment.
   b. Unfamiliar routines and policies.
   c. Uncertain role.
      (1) Confusion due to overlap in parental role and nursing care.
         (a) Routine care, such as feeding, bathing, comforting.
         (b) Discipline and limit setting.
      (2) Unknown expectations of parents by staff.
         (a) Caring for equipment, such as IV pumps, apnea monitors.
         (b) Notifying staff of physical changes.
   d. Unfamiliar personnel entrusted with child's well-being.
      (1) Role of person, such as nurse, respiratory therapist, lab technician.
      (2) Professional level of nurse, such as Registered Nurse, Licensed Visiting Nurse, Certified Nurse Assistant, or Staff Nurse, Clinical Nurse Specialist, Pediatric Nurse Practitioner, or Nurse Manager.

(3) Numbers of persons, due to shift schedules.
(4) Variations in technique among personnel.
(5) Differences in personalities.
3. Type of admission.
  a. Planned admission.
    (1) Will be appraised as stressful due to concern with child's health.
    (2) Stress may be low or under control depending on extent to which parents have been able to prepare for themselves and child for event.
  b. Unexpected admission (i.e., from clinic visit).
    (1) Will generate stress as child's health is altered.
    (2) Family routines must be quickly revised.
  c. Emergency admission (i.e., through ER).
    (1) Will result in high stress as child's life is threatened.
    (2) No time to plan and cope with stress.
4. Length of stay.
  a. Unknown: increases stress due to inability to plan.
  b. Short: may increase stress if parents think child is being discharged too soon, and do not feel ready to care for child at home.
  c. Long: may increase stress, parents face continued altered life routines.
5. Changes in child's behavior.
  a. Loss of developmental milestones (regression).
  b. Changes in child's emotional responses.
    (1) Fear.
    (2) Sadness.
    (3) Crying.
    (4) Confusion.
    (5) Quiet.
    (6) Rebellious/resistant.
  c. Physical changes due to illness, injury, medication, treatment.
    (1) Pain.
    (2) Alteration in appearance.
    (3) Difficulty or inability to communicate.
    (4) Loss of mobility.
    (5) Loss of strength.
    (6) Alteration in mental function.
6. Changes in daily routine of family life.
  a. If rooming-in, altered daily routine.
    (1) Shifting of work responsibilities.
    (2) Arranging for child care for siblings.
    (3) Modifying activities of daily living.
    (4) Canceling social plans.
  b. If visiting, modified daily routine to add time for visit.
    (1) Conflicting priorities occur between parenting and work.
    (2) Attempts to fit it all in by decreasing

sleep or omitting portions of routine.
(3) Disrupts mealtime with family; altered intake.

C. Parental reactions to hospitalization.
1. Anxiety/worry most commonly experienced.
  a. Admission.
  b. Prior to invasive treatments.
  c. Prior to surgery.
  d. Prior to discharge.
2. Guilt relating to diagnosis.
3. Relief sometimes experienced.
  a. If child was too ill to care for easily at home.
  b. If parents were exhausted.
  c. If child's condition frightened parents.
4. Anger.

D. Parental involvement.
1. Needs of parents.
  a. Information about child's condition and treatment.
  b. Hope about the child's condition and outcome.
  c. To be able to trust health care professionals.
  d. To know that child is receiving the best possible care.
  e. To be acknowledged, valued, and trusted by health care professionals as a member of their child's health care team.
  f. Input from staff about what type of involvement in the child's care is appropriate.
  g. To be able to express feelings, receive support, and professional counsel.
  h. To know how to manage personal needs by receiving information about available physical/psychosocial/spiritual resources.
  i. To maintain relationships with family members and others in personal and professional life.
2. Parental desires.
  a. Nearly all desire involvement in normal child caretaking.
  b. Nurse should accommodate parents' desire for involvement as much as possible.

II. PARENTAL COPING WITH ACUTE ILLNESS OF CHILD

◆ ◆ ◆ ◆ ◆ ◆ ◆ ◆ ◆ ◆ ◆ ◆ ◆ ◆ ◆ ◆ ◆ ◆

See Chapter 20: Chronic Conditions: Effects on the Child's Family

A. Coping with hospitalization related to phase of illness.
1. Passivity or acquiescence tends to occur in early phase.
  a. Seen when symptoms develop suddenly.

b. Accepts recommendations of professionals.
2. Information seeking follows passivity.
   a. Asks many different professionals for information.
   b. Seeks additional information from literature.
   c. Analyzes differences in information.
   d. Seeks to clarify differences, fill in gaps in knowledge.
   e. Develops personal "understanding" of diagnosis and management.
3. Child advocacy develops as parents gain comfort with information and environment.
   a. Realize that as parents, they best know child's potential needs and responses.
   b. Reclaim right to determine child's experiences, such as occurrence and timing of invasive procedures.

B. Parental coping behaviors commonly seen during hospitalization of acutely ill child.
1. Seeking support from friends and family.
2. Seeking spiritual support.
3. Continuation of caregiving role.

C. Coping with family life disruption during hospitalization of child.
1. First priority: hospitalized child's needs.
   a. Parents generally believe hospitalized child needs more attention than usual.
   b. Parents generally believe that a parent should be with the child as much as possible during hospitalization.
   c. Mothers spend more time with child than do fathers.
   d. Time spent with child may decrease as child's health improves.
2. Second priority: siblings' needs.
   a. Siblings' needs met without outside help.
   b. Siblings' needs met with outside help.
   c. Parental time spent with siblings may increase as sick child's health improves.
3. Third priority: work responsibilities.
   a. Lower priority placed on mother's work than father's during hospitalization.
   b. Mothers more likely than fathers to take time off from work to be with child.
   c. Fathers who continue routine work may attempt to rearrange work schedule to permit visiting child before or after work.
4. Fourth priority: home responsibilities.
   a. Essentials, such as meals, are delegated to older sibling or substitute caretaker.
   b. Nonessentials, such as cleaning, may be ignored.
5. Fifth priority: parent's needs.
   a. Parent's often ignore own needs.

b. If rooming-in, meeting physical needs may be difficult, depending on availability of services (bed, shower, etc) in the hospital.
c. "Non-essential" activities, such as exercise, interacting with spouse, family, friends may be omitted whether rooming-in or visiting.

III. SIBLING STRESSORS/RESPONSES

A. Sources of stress for siblings.
1. Child's illness as a source of stress.
   a. Fear ill child may die.
   b. Fearful imagining of what might be happening to ill child in the hospital.
   c. Guilt regarding cause of illness or injury.
      (1) Actual guilt, if contagious disease was transmitted or injury was inflicted.
      (2) Actual guilt if sibling might have prevented illness or injury.
      (3) Fantasized guilt if sibling thinks he/she may have caused illness/injury (although untrue).
   d. Separation from ill child.
   e. Fear of developing the same illness or injury.
2. Substitute care arrangements as a source of stress.
   a. Separation from primary care provider.
      (1) Mother generally focuses time on hospitalized child.
      (2) Father generally has less time for siblings while with ill child in hospital.
      (3) Manifestations of separation anxiety differ according to age of sibling.
      (4) Feelings of insecurity, jealousy, and abandonment may develop.
   b. Change in person providing daily care.
      (1) In-home care provided by father, older sibling, relative such as grandmother.
      (2) Out-of-home care provided by relative, neighbor, or friend of family.
      (3) Sibling may not get along well with substitute caregiver.
   c. Change in activities of daily living.
      (1) Changes in eating patterns, type and timing of meals.
      (2) Changes in routines, such as getting up, play activities, bath time, bedtime.
      (3) Changes in behavioral expectations and discipline.
   d. Change in responsibilities.
      (1) Expected to take more responsibility for self, unless infant or young toddler.
      (2) Older siblings may be expected to take care of younger siblings.
      (3) Older siblings may be expected to take on some household responsibilities.

B. Sibling responses to hospitalization.
   1. Negative reactions.
      a. Regression to earlier level of behavior.
      b. Anger toward parents, ill child, substitute caregiver, self.
      c. Anxiety, may be influenced by parental anxiety.
      d. Physical symptoms, similar or dissimilar to sibling who is ill and/or hospitalized.
   2. Positive reactions.
      a. Increased self-confidence.
      b. Increased ability to take on responsibilities within family.
      c. Increased empathy for others.
   3. Factors possibly related to sibling response.
      a. Acuity of illness, i.e., critical illness.
      b. Length of time since new diagnosis of illness.
      c. Socioeconomic level of family, i.e., related to lower income and educational level of parent.
      d. Changes in parents' interaction with sibling, i.e., caregiving, emotional availability.
      e. Age of sibling: between 4 and 11 years increased vulnerability.
      f. Close relationship with ill child.
      g. Out-of home care for siblings.
      h. Little understanding/knowledge regarding ill child's condition.
      i. Parents may underestimate number of changes sibling experiences.

C. Sibling coping.
   1. Repertoire of possible coping behaviors used varies greatly depending on developmental age of child. *For information on coping behaviors of well child, see Chapter 3: Cognitive and Psychosocial Development.*
   2. Visiting ill child.
      a. Supports relationship between sibling and ill child.
      b. Helps to decreases fantasies and fears regarding hospitalization.
      c. Increases communication and support within the family system.
      d. Does not increase rate of infection for hospitalized child.

IV. CULTURAL EXPECTATIONS AND SUPPORT OF FAMILIES DURING ACUTE ILLNESS OF A CHILD

◆ ◆ ◆ ◆ ◆ ◆ ◆ ◆ ◆ ◆ ◆ ◆ ◆ ◆ ◆ ◆ ◆ ◆ ◆

A. Role of culture and family.
   1. Family is the medium of cultural transmission.
   2. Family provides the environment for transmis-sion of beliefs, attitudes, and traditions, including health care patterns. *See Chapter 29: Cultural Influences.*
   3. Each family is a member of a larger cultural/ethnic group.
   4. Each family has unique, individual characteristics differing from the larger cultural group. Differences depend on:
      a. Degree of acculturation.
      b. Length of time family has lived in the host country.
      c. Other factors, such as neighborhood environment, level of education, ability to communicate, etc.
   5. Every family has cultural behaviors and expectations.
      a. Avoid stereotyping.
      b. Be aware that culture of hospital may conflict with culture of family.
      c. Provide culturally congruent care to every family.
      d. Be aware that apparent similarities to dominant culture may mask cultural differences.

B. Cultural assessment process.
   1. Definition: systematic appraisal of cultural beliefs, values, and practices of individuals and families for the purpose of determining nursing needs and providing culturally congruent interventions.
   2. When to do assessment.
      a. Standard cultural assessment should be part of initial hospital admission process.
      b. Further in-depth assessment may need to be carried out at a later time.
   3. How to do assessment.
      a. Use a warm, accepting approach that denotes respect and valuing of the families' cultural uniqueness and differences.
      b. Develop a trusting relationship between the family and caregiver.
         (1) Start with nonthreatening topics, such as language and food preferences.
         (2) Convey to family that the information they provide is considered important.
         (3) Treat the information with respect. For example, avoid behavior that demonstrates the nurse thinks the information is funny, ridiculous, bizarre, or exotically entrancing.
         (4) Record the information for sharing with other members of the health care team.
      c. Use open-ended questions.
      d. Plan 15–20 minutes for assessment with respect to time constraints.
   4. What to include in assessment process.
      a. Communication. *Also see Chapter 30: Communication.*

(1) What language does the family prefer to use when speaking to health care team?
(2) What is preferred language dialect?
(3) If English is not spoken, is there a family member or friend who can speak English and who is willing to interpret?
b. Cultural orientation, national background, immigration history.
(1) What cultural/ethnic group does the family prefer to identify with?
(2) Where was the child born? Where were the parents born?
(a) If outside of the United States, how old were the parents (or the child) when coming to the United States?
(b) How long has the child or the family lived in the United States?
(3) Where has the family/child lived?
c. Family relationships.
(1) Who will be involved with the child's care during hospitalization?
(2) Who will be regularly visiting the child during hospitalization?
(3) Who needs to be present when decisions about the child's care are being discussed and decided?
(4) Who disciplines the child and what are the preferred methods of discipline during illness?
d. Nutritional/diet preferences.
(1) What food preferences does the child/family have?
(2) What foods are encouraged or forbidden during illness or when a child has certain symptoms?
(3) What foods would the family like to bring in for the child to eat?
e. Religious orientation.
(1) What religious practices would the family like to have continued in the hospital?
(2) Are there religious tokens/amulets/pictures that the family would like to have present with the child in the hospital?
(3) Who would the family like to come visit the child for spiritual care during hospitalization?
f. Beliefs about health and illness.
(1) What does the family think caused the child's illness?
(2) What treatments have they already tried at home or in another facility for this illness?
(3) Who else is involved in the health care of the child besides the hospital health care team?
(4) What are the usual remedies used by the family for this illness?

(5) What treatments/remedies would the family like to continue in the hospital?
g. Socioeconomic/educational level.
(1) What is the educational level of the child and the family member?
(2) What are the occupations of the parents?
(3) Based on annual income, family occupations, and type of health insurance, what is the economic level of the family?
h. Need for more in-depth cultural information.
(1) Acute short stay hospitalizations may not require in-depth cultural information.
(2) Factors that may determine a need for a more in-depth cultural assessment.
(a) Lengthy hospitalization.
(b) Severe or life-threatening illness.
(c) Change to category of chronic illness.
(d) Lifestyle changes at home necessary due to long-term care of child.
(e) Extensive patient/family education necessary.
5. Record and collaboratively share cultural information.
a. Include information with admission information.
b. Handle information with professional confidentiality and respect.
c. Refer to pertinent cultural information during patient rounds and while making plans for care.

C. Planning for culturally congruent care.
1. Cultural information resources for planning culturally congruent care.
a. Books that describe selected cultural groups.
b. Health care team member from same cultural group.
c. Member from child's family or child himself or herself (mid to late teens) willing to share cultural information.
2. Use of cultural information resources.
a. Refer to cultural group that family identifies with.
b. Allow for individual differences to avoid stereotyping.
c. Note information specific to health problem of child.
(1) Common explanations for illness within cultural groups.
(2) Alternative treatments that are commonly practiced in a selected ethnic group.
(3) Possible gender role conflicts with members of the health care team.
(4) Religious orientation if an essential component of family's culture.

d. Share cultural information resources with other members of the health care team.

3. Application of cultural information to patient care.

a. Appropriate use of interpreters. *See Chapter 29: Cultural Influences.*

b. Preserving and maintaining cultural beliefs and practices. Examples:

(1) Allowing religious symbols, i.e., amulets, tokens, to be worn by child.

(2) Encouraging a mother to bring in appropriate traditional foods from home.

(3) Allowing cultural symbols believed to promote healing to be present on the child or in the room.

(4) Allowing a traditional healer to be a member of the child's health care team.

c. Accommodating for and negotiating with cultural beliefs and practices. Examples:

(1) Modifying traditional food items to be more adherent to child's dietary restrictions.

(2) Explaining a therapy regimen within the context of their cultural perspective of illness, i.e., balance of factors (hot and cold, yin and yang, etc.)

(3) Allowing a traditional healer to participate in a child's care with the mutual consent that all therapy measures be discussed with health care team.

(4) Accommodating for the extended family by expanding hospital visitation protocols, i.e., allowing a variety of family members to be present with the child in the hospital.

d. Repatterning and restructuring cultural beliefs and practices. Examples:

(1) Discontinuing a home-remedy due to the presence of a harmful substance in the remedy, such as a remedy that contains lead.

(2) Discussing dehydration and oral rehydration therapy with a family who believes that withholding fluids is necessary when an infant or child has diarrhea.

V. FAMILY STRENGTHS

◆ ◆ ◆ ◆ ◆ ◆ ◆ ◆ ◆ ◆ ◆ ◆ ◆ ◆ ◆ ◆ ◆ ◆ ◆

A. Identification of strengths in family support a positive response to acute illness and hospitalization of child.

1. Provides for physical, psychosocial, and spiritual needs of family members.

2. Positive outcomes.

a. Exhibits strong sense of family through rituals, traditions, and unity of purpose.

b. Communicates in a positive, interactive manner within and without family.

c. Demonstrates trust, respect, and appreciation for each other.

d. Gives support, commitment, security, and encouragement to each other.

e. Shares family responsibilities and roles.

f. Recognizes need for help, engages in self-help, and accepts help appropriately.

g. Views crisis as opportunity for growth.

h. Copes through use of humor and play.

i. Uses a variety of coping behaviors.

j. Uses resources both internal and external to the family.

B. Identify reasons to help family recognize strengths.

1. Provides positive input to family during time of crisis.

2. Helps family identify internal resources.

3. Empowers family to cope with situation.

4. Helps family identify existing strengths needed to cope with acute illness.

5. Strengthens the family unit.

VI. FAMILY RESOURCES

◆ ◆ ◆ ◆ ◆ ◆ ◆ ◆ ◆ ◆ ◆ ◆ ◆ ◆ ◆ ◆ ◆ ◆ ◆

A. Informal.

1. Persons.

a. Family, immediate and extended.

b. Neighbors.

c. Friends.

d. Other parents.

2. Groups.

a. Church or religious group members.

b. Social group, such as club.

c. Work group from place of employment.

d. Self-help (support) groups.

B. Formal.

1. Professionals.

a. Health care personnel such as nurses, physicians, social workers, child life.

b. Clergy or other spiritual leaders.

c. Counselors such as psychologists, therapists.

2. Organizations.

a. Hospitals.

b. Public health departments.

c. Clinics.

d. Insurance companies.

e. National Health care (Medicare).

f. State health care programs.

g. Nonprofit charitable agencies, nongovernmental organizations.

BIBLIOGRAPHY

◆ ◆ ◆ ◆ ◆ ◆ ◆ ◆ ◆ ◆ ◆ ◆ ◆ ◆ ◆ ◆ ◆ ◆

Craft, M.J. (1993). Siblings of hospitalized children: Assessment and intervention. *Journal of Pediatric Nursing, 8,* 289–297.

Kristjánsdóttir, G. (1995). Perceived importance of needs expressed by parent of hospitalized two-to six-year-olds. *Scandinavian Journal of Caring Sciences, 9,* 995–103.

Lazarus, R.S., & Folkman, S. (1984). *Stress, appraisal, and coping.* New York: Guilford Press.

Melnyk, B. (1994). Parental coping with unplanned hospitalization: Effects of informational interventions on mothers and children. *Nursing Research, 43,* 50–55.

Melnyk, B. (1995) Parental coping with hospitalization: A theoretical framework to guide research and clinical intervention. *MCN, 23,* 123–131.

Miles, M.S., Carter, M.C., Riddle, I., Hennessey, J., & Eberly, T.W. (1989). The pediatric intensive care unit environment as a source of stress for parents. *Maternal Child Nursing Journal, 18,* 199–206.

Purnell, L.D., & Paulanka, B.J . (1998). *Transcultural health care: A culturally competent approach.* Philadelphia: F.A. Davis Company.

Seidemon, R.Y., Watson, M.A., Corff, K., Odle, P., Haase, J., & Bowerman, J.L. (1997). Parent stress and coping in NICU and PICU. *Journal of Pediatric Nursing, 12,* 169-177.

Society of Pediatric Nurses Family-Centered Care Clinical Practice Guideline. (1998). *Family-centered care: Putting it into action.* Denver: Society of Pediatric Nurses.

Thompson, R.H. (1985). *Psychosocial research on pediatric hospitalization and health care: A review of the literature.* Springfield, IL: Charles C. Thomas.

STUDY QUESTIONS

Mr. and Mrs. Garcia have just admitted Frederico, 2½ years old, to the hospital for an acute illness. It is Frederico's first admission, and neither parent is familiar with the hospital environment. (Questions 1–5).

1. Of the following events, which might the parents find particularly stressful?
   a. Waiting for the diagnostic lab work to be done
   b. Holding Frederico while the nurse obtains the admission history from the parents
   c. Receiving information about the location of the cafeteria, phone, and restroom
   d. Being asked what part of Frederico's daily care the parents would like to do
   e. Being told that visiting hours are unrestricted

2. Which aspect of the hospital environment might NOT be a source of stress for the parents?
   a. Understanding the medical terminology used
   b. Interacting with parents of other ill children
   c. Figuring out which nurse is responsible for which aspect of Frederico's care
   d. Adapting to hospital policies, such as physician accessibility, patient rest periods, etc.
   e. Seeing other sick children receive a variety of treatment

3. All of the following behaviors exhibited by Frederico are likely to be a source of stress for the parents EXCEPT:
   a. limited activity due to IV in his foot.
   b. resisting the restraints needed to keep the IV intact.
   c. less frequent communication about needing the "potty" after being nearly toilet trained.
   d. emotions of sadness and occasionally crying.
   e. desire to be cuddled.

4. Which of the following statements represents the coping behaviors Mr. and Mrs. Garcia would be most likely to exhibit immediately after Frederico's unexpected admission?
   a. "Frederico just went to sleep; come back later to do the blood tests."
   b. "The last time you had a patient with the same problem as Justin's, did he get the same antibiotics? How long did it take for them to work?"
   c. "Please do whatever you think is best to help Justin get well."
   d. "I should have realized sooner that Justin was getting sick, then maybe he wouldn't have to be in the hospital."
   e. "I wish I could wake up and find out this was all a bad dream."

5. Mrs. Garcia tells the nurse that she is having a hard time dealing with the pain and discomfort Frederico is experiencing during blood tests and other diagnostic work. Which of the following actions would best support the mother's needs?
   a. Encourage her to go home and rest.
   b. Help her find ways she can make Frederico more comfortable.
   c. Suggest that she step out of the room when tests are done.
   d. Reassure her that the tests are necessary and the pain is over quickly.
   e. Tell her that her feelings are normal so don't worry about it.

6. Which of the following is TRUE regarding allowing siblings to visit a child in the hospital?
   a. The rate of infection of the hospitalized children will increase.
   b. Seeing the hospital equipment increases the siblings fears.
   c. Communication is unnecessary within the family if all members have visited the sick child.
   d. Visiting supports the relationship between the two children.
   e. Visiting increases the siblings likelihood of "acting sick" to get extra attention from the parents.

7. Jessie, 4 years old, is hospitalized because of an acute illness. When the nurse is 5 minutes late administering her pain medication, Jessie's parents shout at the nurse. The nurse recognizes the parents' behavior is likely:
   a. a denial of their child's illness.
   b. an expression of the anger they feel because of their daughter's illness.
   c. a reaction that prevents development of effective nurse-family communication.
   d. an indication that the parents need more education about their child's condition.
   e. evidence that the parents do not like or trust the nurse.

ANSWERS

1.a   2.b   3.e   4.c   5.b   6.d   7.b

Chapter 13

Acute Illness: Care Technologies

Beth. S. Nachtsheim, MS, RN, PCCNP

Concept

◆◆◆◆◆◆◆◆◆◆◆◆◆◆◆◆◆◆◆◆◆◆◆◆◆◆◆◆

- ◆ Children with acute illnesses or injuries and their families

Objectives

◆◆◆◆◆◆◆◆◆◆◆◆◆◆◆◆◆◆◆◆◆◆◆◆◆◆◆◆

At the completion of this chapter, the reader will be able to:

- ◆ Identify common advantages and disadvantages of various methods of medication administration.
- ◆ Describe the catheter-over-needle insertion procedure.
- ◆ State the effects of immobility and discuss common nursing interventions for prevention of these effects.
- ◆ Calculate the caloric requirements for acutely ill infants/children.
- ◆ Describe the use of common oxygenation/ventilation technologies.
- ◆ Summarize the general care of the postoperative pediatric patient.

Key Points

◆◆◆◆◆◆◆◆◆◆◆◆◆◆◆◆◆◆◆◆◆◆◆◆◆◆◆◆

- ◆ Families should be involved in their child's care whenever possible.
- ◆ Delivery rates of intravenous medications are drug specific.
- ◆ A local anesthetic cream may be beneficial for insertion site anesthesia prior to venipuncture.
- ◆ Untreated, the effects of immobility complicate recovery and prolong convalescence.
- ◆ The intestines function best when nutrition is enteral.
- ◆ Endotracheal tubes are not secure airways and must be closely monitored.

13

Acute Illness: Care Technologies

◆ ◆

I. MEDICATION ADMINISTRATION

A. Overview.
1. There are many methods of medication delivery.
2. Advantages and disadvantages.
   a. Speed of delivery.
   b. Level of comfort.
   c. Dosing reliability.
   d. Toxicity.
   e. Ease of use.
3. Include families and primary caretakers in all aspects of care delivery.
4. Too many options can confuse children.
   a. For children's understanding of illness, injury, and hospitalization, *see Chapter 11: Acute Illness, Injury, and Hospitalization: Effects on the Child.*
   b. Choices should be limited, e.g., "Do you want your medicine in this leg, or that one?"
   c. Be truthful when responding to the children's questions. Do not tell them something does not hurt, or burn, or taste bad, if it clearly does. *See Chapter 30: Communication.*

B. Intravenous therapies.
1. Definition: delivery through peripheral or central vein.
2. Advantages.
   a. Rapid delivery to central circulation.
   b. Avoids first-pass hepatic metabolism.
   c. Reliable dosing.
   d. Ease of delivery once device is in place.
3. Disadvantages.
   a. More rapid onset of toxic effects.
   b. Increased risk of infection.
   c. Inadvertent delivery of medications to surrounding tissues may cause damage.
   d. Insertion of peripheral or central venous access device often may be difficult and/or painful.
   e. Usually requires IV pump for safe delivery in infants and young children.
   f. Difficult to stabilize device in active child.

C. Enteral route of administration.
1. Definition: delivery through the oral/gastric system.
   a. Tips to facilitate delivery.
      (1) Stroking the neck encourages swallowing.
      (2) Pursing lips prevents spitting.
      (3) Deliver ½ cc of liquid by syringe inside cheek at a time and wait for infant to swallow.
   b. Avoid mixing medications in formula.
2. Advantages.
   a. Doesn't require specialized training or equipment.
   b. Reliable dosing.
   c. Ease of use.
3. Disadvantages.
   a. Medication must pass through hepatic metabolism.
   b. Slow onset.
   c. Taste/consistency/odor can affect compliance.
   d. Administration timing may need to be coordinated around meals.

D. Intraosseous infusion.
1. Definition: delivery through the bone marrow to the central circulation via the nutrient veins.
   a. Specially designed needle usually placed in the femur or tibia.
   b. Can be used to deliver any medication/fluid given intravenously including blood products.
2. Advantages.
   a. Rapid delivery to central circulation.
   b. Avoids first-pass hepatic circulation.
   c. Reliable dosing.
   d. Ease of delivery once device is in place.
   e. Can be placed quickly and accurately after minimal training.
3. Disadvantages.
   a. More rapid onset of toxic effects.
   b. Increased risk of infection.
   c. Inadvertent delivery of medications/fluid to surrounding tissues may cause damage.
   d. Requires insertion of intraosseous device.
   e. Stabilization of device can be difficult.
   f. Device should be left in place no longer than 24 hours and should be considered a bridge to other delivery methods only.

E. Ophthalmic route of administration.
1. Definition: delivery through the mucous membranes of the conjunctiva.
   a. May directly pass to the central circulation.
   b. Delivery of drops easier than ointment.
   c. Place medication in lower conjunctival sac avoiding the cornea.
2. Advantages.
   a. Rapid delivery.
   b. Avoids first-pass hepatic metabolism.
3. Disadvantages.
   a. Delivery of medication to active or resistant child difficult.
   b. Blurred vision possible after administration.
   c. Increased risk of spreading infection via contaminated medication container.
   d. Inadvertent systemic effects of medication.

F. Transdermal route of administration.
1. Definition: delivery through the skin.
   a. Affected by variety of factors, including skin thickness, blood flow, surface area, medication pH, lipid solubility, and application dose.
   b. Examples: fentanyl patches, EMLA®, nitroglycerine paste, and TAC (tetracaine, adrenaline, cocaine).
2. Advantages.
   a. Delivery to local or central circulation.
   b. Avoids first-pass hepatic circulation.
   c. Ease of delivery.
   d. 24-hour delivery possible with patches.
3. Disadvantages.
   a. Slow onset and erratic medication distribution.
   b. Inability to control dosing accuracy may increase toxic effects.
   c. Inadvertent systemic effects of medication.
   d. Not to be applied to damaged skin, poorly vascularized areas, or mucous membranes.
   e. Localized allergic responses or skin irritation may occur via patch.

G. Respiratory tract route of administration.
1. Definition: delivery through the mucous membranes of the respiratory tract.
   a. May directly pass to central circulation.
   b. Influenced by many factors, including particle size, lipid solubility, and method/site of administration.
   c. Examples include operative anesthetics, ß-agonists, corticosteroids, antiviral agents, surfactant, resuscitation medications, nitric oxide, helium, and oxygen.
2. Advantages.
   a. Rapid delivery to local or central circulation.
   b. Avoids first-pass hepatic metabolism.
   c. Ease of use.

   d. Can be used in place of intravenous/intraosseous access to deliver medications during resuscitation.
3. Disadvantages.
   a. Delivery of medication to active or resistant child difficult.
   b. More rapid onset of toxic effects.
   c. Taste/consistency/odor affects compliance.
   d. Inadvertent local or systemic effects of medication possible.
   e. Requires trained staff and sophisticated equipment/facilities for delivery of anesthetics/gases.

H. Nasal route of administration.
1. Definition: delivery through the mucous membranes of the nasal passages.
   a. May directly pass to central circulation.
   b. Examples: vasopressin, corticosteroids, narcotics, and sedatives.
2. Advantages.
   a. Rapid delivery to local or central circulation.
   b. Avoids first-pass hepatic metabolism.
   c. Ease of use.
3. Disadvantages.
   a. Delivery of medication to active or resistant child difficult.
   b. More rapid onset of toxic effects.
   c. Smell/taste/discomfort may affect compliance.
   d. Inadvertent local or systemic effects of medication may occur.

I. Oral mucosa as route of administration.
1. Definition: delivery through the tissues of the oral mucosa. Examples: nitroglycerin and fentanyl lozenges.
2. Advantages.
   a. Rapid delivery to central circulation.
   b. Avoids first-pass hepatic metabolism.
   c. Ease of use.
3. Disadvantages.
   a. Taste/consistency affect compliance.
   b. Dosing directly related to mucosal exposure time requires patient cooperation.
   c. Inadvertent systemic effects of medication may occur.

J. Rectal route of administration.
1. Definition: delivery through the rectal mucosa.
   a. May directly pass to central circulation.
   b. Medication absorption depends on a variety of factors: medication form and volume, venous drainage of the rectal vault, and presence or absence of stool.
   c. Examples: antipyretics, analgesics, antiemetics,

sedatives, and enemas.
2. Advantages.
   a. Drugs delivered high in the rectum must first-pass hepatic metabolism; drugs delivered low in the rectum are delivered systemically.
   b. Ease of use.
   c. Can be used in place of intravenous/oral access to deliver medication and fluids.
   d. Generally well tolerated in infants and young children.
3. Disadvantages.
   a. Slow onset.
   b. Absorption erratic; subsequently, dosing may vary.
   c. Inadvertent local or systemic effects of medication may occur.
   d. Use in immunosuppressed children to be avoided as even minimal trauma may lead to bacteremia or abscess.
   e. May require placement of rectal tube; stabilization in active child may be difficult.

K. Intramuscular route of administration.
1. Definition: delivery into muscle mass.
   a. May pass quickly to central circulation.
   b. Historically, needles have been used as the most common delivery device. The jet carbon dioxide injector, however, allows needle-less delivery and enjoys increasing popularity in the pediatric setting.
   c. Gluteus muscles should not be used until children are walking.
   d. Deltoid and vastus lateralis muscles preferred.
   e. Example: antibiotics.
2. Advantages.
   a. Relative speed of delivery to central circulation.
   b. Avoids first-pass hepatic metabolism.
   c. Ease of use.
3. Disadvantages.
   a. Increased risk of infection/abscess.
   b. Inadvertent delivery of medications to subcutaneous tissues damaging.
   c. Inadvertent delivery directly into venous system.
   d. Delivery of medication to active or resistant child can be difficult.
   e. Residual, temporary pain at delivery site; EMLA® may be used prior to injection.
   f. Functional damage with inappropriate site selection/needle insertion.

L. Otic route of administration.
1. Definition: delivery into external auditory canal.
   a. Cotton used to hold medication in canal.
   b. Warm otic solutions between palms prior to administration.
   c. Pull pinna of ear downward and back for infants and young children to straighten canal.
   d. Examples: ceruminolytics and local anesthetics.
2. Advantages.
   a. Delivery to site immediate.
   b. Rapid onset.
3. Disadvantages.
   a. Delivery of medication to active or resistant child can be difficult.
   b. Discomfort may affect compliance.
   c. Cannot be used when tympanic membrane perforated.

II. VASCULAR ACCESS DEVICES

A. Overview.
1. Central venous line access (CVL) can be used to deliver fluids, nutrition, and medications while simultaneously providing valuable information regarding central venous pressure and even cardiac output.
2. CVLs can also be used to obtain blood specimens; this is especially helpful for the small child with limited vascular access.
3. Peripheral venous lines (PVLs) may also be used to deliver fluids, limited nutrition, and medications.
   a. Cannot be used to monitor central venous pressure.
   b. Not large enough to allow for blood sampling.
4. All venous access lines are of increased risk for infection.
   a. Central lines require meticulous attention to site care, dressing integrity, and line entry disinfection if life-threatening infections are to be avoided.
   b. Care of these lines is described in *Chapter 21: Chronic Conditions: Care Technologies*.
5. Arterial lines may be used for blood pressure monitoring and blood sampling.
   a. Risk of infection is less than with central venous access.
   b. Complications, such as arterial spasm and hemorrhage, may occur.

B. Peripheral venous catheter insertion.
1. Indications for use.
   a. Fluid/nutrient administration.
   b. Medication administration.
   c. Blood administration.
   d. Blood sampling.
2. Contraindications.
   a. Cellulitis.
   b. Underlying fracture.

c. Deep vessel insertion for children with uncorrected coagulopathies.
3. Complications.
   a. Phlebitis.
   b. Infiltration.
   c. Tendon/nerve damage.
   d. Air embolus.
   e. Infection.
4. Equipment.
   a. Needle device.
      (1) Butterfly needle: primarily used for blood sampling, difficult to secure for long-term use, lowest risk of infection.
      (2) Catheter-over-needle: most common device for long-term use; risk of infection increases with time.
      (3) Needle-over-catheter: less commonly used; requires greater training to insert; can be used for long-term access; highest risk of infection; care similar to central venous catheters.
   b. Padded arm/leg board (appropriate length).
   c. Cloth tape.
   d. Gauze 2x2.
   e. Betadine solution swab.
   f. Transparent or other dressing.
   g. Protective IV cover.
   h. Tourniquet.
   i. T-connector.
      (1) Allows for entry port at site of insertion.
      (2) Provides for stabilization of tubing in active child.
   j. EMLA®.
      (1) May be used for insertion site anesthesia.
      (2) Apply to insertion site 1-2 hours prior to procedure.
      (3) Place protective covering over site to prevent ingestion by curious child.
5. Keypoints for catheter-over-needle insertion techniques.
   a. Wash hands.
   b. Don nonsterile gloves.
   c. Choose venous access site.
      (1) Scalp veins may be used in the young infant.
      (2) Palpate the site for pulsations as arteries may resemble veins.
      (3) Prepare insertion site by cutting hair and/or shaving small area.
      (4) Save hair for caretakers as this may represent the infant's first hair cut. (Some cultures do not cut the infant's hair until at least 1 year old in a formal ceremony.) Caretaker teaching and preparation are vital.
      (5) The lower extremities may be used in infants and children.
      (6) Transillumination with a small flashlight is often helpful in identifying venous access sites in infants.
   d. Secure site.
      (1) Padded arm/leg boards may be used before or after venous access.
      (2) Back tape with gauze whenever possible to reduce skin irritation.
      (3) Do not use sharp edged tapes such as plastic.
      (4) Do not place tape directly over antecubital space or near axilla as it can become a constrictive tourniquet.
      (5) Do not place tape over vessel proximal to venous access and reduce visibility.
   e. Clean site with betadine solution or according to agency policy.
   f. Place tourniquet.
      (1) For scalp veins, a rubber band with tape tab may be used.
         (a) Lift the rubber band by the tab after insertion and cut with scissors for removal.
         (b) Never allow rubber band to lay over infant's eyes.
      (2) Tourniquets restrict venous return and dilate veins.
         (a) They should not restrict arterial blood flow.
         (b) If tissue discoloration/mottling occur, release tourniquet, allow blood flow to return, and reapply.
   g. Tips for catheter insertion.
      (1) Pull skin taut and insert needle into vein at 45° angle.
      (2) Keep fingers to sides of device rather than under device to keep this angle.
      (3) Advance needle very slowly. Infants may have very slow blood return in needle device.
      (4) Never remove needle from skin or catheter and then reinsert. This can result in:
         (a) Increased risk of infection.
         (b) Risk of catheter shearing.
      (5) Slowly advance catheter over needle into vein.
      (6) Attach t-connector.
         (a) May withdraw blood specimen.
         (b) May infuse normal saline flush.
      (7) Catheter hub may be secured with tape.
         (a) Do not place tape over vessel proximal to catheter.
         (b) Apply transparent dressing or bandage over insertion site.
      (8) Secure tubing to arm/leg board to prevent inadvertent dislodging of catheter.

h. Write date/time on dressing. When possible, venous access devices should be removed within 72 hours to prevent infection.

III. MOBILITY/IMMOBILITY IN THE ACUTELY ILL/INJURED CHILD

A. Overview.
Mobility is quickly impaired even during the mildest illness. With prolonged hospitalizations or chronic illness, the effects of immobility can be profound. Untreated, the effects of immobility complicate recovery and prolong convalescence. These effects, therefore, should be anticipated, and with nursing vigilance be minimized and/or prevented.

B. Causes of immobility in children.
1. Primary injury/disorder (e.g., fractures).
2. Fear.
3. Pain.
4. Secondary to treatment (e.g., surgery, traction, casts, devices).

C. Effects of immobility.
1. Venous stasis/edema.
2. Paresthesia.
3. Constipation.
4. Urinary retention.
5. Skin breakdown.
6. Muscle wasting and protein breakdown.
7. Contractures and bone demineralization.
8. Atelectasis.
9. Depression, isolation, boredom, sensory deprivation, psychosis.

D. Nursing interventions.
1. Allow for mobilization whenever possible.
   a. Specialty beds.
   b. Wheelchairs/wagons.
   c. Overhead pull-up bars/triangles.
   d. Sitting up in chair or parent's arms.
2. Active and passive range of motion.
3. Splints.
4. Skin care/massage.
5. Hydration/nutrition.
6. Pulmonary toilet.
7. Position changes every 1–2 hours.
8. Sparing use of physical and pharmacologic restraints.
9. Toys, videos, mobiles, tapes, touch, telephones, stories, and games for entertainment, distraction, and sensory/social stimulation.
10. Casts and cast care.
    a. Casts may be used to immobilize (fractures,

joints, postspinal fusions, severe sprains/strains).
    b. There are two major types of material used: plaster and fiberglass.
       (1) Plaster/gauze.
           (a) Malleable: excellent medium for fractures requiring delicate resetting maneuvers such as those involving growth plates.
           (b) Stockinette lines the cast and folds over the ends to provide a smooth edge; cotton batting is usually molded over bony prominences.
           (c) Heat produced while drying may be uncomfortable.
           (d) Must wait several hours for curing to complete.
           (e) Water dissolves plaster.
           (f) Significantly less expensive than fiberglass.
       (2) Fiberglass/resin.
           (a) Not very malleable; however, more rigid than plaster, making it an excellent medium for long bone and weight-bearing fractures.
           (b) Usually lined with stockinette and cotton as is plaster; can be unlined, which is more irritating to skin.
           (c) Should not be exposed to water if stockinette or cotton lined; may be dried with a cool hairdryer as water will not affect fiberglass integrity.
           (d) Can be used immediately.
    c. Tips for caring for children in a cast.
       (1) Cast should be elevated for the first 24 hours; elevation increases comfort and decreases swelling.
       (2) Do not use powders or creams inside cast. Use cool hairdryer to treat pruritus.
       (3) Personal hygiene should be meticulous; bedding and chairs kept clean so debris less likely to collect inside cast.
       (4) Note all odors and report immediately.
       (5) Report a broken or loose cast immediately.
       (6) Standard seatbelt restraint devices cannot be used for children in spica casts. Contact orthopedic clinic for assistance in providing alternate restraint options.
    d. Compartment syndrome can be limb threatening. It follows swelling/compression that compromises venous return, arterial flow, and nerve conduction, and most commonly occurs within the first 24 hours after casting swollen wrists or ankles. It is customary for posterior molds/splints to be applied to edematous extremities; they are replaced with casts after the swelling

has subsided. The following signs and symptoms should be reported immediately:
 (1) Worsening pain from ischemia.
 (2) Pallor from arterial compression/venous stasis.
 (3) Paresis from muscle/nerve compression.
 (4) Paresthesia from nerve compression.
 (5) Pulselessness from arterial occlusion.
11. Traction.
 a. When fractures cannot be realigned with casting materials alone, traction is required.
 b. Traction can be applied with skin adhesion products (skin traction) and/or pins placed directly into bone (skeletal traction).
 c. Pulleys and weights provide a mechanism of counterforces that reapproximate the bony ends and can be used with either skin or skeletal traction.
 d. The Ilizarov external fixation device is a form of traction that can be used on an outpatient basis to lengthen long bones or fixate fractures.
 e. Nursing interventions.
  (1) Once skeletal traction device is in place, it must never be discontinued by the nurse. Use manual traction during rewrapping of skin adhesive devices or when repositioning.
  (2) Check for proper body alignment every 1–2 hours.
  (3) Check weight and pulley system every 1–2 hours.
   (a) Keep weights off floor.
   (b) May need to restrain child's upper body to maintain position.
  (4) Examine all extremities for circulatory impairment or pain.
  (5) Examine bedding frequently as lost food, wrinkled sheets, and small objects can irritate and abrade.
  (6) Clean pin sites per protocol.

IV. NUTRITIONAL MANAGEMENT OF THE ACUTELY ILL/INJURED CHILD

◆ ◆ ◆ ◆ ◆ ◆ ◆ ◆ ◆ ◆ ◆ ◆ ◆ ◆ ◆ ◆ ◆ ◆

A. Overview.
 Each child should have his/her nutritional management individualized. Infants and young children should not have their nutrition withheld for longer than 3 days. Malnutrition occurs quickly during serious illness, trauma, or infection as children have little metabolic reserve and increased demand. Inadequate nutritional intake can lead to prolonged convalescence and/or hospitalization.

B. Nutrition can be delivered enterally, parenterally, or as a combination of both methods
 It can be delivered by mouth, nasogastric/gastric tubes, nasojejunal tubes, or peripheral or central veins. Families can be taught to use any of these methods in the home setting.

C. Calculation of nutritional requirements.
 1. Fluid requirement.
  1–10 kg=100 ml/kg/day
  10–20 kg=1000 ml + 50 ml for each kg>10
  >20 kg=1500 ml + 20 ml for each kg>20
 2. Estimating energy needs (see Table 13-1).
  a. Caloric requirement (see Tables 13-2 and 13-3).
  b. Protein requirement. *See Chapter 21: Chronic Conditions: Care Technologies.*

D. Enteral feedings. *Also see Chapter 21: Chronic Conditions: Care Technologies.*
 1. The intestines make up one of the largest immune organs in the body.
  a. When intestinal route not used, the body loses a barrier to infection and allows for bacterial invasion.
  b. Whenever possible, the enteral route should be used for nutritional delivery even if used in combination with parenteral nutrition.
 2. Types of liquid enteral nutrition.
  a. Breast milk: considered best formula for infants as it contains cellular and acellular immunoprotective elements.
  b. Elemental formulas, such as Vivonex®, Pregestimil®, and Alimentum® contain very simple protein, carbohydrate, and fat preparations that are more readily digested when bowel function has been altered.
  c. Nonelemental formulas, such as Enfamil®, Similac®, and Prosobee®, contain proteins, carbohydrates, and fat from traditional sources. May be lactose, casein, or long-chain triglyceride free.
  d. Modular formulas, such as Suplena®, Pulmocare®, and Glucerna®, contain special supplementation that treats specific problems, such as cystic fibrosis.
  e. Hydrating and rehydrating fluids such as Pedialyte® and Rehydralyte® contain glucose and electrolytes.
 3. Tube placement and care. *See Chapter 21: Chronic Conditions: Care Technologies.*
  a. Differences between oral, nasal, and jejunal tubes.
  b. Measurement and placement of OG/NG tubes in infants and children.
  c. Special feeding needs.
 4. Special considerations.

Table 13-1
Energy Source Distribution

	Infants	Older children
Protein	7–16%	7–9%
Carbohydrates	35–65%	35–65%
Fat	30–55%	30–55%

Table 13-2
Caloric Requirements

0–1 years of age	90–120 kcal/kg/day
1–7 years of age	75–90 kcal/kg/day
7–12 years of age	60–75 kcal/kg/day
12–18 years of age	30–60 kcal/kg/day

Table 13-3
Conditions Increasing Caloric Requirements

Fever	12% for each degree above 37°C
Cardiac failure	15-25%
Major surgery	20-30%
Burns	up to 100%
Severe sepsis/infection	40-50%
Long-term growth failure	50-100%
Trauma	10-80%
Energy source distribution	% of total calories (see Table 13-1)

a. Use pacifiers to stimulate nonnutritive sucking.
b. Follow protocol for tube feeding and post-feeding care.
5. Complications of enteral feedings.
a. Aspiration.
b. Tube displacement/erosions.
c. Diarrhea.

E. Parenteral Feedings. *Also see Chapter 21: Chronic Conditions: Care Technologies.*
1. Parenteral nutrition is used to restore or maintain adequate nutritional intake in children who cannot be fed enterally. It is also indicated in any infant or child who is unable to meet his/her requirements enterally for 3 or more days.
2. Common indications for use.
a. Congenital or acquired anomalies of the gastrointestinal tract including:
(1) Short gut syndrome.
(2) Radiation enteritis.
(3) Acute pancreatitis.
(4) Abdominal surgery.
(5) Enteric fistula.
(6) Inflammatory bowel disease.
(7) Intractable vomiting or diarrhea.
(8) Bowel obstruction.
(9) Paralytic ileus.
(10) Necrotizing enterocolitis.
b. Hypermetabolic states (i.e., severe trauma, sepsis, burns, cancer).
c. Chylothorax.
d. Cardiorespiratory disease.
e. Renal/hepatic failure.
f. Inborn errors of metabolism.
g. Low birth weight and high risk infants.

3. Complications of parenteral feedings.
a. Infection: amino acids and dextrose solutions support fungal growth, and fat provides an excellent medium for bacterial and fungal growth. Translocation of bacteria through unused bowel wall can lead to sepsis.
b. Mechanical problems: pneumothorax, thrombus, phlebitis, and vessel wall erosions.
c. Metabolic problems: hyperglycemia, electrolyte imbalances, hyperlipidemia, cholestasis, and chronic liver dysfunction are not uncommon.

F. Nutritional monitoring.
1. Height and weight. While acutely ill, children's weights should be recorded daily and heights weekly, with both documented on a growth chart. After initial weight loss, newborns should gain approximately 25 grams/day.
2. Laboratory studies. Electrolytes and liver function tests should be obtained prior to nutritional supplements and once to twice weekly thereafter. If receiving parenteral fat, triglycerides should also be monitored.
3. Urine should be tested daily for glucose, ketones, and specific gravity.
4. Intake and output should be documented daily.

V. OXYGENATION AND VENTILATION
◆ ◆ ◆ ◆ ◆ ◆ ◆ ◆ ◆ ◆ ◆ ◆ ◆ ◆ ◆ ◆ ◆ ◆ ◆ ◆

A. Overview.
Infants and young children have poorly developed respiratory tracts that mature by the age of 7 to 8 years, yet twice the metabolic need for oxygen. This places them at risk for hypoxemia and hypoventilation when there is additional impair-

ment of respiratory function due to infection, illness, or trauma. *See Chapter 1: Biologic Development.*

1. Respiratory failure is the most common pathway to cardiac arrest in young children.
2. Examples of those at risk include those with upper respiratory infection, head or chest trauma, reactive airway disease, croup, sedatives/analgesics, hydrocarbon ingestion, smoke inhalation, foreign body aspiration, pneumonia, craniofacial abnormality, and endotracheal tubes/tracheostomy.

B. Recognition of respiratory failure.

1. Vital signs: alterations in vital signs may predict impending respiratory failure.
   a. Heart rate: with increased metabolic demand for O_2, heart rate should increase; decreased heart rate is impending sign of failure.
   b. Respiratory rate: with increased metabolic demand for O_2, respiratory rate should increase; decreased respiratory rate not related to therapy is impending sign of fatigue and failure.
   c. Pulse oximetry reports the saturation of hemoglobin with oxygen.
      (1) PaO_2 equals pulse oximeter reading when saturations are >95%.
      (2) Saturations of 90% reflect PaO_2 of approximately 60%.
      (3) Alterations in hemoglobin concentration or form affect accuracy of readings.
      (4) Carbon monoxide binds with hemoglobin more readily than oxygen and will also alter accuracy.
      (5) Readings < 95% support use of supplemental oxygen.
      (6) Readings < 90% in room air represent hypoxemia. If these continue despite appropriate therapy, may represent impending respiratory failure.
   d. End-tidal CO_2 can be measured by nasal prongs or device on endotracheal/tracheostomy tube.
      (1) Usually within 5 mm/Hg of $PaCO_2$.
      (2) Rising readings may represent hypoventilation or CO_2 retention.
      (3) Low readings may represent a displaced endotracheal tube.
2. Signs and symptoms of impending respiratory failure.
   a. Changing level of consciousness: as hypoxemia progresses, irritability and agitation increase.
      (1) Elevations in CO_2 lead to lethargy.
      (2) Sedated patients may not display level of consciousness changes.
   b. Work of breathing: nasal flaring, head bobbing, stridor, grunting, retractions, or paradoxical chest/abdominal movement may develop.
   c. Air entry: decreased chest wall movement or unequal or absent breath sounds are ominous signs.
   d. Color: as hypoxemia and hypoventilation progress, color becomes pale, ashen/gray, then cyanotic.
      (1) Cyanosis can be a very late sign and is not specific to respiratory failure.
      (2) Cyanosis is dependent upon circulating hemoglobin and may also present in shock, cyanotic heart defects, and hypothermia.

C. Nursing interventions for impending respiratory failure.

1. Maintain position of comfort with head of bed elevated or in caregiver's arms if not contraindicated, such as in cervical spine trauma.
2. Maintain normothermia and NPO status as temperature instability and feeding activity increases metabolic demand for O_2.
3. Place on cardiorespiratory and pulse oximetry monitors.
4. Maximize O_2 delivery (see methods listed below).

D. Nursing interventions for respiratory failure.

1. Elevate head of bed if not contraindicated.
2. Maintain normothermia and NPO status.
3. Initiate IV therapy.
4. Place on cardiorespiratory and pulse oximetry monitors.
5. Maximize O_2 delivery and assist ventilation if necessary (see methods listed below).
6. Decompress abdomen if distention impedes ventilation.

E. Oxygen delivery methods.

1. O_2 should be humidified since tachypnea and mouth breathing decrease the water saturation of gases reaching the alveoli, which may impair mucociliary function. Warming should be added for neonates and those with endotracheal/tracheostomy tubes since cool gases may contribute to hypothermia.
2. Blow-by/face tent: one size.
   a. O_2 dependent on gas flow and proximity to face.
   b. Used for minimal signs and symptoms of impending respiratory failure.
3. Simple face mask: infant, pediatric, and adult sizes.
   a. O_2 delivery dependent on minute ventilation, gas flow, mask fit.
   b. Used for minimal signs and symptoms of impending respiratory failure.

4. Nasal cannula: infant, pediatric, and adult sizes.
   a. O_2 delivery dependent on minute ventilation and gas flow.
   b. Rates of up to 3 liters/minute tolerated in children, which is approximately equal to F_iO_2 .3–.4.
   c. Used for minimal to moderate signs and symptoms of impending respiratory failure. Better tolerated than face masks.
5. Venturi masks: pediatric and adult sizes.
   a. High flow system that entrains room air and delivers fixed dilution of O_2 depending on face mask fit.
   b. Can deliver up to F_iO_2 .5.
   c. Used for minimal to moderate signs and symptoms of impending respiratory failure.
6. Nonrebreathing and partial rebreathing masks: come in infant, pediatric, and adult sizes.
   a. High flow systems where delivery of F_iO_2 1.0 to reservoir bag exceeds minute ventilation.
      (1) A one-way valve separates bag from mask. As infant inhales, the valve opens and O_2 is inspired. The valve then closes and CO_2 is exhaled through the side ports.
      (2) Reservoir bag should be inflated approximately ⅔ full.
   b. Limited by infant's inspiratory force. Can deliver F_iO_2 0.7–1.0, depending upon face mask fit.
   c. Used for moderate to severe signs and symptoms of impending respiratory failure.
7. Bag/valve/mask device: neonate, infant, and pediatric sizes.
   a. Bag/mask to face or bag/endotracheal/tracheostomy tube.
   b. Can deliver any O_2 dilution with use of blender.
   c. Available in self-inflating and anesthesia versions.
   d. Used for respiratory failure and ventilation delivery.
   e. Oral airway may improve delivery technique.

F. Airway adjuncts.
1. Oral airways: many sizes.
   a. Produce significant gag response; used in unconscious patient.
   b. Helpful adjunct to bag/valve/mask ventilation.
   c. Sized from the teeth to the ramus of the mandible.
2. Nasopharyngeal airway: many sizes.
   a. Better tolerated by conscious patients.
   b. Sized from the nares to the tragus of the ear.
   c. Can occlude with secretions; therefore, may require frequent suctioning to maintain patency.

3. Endotracheal tubes (ETT): sizes 2.5 mm through adult.
   a. Larger sizes have cuffs. Children approximately 7–8 years of age have cylindrical-shaped tracheas similar to adults.
   b. Smaller sizes are uncuffed as young children have natural narrowing at cricoid cartilage.
   c. Endotracheal tubes do not provide secure airways and should be closely monitored to maintain their stability.
   d. Suction when necessary to keep free of secretions. See agency protocols.
   e. Resecure as often as necessary.
   f. No traction or tension must be placed on the ETT, as minimal tube displacement may result in extubation. This is especially true during suctioning, weighing, and other daily maneuvers.
   g. Inadvertent carinal stimulation may result in bradycardia and/or bronchospasm.
   h. Inadvertent mainstem bronchus intubation may result in atelectasis of the nonventilated lung and hyperexpansion/pneumothorax of the ventilated lung.
   i. Report ETT marking at lip or gum line.
   j. Appropriate size face mask and bag/valve device always must be immediately accessible should inadvertent extubation/obstruction occur.
4. Tracheostomy tubes: neonatal through adult sizes.
   a. Cuffed tubes available as with endotracheal tubes.
   b. Suction when necessary to keep free of secretions.
   c. When first placed, outer cannula must not be changed for at least 7 days or according to agency protocol. During this time the tracheotomy does not provide secure airway and should be closely monitored and carefully suctioned to maintain stability; sutures are usually placed to assist in recannulation, if necessary.
   d. Skin abrasion/erosion can occur under chin, around stoma, and under securing device. Meticulous skin care is required. Many securing devices are available; metal ball chains have been promoted for children as they roll over skin rather than bind.
   e. Care of the inner cannula and trach site must be done frequently. Follow agency protocols.
   f. Appropriate size spare tube must always be immediately accessible should inadvertent decannulation/obstruction occur.

G. Ventilation methods.

The goals of ventilation include to improve gas exchange, treat respiratory muscle fatigue/atrophy, alter lung pressures/volumes, expand airways, and permit lung and airway healing. Disadvantages include barotrauma and intrathoracic pressure changes that can lead to decreased cardiac output and increased intracranial pressure. Families can be taught to use many of these methods in the home setting.

1. CPAP: continuous positive airway pressure.
   a. Constant, external pressure to expand airways during child's own respirations.
   b. Can be applied through a conventional ventilator to an ETT/trach or through nasal prongs/mask.
   c. Disadvantage to nasal prongs/mask is gastric insufflation and occasional agitation.
2. BIPAP: bilevel positive airway pressure. CPAP plus pressure support (see below) delivered during the child's own respirations.
   a. May expand airways and treat respiratory muscle fatigue/atrophy.
   b. Intermediate step to full ventilatory support.
   c. Delivered through face mask.
   d. Disadvantage is gastric insufflation and agitation.
3. Mechanical ventilation.
   a. Pressure control ventilators.
      (1) Deliver a preset pressure above PEEP (see below).
      (2) Deliver higher pressures at the beginning of a breath that decreases by the end of inspiration. Lung compliance and resistance will alter delivered volume of gas.
      (3) Used for neonates and young infants.
   b. Volume control ventilators.
      (1) Deliver a preset volume of gas.
      (2) Maintain constant volume with each respiration regardless of lung compliance or resistance.
      (3) Used for older infants and young children.

H. Mechanical ventilation modes.

1. PEEP: positive end expiratory pressure.
   a. Alveolar distending pressure controlled during mechanical ventilation as a baseline.
   b. Replaces the pressures provided by the nasopharyngeal vault in the spontaneously breathing child.
   c. Baseline physiologic PEEP is approximately 3–4 cm of H_2O.
   d. Higher pressures may be needed to distend airways but also increase intrathoracic pressure, which may decrease venous return.
2. SIMV: synchronized intermittent mandatory ventilation.
   a. Delivers preset number of breaths synchronized with the child's own respirations.
   b. Breaths taken by the child beyond the preset number receive continuous gas flow or pressure support (see below).
3. Assist/control ventilation: preset delivery with every spontaneous breath the child takes. Should the child fail to take a breath, a preset number of breaths will be delivered.
4. Pressure support ventilation: all spontaneous breaths of the infant/child are supported.
   a. The volume, pressure, and duration of flow are all determined by the inspiratory effort of the child.
   b. Used as a weaning method from more traditional ventilation.
   c. Measured as the pressure desired above the baseline PEEP.
5. High frequency oscillator ventilation: increases gas exchange with smaller volumes of gas delivered at rates up to 3,000 breaths/minute. Used to reduce effects of barotrauma in infants and young children.
6. High frequency jet ventilation: jet of gas delivered through special ETT at rates of 60–200 breaths/minute. Also used to reduce effects of barotrauma and treat hypoxemia.
7. Liquid ventilation: replaces gaseous lung volume with perfluorocarbon. Conventional ventilation is then employed.
   a. Reduces alveolar surface tension and improves lung compliance.
   b. Requires maintenance of perfluorocarbon levels in the lung during therapy.
8. ECMO: extracorporeal membrane oxygenation. Gas exchange is provided by an external circuit similar to those used in heart-lung bypass surgery.
   a. Extremely invasive.
   b. Allows for lung and airway healing in select infant/child population with refractory respiratory failure.

I. Gas options.

1. Subambient oxygen: oxygen content less than that of room air (21%), produced by mixing nitrogen with oxygen. Increases pulmonary resistance. Blood diverted to systemic circulation when cardiac shunts are present such as in hypoplastic left heart syndrome.
2. Heliox: combination of helium and oxygen.
   a. Mixed at concentrations of 70% helium and 30% oxygen.
   b. Less dense than air; used when airway resistance is high, such as in croup or status asthmaticus.

3. Nitric oxide: relaxes lung vascular and airway smooth muscle, thus reducing pulmonary resistance.
   a. Usually delivered mixed with oxygen at 20-80 ppm.
   b. Known byproducts include nitrogen dioxide and methemoglobin; both levels require monitoring during therapy.
   c. Used for severe pulmonary hypertension.

VI. POSTOPERATIVE CARE OF THE ACUTELY ILL/INJURED CHILD

◆ ◆

A. Overview.

Care of a child after surgery can be divided into distinct phases. The first phase is the immediate return of the infant or child from the operating room; the second phase is the subsequent 24–48 hours; and the last relates to preparation for maximal wellness.

B. Immediate postoperative period.

1. Ensure that the unit is ready to accept the infant/child from the operating room.
   a. Appropriate size crib or bed; overhead warmers should be used for neonates as cold stress increases oxygen and glucose demands which may lead to hypoxia, hypoglycemia, acidosis, and pulmonary hypertension.
   b. Monitoring equipment for heart rate, respiratory rate, blood pressure, oxygen saturation, and end-tidal CO_2 is needed. If other parameters are to be monitored such as pulmonary artery or central venous pressures, this equipment will also be needed.
   c. Pumps to deliver fluids and medications.
   d. Airway equipment includes bag/valve/mask, oxygen, suction, and readily available reintubation equipment. Ventilator if intubated; extra tracheostomy setup if appropriate.
   e. List of emergency drug doses by the infant/child's weight by bedside.
   f. Extra suction setup for chest tube drainage if applicable.
2. Report from the operative staff should include:
   a. Type and duration of anesthesia.
   b. Untoward events.
   c. Blood loss.
   d. Length of time on heart/lung bypass, aortic cross-clamp time, or cold arrest time if applicable.
   e. Intake/output during surgery.
   f. Size of endotracheal/tracheostomy tube and ventilator settings if applicable.

3. When transferring child to postoperative crib/bed and pumps (varies with institution):
   a. Support/secure ETT during transfer, if present.
   b. Secure all lines/tubes prior to transfer.
   c. Assess airway status immediately after transfer especially if ETT present.
   d. Untangle/secure all lines/tubes after transfer.
   e. Smooth all bedding under child and view back for intraoperative injury. Prolonged surgeries and those with cautery or cold arrest increase the risk for burns, abrasions, and skin breakdowns.
4. Obtain a complete set of vital signs and perform nursing assessment every 5 minutes for the first 30 minutes, then every 15 minutes until stable. Assessment to include:
   a. Neuro status.
      (1) Movement/sensation in all extremities.
      (2) Level of consciousness.
      (3) Pupillary response.
   b. Cardiovascular status.
      (1) Heart rate, blood pressure.
      (2) Distal/proximal pulses, skin temperature/color, capillary refill all extremities.
      (3) Shunt/valve murmurs if applicable.
   c. Respiratory status.
      (1) Airway patency.
      (2) Spontaneity of respirations.
      (3) Depth, regularity, and equality of respirations.
   d. Body temperature status.
      (1) Elevated body temperatures can represent a normal variant following cardiovascular surgery, decreased cardiac output syndrome, or infection. May predispose infant/child to junctional ectopic tachycardia in those with preexisting rhythm abnormalities. Increases metabolic demand.
      (2) Depressed body temperatures, especially in the neonate, may lead to cold stress.
5. Check all fluids/blood and medications being administered for correct drug/fluid/blood type and dose.
6. Obtain blood specimens (varies with surgical procedure). Record specimen sample size on output sheet for neonates as this can accumulate to significant loss for body size.
7. Obtain chest x-ray (varies with surgical procedure).
8. Check placement/patency of all lines and tubes.
   a. ETT by auscultation and chest x-ray, note location marking on tube at lip or gum line.
   b. Central lines and chest tubes on chest x-ray.
   c. Nasogastric tubes by auscultation or chest x-ray.

    d. Indwelling urinary catheters by drainage.
9. Monitor bleeding. Report immediately drainage that increases or becomes more sanguinous from:
    a. Surgical site.
    b. Drainage tubes.
10. Keep accurate intake and output of all fluids.
11. Evaluate pain and sedation needs. *See Chapter 22: Chronic Conditions: Symptom Management.*
12. Allow caretakers to visit even if visit must be limited to a few minutes as this will facilitate family coping. Orient parents to child's care. *See Chapter 20: Chronic Conditions: Effects on the Child's Family* and *Chapter 23: Chronic Conditions: Intervention Strategies.*

C. The next 24–48 hours of the postoperative period.
1. Continuously evaluate pain and sedation needs. The effects of pain are deleterious to recovery and include catecholamine surges, splinting, increased metabolic demands, and mental discomfort/anguish.
2. Monitor vital signs every 1–4 hours depending on the surgical procedure. Report sudden increases/decreases and trends. Report all temperature elevations.
3. Monitor bleeding from:
    a. Surgical site.
    b. Drainage tubes if applicable.
4. Monitor for infection related to surgical procedure, immobility, or lines/tubes.
    a. Atelectasis; especially if thoracic/abdominal surgery.
    b. Surgical site.
    c. Phlebitis; in older children.
    d. Urinary tract; especially if indwelling catheter.
    e. Blood; especially if central venous access.
5. Provide pulmonary toilet as atelectasis is common with immobility and splinting.
6. Wean oxygen/ventilation as tolerated.
7. Provide wound care that may include:
    a. Surgical site.
    b. Drainage tubes.
    c. Central venous access sites.
8. Check security of line/tubes/catheters.
    a. Chest tubes are extremely painful when manipulated.
    b. Indwelling urinary drainage devices can traumatize urethral tissue and increase risk of infection; they are extremely painful when under tension.
    c. Nasogastric tubes can migrate with time, which allows for increased risk of aspiration or decreased drainage.
    d. Central venous access devices can be displaced; trauma to insertion site can increase risk of infection.
    e. Endotracheal tubes can be displaced easily, which allows for inadvertent extubation, carinal irritation, or mainstem bronchus intubation.
9. Monitor return of bowel function and provide for nutrition.
    a. Immobility, anesthesia, analgesics/sedatives, electrolyte abnormalities, and bowel ischemia may produce an ileus.
    b. Bowel sounds auscultation is an inexact method of determining bowel function.
    c. Evaluate abdominal distention, flatus, and nasogastric secretions, as well as bowel sounds for return of function.
    d. Provide nutrition enterally when possible and advance feedings as tolerated; if bowel function delayed more than 3 days, provide nutrition parenterally.
10. Obtain blood specimens and x-rays specific to surgical procedure.
11. Involve caretakers in daily care. Family members are often able to identify their children's needs more readily than medical professionals. Allow the family to touch, play, and even hold their child if possible during this time.

D. Preparation for maximal wellness.
1. Prepare child and family for discharge.
    a. Home/extended care facility.
    b. Caregiver prepared to support child's care needs. See *Chapter 11: Acute Illness, Injury, and Hospitalization: Effects on the Child* and *Chapter 17: Acute Illness: The Continuum of Care.*
    c. Appropriate referrals and return visits.
    d. Modifications needed in home/school environment based on adaptations to current acute illness/injury.
2. Plan for maintenance of maximal wellness.

BIBLIOGRAPHY

American Academy of Pediatrics Committee on Drugs. (1997). Alternative routes of drug administration—Advantages and disadvantages (subject review). *Pediatrics, 100*(1), 143–152.

Bernardo, L.M., & Bove, M. (Eds.). (1993). *Pediatric emergency nursing procedures.* Boston: Jones and Bartlett.

Connors, C.A., & Rosenthal-Dichter, C. (1997). Components of breathing: Pediatric ventilatory challenges. *Critical Care Nurse, 17*(1), 60–70.

Curley, M.A., Bloedel Smith, J., & Moloney-Harmon, P.A.

(Eds.). (1996). *Critical care nursing of infants and children.* Philadelphia: Saunders.

Del Valle, R.M., & Hecker, R.B. (1995, Jan/Feb). A review of ventilatory modalities used in the intensive care unit. *The American Journal of Anesthesiology,* 23–30.

Dieckmann, R.A., Fiser, D.H., & Selbst, S.M. (Eds.). (1997). Pediatric emergency and critical care procedures. St. Louis: Mosby.

Maneker, A.J., Petrack, E.M., & Krug, S.E. (1995). Contribution of routine pulse oximetry to evaluation and management of patients with respiratory illness in a pediatric emergency department. *Annals of Emergency Medicine, 25*(1), 36–40.

The Neonatal Inhaled Nitric Oxide Study Group. Roberts, J.D., Fineman, T.R., Morin, F.C., Shaul, P.W., Rimar, S., Schribner, M.D., Polin, R.A., Zwass, M.S., Zayek, M.M., Gross, I., Heymann, M.A., & Zapol, W.M. (1997). Inhaled nitric oxide in full-term and nearly full-term infants with hypoxic respiratory failure. *The New England Journal of Medicine, 336*(9), 597–604.

Padman, R., Lawless, S., & Von Nessen, S. (1994). Use of bipap by nasal mask in the treatment of respiratory insufficiency in pediatric patients: Preliminary investigation. *Pediatric Pulmonology, 17,* 119–123.

Roberts, J.D., Fineman, T.R., Morin, F.C., Shaul, P.W., Rimar, S., Schribner, M.D., Polin, R.A., Zwass, M.S., Zayek, M.M., Gross, I., Heymann, M.A., & Zapol, W.M. (The Neonatal Inhaled Nitric Oxide Study Group) (1997). Inhaled nitric oxide and persistent pulmonary hypertension of the newborn. *The New England Journal of Medicine, 336*(9), 605–610.

Rogers, M.C. (Ed.). (1996). *Textbook of pediatric intensive care.* Baltimore: Williams & Wilkins.

Sinclair Hart, L., Berns, S.D., Houck, C.S., & Boenning, D.A. (1997). The value of end-tidal CO_2 monitoring when comparing three methods of conscious sedation for children undergoing painful procedures in the emergency department. *Pediatric Emergency Care, 13*(3), 189–194.

Wong, D.L. (1995). *Whaley & Wong's nursing care of infants and children* (5th ed.). St. Louis: Mosby.

STUDY QUESTIONS

◆ ◆

1. Medications delivered by which route must first be metabolized by the liver to be effective?
   a. Intravenous
   b. Enteral
   c. Intraosseous
   d. Oral mucosa
   e. Rectal

2. Which of the following is NOT a complication of peripheral venous catheters?
   a. Phlebitis
   b. Infiltration
   c. Air embolus
   d. Fracture
   e. Tendon/nerve damage

3. Which of these nursing actions is/are appropriate when a peripheral venous access catheter is placed in an infant's scalp?
   a. Palpate the site for pulsations.
   b. Save hair, if cut, for caretakers.
   c. Never allow tourniquets to lay over the infant's eyes.
   d. Prepare the family for the device location.
   e. All of the above

4. Which of the following is NOT considered an effect of immobility?
   a. Edema
   b. Atelectasis
   c. Incontinence
   d. Muscle wasting
   e. Constipation

5. A 6-month-old child hospitalized for osteomyelitis requires approximately how many kcal/kg/day?
   a. 150
   b. 75
   c. 50
   d. 250
   e. 325

6. Which of these ingredients constitute elemental formulas?
   a. Special supplements for specific diseases
   b. Traditional proteins, carbohydrates, and fats
   c. Glucose and electrolytes
   d. Cellular and acellular immunoprotective elements
   e. Simple proteins, carbohydrates, and fats

7. Which of the following oxygen delivery methods should be used for infants/children with moderate to severe signs of impending respiratory failure?
   a. Venturi mask
   b. Nonrebreather or partial rebreather mask
   c. Nasal cannula
   d. Blow-by
   e. Simple face mask

8. ETT displacement may result in which of the following?
   a. Bronchospasm
   b. Pneumothorax
   c. Atelectasis
   d. Bradycardia
   e. All of the above

9. The effects of cold stress in the neonate include which of the following?
   a. Hyperglycemia
   b. Hypoxia
   c. Hypoglycemia
   d. b and c
   e. a and b

10. Pain induces which response in children?
    a. Catecholamine surges
    b. Mental alertness
    c. Decreased metabolic requirements
    d. "No pain – no gain.
    e. Respiratory depression

ANSWERS

◆ ◆ ◆ ◆ ◆ ◆ ◆ ◆ ◆ ◆ ◆ ◆ ◆ ◆ ◆ ◆ ◆ ◆ ◆

1.b 2.d 3.e 4.c 5.a 6.e 7.b 8.e 9.b 10.a

Chapter 14

Acute Illness: Symptom Management

Deborah G. Loman, PhD, RN, CPNP

Concept

◆◆◆◆◆◆◆◆◆◆◆◆◆◆◆◆◆◆◆◆◆◆◆◆◆◆◆

◆ Children with acute illness or injuries and their families

Objectives

◆◆◆◆◆◆◆◆◆◆◆◆◆◆◆◆◆◆◆◆◆◆◆◆◆◆◆

At the completion of this chapter, the reader will be able to:

◆ Describe the assessment of symptoms in young children.

◆ Identify both nonpharmacologic and pharmacologic interventions appropriate for the child with nausea.

◆ Identify key risk factors associated with the development and management of altered skin integrity in children.

◆ Discuss fever phobia and key teaching areas for parents.

◆ Discuss strategies to decrease fear in children.

◆ Describe general principles of pain management in children.

Key Points

◆◆◆◆◆◆◆◆◆◆◆◆◆◆◆◆◆◆◆◆◆◆◆◆◆◆◆

◆ A symptom refers to a feeling, a subjective response or cue, which is perceived by the child, and is not directly measurable by others.

◆ Children are twice as likely as adults to experience postoperative nausea and vomiting.

◆ A number of factors contribute to skin breakdown in hospitalized children including: immobility, prolonged pressure, hypoxia-hypoperfusion, decreased sensory perception, exposure to friction and moisture, and poor nutrition.

◆ Parents should be taught to look beyond the child's level of fever and assess comfort, activity, behavior, and nutritional intake to evaluate degree of illness.

◆ Nurses must not only be knowledgeable about pain assessment and management in children but also participate in the institution's efforts to evaluate and improve the care.

14

Acute Illness: Symptom Management

I. ASSESSMENT OF SYMPTOMS IN CHILDREN

A. Nurses use both symptoms and signs in the assessment of children and the planning and evaluation of care.
1. Definitions (McDaniel & Rhodes, 1995; Selekman & Malloy, 1995).
   a. A symptom refers to a feeling, a subjective response, or a perception that is not directly measurable by others, e.g., fatigue, nausea.
   b. A sign refers to an objective finding that can be observed and measured by others, e.g., elevated temperature, vomiting.
2. Factors that affect symptom recognition in young children.
   a. Cues sent by the child will be influenced by:
      (1) Child's developmental and cognitive level and previous experiences.
      (2) Pain and nausea in infants may be experienced as more generalized sensations than specific ones. Infant's symptoms may be communicated via subtle behavioral cues that require careful observation.
      (3) Children may not have the ability to identify the sensation nor to verbally communicate what they feel.
   b. Ability of the parent/nurse to interpret the cues correctly will be influenced by:
      (1) Parental anxiety, which may alter the parent's ability to identify the child's symptoms.
      (2) Nurse's knowledge of child development and pathophysiology.
      (3) Personal biases and experiences of parents and nurses.
      (4) Child's temperament, which may affect the attitudes and practices of care givers.
      (5) Differences between the parent's and nurse's education, cultural beliefs, and/or health care beliefs/practices.

B. Assessment of illness or distress in young children.
1. Crying in young children is difficult to interpret as it can indicate hunger, pain, nausea, fear, fatigue, general distress, illness, or other states.
2. Fussiness/irritability, a decrease in activity and in eating are associated with a child not feeling well.
3. Degree of illness is derived through a combination of signs and interpretation of behavioral cues.
   a. Mild illness: alert, active, smiles, feeds well, cries strongly but is easily consoled.
   b. Moderate illness: irritable with crying but continues to feed, consolable, smiles briefly, less playful and active than usual.
   c. Severe illness: lethargic, poor eye contact, irritable, not easily consoled, feeds poorly, may have signs of severe dehydration or poor perfusion or respiratory distress.

II. NAUSEA

A. Definitions.
1. An "unpleasant sensation vaguely referred to the throat or abdomen with an inclination to vomit" (Wong, 1995, p. 450).
2. An "awareness of discomfort in the gut accompanied by the feeling that vomiting would make it feel better" (Wickham, 1989, p. 564).
3. Child may verbalize "I feel sick to my stomach" or a similar statement.

B. Etiology.
1. The sensation is mediated by the autonomic nervous system and may be accompanied by perspiration, pallor, gastric stasis, and tachycardia.
2. It is difficult to separate nausea from vomiting since they are often associated with one another.
3. In children nausea/vomiting (N/V) most often occurs postoperatively from side effects of anesthesia and from chemotherapy as well as from gastroenteritis or motion sickness.
4. Vomiting occurs from stimulation of the vomiting center (VC) in the brain via:
   a. Cerebral cortex and limbic system.
   b. Vestibular system.

Table 14-1
Behavioral Interventions to Decrease Nausea and Vomiting in Children

TECHNIQUE	DESCRIPTION	METHODS
Distraction	Divert attention from a threatening situation or distressing procedure	Touching, stroking, rocking, breathing, counting, storytelling, puppet play
Guided Imagery	Concentrated focusing on images formed in one's mind	Visual – favorite place, TV show. Auditory – favorite song, instrument. Movement – flying, swimming, running (any activity)
Muscle Relaxation	Systematic, progressive method of diversion through contracting and relaxing various muscle groups	Tightened and relax muscles, beginning with the feet and moving toward the head
Self-Hypnosis	Increased attention, receptiveness, and responsiveness to an idea or set of ideas	Combined use of distraction, guided imagery, and muscle relaxation

Used with permission from Hockenberry-Eaton, M., & Benner, A. (1990). Patterns of nausea and vomiting in children: Nursing assessment and interventions. *Oncology Nursing Forum, 17*(4), p. 580.

c. CTZ: chemoreceptor trigger zone.
d. Afferent vagus and visceral nerves.
5. Examples of stimuli that may stimulate the VC.
  a. Psychologic stimuli as stress, fear, and anticipation.
  b. Motion: via the vestibular system, which originates from the labyrinth of the inner ear.
  c. Chemical signals from either the cerebrospinal fluid (e.g., neurochemicals) or the bloodstream.
  d. Vagal and/or visceral nerves stimulation by gastrointestinal irritation or distention or delayed gastric emptying.
6. Postoperative nausea/vomiting (PONV) (Shende & Mandal, 1997).
  a. A number of anesthetics and opiodes are associated with PONV.
  b. Children are twice as likely as adults to experience PONV (but infants less so than children or adults).
  c. Previous history of PONV or motion sickness is a risk factor.
  d. High incidence occurs after strabismus surgery (from either visual image distortion or from stimulation of oculoemetic reflex) and after tonsillectomy (irritant effect of blood).

C. Assessment.
1. Assess child's attitudes and previous experience with nausea and the degree of distress experienced.
2. Ask what words the child uses for nausea and vomiting.
3. Rely on self-report of nausea by the child, parental perceptions, and behavioral cues.

4. Assess for behavioral cues.
  a. Holding a hand over the stomach or mouth.
  b. Refusal to eat or drink.
  c. Decreased activity.
  d. Crying or irritability.
5. Assess for autonomic signs/symptoms.
  a. Faintness.
  b. Diaphoresis.
  c. Pallor.
  d. Tachycardia.
6. Consider use of a rating scale for nausea for children undergoing chemotherapy.
7. Assess nature of vomiting and emesis
  a. Presence of nausea.
  b. Projectile or nonprojectile emesis.
  c. Amount and color of emesis.
  d. Patterns and triggers.
  e. Methods that decrease N/V.
8. Assess for associated problems: dehydration, weight loss, presence of bowel sounds and abdominal distention, fluid and electrolyte imbalances, decreased nutritional status, feelings of anxiety, hopelessness, and loss of control (Keller, 1995).
9. Since nausea is a symptom, note carefully any other characteristics that may provide data to help determine the etiology if unknown.
  a. Many conditions produce nausea and/or vomiting.
  b. Examples include pyloric stenosis, GI obstruction, metabolic disorders, increased ICP, and pregnancy.

D. Nursing interventions.
The two types of interventions are more effective if used together to decrease persistent nausea and

Table 14-2
Antiemetics Used for Nausea/Vomiting in Children

Type	Action	Comments
Phenothiazines promethazine (Phenergan) prochlorperazine (Compazine) trimethobenzamide (Tigan)	Block dopamine receptors in CTZ	Risk of extrapyramidal side effects, (i.e. dystonic reactions) in young children (Morrow, 1989) children Effectiveness varies; Used for persistent vomiting of known etiology Use Tigan only in children > 10 kg or > 2 years
Metoclopramide (Reglan)	Affects vagal and visceral nerves Stimulates motility of upper GI tract and increases gastric emptying Blocks dopamine receptors	Usually well tolerated although can cause dystonic reactions
Ondansetron (Zofran)	Blocks serotonin at 5-HT$_3$ receptor sites in CTZ and vagal nerve	Effective in preventing and/or reducing N/V associated with anesthesia and chemotherapy Minimal side effects Expensive
Antihistamines cyclizine (Marezine) meclizine (Antivert, Bonine) dimenhydrinate (Dramamine)	Affects the vestibular system	One side effect is sedation Not recommended < 6 years Not recommended < 12 years Not recommended < 2 years (Benitz, 1995)
Lorazepam (Ativan)	CNS depressant Reduces anxiety and affects VC	Sedation

vomiting as they may affect the VC through more than one route.

1. Nonpharmacologic interventions.
   a. Decrease anxiety by providing information.
   b. Have children/families identify triggers and methods that have helped in the past.
   c. Use guided imagery, relaxation, self-hypnosis, and distraction techniques such as music, stories, video games (Hockenberry-Eaton & Benner, 1990) (see Table 14-1).
   d. Promote sleep.
   e. Encourage family support.
   f. Provide calm and pleasant atmosphere, especially at mealtime and eliminate stress.
   g. Encourage fluids and a light diet of small, frequent meals.
   h. Avoid fluids of high osmolality and foods with long chain triglycerides since they slow gastric emptying (Hoekelman, 1992).
   i. Avoid food with strong odors.
   j. Avoid favorite foods when nauseated to prevent child from becoming conditioned stimuli that can trigger N/V in the future.
   k. Have child eat slowly so as to help avoid gastric distention, which may induce vomiting by stimulating afferent nerve pathways.
   l. Monitor weight and urine output if child has persistent nausea.
2. Pharmacologic interventions.
   a. Indications.
      (1) To prevent or reduce postoperative nausea and vomiting (PONV).
      (2) To prevent or reduce N/V associated with chemotherapy.
      (3) To reduce persistent N/V of known etiology.
   b. Location of action of antiemetics (Benitz & Tatro, 1995).
      (1) Chemotrigger receptor zone (CTZ).
      (2) Vagal and visceral nerves.
      (3) Vestibular system.
      (4) Cerebral cortex/limbic system.
   c. Types of antiemetics (see Table 14-2).
      (1) Phenothiazines – including promethazine (Phenergan), prochlorperazine (Compazine) and trimethobenzamide (Tigan).

(2) Metoclopramide (Reglan).
(3) Ondansetron (Zofran).
(4) Antihistamines – cyclizine (Marezine), meclizine (Antivert, Bonine), and dimenhydrinate (Dramamine).
(5) Lorazepam (Activan).

d. Route of administration for antiemetics.
(1) IV route preferred if available.
(2) Rectal route preferable to oral as nausea is associated with gastric atony; children often prefer oral to rectal route.

e. Dose: the recommended dose for weight and age should be given to be effective.

f. Special situations.
(1) Chemotherapy: give antiemetic before the chemotherapy begins and around the clock.
(2) N/V of unknown etiology: the use of antiemetics is generally discouraged because of the possible side effects and the risk of masking the underlying problem, i.e., GI obstruction or pregnancy.
(3) Acute gastroenteritis: consensus is that antiemetic drugs are not needed; use small amounts of oral glucose-electrolyte solution frequently, i.e. as often as 5 ml every 1–2 minutes, to maintain hydration (American Academy of Pediatrics [AAP], 1996).

III. FATIGUE

◆ ◆ ◆ ◆ ◆ ◆ ◆ ◆ ◆ ◆ ◆ ◆ ◆ ◆ ◆ ◆ ◆ ◆ ◆

A. Overview.
1. Definition.
a. A complex, multicausal, nonspecific, and subjective phenomenon for which not one definition is accepted (Tiesinga, Dassen, & Halfens, 1996).
b. A feeling of weariness with increasing discomfort and decreasing efficiency for which there may be a biochemical basis associated with:
(1) Physical or mental overwork.
(2) A somatic illness.
(3) An emotional condition characterized by boredom, lack of energy and initiative, absence of a sense of well-being.
c. Reflected by a decrease in normal physical activity in children.
2. Etiology.
a. In young children fatigue is more often due to an organic cause that could include moderate- to-severe anemia, head trauma, lead poisoning, dehydration, hypothyroidism, pregnancy, mononucleosis, chronic renal failure, diabetes mellitus, leukemia, congenital heart disease, and/or congestive heart failure.
b. In older children, there may be a psychologic

source, such as depression, anxiety, or difficulty with peers, school, or family.

B. Assessment.
1. Review with child and parents:
a. Any changes in growth and development.
b. Ability to play, eat, and interact.
c. Day and nighttime rest and sleep patterns.
d. Extent of involvement in sports and extracurricular activities as age appropriate.
e. Level of functioning in school and with peers.
f. Use of over-the-counter drugs containing antihistamines for colds or allergy symptoms.
g. Use of illicit drugs such as alcohol or barbiturates.
h. Exposure to environmental toxins (such as carbon monoxide).
2. Examine the child for:
a. Presence of pallor, bruising, unusual color.
b. Muscle tone.
c. Type of skin turgor and presence of edema.
d. Lymphadenopathy.
e. Status of cardiac and respiratory systems including heart rate, blood pressure, peripheral pulses, respiratory rate, and respiratory distress.

C. Nursing interventions.
1. Encourage rest and activity as tolerated.
2. Promote quiet activities.
3. Allow for periods of uninterrupted rest and sleep.
4. Encourage a nutritious, balanced diet.
5. Discuss with the family ways to minimize emotional distress.
6. Encourage relaxation.
7. Reduce stressors in the hospital setting such as noises, lights, frequent activity by staff in child's room, which all contribute to sleep deprivation.

D. Nursing interventions for the infant with fatigue related to activity intolerance, from imbalance between oxygen supply and demand (e.g., appropriate for some infants with congenital heart disease).
1. Provide feeding and diaper changes before infant cries.
2. Respond promptly to crying or other signs of distress.
3. Use a pacifier during fussy times to decrease crying.
4. Offer small, frequent feedings.
5. Allow frequent rest periods during feeding.
6. Use a soft nipple, with large opening.
7. Discuss high calorie formulas if poor weight

gain.

8. Discuss gavage feedings if poor intake and weight gain.
9. Ensure periods of uninterrupted sleep and rest.
10. Schedule activities after rest but not before feeding.
11. Skip the bath and other unnecessary activities if infant is tired.

IV. SKIN INTEGRITY

◆ ◆ ◆ ◆ ◆ ◆ ◆ ◆ ◆ ◆ ◆ ◆ ◆ ◆ ◆ ◆ ◆ ◆ ◆ ◆

A. Overview.

Although alteration in skin integrity primarily has been associated with adults, it also occurs in children. In a recent study of 271 children in the PICU, altered skin integrity occurred in 26% of admissions and 7% had skin breakdown (partial thickness skin loss or greater) (Zollo, Gostisha, Berens, Schmidt, & Weigler, 1996). In addition, children sustain abrasions, burns, and wounds, and are at risk for altered skin integrity from diaper dermatitis, ostomies, and IV infiltrations.

1. Factors contributing to skin breakdown (Quigley & Curley, 1996; Zollo et al., 1996).
   a. Prolonged pressure.
   b. Decreased sensory perception.
   c. Decreased mobility and activity.
   d. Extrinsic factors: moisture, friction, and shear.
   e. Intrinsic factors: nutrition, tissue perfusion, and oxygenation.
2. Common locations of skin breakdown in children (Quigley & Curley, 1996; Zollo et al., 1996).
   a. Occiput in infants and toddlers (greater proportion of body weight and surface area of the head).
   b. Sacrum (increased pressure as child gets older).
   c. Nose, buttocks, diaper area, taped areas, and incision sites.

B. Recommended method of grading skin damage or pressure ulcers (Panel for the Prediction and Prevention of Pressure Ulcers in Adults, 1992).

1. Staging of skin breakdown.
   a. Stage 1: nonblanchable erythema of intact skin.
   b. Stage 2: partial-thickness skin loss involving the epidermis and/or dermis. May be an abrasion, blister, or shallow crater.
   c. Stage 3: full-thickness skin loss involving damage to subcutaneous tissue. Will have deep crater.
   d. Stage 4: full-thickness skin loss with tissue necrosis or damage to muscle, bone, or supporting structures. May also have a sinus tract.
2. Additional comments.
   a. Stage 1 should not be confused with reactive hyperemia, which is blanchable. This may be present for ½ to ¾ as long as the initial pressure to the area existed.
   b. The presence of eschar prevents accurate staging of the pressure ulcer.

C. Prevention of pressure ulcers.

1. Identify early those children at-risk. Assess all who have skin breakdown or are immobile on admission and reassess every 24 hours.
2. Consider use of the Modified Braden Q to predict children at risk (Quigley & Curley, 1996) (see Table 14-3).
   a. Developed for use with children. Modified from Braden Scale for Predicting Pressure Ulcer Risk used with adults.
   b. Has 7 subscales: mobility, activity, sensory perception, skin moisture, friction and sheer, nutrition, and tissue perfusion.
   c. Range of possible scores for the Braden Q is 7 to 28 with < 23 points indicating risk for altered skin integrity.
3. Prevent friction injury.
   a. Use protective sheepskin over the elbows or heels.
   b. Apply transparent dressings over susceptible areas.
   c. Use soft, smooth bed linens.
   d. Apply absorbent powder to keep the skin dry. Be careful to keep powder away from mouth and nose.
4. Prevent shear injury.
   a. Use draw sheets or trapeze bar to reposition.
   b. Elevate the bed not more than 30° for short periods.
   c. Use the knee gatch or elevate knees with pillow to reduce pressure on the sacrum.
5. Prevent epidermal stripping.
   a. Use minimal tape.
   b. Use porous tape.
   c. Remove tape by slowly peeling the tape away while stabilizing the skin.
   d. Use water or adhesive remover to break the adhesive bond.
   e. Quickly rinse off any adhesive remover used.
   f. Use solid wafer skin barriers, transparent dressings, or laced binder instead of tape on skin next to wounds.
6. Reduce exposure to chemical substances such as urine, feces, wound, or stoma drainage. Use moisture barriers and gently cleanse skin after exposure.

Table 14-3
Modified Braden Q Scale

Intensity and Duration of Pressure					Score
Mobility The ability to change and control body position	**1. Completely immobile:** Does not make even slight changes in body or extremity position without assistance.	**2. Very limited:** Makes occasional slight changes in body or extremity position but unable to completely turn self independently.	**3. Slightly limited:** Makes frequent though slight changes in body or extremity position independently.	**4. No limitations:** Makes major and frequent changes in position without assistance.	
Activity The degree of physical activity.	**1. Bedfast:** Confined to bed	**2. Chairfast:** Ability to walk severely limited or nonexistent. Cannot bear own weight and/or must be assisted into chair or wheelchair.	**3. Walks occasionally:** Walks occasionally during day, but for very short distances, with or without assistance. Spends majority of each shift in bed or chair.	**4. All patients too young to ambulate:** **OR, walks frequently:** Walks outside the room at least twice a day and inside room at least once every 2 hours during waking hours.	
Sensory perception The ability to respond in a developmentally appropriate way to pressure-related discomfort.	**1. Completely limited:** Unresponsive (does not moan, flinch, or grasp) to painful stimuli due to diminished level of consciousness or sedation; OR, limited ability to feel pain over most of body surface.	**2. Very limited:** Responds only to painful stimuli. Cannot communicate discomfort except by moaning or restlessness; OR, has sensory impairment that limits the ability to feel pain or discomfort over half of body.	**3. Slightly limited:** Responds to verbal commands, but cannot always communicate discomfort or need to be turned; OR, has some sensory impairment that limits ability to feel pain or discomfort in one or two extremities.	**4. No impairment:** Responds to verbal commands. Has no sensory deficit that would limit ability to feel or communicate pain or discomfort.	

Table 14-3 continues on opposite page

D. Interventions for children with altered skin integrity (Panel for the Prediction and Prevention of Pressure Ulcers in Adults, 1992).

1. Encourage a diet that promotes wound healing: protein, calories, Vitamin C, and zinc.
2. Do not massage reddened areas over bony prominences because it can cause deep tissue damage.
3. Change child's position or turn frequently if possible; use pressure relief device such as a 4″ eggcrate foam overlay (2″ in infants) in children on bed rest.
4. Consult with clinical nurse specialist (CNS) regarding use of specialty beds or pillows for immobilized children.
5. Document color, size, location, presence of sinus tracts, odor, and drainage.
6. Do not use hydrogen peroxide or betadine (povidone-iodine) on wounds as they are cytotoxic to healthy cells.
7. Place pectin-based or hydrocolloid skin barrier directly over excoriated skin. Leave barrier undisturbed until it begins to peel off.
8. Maintain a moist environment to promote faster healing in a wound.
9. Consult with CNS as appropriate regarding type of dressing to use based upon type of wound, presence of infection or drainage, and products available. Dressing may be dry or moist; adherent or nonadherent; protective, absorbent, and/or debriding (Quigley & Curley, 1996; Wong, 1995).

E. Interventions for use with neonates (Malloy-McDonald, 1995).

1. Preventive skin care.
   a. Bathe 2–3 times per week with plain water.
   b. Cleanse diaper area daily with mild, nonfragrant soap.
   c. Avoid skin care products with chemicals that are harmful to children such as diaper wipes, lotions, shampoos, and powders.
   d. Use a bland vegetable oil or safflower oil rather than perfumed lotion or oils.
   e. Avoid use of baby powder because of the risk of aspiration.
2. Management of skin excoriation (Malloy & Perez-Woods, 1991).

Table 14-3 (continued)
Modified Braden Q Scale

Tolerance of the Skin and Supporting Structure				Score
Moisture: Degree to which skin is exposed to moisture.	**1. Constantly moist:** Skin is kept moist almost constantly by perspiration, urine, drainage, etc. Dampness is detected every time patient is moved or turned.	**2. Very moist:** Skin is often, but not always, moist. Linen must be changed at least every 8 hours.	**3. Occasionally moist:** Skin is occasionally moist, requiring linen change every 12 hours.	**4. Rarely moist:** Skin is usually dry, routine diaper changes; linen requires changing only every 24 hours.
Friction – Shear Friction: Occurs when skin moves against support surfaces. **Shear:** Occurs when skin and adjacent bony surface slide across one another.	**1. Significant problem:** Spasticity, contracture, itching or agitation leads to almost constant thrashing and friction.	**2. Problem:** Requires moderate to maximum assistance in moving. Complete lifting without sliding against sheets is impossible. Frequently slides down in bed or chair, requiring frequent repositioning with maximum assistance.	**3. Potential problem:** Moves feebly or requires minimum assistance. During a move, skin probably slides to some extent against sheets, chair, restraints, or other devices. Maintains relatively good position in chair or bed most of the time but occasionally slides down.	**4. No apparent problem:** Able to completely lift self during a position change; moves in bed and in chair independently and has sufficient muscle strength to lift up completely during move. Maintains good position in bed or chair at all times.
Nutrition: Usual food intake pattern.	**1. Very poor:** NPO and/or maintained on clear liquids, or IVs for more than 5 days OR albumin<2.5 mg/dl OR never eats a complete meal. Rarely eats more than half of any food offered. Protein intake includes only 2 servings of meat or dairy products per day. Takes fluids poorly. Does not take a liquid dietary supplement.	**2. Inadequate:** Is on liquid diet or tube feedings/TPN, which provide inadequate calories and minerals for age OR albumin <3 mg/dl OR rarely eats a complete meal and generally eats only about half of any food offered. Protein intake includes only 3 servings of meat or dairy products per day. Occasionally will take a dietary supplement.	**3. Adequate:** Is on tube feedings or TPN, which provide adequate calories and minerals for age OR eats over half of most meals. Eats a total of 4 servings of protein (meat, dairy products) each day. Occasionally will refuse a meal, but will usually take a supplement if offered.	**4. Excellent:** Is on a normal diet providing adequate calories for age. For example, eats most of every meal. Never refuses a meal. Usually eats a total of 4 or more servings of meat and dairy products. Occasionally eats between meals. Does not require supplementation.
Tissue Perfusion and Oxygenation.	**1. Extremely compromised:** Hypotensive (MAP <50mmHg; <40 in a newborn) or the patient does not physiologically tolerate position changes.	**2. Compromised:** Normotensive; oxygen saturation may be <95%; hemoglobin may be <10 mg/dl; capillary refill may be >2 seconds; serum pH is <7.40.	**3. Adequate:** Normotensive; oxygen saturation may be <95%; hemoglobin may be <10 mg/dl; capillary refill may be >2 seconds; serum pH is normal.	**4. Excellent:** Normotensive; oxygen saturation >95%; normal Hgb; capillary refill <2 seconds.

From Quigley, S.M., & Curley, M.A.Q. (1996). Skin integrity in the pediatric population: Preventing and managing pressure ulcers. *Journal of the Society of Pediatric Nurses, 1*, 11-12. Reprinted with permission from Nursecom, Inc.

a. Keep area clean and dry.
b. Wash with mild soap and water.
c. Protect the area with transparent elastic film dressing like Tegaderm or OpSite.
d. Use hydrogel dressings to protect the skin and promote healing of skin excoriation.
e. Avoid any substance that may be absorbed through immature or excoriated skin such as adhesive removers, alcohol, povidone-iodine, hexachlorophene, topical antibiotics, steroids, tincture of benzoin, or silver sulfadiazine cream.
3. Avoidance of mechanical and thermal injury.
a. Remove and rotate electrodes every 24 hours.
b. Use a protective/pectin-based skin barrier between the neonate's skin and adhesives for endotracheal tubes, IVs, NG tubes, surgical dressings, etc.
c. Avoid heat lamps.
d. Use pulse oximetry instead of transcutaneous monitoring when possible.
e. Keep heating pads below 40°C as well as temperature when prewarming for heelsticks
f. Assess fingers or toes hourly if IV site is on an extremity.
g. Tape IV catheter to allow for viewing of the site.
h. Have hyaluronidase available for use in IV infiltrations to prevent tissue necrosis.

V. FEVER

◆ ◆ ◆ ◆ ◆ ◆ ◆ ◆ ◆ ◆ ◆ ◆ ◆ ◆ ◆ ◆ ◆ ◆ ◆ ◆

A. Etiology and definition.
1. Natural physiologic response to infection or stressors.
2. Result of a up-regulation of the temperature set point in the hypothalamus as a response to circulating pyrogens.
3. Elevated body temperature, often with 100.4°F or 38°C (rectal) (Baraff et al., 1993) or 100°F (oral) as the lower limit.

B. Assessment of the child with fever.
1. Several different routes are used to measure fever.
a. Rectal: traditionally viewed as most accurate, but may be inaccurate from stool in rectum; intrusive, not acceptable to children; could be damaging to rectum if thermometer inserted too far, or in a uncooperative child, or if rectal insertion is contraindicated as with rectal surgery.
b. Oral: acceptable to most; cannot use in young children (< 4) until they learn to hold a thermometer in the mouth; affected by eating and drinking cool or warm fluids and mouth breathing.
c. Axillary: viewed as least accurate, except in neonates, especially if temperature is elevated; safe; acceptable route children.
d. Tympanic: rapid; nonintrusive; acceptable; more expensive; can be affected by extremes in ambient temperature; less accurate when temperature is elevated (may read higher than rectal temperature) (Selfridge & Shea, 1993). Need to know proper technique; varies with age of child.
2. In general, rectal temperature > than oral > axillary but the exact difference varies within and between individuals (Haddock, Merrow, & Swanson, 1996).
3. Observe other behaviors of the child: level of comfort and activity, eye contact, appetite, alertness, and fontanel status.
4. Assess hydration status and expect an increase in pulse rate (10 beats/minute/degree of fever) and respiratory rate in younger children.

C. Interventions.
1. Give an antipyretic if child is uncomfortable or has a fever of 102° or greater.
2. Use the appropriate type of antipyretic.
a. In general, use acetaminophen for fever.
b. In general, avoid aspirin because of concern about the possible association with Reye's syndrome, especially if child has viral infection.
c. May give ibuprofen to children if > 6 months, unless dehydrated.
3. Use the appropriate dose of antipyretic.
a. Acetaminophen: 10–15 mg/kg up to 650 mg/4 hrs.
b. Ibuprofen: 5–10 mg/kg every 6 hours up to 400 mg per dose (not to exceed 40 mg/kg/day).
4. Question the use of sponging as it has limited if any benefits (Berlin, 1996).
a. Never use alcohol for sponging (child could absorb toxic levels).
b. Never sponge with cold water but only warm water (to prevent shivering).
c. Give an antipyretic first, then sponge 30–45 minutes later to allow time for lowering of the temperature set point.
d. Stop sponging if the child starts to shiver.
5. Encourage fluids as fluid loss increases with each degree of fever (Berlin, 1996).
6. Do not push foods as peristalsis often decreases.
7. Dress the child in light clothing and cover with a light sheet; keep room temperature comfortable.
8. If an infant with a low grade fever has been bundled, unbundle and recheck temperature in 15–30 minutes.

9. Any child less than 3 months with a fever needs to be evaluated by a physician or a nurse practitioner (unless the fever occurs immediately after a DTP immunization).
10. Observe for any changes in behavior that might indicate a source for infection. A higher fever (>102) or a persistent fever in a child 3–36 months is more likely associated with systemic illness (Baraff et al., 1993).
11. Provide teaching to parents/caregivers.
    a. Teach how to measure temperature.
    b. Discuss age and weight appropriate antipyretic dose as many children have outgrown a previous dose.
    c. Describe differences in mg dosages of drops, elixirs, and tablets.
    d. Discuss purpose of fever and dispel fever phobia (Berlin, 1996).
       (1) Only a very high fever (106–107°) will cause neurologic sequela.
       (2) There may be a benefit to the body of not suppressing a fever.
       (3) Few children have febrile seizures and those that do may develop them from the rapid rise in temperature rather than the absolute level of elevation.
       (4) Look beyond the fever and assess other aspects of behavior: activity, drinking, eating, sleeping, discomfort.

VI. FEAR

◆ ◆ ◆ ◆ ◆ ◆ ◆ ◆ ◆ ◆ ◆ ◆ ◆ ◆ ◆ ◆ ◆ ◆ ◆

A. Overview.

Children have fears of the known, the unknown, and of the imagined. When they become ill, fears can become intensified by stress, hospitalization, and pain.
1. Defined as an unpleasant often strong emotion caused by anticipation or awareness of danger; implies anxiety.
2. Factors that influence type of fear.
   a. Age and cognitive development of the child: fears become better articulated, more varied, and more realistic as child gets older.
   b. Environment.
   c. Social: family and peer influences.
   d. Media.
   e. Previous experiences.
3. General types of fear in nonhospitalized and hospitalized children.
   a. Fear of needles especially in preschool and school-age children.
   b. Supernatural (including the dark) and natural phenomena.
   c. Home, school, and peer related.

d. Safety.
e. Drugs.
f. Political, ecologic.
4. Types of fear associated with hospitalization. and illness (Hart & Bossert, 1994).
   a. Fear of separation from family, peers, familiar activities.
   b. Intrusive procedures (injections, finger sticks, surgery).
   c. Confinement to hospital or bed.
   d. Being told that something is wrong with them.
5. Characteristics of fears in hospitalized children.
   a. Hospitalized children have more intense fears than nonhospitalized children.
   b. Presence of fear not related to age in children, but their means of coping with fear is related to cognitive maturity.
   c. Children with higher trait anxiety have reported a significantly greater amount of fear (Hart & Bossert, 1994.
6. Fears of school-age children who had undergone surgical procedures.
   a. Perceived threat to body integrity, of the integrity of the surgical scar, of physical well-being.
   b. Fear of the cause of pain (tumor, infection).
   c. Fear of permanent crippling because of pain.
   d. Fear that pain would be unbearable, permanent.

B. Strategies to help children deal with fears.
1. Establish rapport with the child and encourage expression of feelings and anxieties.
2. Assess specific fears of child and plan appropriate interventions (e.g., fear of dark— keep nightlight on).
3. Provide developmentally appropriate information (fear of the unknown is more upsetting than that which is known and understood) (see Table 14-4 for preparation guidelines).
4. Provide information about any sensory experience the child will encounter; (children may have less distress if they receive both sensory and procedural information).
5. Encourage the use of stories and play to describe, draw, or act out events that they have experienced or will experience. This promotes a way to resolve fears or rehearse alternatives for stressful situations in the presence of a supportive adult.
6. Encourage parents to stay with young children during hospitalization and procedures.
7. Avoid the use of any unnecessary injections.
8. When a syringe or needle is to be used for procedures or medications, inform the child first

Table 14-4
Guidelines for Preparation

1. Younger children respond better to preparation involving play materials. Older children will benefit from viewing peer-modeling films.

2. The cognitive level of the child should structure the preparation. Prepare the school-age child (concrete operations) several days in advance. Preschool children (preoperational) benefit from preparation closer to the actual event.

3. The child's psychosocial stage of development (Erikson, 1963) should be reflected in the choice of preparation techniques. Allowing a toddler to play with hospital equipment with an adult will aid in decreasing anxiety and in increasing a sense of autonomy.

4. For children with previous hospital experience, information formats with coping procedures built in will be more beneficial in decreasing anxiety.

5. Each child and parent needs an individualized explanation of the type of surgery that will be performed regardless of the type of preparation used.

6. Facilitate the communication of information and allow the child and parents the freedom to verbalize fears, anxieties, and questions. This will aid in decreasing the anxiety level of the parents and may also help to decrease the anxiety level of the child.

From Bates, T. & Broome, M. (1986). Preparation of children for hospitalization and surgery: A review of the literature. *Journal of Pediatric Nursing, 1*, p. 237. Used with permission from W.B. Saunders Company.

of its purpose. *See Chapter 30: Communication.*

9. Encourage syringe play in children who have experienced procedures with needles.

10. Assess and promote pain reduction measures as pain can increase fear and fear can increase pain.

11. Realize that even with preparation, young children (3–6 years) are more upset and less cooperative with procedures than older children (7–14 years).

12. If child seems excessively fearful, explore the possibility of physical, emotional, or sexual abuse or exposure to a traumatic event

VII. Pain

◆ ◆ ◆ ◆ ◆ ◆ ◆ ◆ ◆ ◆ ◆ ◆ ◆ ◆ ◆ ◆ ◆ ◆ ◆

A. Overview.
1. Definitions.
   a. An unpleasant sensory and emotional experience arising from actual or potential tissue damage.
   b. Pain is whatever the person says it is and exists whenever the person says it does. This definition acknowledges the subjective nature of pain.

2. Status of pain management in children.
   a. There is a need for more pain management information of neonates and infants (McRae, Rourke, Imperial-Perez, Eisenring, & Ueda, 1997).
   b. Infants often receive less than the minimum recommended dosage for morphine and some receive no analgesics after surgery.
   c. A national survey of nurses and doctors at teaching hospitals revealed:
      (1) 27% do not use any self-report pain assessment scales.
      (2) 50% reported using the DPT cocktail often or sometimes.
      (3) Effectiveness of pain assessment and management was lower with infants and younger children (Broome, Richtsmeier, Maikler, & Alexander, et al., 1996).

B. Assessment of acute pain in children.
1. Obtain a pain history from the child and/or parents upon admission. Find out what words the child uses for pain, previous experience with pain, pain management and medication, and any allergies.
2. Assess the family's cultural beliefs about pain and health care.
3. Assess pain level and pain relief at regular intervals. Use a visible flow sheet for documentation.
4. Evaluate the effectiveness of pain assessment and management within the institution. Assess and dispel myths about pain in children.
5. Involve the child and family in pain assessment and management and discuss their preferences.
6. Measure the child's pain using self-report and/or behavioral observations.
7. Use self-report tools that are reliable and valid as well as simple for the child and practical for the nurse. Use self-report tools for children 3–4 years and older (See Table 14-5 for example of tools).
8. Use behavioral observations especially with preverbal children: vocalizations, facial expressions, motor responses, body posture, activity, and appearance.
9. Interpret behaviors cautiously since the behaviors may be ways of coping with pain (e.g., watching TV, lying still, sleeping).
10. Use the parent's report of pain if child is unable to give a self-report.
11. Use physiologic measures (i.e., heart rate, respiratory rate and blood pressure) only as adjuncts to self-report and behavioral observation as they are not sensitive, specific, or consistent for pain.
12. Maintain a high level of suspicion of possible pain, since children often cannot or will not report pain. Assume that anything painful to

Table 14-5
Self-Report Measures of Pain in Children

Tool or Scale	Descriptions	Comments
Oucher	6 vertical photographs of a child. Bottom one with no hurt and top one with biggest hurt. Numbers ranging from 1 to 100 (by tens) opposite the photos.	Ages 3–12 years. 3 ethnic versions (African-American, Caucasian, Hispanic) (Beyer, Denyes, & Villarruel, 1992)
Poker Chip Tool	4 red poker chips, with 1 chip as a little bit of hurt and 4 chips as the most hurt.	Ages 4 years and older. Must be able to count. Instructions also available in Spanish (Acute Pain, 1992).
Wong-Baker FACES Scale	6 cartoon faces with range from smiling to crying for no pain to worst pain.	Ages 3 years and older. Translations of scale explanations available in eight languages (Wong, 1996).
Word-Graphic Rating Scale	Horizontal line with no pain at left side and worst possible pain on right side. Five-word descriptors placed at equidistant points along the line.	Ages 4 years and older (Acute Pain, 1992)

adults will be painful to infants and young children.

C. General principles of acute pain management in children (Acute Pain, 1992).
1. Provide adequate preparation (developmentally appropriate) for the child and family about procedures.
2. Emphasize the importance of communicating about pain and treating pain early.
3. Do not perform procedures in the child's bed or room unless absolutely necessary.
4. Allow parents to be with the child before, during, and after the procedure. Prepare the parents to be supportive.
5. If the child is to have repeated procedures, provide maximum treatment for any pain and anxiety with the first procedure to minimize the development of anticipatory anxiety before subsequent procedures.
6. If uncertain about assessment of pain in young children, administer a trial of analgesics.

D. Pharmacologic management of pain in children
1. Be sure that analgesics are ordered and given for the prevention and relief of pain.
2. Recognize that analgesics and/or local anesthetics are used to reduce pain. Anxiolytics and sedatives (e.g., benzodiazepines and barbiturates) may be used to relieve associated anxiety and provide sedation but not to relieve pain.
3. Administer medications, including preoperative medication, via a painless route. Intramuscular injections should rarely be given because most are painful and children are afraid of them.
4. Use ordered oral or intravenous opiates for analgesic effects. Morphine is usually used for management of moderate to severe acute pain.
5. Recognize that physiologic or psychologic dependency rarely results from the brief use of opioids for acute pain management.
6. Use the recommended dosage of analgesia (based on weight and age) as a starting point although individual children vary in their dose requirements.
7. Avoid the use of DPT (Demerol, Phenergan, and Thorazine). The safety and efficacy of DPT does not compare favorable with opioids and benzo-diazepines because of adverse effects (Acute Pain, 1992).
8. Question the use of meperidine (Demerol) because of accumulation of normeperidine, a toxic metabolite. Meperidine may be used for very brief courses in those who have demonstrated an allergy to morphine but is contraindicated in patients with impaired renal function (Acute Pain, 1992).
9. Provide opioids around the clock (ATC) or by continuous infusion rather than as needed (PRN). A PRN schedule produces delays in administration and promotes intervals of inadequate pain control.
10. Consider the use of PCA (patient-controlled analgesia) as children have less pain, less seda-

Table 14-6
Guidelines for Use of EMLA Cream

1. Refers to eutectic mixture of local anesthetics (lidocaine 2.5% & prilocaine 2.5%).

2. Reduces the pain associated with skin puncture and superficial skin procedures, including venapuncture, IM injection, accessing central ports, and lumbar punctures.

3. Is labeled for use for infants and children 1 month and older.

4. Should be applied for a minimum of 1 hour for effect and a maximum of 4 hours.

5. May produce side effects of mild, local skin pallor, erythema, or edema.

6. Is contraindicated in those with history of sensitivity to local anesthetics.

7. Should not be used in infants < 12 mos. who are receiving methemoglobin-inducing agents (e.g., sulfonamides, acetaminophen, nitrates or nitrites, nitrofurantoin, phenobarbital, phenytoin, and others).

8. Should be kept away from contact with the eyes, mucus membranes or oral ingestion.

9. Has a maximum skin area coverage based upon weight of the child.

From EMLA product insert.

tion, greater satisfaction, and no increase in opioid-related complications. Monitor the PCA pump frequently for potential problems.

11. Monitor for side effects and record effectiveness of the pain medication.

12. Devise a bowel management plan early to handle constipation associated with use of opioids.

13. Participate in conscious sedation only if there is adequate support and appropriate monitoring.

14. Avoid giving NSAIDs to children at risk for bleeding or gastric ulceration. Aspirin is generally avoided because of association with Reyes syndrome but may be used if child does not have a viral illness or fever.

15. Request to use EMLA cream as a topical anesthestic before a variety of procedures (see Table 14-6).

E. Nonpharmacologic management of pain in children (Kachoyeanos & Friedhoff, 1993; Vessey, Carlson, & McGill, 1994).

1. Encourage parents or significant others to be with the child.

2. Use sensorimotor approaches with infants and young children such as pacifiers, swaddling, holding, and rocking.

3. Encourage the presence of familiar toys or blankets or other objects.

4. Maintain a quiet, calm environment.

5. Use cognitive/behavioral strategies such as imagery, relaxation, distraction, preparatory information, rehearsal, music, and positive reinforcement before and/or during painful procedures. For example, the use of blowing away the pain or blowing bubbles or watching a kaleidoscope during a painful procedure may result in fewer pain behaviors (Kachoyeanos & Friedhoff, 1993).

6. Evaluate if physical strategies including the application of heat or cold, massage, exercise, or rest are helpful.

7. Allow older children control over management as they may prefer nonpharmacologic strategies over medication for procedures that are not excessively painful.

8. For children exposed to numerous painful procedures, devise "safe" periods, during which nothing painful is done.

F. Special considerations for the nursing care of neonates and infants.

1. Be proactive in the assessment and management of pain in hospitalized infants.

2. Inform parents that pain relief is an important part of infant care and encourage parents to participate in pain assessment and management (National Association of Neonatal Nurses [NANN], 1995).

3. Promote interdisciplinary collaboration for optimal care.

4. Examine personal and/or unit beliefs that may be barriers to improving infant pain management practices.

5. Dispel common myths about infant pain (National Association of Neonatal Nurses, 1995):
   a. Infants are unable to experience pain because of an immature nervous system.
   b. Infants may not experience pain because they do not always show responses to presumed painful procedures.
   c. Newborns are incapable of remembering pain.
   d. Infants will develop side effects from pain medications as well as possible addiction.

6. Recognize that the physiologic stress of pain in the infant may have negative consequences.

7. Assess for subtle neonatal behavioral pain responses such as a grimace, light cry, or body movement.

8. Realize that infants have a varied and inconsistent response to painful stimuli based upon developmental maturity, behavioral state, clinical stability, and environmental factors.

9. Consider the use of a preverbal scale for pain assessment (Schade, Joyce, Gerkensmeyer, &

Keck, 1996; Lawrence, Alcock, McGrath, Kay, MacMurray, & Dulberg, 1993).
   a. RIPS: Riley Infant Pain Scale.
   b. NAPI: Nursing Assessment of Pain Intensity.
   c. POPS: Postoperative Pain Score.
   d. NIPS: Neonatal Infant Pain Scale.
10. Recognize the value of a scale is it provides an objective measure of intensity of response that can be used to compare pain relief measures.
11. Use nonpharmacologic measures for procedures that involve mild, limited pain.
12. Use ordered analgesics for prolonged or more severe pain in young infants.
   a. Monitor infants for apnea and respiratory depression, especially those who are premature or have neurologic or pulmonary problems.
   b. Start with a smaller dose (mg/kg) but avoid underdosing by observing response for optimal dose and interval of administration.

BIBLIOGRAPHY

◆ ◆ ◆ ◆ ◆ ◆ ◆ ◆ ◆ ◆ ◆ ◆ ◆ ◆ ◆ ◆

Acute Pain Management Guideline Panel. (1992). *Acute pain management in infants, children, and adolescents: Operative or medical procedures and trauma, quick reference guide for clinicians.* AHCPR Pub. No. 92-0020. Rockville, MD: Agency for Health Care Policy and Research, Public Health Service, U.S. Department of Health and Human Services.

American Academy of Pediatrics. Subcommittee on Acute Gastroenteritis. (1996). Practice Parameter: The management of acute gastroenteritis in young children. *Pediatrics, 97,* 424–435.

Baraff, L.J., Bass, J.W., Fleisher, G.R., Klein, J.O., McCracken, G.H., Powell, K.R., & Schriger, D.L. (1993). Practice guideline for the management of infants and children 0–36 months of age with fever without source. *Pediatrics, 92,* 1–12.

Bates, T.A., & Broome, M. (1986). Preparation of children for hospitalization and surgery: A review of the literature. *Journal of Pediatric Nursing, 1,* 230–239.

Benitz, W.E., & Tatro, D.S. (1995). *The pediatric drug handbook* (3rd ed.) St. Louis: Mosby.

Beyer, J., Villaruel, A., & Denyes, M. (1995). *The Oucher: User's manual and technical report.* Mount Royal, NJ: Association for Care of Children's Health.

Broome, M.E., Richtsmeier, A., Maikler, V., & Alexander, M. (1996). Pediatric pain practices: A national survey of health professionals. *Journal of Pain and Symptom Managmeent, 11,* 321–320.

Hart, D., & Bossert, E. (1994). Self-reported fears of hospitalized school-age children. *Journal of Pediatric Nursing, 9,* 83–90.

Hockenberry-Eaton, M., & Benner, A. (1990). Patterns of nausea and vomiting in children: Nursing assessment and intervention, *Oncology Nursing Forum, 17,* 575–584.

Kachoyeanos, M.K., & Friedhoff, M. (1993). Cognitive and behavioral strategies to reduce children's pain. *American Journal of Maternal Child Nursing, 18,* 14–19.

Keller, V.E. (1995). Management of nausea and vomiting in children. *Journal of Pediatric Nursing, 10,* 280–286.

Lawrence, J., Alcock, D., McGrath, P., Kay, J., MacMurray, S.B., & Dulberg, C. (1993). The development of a tool to assess neonatal pain. *Neonatal Network, 12*(6), 59–66.

Malloy, M.B., & Perez-Woods, R.C. (1991). Neonatal skin care: Prevention of skin breakdown. *Pediatric Nursing, 17,* 41–48.

Malloy-McDonald, M.B. (1995). Skin care for high-risk neonates. *Journal of Wound, Continence and Ostomy Nursing, 22,* 177–182.

McRae, M.E., Rourke, D.A., Imperial-Perez, F.A., Eisenring, C.M., & Ueda, J.N. (1997). Development of a research-based standard for assessment, intervention, and evaluation of pain after neonatal and pediatric cardiac surgery. *Pediatric Nursing, 23,* 263–271.

National Association of Neonatal Nurses (NANN). (1995). Position statement on pain management in infants. *Neonatal Network, 14*(5), 54–55.

Panel on the Prediction and Prevention of Pressure Ulcers in Adults. (1992). *Pressure ulcers in adults: Prediction and prevention. Clinical Practice Guideline.* Number 3. AHCPR Publication No. 920047. Rockville, MD: Agency for Health Care Policy and Research, Public Health Service, U.S. Department of Health and Human Services.

Quigley, S.M., & Curley, M.A.Q. (1996). Skin integrity in the pediatric population: Preventing and managing pressure ulcers. *Journal of the Society of Pediatric Nurses, 1,* 7–18.

Schade, J.G., Joyce, B.A., Gerkensmeyer, J., & Keck, J.F. (1996). Comparison of three preverbal scales for postoperative assessment in a diverse pediatric sample. *Journal of Pain and Symptom Management, 12,* 348–359.

Selekman, J., & Malloy, E. (1995). Difficulties in symptom recognition in infants. *Journal of Pediatric Nursing, 10*(2), 89–92.

Selfridge, J., & Shea, S. (1993). The accuracy of the tympanic membrane thermometer in detecting fever in infants aged 3 months and younger in the emergency department setting. *Journal of Emergency Nursing, 19,* 127–130.

Tiesinga, L.J., Dassen T.W.N., & Halfens, R.J.G. (1996). Fatigue: A summary of the definitions, dimensions, and indicators. *Nursing Diagnosis, 7,* 51–62.

Wickham, R. (1989). Managing chemotherapy – Related nausea and vomiting: The state of the art. *Oncology Nursing Forum, 16,* 563-574.

Wong, D. (1995). *Whaley & Wong's nursing care of infants and children* (5th ed.). St. Louis: Mosby.

Wong, D.L. (1996). *Wong and Whaley's clinical manual of pediatric nursing* (4th ed.). Mosby: St. Louis.

Zollo, M.B., Gostisha, M.L., Berens, R.J., Schmidt, J.E., Weigler, C.G.M. (1996). Altered skin integrity in children admitted to a pediatric intensive care unit. *Journal of Nursing Care Quality, 11,* 62–67.

STUDY QUESTIONS

1. In assessing children for symptoms, an important aspect is to:
   a. rely only on objective signs.
   b. rely primarily on one's intuition about child's feelings.
   c. disregard crying since it is nonspecific.
   d. interpret both signs and subtle behavioral clues.
   e. minimize parents' description of child's usual temperament.

2. An appropriate intervention for the school-age child with nausea would be to:
   a. encourage small bites of favorite foods.
   b. give sips of fluids with high osmolality and glucose content.
   c. provide information to decrease anxiety.
   d. encourage rocking and movement for distraction.

3. Which of the following statements is accurate regarding pharmacologic management of nausea and vomiting in children?
   a. The use of phenothiazines is the drug of choice in children with minimal side effects and no age restrictions.
   b. Antiemetics are underused in children and should be used more freely in anyone with persistent nausea/vomiting.
   c. The oral route for antiemetics is most effective.
   d. Antiemetics should be avoided when the etiology of nausea/vomiting is unknown since symptoms could be masked.

4. The risk of altered skin integrity and/or development of pressure ulcers in hospitalized children:
   a. is very low and occurs primarily in children with paralysis.
   b. occurs primarily in incontinent infants.
   c. can be minimized by massaging reddened areas over bony prominences.
   d. is increased by friction and hypoperfusion.

5. The most common site of pressure ulcers in infants is the:
   a. knee.
   b. nose.
   c. occiput.
   d. sacrum.

6. In a healthy preschooler with a fever of 103° axillary with a viral syndrome, the most appropriate nursing intervention would be to:
   a. give acetaminophen based upon the child's weight and the sponge immediately with tepid water for 15 minutes.
   b. give aspirin based upon weight and assess activity and comfort level.
   c. give acetaminophen based upon weight and encourage fluids.
   d. give ibuprofen based upon weight on an empty stomach to promote absorption.

7. When providing teaching to parents about caring for a child with a fever, which of the following information should be included?
   a. A fever should be viewed as potentially harmful.
   b. The child's level of comfort and activity, and ability to drink should be assessed.
   c. A child under 2 years with a fever should be seen by a physician.
   d. The tympanic route for measuring temperature is the most accurate.

8. When considering appropriate interventions to reduce fear in hospitalized children, the nurse should remember:
   a. with proper preparation, a preschooler will not fear unfamiliar intrusive procedures.
   b. school-age children have no need for syringe play since they have usually outgrown their fear of needles.
   c. information about the sensory experience of a procedure along with the knowledge component will increase the child's level of fear.
   d. early assessment and management of pain can decrease fear in children.

9. When providing interventions for pain in infants, which of the following is correct?
   a. Opioids should be avoided because of the risk of respiratory depression.
   b. Holding and rocking should be used for an episode of mild, limited pain.
   c. If an intervention is effective, it should be reflected by a corresponding decrease in physiologic response (pulse, BP).
   d. It is better not to have parents present during a painful procedure but rather involved only in comforting afterwards.

10. General principles of acute pain management in children include:
   a. using mild analgesics as much as possible to avoid the risk of addiction.
   b. observing the child's response to a procedure the first time to gauge the need for additional treatment for pain reduction with future repeated procedures.
   c. giving pain medication PRN (as needed) rather than ATC (around the clock) to reduce sedation and constipation.
   d. assessing the child's self-report of pain before and after medication to document and evaluate response.

ANSWERS

◆◆◆◆◆◆◆◆◆◆◆◆◆◆◆◆◆◆◆◆◆◆◆◆

1.d 2.c 3.d 4.d 5.c 6.c 7.b 8.d 9.b 10.d

Chapter 15

Acute Illness: Intervention Strategies

Barbara C. Woodring, EdD, RN
Marion E. Broome, PhD, RN, FAAN

Concept

◆◆◆◆◆◆◆◆◆◆◆◆◆◆◆◆◆◆◆◆◆◆◆◆◆◆◆

◆ Children with acute illnesses or injuries and their families

Objectives

◆◆◆◆◆◆◆◆◆◆◆◆◆◆◆◆◆◆◆◆◆◆◆◆◆◆◆

At the completion of this chapter, the reader will be able to:

◆ Describe four general principles for planning interventions for acutely ill children.

◆ Evaluate appropriate outcomes after preparing a child and family for hospitalization or procedures.

◆ Describe critical content for teaching a child and family about the disease, diet, and medications.

◆ Integrate concepts of atraumatic nursing care into plans for the child who is acutely ill.

◆ Define the concept of surveillance as applied to the nursing care of a child who is acutely ill.

◆ Analyze the physical environment in which care is provided and suggest methods for making it safer for the child.

Key Points

◆◆◆◆◆◆◆◆◆◆◆◆◆◆◆◆◆◆◆◆◆◆◆◆◆◆◆

◆ Both a child and parent should be involved in teaching sessions about disease, diet, and medications.

◆ Interventions should be age-appropriate, culturally sensitive, and cost-effective.

◆ Both short- and long-term outcomes associated with interventions should be measured.

◆ Specific observations related to biophysiologic changes occurring in the child who is acutely ill must be made and reported, in a timely, sequential manner.

◆ The environment must be altered to protect the child from accidental injuries.

◆ Outcomes should be directed toward providing atraumatic care based on data obtained through various methods of surveillance.

15

Acute Illness: Intervention Strategies

◆◆◆◆◆◆◆◆◆◆◆◆◆◆◆◆◆◆◆◆◆◆◆◆◆◆◆◆◆◆◆

I. OVERVIEW

When a child becomes acutely ill, and the intervention of a health care provider is required, the entire family is affected. Families respond in a variety of ways to the stress of a child's acute illness; however, the nurse who is caring for the child and his or her family must strive to keep that family unit intact for as much of the acute care cycle as possible. It is the family that provides stability, normalcy, and comfort to a child who is acutely ill. Therefore, every effort must be made to support and integrate concepts of family-centered care. *See Chapter 28: Family-Centered Care.* This may require that the nurse and parent quickly negotiate/renegotiate caregiving roles, especially in emergent and/or life-threatening situations.

The notion of atraumatic care has recently been redefined and has found a place in the repertoire of those who provide care for children who are acutely ill (Wong, 1996). It is readily acknowledged that some interventions are traumatic and/or painful; nonetheless, these interventions are necessary for progression toward wellness. Alterations can make the interventions less stressful, traumatic, and/or painful (see Table 15-1). Pediatric nurses must strive to incorporate atraumatic principles into every aspect of care.

II. GENERAL PRINCIPLES FOR PLANNING, IMPLEMENTING, AND EVALUATING INTERVENTIONS FOR ACUTELY/CRITICALLY ILL CHILDREN AND ADOLESCENTS

A. Planning.
1. The child and family should be involved in planning from the beginning.
2. The child and family's input should be actively solicited.
3. Interventions should be planned, when at all possible, in anticipation of an event.
4. Interventions should be built upon child and family's strengths and resources.
5. Interventions are based on the developmental level of the family as well as the developmental capabilities of the child.
6. As many members of the multidisciplinary team as possible should be involved in planning for intervention.
   a. Intervention should be child-focused, not provider-centered.
   b. Interventions should be planned to overlap minimally to provide adequate rest time.
7. Outcomes should be decided on as planning begins.

B. Implementation.
1. The intervention must be sensitive to cultural, religious, and gender differences.
2. Principles of family-centered care must be evident in each intervention; maintainence of the intact family is essential.
3. Implementation strategies should be cost-effective.
4. Multiple opportunities for the family to learn new strategies and to adapt planned interventions must be provided.
5. The resources of the interdisciplinary health care team may be used to provide a full range of interventions necessary to achieve the child's maximum state of well-being.

C. Outcomes and evaluation.
1. Evaluation of effectiveness should be ongoing and shared by the family and all health care team members.
2. Outcomes must be documented and communicated on a regular basis with all team members — preferably in a care conference.
3. Outcomes should reflect both short-term and long-term measurements.

III. PREPARATION FOR HOSPITALIZATION, SURGERY, AND PROCEDURES

A. General principles of preparation.
1. Use preparation methods that are age-appropriate (see Table 15-2). *Also see Chapter 3:*

Table 15-1
Examples of Atraumatic Care

Aspects of Care	Intervention
Psychologic	Always explain what is happening to the child in language she/he will understand, not in adult/medical terms. Keep communications simple and direct; provide only as much detail as child needs to understand. Be honest; do not tell the child a procedure is not going to hurt if it is, but do not dwell on the pain factor. Use topical anesthesia and medications to assist in obtaining the child's cooperation during procedures. Ask the child to draw a picture of what is going to happen — use the opportunities for discussion, clarification, and/or education. Keep the parents involved as much as possible; encourage nurture and support of the child. Do not isolate the child from the parent. The parent's absence may be more traumatic to the child than the procedure.
Environment	Keep the child's environment as nonthreatening as possible. Interpret the surroundings from the child's perspective: What does that large machine look like — possibly a monster? Is the room very sterile with no familiar or friendly items around? Could the equipment be draped or placed in other areas and/or the implements be moved out of sight? Use child-size furniture/fixtures and colorful wall hangings or child-drawn pictures of toys, flowers, rainbows, etc., to brighten environment.
Restraints	Use restraints as minimally as possible and use the least restrictive one that provides safety (e.g., use mittens before applying a full arm restraint). If a restraint is absolutely necessary, provide frequent unrestrained movement under supervision.
Pain	Medicate appropriately and frequently. Do not withhold medication after painful procedures/surgery. Assess for pain responses such as fretfulness, irritability, grimace, shallow/rapid respirations, thrashing, crying. Use subjective pain scales when appropriate. Administer medication via oral and intravenous (IV) routes when possible; use intramuscular or subcutaneous routes as last alternatives.
Drawing blood/IV fluids	Use EMLA or similar preparation to numb area prior to needle stick. Use a nontraumatic lancet for heelsticks; use smallest gauge needle possible to obtain/maintain venous access. Consolidate lab studies to draw as small amount of blood as infrequently as possible. Insert IV in site that allows mobility without restraint, when possible. Use air-filled or well padded, appropriate length arm board, if restraint needed. Allow older child to become familiar with equipment by playing with tubing (needleless). Use brightly colored band-aids to cover needle stick sites.

Adapted with permission from Bowden, V., Dickey, S., & Greenberg, C. (Eds). (1998). *Children and their families: The continuum of care*, p. 474. Philadelphia: Saunders.

Cognitive and Psychosocial Development.
2. Consider child and family's resources (cognitive, financial, and cultural) when preparing them.
3. Assess parent's desired level of involvement prior to preparation session.
4. Provide information about the process and structure of the impending event, as well as about how the child could be expected to feel.
5. Include parents and/or siblings as appropriate.
6. Include skills training such as relaxation, distraction, and/or imagery. *See Chapter 14: Acute Illness: Symptom Management.*
7. Build on prior experiences, understanding, and skills.

B. **Adverse medical experiences: hospitalization, procedures, and surgery. Examples of media used to prepare child and prevent adverse experiences include:**
1. Tours of units, OR, lab, etc.
2. Play sessions for younger children.
3. Videotape depicting actual child experiencing event.
4. Demonstration of simple procedures.
5. Provide written materials reinforcing concepts and use pictures to illustrate and enhance understanding by children, adolescents, and parents.

Table 15-2
Preparation Techniques for Infants – Adolescents

Preparation Technique	Infant	Toddler	Preschooler	School-age	Adolescent
Focus on parent	X	X	X		
Focus on child			X	X	X
Prepare immediately before event	N/A	Yes	Yes	No	No
Videotape; written instructions	Yes (parent)	Yes (parent)	Yes	Yes	Yes
Coping skills (i.e. relaxation)			Yes	Yes	Yes
Demonstrate medical equipment	Yes (parent)	Yes (parent)	Yes	Yes	Yes
Encourage diary of event	No	No	No	Yes	Yes
Involve in decision making	Yes (parent)	Yes (parent)	Yes	Yes	Yes

C. Outcomes of preparation (see Figure 15-1).
1. Parent's ability to reinforce preparation is improved.
2. Parent understands and is comfortable with role during hospitalization.
3. Anxiety levels of child and parent are decreased when discussing impending event.
4. Child and parent can explain care and treatment in their own words.
5. Child and parents' ability to demonstrate coping skills to deal with stressor of hospitalization and/or surgery improves.
6. Parent and child verbalize satisfaction with the amount of preparation they received.

IV. TEACHING CHILD AND FAMILY ABOUT ILLNESS AND TREATMENT

◆ ◆ ◆ ◆ ◆ ◆ ◆ ◆ ◆ ◆ ◆ ◆ ◆ ◆ ◆ ◆ ◆ ◆ ◆

A. General principles of teaching.
1. Assessment of the child and parents' understanding must precede any teaching episode.
2. Teaching must begin prior to discharge.
3. Teaching sessions should be done with both child and parents present.
   a. Determine the cognitive level of the child.
   b. Determine the reading/comprehension of the parent(s).
   c. Provide simple, jargon-free explanations.
4. Multiple mediums or teaching stategies (verbal instructions, videos, written instructions or pamphlets, visual aids, pictures, etc.) enhance the probability of the individual retaining the information taught.
5. Skills that are essential for care at home (e.g., suctioning, insulin injections) need to be taught first; thorough understanding of concepts of illness and care may come much later for most children and families.
6. Parents and children assimilate knowledge and skills best when they perceive they need the information, not before.

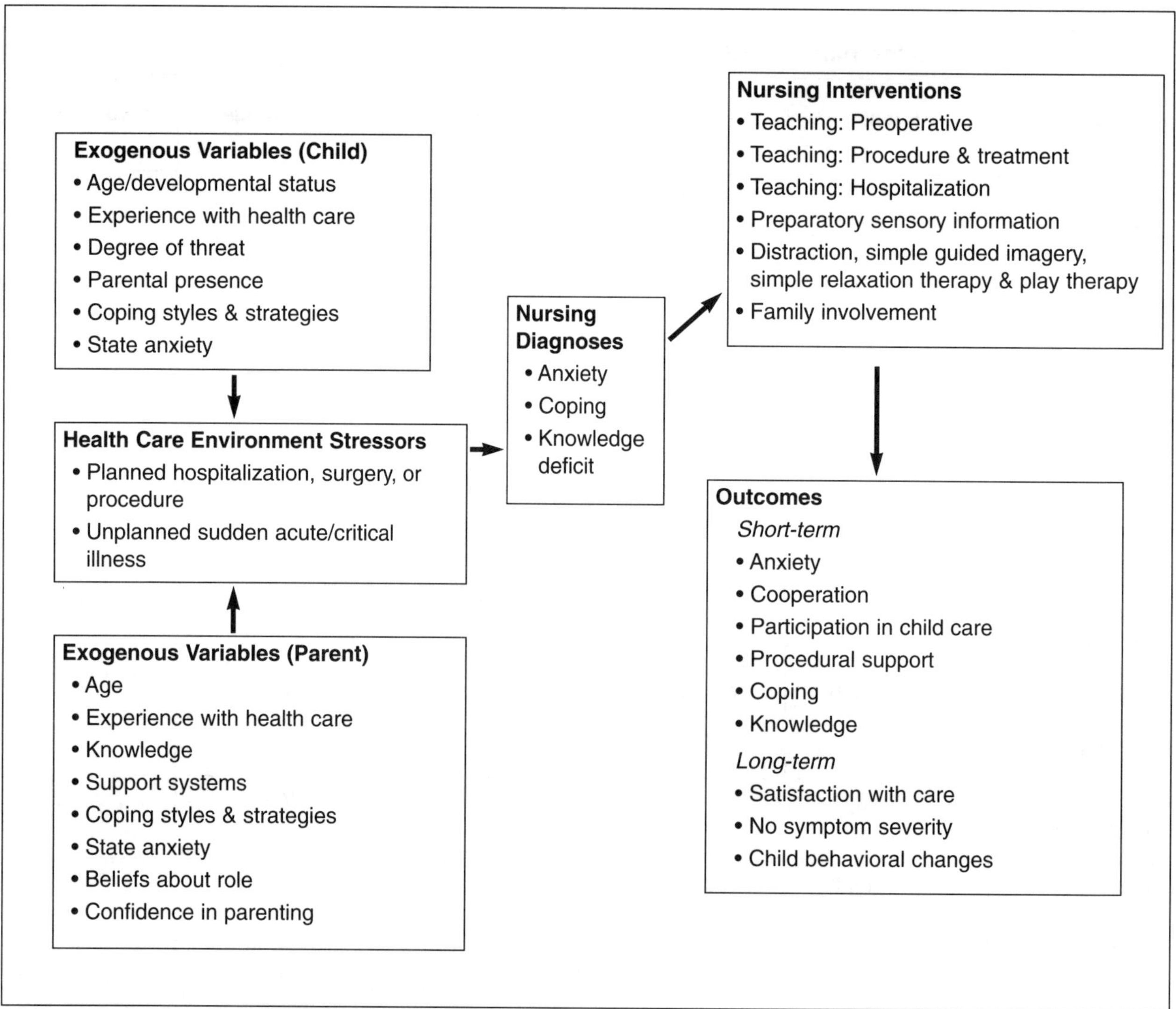

Figure 15-1
Preparation Model for Stressful Health Care Experiences

Used with permission from Broome, M., & Huth, M. (In press). Preparation for hospitalization, surgery, and procedures. In M. Craft & J. Denehy (Eds.), *Nursing interventions with children and families*. Thousand Oaks, CA: Sage Publications.

7. Return demonstration of skills taught should be observed several times or until child or parent is comfortable performing skill.
8. When discharged, parents and child should be given a resource person to call to ask questions.

B. Disease process.
1. Definition: assisting the child and family to understand information related to a specific disease process.
2. Determine child and parents readiness to hear about disease process.
   a. Anxiety level.
   b. Cognitive abilities.
3. Elicit their current beliefs about the illness: etiology, status, care, and treatment plans.
4. Content should include:
   a. Etiology: identify possible sources and/or causes.
   b. Symptom management options: discuss in terms understood by family.
   c. Diagnostic tests and procedures.
   d. Therapy/ treatment options: consider cultural/ethnic/religious background of family.
   e. Alternative treatments, as appropriate.
   f. Potential complications and/or side effects of treatment or disease.
   g. Self-care requirements.
   h. Measures to prevent/minimize side effects or reoccurrence.
   i. Available resources/support groups.
5. Help family to process data related to child's condition, progress, and prognosis.
6. Provide written explanations about self-care and

follow-up requirements, as well as a phone number for questions.

C. Medications.
1. Definition: preparing a patient to safely take the prescribed medication and monitor side effects.
2. Determine child and parents readiness to hear about medication.
   a. Anxiety levels.
   b. Cognitive abilities.
3. Elicit their current beliefs about medication: purpose, action, and adherence to prescription.
4. Content should include:
   a. Purpose and name of medication (generic and brand).
   b. Action and side effects.
   c. Dosage, route, and duration of medication; need for regular administration, as prescribed.
   d. Management of side effects.
   e. Symptoms indicating need to discontinue medication and notify health care provider.
   f. Potential consequences of discontinuing medication abruptly and how to manage missed doses.
   g. Food/drug interactions.
   h. Proper mixing and storage of medication.
   i. Use of devices and techniques to administer medication, if appropriate.
   j. Disposal of needles and unused medication.
   k. Development of a written schedule of medications to be taken.
   l. Procedures for refilling prescriptions.

D. Diet.
1. Definition: preparing a patient to correctly follow a prescribed diet.
2. Explain the purpose of the diet and relate purpose to child's condition.
3. Assess child and family's current level of understanding about prescribed diet.
4. Assess family's resources (money, transportation) needed to obtain food; provide suggestions to augment resources.
5. Assess child's willingness to eat food on diet.
   a. Encourage child to choose from menu of allowable foods; use food models for visual reinforcement.
   b. Measure intake: involve child in measuring and recording.
   c. Obtain child's opinion about foods allowed and methods of preparation.
6. Instruct child/parent about reading content labels.
7. Refer to dietitian, as appropriate.

E. Outcomes evaluation.

Parent and or child should be able to:
1. Describe their illness: basic causes.
2. Discuss the management of symptoms associated with the illness.
3. Explain simple diagnostic tests child will experience.
4. Describe actions and side effects of medications taken, as well as dosage and schedule.
5. Discuss how they will document and report changes in child's condition.
6. Have parent and child demonstrate skills needed to implement diet preparation.
   a. Develop a daily meal plan from menu of choices based on prescribed diet.
   b. If necessary, measure prescribed amounts.
   c. Read food labels on packaging and interpret correctly.
7. Demonstrate selected techniques and psychomotor skills necessary to care for child.
   a. Insulin injection.
   b. Glucometer readings.
   c. Suctioning.
   d. Respiratory treatments.
   e. Dressing changes.

IV. ENVIRONMENTAL SAFETY AND SURVEILLANCE

◆ ◆ ◆ ◆ ◆ ◆ ◆ ◆ ◆ ◆ ◆ ◆ ◆ ◆ ◆ ◆ ◆ ◆ ◆

A. Surveillance.
1. Definition: purposeful and ongoing acquisition, interpretation and synthesis of child-related data for clinical decision making.
2. General principles of surveillance.
   a. Obtain a history of normal behaviors, activities, and routines; identify possible areas of risk.
   b. Facilitate collection of diagnostic data; maintain safety of child's own room by use of treatment room for painful procedures.
   c. Analyze, interpret, and report diagnostic data as appropriate.
   d. Interpret diagnostic data to parent/child as appropriate.
   e. Monitor changes in the biophysiologic status of child (e.g., neurologic signs, vital signs, sleep patterns, tissue perfusion, behavioral changes, type and amount of drainage from tubes and/or orifices, etc.) and report significant alterations.
   f. Collaborate with health care team to prevent and/or monitor progress of infectious processes.
      (1) Evaluate possibility of child/family exposure to airborne, transmittable diseases (e.g., measles, chicken pox, meningitis,

Table 15-3
Ensuring Environmental Safety for the Hospitalized Child

Suggestions for Assuring a Child-Safe Environment	
• Security procedures are in place that preclude unauthorized removal of a child from the unit.	• The bed should be as close to floor level as possible when not delivering direct care.
• Trash cans with locking lids, or those that do not have easily removable plastic liners should be used in all areas accessible to the young child. (Plastic bags could suffocate a child.)	• Breakable drinking glasses, bottles, thermometers, and equipment must be stored above the child's reach.
• Do not leave any empty plastic bags in child's room, play room, or rooms accessible to child.	• Electrical cords must be placed out of the child's walking path.
• Inspect toys for removable parts that could be aspirated; no latex or breakable balloons allowed.	• Medications, ointments for diaper rash, cleaning supplies, etc. CANNOT be left within the reach of the child. Be alert to leaving tray/carts of medications and solutions in halls or near child's room.
• Electrical outlets within the child's room or walking path must have child-proof, occlusive covers in place.	• Doors to adjoining bathrooms must be locked when an adult is not in room; toilet seat locks are also desirable. (Children can drown in 1 inch of water.)
• Electrical beds must be disconnected from their power source or in "off" position. (Children have been killed or severely disabled by becoming entrapped between the metal bed frame and descending mattress frame.)	• Drawers must be closed tightly to prevent the child from being injured by walking into sharp corners.
• Infants, toddlers, and preschool-age children should not have access to electrical hand-operated bed controls.	• Cords from drapes or window coverings must be out of reach of child (may lead to strangulation).
• The child's bed has appropriate bed rails on sides/head/foot of bed. If child is a climber, a protective bubble, shell, or net over top of the crib may also be needed to prevent falls.	• Restraints should be used sparingly, but if applied they must be removed from the child's bed when not in use. (Toddlers have hung themselves from cloth wrist and chest restraints that were left attached to bedsides, but not in place on the child.)

Adapted with permission from Woodring, B (1998). The child with a medical-surgical condition. In M. Broome (Ed.), *Comprehensive care of the pediatric patient: Prehospitalization through rehabilitation* (pp. 157–164). Park Ridge, IL: Emergency Nurses Association.

tuberculosis) prior to admission.
  (2) Reinforce hand-washing at every opportunity.
  (3) Implement and enforce appropriate isolation techniques/infection control precautions.
  g. Consult with appropriate health care professionals to alter plan of care based on objective/subjective data collected.
3. Outcomes of surveillance.
  a. Changes in child's condition will be observed and reported quickly.
  b. Plan of care will be altered rapidly, based upon accurately observed/reported data.
  c. Nosocomial infections will be averted.
  d. Infectious processes will be contained, preventing spread within child or to other children.

B. Safety.
1. Definition: purposeful and ongoing collection and analysis of information about the child and the environment for use in promoting and maintaining an accident-free environment.
2. General principles of safety.
  a. Place child in the least restrictive environment that allows for necessary protection and observation.
  b. Know institutional policies related to use and monitoring of restraints.
  c. Identify safety hazards that exist within the physical environment (see Table 15-3).
  d. Monitor child for impaired physical or cognitive functions that might lead to unsafe behaviors/conditions.
  e. Provide appropriate supervision/surveillance, based on child's cognitive and developmental levels.
3. Anticipated outcome.
  a. Child will be able to move and play in a safe, minimally restricted environment.
  b. No injuries will result from nursing care or treatment interventions.

BIBLIOGRAPHY

Bar-Mor, G. (1997). Preparation of children for surgery and invasive procedures: Milestones on the way to success. *Journal of Pediatric Nursing, 12*(4), 252–255.

Bowden, V., Dickey, S., & Greenberg, C. (Eds.). (1998). *Children and their families: The continuum of care.* Philadelphia: Saunders.

Broome, M., & Huth, M. (in press). Preparation for hospitalization, surgery and procedures. In M. Craft, & J. Denehy (Eds.), *Nursing interventions with children and families.* Thousand Oaks, CA: Sage Publications.

Melnyk, B. (1995). Parental coping with unplanned childhood hospitalization: A theoretical framework to guide research and clinical interventions. *MCN, 23,* 123–131.

Ryan-Wenger, N. (1996). Children, coping and the stress of illness: A synthesis of the research. *Journal of the Society of Pediatric Nurses, 1*(3), 126–138.

Smith, D., Nix, K., Kemper, J., Liguori, R., Brantly, D., Rollins, J., Stevens, N., & Clutter, L. (1991). *Comprehensive child and family nursing skills.* St. Louis: Mosby.

Wong, D. (1995). *Whaley and Wong's nursing care of infants and children* (5th ed.). St. Louis: Mosby.

Woodring, B. (1998). The child with a medical-surgical condition. In M. Broom (Ed.), *Comprehensive care of the pediatric patient: Prehospitalization through rehabilitation* (pp. 157–164). Park Ridge, IL: Emergency Nurses Association.

Editor's Note

The guiding source for all the interventions and activities listed were McCloskey, J., & Bulecheck, G. (1996). *Nursing interventions classification (NIC): The Iowa Intervention Project.* St. Louis: Mosby.

The outcome evaluation was guided by material from Johnson, M., & Maas, M. (1997). *Nursing outcomes evaluation* (NOC). St. Louis: Mosby.

STUDY QUESTIONS

1. The most important factor to consider when developing a preparation session for a child who has been hospitalized is:
   a. previous experience.
   b. the child's developmental age.
   c. the parent's anxiety level.
   d. the type of procedure planned.
   e. the number of siblings.

2. Content that is essential to include when teaching a family about the child's disease is:
   a. etiology.
   b. symptoms to expect and methods to manage them.
   c. therapy and treatment options.
   d. laws protecting the child from discrimination.
   e. a, b, c.

3. Outcomes to evaluate after teaching a child and parent about medications should include:
   a. understanding of action.
   b. ability to describe side effects.
   c. understanding of who to call for further information.
   d. ability to describe food, medication interactions.
   e. all of the above.

4. Outcomes evaluation of interventions for an acutely ill child should be:
   a. both short-term and long-term.
   b. directly associated with the assessment.
   c. documented by the parent.
   d. collected by an external agency.
   e. documented by the nurse.

5. Marco, 26 months old, has been admitted to the hospital with a diagnosis of bacterial meningitis. The only rooms available in the hospital are located on an adult medical-surgical nursing unit. Which of these factors is MOST important to consider when preparing the room for Marco's admission?
   a. The room is located on the end of the hall so the child's crying would not disturb the adult patients.
   b. The adult bed is replaced by a crib.
   c. The nursing staff is prepared to deal with the developmental needs of this age child.
   d. All cleaning products are removed from countertops and/or under the sink.
   e. Family members are encourage to remain with the child and participate in his care.

6. Sandy, 6½ years of age, is the roommate of 4-year-old Angie. Sandy is upset that she cannot have her bed's remote control box at her bedside. What is the most appropriate explanation to be given to Sandy?
   a. You are too young and may injure yourself by raising/lowering the bed.
   b. The remote control is broken.
   c. You will probably use the electric bed as a toy, so we'll just keep the remote control at the nurses station to remove that temptation.
   d. Angie might get hurt on the bed if she were to get hold of the remote control to your bed.
   e. None of the above is appropriate for this age child.

7. You are assigned to provide care for 24-month-old Collen, admitted with asthmatic bronchitis, and 8-year-old Tom, who is in skeletal suspension traction for a fractured leg. Both children want to go to the playroom, but there is no Child Life Specialist available. To provide appropriate surveillance/supervision for both children, how will you handle this situation?
   a. Take Collen to the playroom and get him started playing with a large piece puzzle so he won't miss you while you return to bring Tom to the play room .
   b. Take Tom in a wheel chair to the playroom, when he has started building one of the models, bring Collen in, then remain with both children.
   c. Take Tom's bed into the playroom and arrange it so he can begin a video game, then bring in Collen and help him play with the crayons and drawing paper.
   d. Explain that since a Child Life Specialist is not available, the children will have to play in their rooms today.
   e. Take Collen to the playroom in the morning and Tom in the afternoon.

8. Ten-year-old Tameka is about to be discharged. Tameka has an immune-deficiency disorder and was admitted last week with a lung infection. In teaching Tameka to take care of herself, which of these concepts is MOST important?
   a. Wash your hands after you cover a sneeze, when you come in from school or play, and/or before you eat anything.
   b. Avoid children who have colds.
   c. Take your antibiotic before you eat.
   d. Tell your play mates that you need to rest frequently so you should play in only short intervals.
   e. Avoid participation in any type of athletic activities where you could become injured.

9. Fourteen-year-old Jason was admitted to the observation unit following a fall from his "dirt bike." Jason was wearing a helmet, which was badly damaged in the fall. Which of the following nursing interventions would initially be most important for Jason?
   a. Determine Jason's past history of falls and trauma..
   b. Check vital signs and neurologic signs to obtain baseline data.
   c. Assess Jason's understanding of bike safety and determine cause of the fall.
   d. Consult with the dietitian since Jason says he never eats meat products.
   e. Assess Jason's family situation since no parent has visited since his admission.

10. The mother of 6-year-old Sammy, admitted with neutropenia and fever, complains that Nurse Smith does not follow the procedure by washing her hands every time she enters Sammy's room. The most appropriate nursing intervention would be to:
    a. remove Nurse Smith from caring for Sammy.
    b. observe Nurse Smith and determine if the mother's comments are accurate.
    c. question Nurse Smith about the situation.
    d. provide an inservice for the staff related to the importance of hand washing, especially for compromised children.
    e. b and c.

ANSWERS

1.b 2.e 3.e 4.a 5.d 6.d 7.c 8.a 9.b 10.e

Chapter 16

Acute Illness: Outcomes of Care

Lois Van Cleve, PhD, RN

Concept

◆◆◆◆◆◆◆◆◆◆◆◆◆◆◆◆◆◆◆◆◆◆◆◆◆◆

◆ Children with acute illnesses or injuries and their families

Objectives

◆◆◆◆◆◆◆◆◆◆◆◆◆◆◆◆◆◆◆◆◆◆◆◆◆◆

At the completion of this chapter, the reader will be able to:

◆ Identify outcomes of care for families with acutely ill children.

◆ Discuss limitations and sequelae a child may experience from their illness and hospitalization and their impact on the child and family.

◆ Recognize the importance of patient/family care practice outcomes and their long-term impact on health.

◆ Consider the direct and indirect costs of acute illness to the child/family.

◆ Describe the usefulness of using outcomes on a critical pathway to guide and evaluate care during hospitalization and acute illness.

Key Points

◆◆◆◆◆◆◆◆◆◆◆◆◆◆◆◆◆◆◆◆◆◆◆◆◆◆

◆ The product of nursing is outcomes of care.

◆ Nurses have a responsibility to develop strategies for evaluating the outcomes of their patient care.

◆ Key child/family outcomes of care have been identified in nursing practice.

◆ Clinical/critical pathways are widely used in practice for tracking and evaluating outcomes of clients.

◆ There is a critical need for clinically sensitive, useful measures to evaluate the efficacy and cost-effectiveness of nursing care.

16

Acute Illness: Outcomes of Care

I. OVERVIEW

Nurses must demonstrate their care as essential and cost effective in an environment of cost containment. Outcomes of care for nursing practice are emerging with few measures developed that arise from a nursing science base. Current outcomes are measures of nursing practices during an acute illness and focus on staffing costs and quality indicators such as patient falls, infection control, medication errors, and documentation compliance. Often, direct correlations between nursing care and outcomes cannot be drawn. Outcomes of care in the child with an acute illness, therefore, are few but developing.

II. FACTORS DRIVING THE OUTCOMES

A. The escalation of health care costs have resulted in the need for:
1. Prospective payment systems.
2. Cost containment.
3. Medicare/Medicaid regulations related to improvement of care.

B. Existing variability in health care practices result in concerns regarding the quality and cost of nursing care.

C. Evolving health care delivery systems require cost accountability.
1. Differentiated nursing practice (i.e., assistive personnel, professional nurses) in patient settings.
2. Case management.
3. Health management organizations.
4. Increase of monitoring by private insurance companies.

D. Health care providers are now held accountable for their therapeutic actions by the public.
1. High acuity level and high ratio of RN staff to patient increases cost.
2. Nurses must demonstrate products of care resulting from nursing intervention.

III. EXAMPLES OF POTENTIAL OUTCOMES IN PEDIATRIC ACUTE CARE NURSING PRACTICE

A. Decreased length of stay during the hospitalization of the child:
1. Decreases the risk for long-term medical and psychosocial complications.
2. Increases the need to prepare parents and the home environment to receive and care for acutely ill children.
3. Focuses the need to teach parents initial and ongoing assessment and management of acutely ill infant/child at home.

B. Repeated measures of changes in the child's status during an acute illness can demonstrate effect of nursing intervention on selected outcomes.
1. Physical outcomes.
   a. Eating, weight gain/loss.
   b. Sleep states.
   c. Energy retention/expenditure.
   d. Physiologic variables of heart rate, oxygen saturation, blood pressure (cardiopulmonary stability or instability).
   e. Cerebral function (see Table 16-1).
   f. Symptom distress.
      (1) Pain ratings.
      (2) Nausea and vomiting.
      (3) Degree of dypsnea.
2. Psychologic outcomes.
   a. Developmental regression such as thumb sucking, bed wetting.
   b. Separation anxiety.
   c. Irritability, mood changes.
3. Social outcomes.
   a. Interest or lack of interest in the environment.
   b. Changes in ability to communicate.
   c. Change in response to personal attention from others.

C. Assessing child's health status after an acute illness/hospitalization.
1. Sensory performance (e.g., speech, hearing sight,

Table 16-1
Pediatric Cerebral Performance Category Scale

Score	Category	Description
1	Normal	Normal, at age-appropriate level; healthy, alert, and capable of normal activities of daily life. School-age child attending regular school classroom.
2	Mild Disability	Conscious, alert, and able to interact at age-appropriate level. Possibility of minor physical problem that is still compatible with normal life; able to function independently. School-age child attending regular school classroom but grade perhaps not appropriate for age; possibility of mild neurologic deficit.
3	Moderate Disability	Conscious, sufficient cerebral function for age-appropriate, independent activities of daily life. Possibility of moderate disability from noncerebral systems dysfunction alone or with cerebral system dysfunction. Performs independent activities of daily life but is disabled for competitive performance in school. School-age child attending special education classroom and/or learning deficit present.
4	Severe Disability	Conscious but dependent on others for daily support because of impaired brain function. Possibility of severe disability from noncerebral systems dysfunction alone or with cerebral system dysfunction.
5	Coma or Vegetative State	Any degree of coma without the presence of all brain death criteria. Unawareness, even if awake in appearance, without interaction with environment. Cerebral unresponsiveness and no evidence of cortex function (not aroused by verbal stimuli). Possibility of some reflexive response, spontaneous eye-opening, and sleep-wake cycles. Possibility of severe disability from noncerebral systems dysfunction alone or with cerebral system dysfunction. Dependent on others for activities of daily living support.

Reprinted with permission from Fiser, D.H. (1992). Assessing the outcome of pediatric intensive care. *Journal of Pediatrics, 121*(1), 69.

2. Mobility.
3. Emotional status (happiness, free from worry, anxious); increased anxiety/distress during subsequent health care experiences.
4. Cognition (ability to learn).
5. Self-care abilities.
6. Interaction with others (peers, siblings).
7. School performance.

D. The child's/family's satisfaction with care interventions.
1. The child and parents' satisfaction with care should be assessed at regular intervals regardless of setting, (i.e., hospital, home, or clinic).
2. Elements of satisfaction.
   a. Does nursing care (assessment/intervention) promote/hinder the development of social, cognitive, communication, and motor skills?
   b. Does the nursing care provide the child with acceptable and appropriate means of expressing or acting out feelings?
   c. Does the nursing care strengthen the child's positive self-concept?
   d. Does the nursing care facilitate, strengthen, and encourage family involvement with the child and health professionals?
   e. Has the child been encouraged to interact with peers as appropriate?
   f. Has the transition from hospital to home or home to hospital been facilitated?
   g. Have normalizing experiences been encouraged?

E. The child's/family's ability to cope with the stressors of acute illness. *See Chapter 11: Acute Illness, Injury, and Hospitalization* and *Chapter 12: Acute Illness: Effects on the Child's Family.*

F. The child's/family's quality of life.
1. Effect of acute illness on child's emotional state.
   a. Anxiety regarding illness outcomes.
   b. Threats to self-esteem.
2. Effect of acute illness on the child's physical state.
   a. Changes in physical appearance.
   b. Changes in physical activity.

3. Social involvement during acute illness.
   a. Change in relationships with friends and family.
   b. Change in school performance.
   c. Change in cognitive development.
   d. Change in spiritual development.
   e. Change in sibling responses to parent/child.

G. The cost to the family.
   1. Direct and measurable cost of treatment and health services during acute illness.
      a. Payment by third party payer (e.g., health insurance).
      b. Cost of follow-up care.
      c. Travel and housing costs during hospitalization.
      d. Child care costs for other siblings during the acute illness.
      e. Increased living expenses.
      f. Missed work time of parents.
      g. Threat of parent job loss due to acute illness of a child.
   2. Indirect and difficult to measure outcomes.
      a. Parent concerns related to separation from child during hospitalization.
      b. Neglect of other family members, siblings, and friends.
      c. Quality of life.
      d. Loss of private time for parents increasing risk to well-being and health.
      e. Loss of time to manage complex family responsibilities.

IV. FACTORS THAT INFLUENCE THE MEASUREMENT OF OUTCOMES IN ACUTE CARE

A. Developmental factors.
   1. Age of child: i.e., premature, infant, child, adolescent.
   2. Cognitive ability of the child to communicate and understand.
   3. Ability of child to care for self physically.
   4. Separation, attachment, and identity concerns.
   5. Family structure: i.e., only child, large family, teenage parents, blended.
   6. Family function.
      a. Open or closed family system affects use or nonuse of resources.
      b. Family cohesion, expression, conflict.

B. Diverse families: impact of acute illness.
   1. Cultural differences may require specific tools for measuring outcomes. (i.e., words to describe pain in the English language may have different meanings in Spanish).
      a. Differences in response to illness and its meaning
         (1) Beliefs and values affect the meaning of illness.
         (2) Customs and practices related to illness differ.
      b. Family and cultural support during acute illness. *See Chapter 12: Acute Illness: Effects on the Child's Family.*
   2. Socioeconomic differences.
      a. Expectations of care and outcomes may differ.
      b. Educational level of child/family may affect their understanding of illness.
   3. Alternative lifestyles.
      a. Different parenting styles.
      b. Social acceptance and support.

V. USING CRITICAL PATHWAYS FOR MONITORING OUTCOMES

A. Clinical/critical pathways are used to track and evaluate patient outcomes.

B. Definition: a structured, multidisciplinary client care plan in which therapeutic interventions are performed for a defined problem and are sequenced on a timeline.

C. Purpose of pathways.
   1. Delineates daily the expected patient outcomes necessary to reach discharge goals.
   2. Requires evaluation of patient's progress daily or periodically.
   3. Provides process for tracking the quality of care.
      a. Use goals as standards.
      b. Assess symptom management outcomes over time.
   4. Pathways identify patients who vary from the standard response.
      a. Individualize the plan for care when child does not meet the expected outcome for the day.
      b. Link interventions to outcomes.
   5. Decreases the length of hospital stay and financial outcomes.
   6. Decreases the cost while maintaining or improving quality.

VI. CHALLENGES IN MEASURING PATIENT CARE OUTCOMES FOR THE ACUTELY ILL CHILD

A. Lack of clinically sensitive, easily used outcome measures for pediatric populations.
1. Often difficult to link interventions to outcomes.
2. Valid and reliable research measures need to be adapted and tested for clinical use.

B. Resocialization of nurses in practice, management, leadership, and education to "think" in terms of outcomes in pediatric acute care.
1. Assessment tools must target specific factors known to respond to intervention.
2. Interventions must be directly linked to assessment and outcome.
   a. Documentation reflects type and strength of intervention.
   b. Intervention must be monitored for consistency of implementation.
3. Outcomes.
   a. Documentation reflects measurement of targeted outcomes.
   b. Outcomes assessment links to baseline assessment to validate change.

C. Additional appropriate nursing care outcomes must be identified for acutely ill children and their families across a variety of settings.
1. Acute care inpatient setting.
2. Intensive care setting.
3. Emergency setting.
4. Primary care setting.
5. Home setting.

VII. A SYSTEMS MODEL FOR NURSING CARE OUTCOMES (see Tables 16-2 & 16-3)

A. Child.
1. Inputs (i.e., child's health status).
2. Process (i.e., delivery of care).
3. Outcomes (i.e., indicators of physiologic status).

B. Nurses.
1. Inputs (i.e., all registered nurses).
2. Process (i.e., nursing interventions).
3. Outcomes (i.e., child outcomes).

C. Setting (e.g., hospital, home, clinic, school).
1. Inputs (i.e., values, attitudes, beliefs, available resources, sufficient providers).

Table 16-2
The Outcomes Model for Health Care Research

	Inputs	Processes	Outcome
Client			
Provider			
Setting			

Reprinted with permission from Holzemer, W.L. (1994). The impact of nursing care in Latin America and the Caribbean: A focus on outcomes. *Journal of Advanced Nursing, 20*, 5–12.

Table 16-3
An Example of the Process Model in Pediatric Pain Management

	Inputs	Processes	Outcome
Child	pain location, intensity quality, duration	change in pain over time	pain relief
Nurse	assessment	monitor/manage non-pharmacologic and pharma-cologic (analgesic) intervention/instruction	reassess document reports
Setting	tertiary hospital	provision of appropriate equipment monitors	percent outside analgesic cycle

2. Process (i.e., staff mix, patient acuity, satisfaction of staff).
3. Outcomes (i.e., provider turnover, morbidity, mortality, readmissions).

BIBLIOGRAPHY

Brooten, D., & Naylor, M.D. (1995). Nurses' effect on changing patient outcomes. *Image: Journal of Nursing Scholarship, 27*(2), 95–99.

Fiser, D.H. (1992). Assessing the outcome of pediatric intensive care. *The Journal of Pediatrics, 121*(l), 68–74.

Holzemer, W.L. (1994). The impact of nursing care in Latin America and the Caribbean: A focus on outcomes. *Journal of Advanced Nursing, 20*, 5–12.

Holzemer, W.L., & Tierney, A. (1996). Variables, variability, and variations research: Implications for medical informatics. *Journal of the American Medical Informatics Association, 2*(3), 183–190.

Moritz, P. (1991). Innovative nursing practice models and patient outcomes. *Nursing Outlook, 39*(3), 111–114.

STUDY QUESTIONS

◆ ◆

1. The most important reason to assess patient outcomes related to nursing interventions is:
   a. to save on health care costs.
   b. to demonstrate nursing knowledge.
   c. to be considered equal partners on the health care team.
   d. to measure changes in the patient status due to nursing care.
   e. to decrease length of hospital stay.

2. Six-year-old Anne is recovering from an emergency appendectomy and is on a pediatric acute care unit of the hospital. One of her parents has been staying with her at all times. Among other symptoms, Anne is being carefully monitored and assessed for pain. When considering outcomes of pain management for Anne, which of the following is accurate?
   a. Fluid intake decreased.
   b. Provides pain score of 8 on 10-point scale.
   c. Displays guarding of abdomen.
   d. Ambulates to hallway with minimal assistance.
   e. Refuses to move in bed.

3. Patient outcomes assessment has become essential in nursing practice because:
   a. there is considerable variability in health care delivery.
   b. nurses are accountable to the public.
   c. patient care outcomes are nursing products.
   d. there have been increases in health care costs.
   e. all of the above

4. In considering the costs of acute care illness to a family, the following are important areas:
   a. The quality of family life
   b. The value of lost income of parents
   c. The problem of decreased mobility of the child
   d. The direct costs of treatment for the child
   e. all of the above

5. Challenges for nurses in using patient care outcomes in their practice are:
   a. the availability of clinically sensitive measures.
   b. the support of the medical centers for more nurses.
   c. changing the mindset of nurses regarding outcomes care.
   d. the availability of easily used outcome measures.
   e. all of the above except b.

6. Modification of nursing outcomes measures may be necessary when there are differences in:
   a. the cause of illness.
   b. the age of the child.
   c. the income of the family.
   d. ethnicity.
   e. all of the above.

ANSWERS

◆ ◆

1.d   2.d   3.e   4.e   5.e   6.e

Chapter 17

Acute Illness: The Continuum of Care

Christine K. Olson, MSN, RN

Concept

◆◆◆◆◆◆◆◆◆◆◆◆◆◆◆◆◆◆◆◆◆◆◆◆◆◆◆◆

◆ Children with acute illnesses or injuries and their families

Objectives

◆◆◆◆◆◆◆◆◆◆◆◆◆◆◆◆◆◆◆◆◆◆◆◆◆◆◆◆

At the completion of this chapter, the reader will be able to:

◆ Describe the continuum of care and potential phases of care.

◆ Recognize transition points in the care of children with acute illness or injury.

◆ Identify common strategies to ease transitions across the continuum of care.

◆ Recognize available resources to assist in planning for transitions.

Key Points

◆◆◆◆◆◆◆◆◆◆◆◆◆◆◆◆◆◆◆◆◆◆◆◆◆◆◆◆

◆ Children often progress rapidly through phases of care in acute illness and injury.

◆ Entry into the continuum of care can occur at any phase of care.

◆ Families need anticipatory guidance to most efficiently manage transitions in care.

◆ Coordination of available resources around child and family needs supports the smoothest transition across the continuum of care.

Acute Illness: The Continuum of Care

I. PHASES OF CARE

Children with acute illness or injury often progress rapidly through the continuum of care requiring careful assessment and planned intervention to make the transitions between phases seamless. The progression through and between the various phases of care is the continuum of care. It varies by diagnosis and with each individual; the continuum need not include all phases of care.

A. Identification of illness/injury.
1. Recognition may be sudden as with the onset of fever, pain.
2. Identification and diagnosis may occur as part of routine health exam.
3. Injury can be traumatic, requiring urgent/emergent intervention.
4. Identification and diagnosis may be prolonged due to insidious onset.

B. Urgent care.
1. May involve primary care provider in familiar surroundings for family and child.
2. May involve visit at a designated urgent care facility or emergency department with less familiar surroundings and procedures.

C. Emergent care.
1. Transportation may be by ambulance, fixed wing aircraft, or helicopter with unfamiliar health care providers.
2. Family may not be available to child and/or care providers for history.
3. Transfer to another facility with specialty or pediatric expertise may be required.

D. Acute care setting within a hospital.
1. Surroundings can vary based on:
   a. Placement criteria (with age mates or by diagnosis).
   b. Facility (pediatric or adult hospital).
2. Accommodations may or may not reflect consideration of family members (e.g., family waiting rooms, sleeping accommodations, proximity to child).

3. Families may be asked to provide history by multiple providers.
4. Admission may be emergent or planned.

E. Intensive care.
1. Facility will dictate availability of pediatric specialists.
2. Technology can be intimidating for both family and patients.
3. Visitation may be restricted or regimented.
4. Level of care provided includes almost constant observation with frequent interventions/procedures.
5. Transfer to this level of care may or may not have been planned for by either family or health care providers.
6. Family's primary care provider may/may not be included as part of health care team, which increases unfamiliarity of staff with family and comfort of family.

F. Intermediate care.
1. Level of care may be dictated by the facility.
2. Level of care provided includes frequent observation and interventions/procedures.
3. Transfer to this type of care from the intensive care unit (ICU) often generates anxiety on part of family who are used to close monitoring of child's status by nurses and physicians.

G. Rehabilitation.
1. Transfer to another facility or area may be necessary.
2. Level of care requires at least 3 hours of therapy each day (speech, physical, and/or occupational).
3. Medical insurance may not include rehabilitation benefits for children.

H. Outpatient specialty care.
1. May occur as part of diagnostic workup or recovery and follow-up care.
2. May involve surgical/invasive procedures requiring anesthesia or sedation.
3. Preparation/instructions for procedures may be required.

I. Home care.
1. May be initiated with or without previous hospitalization.
2. May include multiple providers for care.

J. Transition from acute to chronic illness.
1. May occur over time due to recurrence of health problem, natural course of disease process, or complications of illness/injury.
2. Treatment focus and acceptance of diagnosis by patient and family may be very different from their response to acute illness.

II. TRANSITION POINTS

◆ ◆ ◆ ◆ ◆ ◆ ◆ ◆ ◆ ◆ ◆ ◆ ◆ ◆ ◆ ◆ ◆ ◆

A. Multiple phases result in several transitions.
1. Within the continuum of care for each individual child and family, multiple phases may be encountered for each occurrence of illness/injury.
2. Movement between phases can be identified as transition points.

B. Difficulties of transition.
1. Smooth transfer from one phase of care to another requires frequent, clear communication. Whether written or verbal, details of the plan of care need to be made available for all providers as well as the patient and family.
2. Providers and family may not anticipate transfers/transitions.
   a. A child's rapid progression to wellness or more serious illness may take providers and family by surprise.
   b. Inexperience with disease process/recovery may hinder recognition of impending transition.
   c. Insurance review may require more rapid transfer than desired by providers and/or family.
3. Providers and family have different understandings of the impact of transfers.
   a. Knowledge of another facility and/or area may be limited.
   b. Knowledge of various phases of care may be limited.
   c. Patients and families may be comfortable with level of care provided in one phase and have expectations of similar levels in other phases. Transition from intensive care to either intermediate or acute care settings has been identified as a stressor for families who come to rely on almost constant observation as a measure of security for their child.
4. Insurance requirements may complicate or limit options available.

5. Multiple transfers may be necessary for just one illness/injury.
6. Transfers between phases involve multiple providers.
   a. Expectations and requirements for communication and involvement in decision making are complicated.
   b. Family/child may hear various versions of same "truth," which can cause confusion and erode trust.
7. Hospital systems may speed up or slow transfers between phases depending on:
   a. Availability of beds and resources.
   b. Regulatory or insurance requirements.
8. Providers and family may disagree about the plan of care.
   a. Expectations of outcome may be an issue.
   b. Ethical questions can be raised by one or both.

III. BARRIERS TO ACCOMPLISHING A SMOOTH TRANSITION

◆ ◆ ◆ ◆ ◆ ◆ ◆ ◆ ◆ ◆ ◆ ◆ ◆ ◆ ◆ ◆ ◆ ◆

A. Financial barriers.
1. Quality and quantity of care depends upon insurance coverage.
2. Impact of managed care.
   a. Limited sites/ providers/time frames for visits in which transitions are possible.
   b. Decreased availability of specialty services.
   c. Length of time needed to accomplish transitions within systems.
3. The number of uninsured Americans is rising four times as rapidly as population growth, producing significant numbers of uninsured children.
4. Uninsured – need specific procedures to transition:
   a. Homeless and immigrant children/families.
   b. Working poor.
5. Coverage of equipment and services to ease transitions for children who are acutely and chronically ill often not included in basic insurance policies (e.g., provision and maintenance of lifts, electric wheelchairs, rehabilitation equipment).

B. System barriers.
1. Lack of uniformity in paperwork (forms) for agencies and insurance companies.
2. Lack of agreement in institutional policies.
3. Lack of collegial support and interactions among multiple health care providers involved in transition.

C. Knowledge barriers.
1. Agency-based and insurance-based jargon inhibits clarity of communication between parents/child and health care providers.
2. Lack of understanding by caregivers about child's developmental level, knowledge base, need for control, and feelings about leaving one system of care and moving into unknown.
3. Variations in child's ability to express opinions/ alternate opinions related to transitioning.
4. Lack of understanding on child and family's part about what to expect in caregiving policies and practices in new environment.

IV. STRATEGIES TO EASE TRANSITION

A. RN as care coordinator/manager.
1. Essential that someone act as coordinator when multiple disciplines and/or providers involved.
2. Coordinating role includes communication/ teaching, contacting/arranging resources, clarifying expectations/requirements, assessing essential outcomes, and scheduling around the needs of patient and family.

B. Widespread communication of plan of care.
1. Written documentation systems need to support ready access to information.
   a. Include records of family/child educational sessions.
   b. Document educational content skills/ demonstrated/attained.
   c. Include written plan for family assuming home care of child.
2. Verbal communication should be followed up with written documentation for:
   a. Clarification of expectations.
   b. Record of expectations.
   c. Legal/regulatory requirements.
3. Child's response to interventions done by health care providers, self, family should be documented.

C. Anticipatory guidance of family and child.
1. Preparation should include consideration of:
   a. Reason/rationale for transition.
   b. What to expect both physically and emotionally.
   c. How the child/family/provider can help ease transition.
   d. Outcome.
   e. Expected timeline.
   f. Introductions to new providers if necessary.
2. Follow-up should be ongoing and include information on:
   a. Reason for delays, if any.

b. Options/choices available.
c. Reinforcement of original information.
d. Availability of providers for future questions/concerns.

D. Involve advanced practice nurses (APN).
1. Experience with illness across the continuum of care can be valuable.
2. Knowledge of available resources is extensive.
3. May be case manager.

E. Notify available resources as soon as possible.
1. Include discharge planners, social workers, clergy, etc., as soon as possible.
2. Notification at time of entry to continuum can afford other professionals time to plan and help in the identification of potential transition points.
3. Describe details of management plan and child's response.
4. Be certain local EMS is alerted to presence of technologically dependent child (if appropriate).

F. Case management plans/critical paths.
1. Documented guides to the typical plan of care and response to treatment.
2. Can be individualized based on patient/family needs.
3. May be institution-specific but can be shared with receiving areas/facilities.

G. Home visits/passes.
1. Home assessment for access issues, space needs, etc.
2. Family experience can identify new learning needs and/or equipment needs.

H. Involvement of family and child in the development of the plan of care.
1. Enables individualization of plan.
2. Serves as tool for anticipatory guidance and teaching.
3. Minimizes conflicts of expectations.
4. Is a patient/family right.

V. AVAILABLE RESOURCES TO ASSIST TRANSITIONS

A. Discharge planners.
1. Usually have specialized knowledge of insurance requirements and providers.
2. Require early notification and direction of needs upon discharge.

B. Social workers.
1. Can assist with the emotional support needs of

the family/child.
2. Can arrange for services available beyond health needs.

C. Case managers.
1. May be employees of the insurance provider and/or the providing organization.
2. Have experience in typical progression patterns through the continuum and accompanying needs.

D. Insurance company.
1. Usually require early notification and/or approval of treatment needs.
2. May require additional information/rationale for authorization of care.
3. May have reviewers onsite to monitor progress and plan of care.

E. Public health departments.
1. Some disease notification is required for tracking and follow-up.
2. May assess home situation for follow-up and reinforce teaching and progression within the plan of care.

F. Other disciplines (physical, occupational, speech therapists).
1. Knowledge and experience can be vital to complete care planning.
2. Provide another perspective of care needs and response to treatment.

G. School districts.
1. Required to meet the specialized learning needs of children.
2. Involvement may be directed by a thorough evaluation of learning needs.

H. Community agencies.
1. Broadens network of support for child/family.
2. Able to provide various services for assistance including financial, technical, educational, and emotional.

BIBLIOGRAPHY

Belter, D.M. (1995). Seven steps to managing outcomes across settings. *Nursing Quality Connection, 4*(6), 6.

Blau, J.D. (1997). Clinical pathways. Designing road MAPs for outcomes management across the continuum of care. *Orthopaedic Nursing, 16*(2, Suppl.), 55.

Haggerty, R.J. (1993). Continuum of care system development. *Clinical Pediatrics, 32*(10), 592–596.

Lumsdon, K. (1994). Beyond four walls. Case management evolves into the management of a continuum of care. *Hospitals and Health Networks, 68*(5), 44–45.

Martin, K. (1997). Assessing the continuum of care. *Journal of Nursing Care Quality, 11*(4), 3.

McHugh, M., West, P., Assatly, C., Duprat, L., Howard, L., Niloff, J., Waldo, K., Wandel, J., & Clifford, J. (1996). Establishing an interdisciplinary patient care team: Collaboration at the bedside and beyond. *Journal of Nursing Administration, 26*(4), 21–27.

McNamara, S.T., & Sullivan, M.K. (1995). Patient care coordinators: Successfully merging utilization management and discharge planning. *Journal of Nursing Administration, 25*(11), 33–38.

Nelson, J.M. (1993). Interinstitution coordination smooths transitions. *Oncology Nursing Forum, 20*(1), 117.

Patterson, P.K., Blehm, R., Foster, J., Fuglee, K., & Moore, J. (1995). Nurse information needs for efficient care continuity across patient units. *Journal of Nursing Administration, 25*(10), 28–36.

Sullivan, M.K. (1995). Facilitating continuity of care. The role of the patient care coordinator. *Nursing Clinics of North America, 30*(2), 221–230.

STUDY QUESTIONS

Elizabeth, age 4, was admitted to the intensive care unit from the emergency department, following a motor vehicle accident in which she sustained a fractured femur and a closed head injury. She is now conscious and ready for transfer to a general pediatric unit.

1. If Elizabeth arrived in the emergency department via an ambulance, how many transitions and transfers of care has she experienced thus far?
   a. None yet
   b. Only one
   c. Two
   d. At least three
   e. Several

2. Which of the following is a possible phase of care that Elizabeth could encounter in her recovery, considering her injury?
   a. Emergent care
   b. Outpatient specialty care
   c. Rehabilitation
   d. Home care
   e. All of the above

3. What strategy would best facilitate Elizabeth's care if multiple disciplines are involved?
   a. A care conference with the parents
   b. A clinical path
   c. Ongoing written and verbal communication between team members
   d. Consistent educational materials for all disciplines
   e. A case manager

John is a 9-year-old child admitted to an inpatient pediatric unit with acute abdominal pain. The family's physician admitted John following an office visit. The primary physician suspects acute appendicitis and has informed the family of his concern. On admission to the room, the nurse observes that the family is extremely anxious and attempts to calm their fears by stating that John's symptoms are probably the result of the flu. A resident describes John's admission as necessary to "just run some tests."

4. What result may be produced by the efforts of the nurse and resident to calm the family?
   a. Decreased anxiety and increased confidence in the health team
   b. Increased anxiety and decreased confidence in the health team
   c. Decreased anxiety and decreased confidence in the health team
   d. Increased anxiety and increased confidence in the health team
   e. Initial decrease in anxiety but resultant hostility

5. As John is being prepared for surgery, what strategies would be most helpful to John and his family?
   a. Introductions to the new set of caregivers
   b. Explanations of the impending surgical experience
   c. Communication to the surgical team of John's special needs
   d. All of the above
   e. b and c only

6. John is discharged to his home on intermittent intravenous antibiotics. A home health nurse is scheduled to administer the medications. What information would the home health nurse need to ease the transition from hospital to home?
   a. Activity level, tolerance of diet, and pain control at time of discharge
   b. Reaction to medication in the hospital
   c. Arrangements for supplies and medications
   d. All of the above
   e. a and b only

7. Which of the following best describes a phase of care?
   a. A treatment location
   b. An episode of illness
   c. A step in the continuum from illness to wellness
   d. A plan for each discipline's involvement
   e. Normalization based on disease/disorder

8. At which point or phase do patients enter the continuum of care?
   a. Upon admission to hospital
   b. Upon diagnosis
   c. At any phase
   d. Upon discharge from hospital
   e. None of the above

9. What is the most important role of the nurse in the care of patients along a continuum?
   a. Coordination of plan of care activities
   b. Adherence to medical orders
   c. Arranging for care conferences
   d. Discharge teaching
   e. Involvement of family

10. Resources available to the nurse in the care of a child include:
    a. the insurance company, case managers, and discharge planners.
    b. advanced practice nurses, social workers, and the clergy.
    c. the family, school officials, and support groups.
    d. community agencies, outpatient services, public health care department.
    e. all of the above.

ANSWERS

1.c 2.e 3.c 4.b 5.d 6.d 7.c 8.c 9.a 10.e

Chapter 18

Acute Illness: Selected Acute Illnesses and Injuries

Patricia A. Moloney-Harmon, RN, MS, CCRN

Concept

◆◆◆◆◆◆◆◆◆◆◆◆◆◆◆◆◆◆◆◆◆◆◆◆◆◆◆

◆ Children with acute illnesses or injuries and their families

Objectives

◆◆◆◆◆◆◆◆◆◆◆◆◆◆◆◆◆◆◆◆◆◆◆◆◆◆◆

At the completion of this chapter, the reader will be able to:

◆ Discuss the pathogenesis of gastroenteritis, otitis media, bacterial meningitis, fractures, toxic ingestions, and firearm injuries in children.

◆ Identify risk factors for toxic ingestions in children.

◆ Describe the incidence of firearm injury in the pediatric population.

◆ Discuss therapeutic interventions to treat gastroenteritis, otitis media, bacterial meningitis, fractures, toxic ingestions, and firearm injury in children.

◆ Discuss home care considerations for the child with gastroenteritis, otitis media, bacterial meningitis, fractures, toxic ingestion, and firearm injury.

Key Points

◆◆◆◆◆◆◆◆◆◆◆◆◆◆◆◆◆◆◆◆◆◆◆◆◆◆

◆ Many of the acute infectious processes in children occur with crowded conditions, either in the home or in daycare settings.

◆ "Accidents" such as toxic ingestion and firearm injury in children are preventable.

◆ Patient and family education must stress prevention of future occurrences of acute illness or injury.

◆ Initial assessment of acute illness or injury focus on airway, breathing, and circulation.

◆ Definitive treatment occurs after stabilization of the cardiorespiratory status.

◆ The care of any child with an acute illness or injury will involve collaborative management across the health care team.

18

Acute Illness: Selected Acute Illnesses and Injuries

I. GASTROENTERITIS

A. Overview. Gastroenteritis or acute infectious diarrhea is a common illness in childhood. Children can develop dehydration and malnutrition as a result of diarrhea.

1. Definition: an infectious process of the gastrointestinal tract caused by bacterial, viral, and parasitic agents, resulting in increased movement and rapid emptying of intestinal contents. The rapid excretion prevents absorption and results in the loss of nutrients, electrolytes, and water.
2. Etiology.
   a. Because infants have an immature immune system and have not been exposed to a variety of pathogens and therefore have not developed antibodies, they are more susceptible.
   b. Mostly spread from feces to mouth by contaminated food or water.
   c. May also spread by person to person contact, especially in areas where there are crowded conditions, such as daycare centers.
   d. Poor living conditions, where overcrowding and poor sanitation exists is a major risk factor. It is the most frequent cause of death in children in developing countries.
   e. Rotavirus, a virus, is the most common pathogen associated with gastroenteritis; *Escherichia coli (pathogenic), Salmonella, Shigella, Staphylococcus aureus* are frequently associated bacterial pathogens; *Giardia* and *Cryptosporidium* are common parasitic agents (Wong, 1995).
3. Pathophysiology.
   a. An infectious agent in the GI tract produces acute diarrhea.
   b. Depending on the pathogen, a variety of pathogenic changes may occur.
      (1) Viral agents such as rotavirus will attack the epithelium of the small bowel mucosa causing severe inflammation and decreased absorption of water and sodium.
      (2) Bacterial pathogens usually produce enterotoxins that invade the epithelium of the bowel mucosa causing inflammation and decreased absorption of fluids and electrolytes.
      (3) Parasitic agents cause inflammation and decreased absorption of fluid and electrolytes.
   c. Diarrhea produces several consequences as fluids and electrolytes are lost.
      (1) Dehydration due to loss of fluid in stools, vomiting, decreased fluid intake, and increased insensible losses.
      (2) Electrolyte imbalance due to sodium, chloride, potassium, bicarbonate losses, and insufficient electrolyte replacement.
      (3) Metabolic acidosis due to loss of bicarbonate in stools, accumulation of lactic acid resulting from hypoxemia, which produces tissue hypoxia, and ketosis.
4. Incidence.
   a. Leading cause of illness in children less than 5 years of age.
   b. The incidence is approximately 2½ episodes per person per year.
   c. Accounts for 3% to 5% of hospital admissions for children (Cusson, 1992).

B. Assessment.
1. History and physical exam.
   a. History.
      (1) Potential cause.
      (2) Onset.
      (3) Severity.
      (4) Duration.
      (5) Presence of another infection.
   b. Physical examination.
      (1) Frequent, watery stools.
      (2) Vomiting.
      (3) May have fever, abdominal pain.
      (4) Signs of dehydration.
         (a) Tachycardia.
         (b) Tachypnea.
         (c) Irritable or lethargic.
         (d) Poor skin turgor.
         (e) Slightly moist to dry mucous

Table 18-1
Treatment of Acute Diarrhea

Degree of Dehydration	Signs/Symptoms	Rehydration Therapy	Replacement of Stool Losses	Maintenance Therapy
Mild (5%–6%)	Increased thirst Slightly dry buccal mucous membranes	Oral rehydrating solution (ORS) 50 ml/kg within 4 hours	ORS 10 ml/kg (for infants) or 150–250 ml at a time (for older children) for each diarrheal stool	Breastfeeding, if established, should continue; regular infant formula if tolerated. If lactose intolerance suspected, give undiluted lactose-free formula (or half-strength lactose-containing formula for brief period only); infants and children who receive solid food should continue their usual diet
Moderate (7%–9%)	Loss of skin turgor, dry buccal mucous membranes, sunken eyes, sunken fontanel	ORS 100 ml/kg within 4 hours	Same as above	Same as above
Severe (>9%)	Signs of moderate dehydration plus one of the following: rapid thready pulse, cyanosis, rapid breathing, lethargy, coma	Intravenous fluids (Ringer's lactate), 40 ml/kg/hour until pulse and state of consciousness return to normal; then 50–100 ml/kg of ORS	Same as above	Same as above

*If no signs of dehydration are present, rehydration therapy is not necessary. Proceed with maintenance therapy and replacement of stool losses.

From Wong, D., & Mattis, L. (1995). Conditions that produce fluid and electrolyte imbalance. In D.L.Wong (Ed.), *Whaley and Wong's nursing care of infants and children* (5th ed.) St. Louis: Mosby–Year Book, p. 1238.

membranes.
(f) Sunken eyeballs and fontanels.
2. Diagnostic tests.
 a. Comprehensive laboratory tests are not indicated in a child with simple diarrhea and no signs of dehydration.
 b. Laboratory tests that should be obtained when indicated:
  (1) Stool specimens.
   (a) WBC count.
   (b) Cultures.
   (c) ELISA for rotavirus.
   (d) Ova and parasites if bacterial and viral cultures are negative.
  (2) Reducing substances.
  (3) Stool electrolytes.
  (4) If dehydration is suspected:
   (a) Urine specific gravity.
   (b) CBC, serum electrolytes, BUN.

C. Therapeutic Management
 1. Primary goal is to correct the fluid and electrolyte imbalance and prevent malnutrition. Additional goals include:
  a. Restoring bowel to normal function.
  b. Preventing the spread of infection to others in contact with the child.
 2. Mild cases can be treated at home by parents. Parents are recommended to provide soft drinks, clear juices, or an oral electrolyte solution such as Pedialyte.
 3. Initial treatment for acute diarrhea and dehydration is with oral rehydration therapy (ORT) (see Table 18-1).
  a. Ongoing stool losses are replaced 1:1 with oral rehydrating solution (ORS).
  b. ORS is given frequently in small amounts to these children, even in the presence of emesis.
 4. Normal diet should be given to the child as early as possible.

5. Intravenous fluids are necessary for the child with severe dehydration and vomiting.
   a. Initial volume is 20 m/kg as a bolus.
   b. Subsequent fluid therapy is directed toward correcting the fluid and sodium losses and replacing ongoing losses.
6. Antibiotics are indicated only for bacterial or parasitic causes that have been proven by culture.
7. Antidiarrheal drug therapy generally is not indicated.

D. Common nursing diagnoses, outcomes, and interventions.
1. Fluid volume deficit related to acute infectious diarrhea.
   a. Outcome: Patient will demonstrate signs of normal hydration.
   b. Nursing interventions.
      (1) Give oral rehydration solutions for rehydration and for replacement of lost stool volume.
      (2) Give intravenous fluids as indicated.
      (3) Administer antibiotics if indicated.
      (4) Monitor intake and output.
      (5) Monitor for signs of adequate hydration: vital signs, mucous membranes, skin turgor, mental status, urine output, and urine specific gravity.
      (6) Monitor stools for blood.
      (7) Weigh child daily.
2. Impaired skin integrity related to stools in contact with skin.
   a. Outcome: Patient will have no signs of skin breakdown.
   b. Nursing interventions.
      (1) Change diaper frequently.
      (2) Clean areas in contact with stool with water and mild, nonalkaline soap.
      (3) Apply ointment to areas in contact with stool.
      (4) Closely monitor areas in contact with stool for signs of infection/breakdown.
3. Altered nutrition: less than body requirements related to inadequate intake.
   a. Outcome: Patient will maintain and/or gain weight as appropriate.
   b. Nursing interventions.
      (1) Continue breast-feeding after rehydration if mother is breast-feeding infant.
      (2) Offer normal diet as early as possible.
      (3) Observe feeding patterns (Wong, 1995).

E. Home care considerations.
1 Provide family with instructions about appropriate therapy and observe for signs of dehydration.
2. Discuss with family the appropriate diet for child.

3. Teach parents about basic hygiene measures if appropriate.

II. OTITIS MEDIA

A. Overview. Otitis media (OM) is a common disease of early childhood.
1. Definition: inflammation of the middle ear that may occur with or without effusion.
   a. Acute otitis media has a rapid onset of symptoms and is about 3 weeks in duration
   b. Otitis media with effusion refers to an inflammation of the middle ear with a collection of fluid in the middle ear space.
   c. Subacute otitis media is a middle ear effusion lasting for 3 weeks to 3 months.
   d. Chronic otitis media with effusion is a middle ear effusion that persists beyond 3 months (Wong, 1995).
2. Etiology.
   a. *Streptococcus pneumoniae* and *Haemophilus influenzae* are the organisms that most commonly cause OM.
   b. Daycare centers have been identified as a high risk area for the development of OM.
   c. Secondary smoke has also been identified as a factor in the development of OM.
   d. Breast-fed babies show a lower incidence of OM.
3. Pathophysiology.
   a. Obstruction of the middle ear cause secretions to collect in the middle ear.
   b. Obstruction results in negative middle ear pressure and eventually produces an effusion.
   c. Negative pressure and diminished ciliary transport inhibits drainage.
   d. Complications can occur, which include:
      (1) Tympanic membrane retraction, which results from the negative pressure drawing the tympanic membrane inward. This may cause decreased sound transmission, perforation, and further infection.
      (2) Tympanosclerosis or scarring of the eardrum.
      (3) Perforation, which often occurs with chronic disease.
      (4) Adhesive otitis media occurs due to a thickening of the mucous membrane resulting from the growth of fibrous tissue. This may cause fixation of the ossicles causing hearing loss.
      (5) Cholestcatoma develops when the epithelial lining forms scales that disintegrate the structures in the ear, including bone

and ossicles. It can enter the inner ear and the meninges.

   (6) Inner ear and mastoid sinus infections, and meningitis are rare complications if antibiotic therapy is used.

   e. Primary factor in recurrent otitis media is abnormal function of the eustachian tube. Normally, the eustachian tube equalizes pressure between the middle ear and the atmosphere. When there is an obstruction, trapped air is absorbed and a vacuum is created. Secretions collect within the middle ear, resulting in otitis media with effusion.

4. Incidence.
   a. Highest in children between 6 months and 2 years of age.
   b. Gradually decreases though there is a slight increase at time of school entry (Wong, 1995).
   c. Before school age, boys are affected more than girls; later, both ages are affected equally.
   d. Highest in winter months.

B. Assessment.
1. History and physical examination.
   a. History is consistent with development of OM.
   b. Clinical manifestations.
      (1) Irritability with pulling at the ear.
      (2) Complaints of ear, face, and/or jaw pain.
      (3) Fever.
      (4) Loss of appetite.
      (5) Rhinorrhea.
      (6) Vomiting and diarrhea.
      (7) Upper respiratory infection.
   c. With OM external (OME), child may not complain of pain or may have a fever. Instead, there may be complaints of a popping feeling during swallowing, a full feeling, and a feeling of movement in the ear.
2. Diagnostic tests.
   a. The diagnosis is usually based on symptomatology.
   b. Otoscopy will reveal a tympanic membrane that is red and bulging.
   c. With OME, the tympanic membrane may appear dull gray, the landmarks are hidden, and fluid may be present behind the eardrum.
   d. A culture is done if purulent drainage is noted.

C. Therapeutic management.
1. Acute otitis media.
   a. Antibiotic therapy is the major therapeutic intervention.

   b. Antipyretics are given to control fever.
   c. Once antibiotic therapy has been completed, the child is evaluated for the effectiveness of the therapy and/or for the development of complications.
2. Recurrent otitis media.
   a. Antibiotics are indicated. With long-term antibiotic use, the child should be evaluated once a month to determine if an effusion is developing.
   b. Steroids are not recommended to treat recurrent OM.
   c. If medical treatment is not effective, a myringotomy with insertion of tubes may be performed.
3. Otitis media with effusion.
   a. The goal of therapy is to ensure a fluid-free middle ear and to restore normal hearing.
   b. Medical management is the same as for acute and recurrent OM.
   c. Myringotomy with tube placement is indicated when medical management is not successful.
   d. Most cases of OM resolve; the most common complication, when it does occur, is hearing loss.

D. Common nursing diagnoses, outcomes, and interventions
1. Potential for injury related to infection.
   a. Outcome: Patient will not experience complications related to the infectious process.
   b. Nursing interventions.
      (1) Administer antibiotics as prescribed.
      (2) Administer fluids to prevent dehydration.
2. Pain related to inflammation and pressure in ear.
   a. Outcome: Patient will not experience pain or will have pain diminished to a level that is tolerable to the child.
   b. Nursing interventions.
      (1) Administer pain medication/antipyretics.
      (2) Apply heat to affected side.
      (3) Provide child with soft food or liquid to avoid chewing.
      (4) Place child, or have child lie on affected side (Wong, 1995).

E. Home care considerations.
1. Teach parents that antibiotics must be given for the full course to prevent recurrence.
2. Discuss with parents that temporary hearing loss may occur and to speak directly to their child.
3. Discuss with parents the care of tympanostomy tubes.

III. COMPLEX FRACTURES

◆ ◆ ◆ ◆ ◆ ◆ ◆ ◆ ◆ ◆ ◆ ◆ ◆ ◆ ◆ ◆ ◆ ◆ ◆

A. Overview. Fractures are a common injury in children; they occur whenever the stress force exceeds the resistance of the bone. Children's limited gross motor coordination and high mobility level make them highly susceptible to fractures.

1. Definition: a complex fracture occurs when the bone protrudes through an open wound or when bone fragments damage surrounding tissue.
2. Etiology.
   a. Fractures in childhood have a variety of causes; the causes are the same as those for traumatic injuries in children.
   b. Birth trauma is the usual cause in newborns; fractures occurring in infancy other than those related to birth trauma often indicates physical abuse.
   c. Fractures in children result from motor vehicle and bicycles accidents, falls, and child abuse.
3. Pathophysiology.
   a. Bone injury occurs when external forces act on the body or the bony structure (direct impact) or internal forces (muscle contraction, ligament stress) cause stress (bending forces) (Moloney-Harmon, Srnec, & Muir, 1996).
   b. Fractures occur when loading forces exceed the ability of the bone to store and dissipate energy by temporary deformation.
   c. Loading forces include bending, tension, compression, torsion, and combined loading.
   d. The forces can be applied along the bone's long axis or along the traverse axis.
   e. The magnitude and rate of loading will determine the extent of bone injury.
4. Incidence.
   a. Fractures that occur during the first 2 years of life may be an indication of skeletal abnormalities, bone disease, or child abuse.
   b. Upper extremity fractures are more common in children older than 2 years of age through adolescence (Thomas, 1993).
   c. Osteomyelitis due to an open fracture or an open reduction from a closed fracture is often more extensive in a child.
   d. Torn ligaments and dislocation are less common in children.
   e. Children's fractures heal more rapidly due to osteogenic activity of the periosteum and endosteum.

B. Assessment.

1. History and physical examination.
   a. If the history is not consistent with the injury, child abuse must be considered.
   b. The typical signs of injury include swelling, deformity, pain, and decreased function of the affected part.
   c. Ecchymosis, intense muscular rigidity, and crepitus may be present.
   d. A bone part may be visible through an open wound; bleeding or decreased sensation distal to fracture site may be present in addition to vascular or nerve damage.
   e. The 5 P's of ischemia due to vascular injury should be considered when assessing the affected part: **p**ain, **p**ulselessness, **p**allor, **p**aresthesia, **p**aralysis.
2. Diagnostic evaluation.
   a. Radiographic evaluation.
   b. Laboratory studies (e.g., a decreased hematocrit if the child is bleeding).

C. Therapeutic management.

1. The first priority for treatment is restoration of airway, breathing, circulation.
2. Following assessment of neurovascular status, a splint or traction can be applied. The broken and adjacent bones must be kept from moving. Once the splint or traction is applied, assess neurovascular status to compare to baseline findings.
3. Wound irrigation, debridement, fracture alignment, and stabilization will take place for a complex fracture. Stabilization may include plaster cast, internal or external fixation. Stabilization will depend on fracture pattern, location, degree of soft tissue injury, and type and severity of other injuries.
4. The child must be closely monitored for the development of compartment syndrome.
   a. Compartment syndrome occurs when there is an increase in pressure within an anatomic space. Progressive vascular compromise is the result, which produces circulatory impairment and compromised tissue function.
   b. Direct bleeding, inflammation, or constriction by a splint or a cast may produce compartment syndrome.
   c. The 5 P's (listed above) are signs of compartment syndrome.
   d. Interstitial pressures of 30 to 35 mmHg are indicative of compartment syndrome (Moloney-Harmon, Srnec, & Muir, 1996).
   e. Compartment syndrome requires immediate treatment.
      (1) The limb is placed in a neutral position to avoid further compromise of arterial flow.

(2) Casts are removed.
(3) If symptoms continue, a fasciotomy may be required in order to release pressure and maintain extremity circulation.

D. Common nursing diagnoses, outcomes, and interventions.
1. Potential for injury related to fracture.
   a. Outcome: Patient will not experience complications related to bone injury.
   b. Nursing interventions.
      (1) Observe and palpate each bone to identify abnormalities. Assess the presence of spontaneous movement before moving the extremity.
      (2) Immobilize the affected bone once bleeding is controlled and an initial neurovascular assessment takes place. Immobilize bone *and* joint above and below the injury.
      (3) A detailed neurovascular assessment takes place during the secondary survey and includes assessment for circulation, sensation, and motion. Repeat neurovascular assessments often and compare to baseline.
2. Alteration in physical integrity.
   a. Outcome: Patient will not experience complications related to treatment for bone injury.
      (1) Maintain external fixation devices by cleaning as ordered. Pins should be cleaned with antiseptic solution.
      (2) Perform neurovascular assessments on a regular basis and report any changes from baseline.
      (3) Administer antibiotics as ordered.
3. Alteration in comfort: pain.
   a. Outcome: Patient will report minimal/reduced occurrence of pain. *See Chapter 14: Acute Illness: Symptom Management and Chapter 22: Chronic Conditions: Symptom Management.*
   b. Nursing interventions.
      (1) Assess for indicators of pain. If the child is unwilling or unable, assessment of the physical indicators of pain may be necessary.
      (2) Provide pain medication at regular intervals or consider the use of patient-controlled analgesia (PCA).
      (3) Consider use of nonpharmacologic methods of pain management appropriate to child's developmental level.

E. Home care considerations.
1. Provide parent education.
   a. Keep leg elevated on a pillow above the level of the heart when the child is resting to prevent swelling.
   b. Observe for signs of circulatory compromise, especially after the extremity has been in a dependent position.
   c. Clean pin/fixator devices sites daily with hydrogen peroxide.
2. Discuss with parents methods to loosen and reapply constrictive bandages or splints (Campbell & Campbell, 1991).

IV. ACUTE BACTERIAL MENINGITIS

A. Overview. Acute bacterial meningitis is the most common neurologic infection of early childhood. Rapid, accurate diagnosis and treatment are critical to prevent the unnecessarily high death rates and residual damage that still occur.
1. Definition: an acute inflammation of the meninges that is identified by an abnormal number of WBCs in the cerebrospinal fluid.
2. Etiology/incidence.
   a. Newborn.
      (1) Most cases are the result of organisms acquired at delivery, in the nursery, or even in the household.
      (2) Most common organisms: Group B streptococci, *E. coli.*
   b. Infants.
      (1) Infants less than 3 months are probably protected by passively acquired antibodies.
      (2) Incidence remains high up to 2 years.
      (3) Unimmunized infants at higher risk.
      (4) Most common organisms: *H. influenza* type B, *Neisseria meningitides, Streptococcus pneumonaie.*
   c. Toddlers.
      (1) Incidence decreases after 2 years; beyond 5 years children begin to acquire the protection of antibodies.
      (2) Most common organisms: *H. influenza* type B, *Neisseria meningitides, Streptococcus pneumonaie.*
   d. School-age children and adolescents.
      (1) Incidence sharply reduced after 2 years.
      (2) The same organisms that affect infants and toddlers occur in school-age children, however, meningococcal meningitis occurs predominantly in this age group. This is the only type of meningitis that is spread by droplet transmission and the risk increases with the number of contacts, therefore, affecting primarily this age group though it can occur at any age.
   e. Seasonal variations.

(1) *H. influenza* meningitis primarily occurs in autumn or early winter

(2) Pneumococcal and meningococcal meningitis primarily occur in the late winter or early spring though they may occur at any time.

  f. Predisposing factors.

(1) Males are affected more than females, especially in neonates.

(2) Major causes of neonatal meningitis are premature rupture of membranes and maternal infection during the last week of pregnancy.

(3) Meningitis seems to happen as an extension of a variety of bacterial infections.

(4) CNS anomalies, neurosurgical injuries or procedures, sickle cell disease, and infections elsewhere in the body appear to increase susceptibility.

3. Pathophysiology.

  a. The most common route of infection is pathogens entering CNS indirectly from a distant site. Direct invasion of pathogens from penetrating trauma or from ruptured abscess is less common.

  b. Colonization usually occurs in the upper respiratory tract and enters the small blood vessels.

  c. The bloodborne organisms seed in the meninges and colonize the CSF, producing inflammation of the brain and meninges, which eventually results in invasion and replication in the CSF.

  d. The bacteria and subsequent inflammation produce a series of events that if untreated can lead to cerebral edema, increased ICP, and herniation.

4. Prognosis.

  a. Mortality.

(1) Neonatal meningitis has the highest mortality rate.

(2) β–hemolytic streptococcal, meningococcal, and pneumococcal meningitis are also associated with poor outcomes.

  b. Morbidity highest when disease occurs in first 2 months of life.

B. Assessment.

1. History and physical exam.

  a. Clinical manifestations vary and result from the host response to the pathogen invasion.

  b. Infants tend to have nonspecific symptoms: fever, lethargy, poor feeding, vomiting, diarrhea, bulging fontanel, hypothermia or hyperthermia, hypoglycemia or hyperglycemia.

  c. Children and adolescents may exhibit fever, vomiting, lethargy, headache, altered level of consciousness (LOC), photophobia, back pain, nuchal rigidity, Brudzinski's sign (flexion of the hips with passive flexion of the knees), and/or Kernig's sign (back pain and resistance after passive extension of the lower legs).

  d. Seizures may occur in all age groups.

  e. Petechial rash, most pronounced on the extremities, seen with *N. meningitidis*.

2. Diagnostic tests.

  a. The definitive diagnosis is made after lumbar puncture (See Table 18-2).

  b. Cerebrospinal fluid (CSF) culture and gram stain will identify the causative organism.

  c. Serum glucose should be drawn about approximately ½ hour before the lumbar puncture.

  d. Blood cultures are recommended for all children suspected of meningitis; sometimes the blood culture will be positive even with a negative CSF culture (Eagan, 1995).

  e. Nose and throat cultures may prove helpful.

C. Therapeutic management.

1. Requires early recognition and immediate treatment to prevent mortality and morbidity.

2. Child is isolated and antibiotic therapy initiated.

  a. Before CSF results are returned, broad spectrum antibiotics are given based on most likely etiologic agent.

(1) Newborn empiric therapy: includes aminoglycoside with ampicillin and sometimes cefotaxime.

(2) In child > 6 weeks: cefotaxime or ceftriaxone with or without ampicillin.

  b. Once CSF results are obtained, specific antibiotics are given based on bacterial sensitivity and age of patient.

3. Dexamethasone (0.6 mg/kg/day) is given IV every 6 hours for the first 4 days of therapy.

4. Hydration: the type and amount of IV fluid is determined by patient's condition.

5. Increased intracranial pressure (ICP) is controlled, if appropriate.

  a. Administer osmotic diuretics.

  b. Position to avoid neck compression midline.

  c. Elevate head 15–20°.

  d. Minimize noise.

  e. Avoid suctioning.

  f. Avoid stressful procedures.

  g. Minimize or decrease pain.

6. Complications are treated accordingly.

  a. Subdural effusion.

  b. Disseminated intravascular coagulation.

Table 18-2
Definitive Diagnosis of Meningitis Obtained from a CSF Culture

Parameter	Normal Value	Abnormal Value Associated with Meningitis
Pressure	60–100	increased
Color	clear, no odor	cloudy
WBC	≤ 5	100–60,000 mm³
Predominant WBC type	mononuclear	polymorphonuclear
Glucose	> ⅔ blood glucose > 60 mg/dl	< ½ to ⅔ of blood gluclose < 40 mg/dl
Protein	15–45	>100
Gram stain	negative	positive

    c. Septic shock.
    d. Seizures.

D. Common nursing diagnoses, outcomes, and interventions.
  1. Potential for injury related to infectious process.
    a. Outcome: Patient will not experience complications related to infection.
    b. Nursing interventions.
      (1) Place patient in appropriate isolation.
      (2) Obtain cultures (CSF, blood).
      (3) Administer antibiotics.
        (a) Initiate therapy as soon as ordered.
        (b) Administer doses on time.
      (4) Monitor for signs of respiratory distress, shock, and increased intracranial pressure.
      (5) Initiate emergency treatment for complications, as appropriate.
      (6) Administer intravenous fluids, as ordered.
      (7) Monitor intake and output.
      (8) Decrease environmental stimuli, such as noise and light.
      (9) Implement seizure precautions.
  2. Alteration in comfort: pain related to inflammation of meninges.
    a. Outcome: Patient will not experience pain or pain will be at level acceptable to the child.
    b. Nursing interventions.
      (1) Permit child to assume position of comfort.
      (2) Administer analgesics, as ordered.
      (3) Monitor child's response to analgesics.

E. Home care considerations.
  1. Instruct parents about appropriate vaccinations.
  2. Help parents identify other close contacts who may require vaccinations.
  3. Instruct parents about the importance of follow-up care.

V. POISONING

A. Overview. Accidental poisoning continues to be a major problem for the pediatric population in spite of many prevention efforts. Immediate intervention is necessary to prevent further injury or death.
  1. Definition: a state created when a substance is ingested, inhaled, injected, applied to skin, or absorbed causing structural damage or disturbed function.
  2. Etiology.
    a. Children, especially toddlers, have developmental characteristics that make them susceptible to poisoning.
    b. They are naturally curious, use taste to explore their environment, and are mobile.
    c. Other risk factors for poisoning are access to poisons, lack of proper supervision, recent move, pregnancy, unemployed or single parent household (Longo & Dickenson, 1996).
  3. Pathophysiology: depends upon agent ingested.

B. Assessment (See Table 18-3).

C. Therapeutic management.
1. Emergency management.
   a. Initial management includes establishing stable cardiorespiratory status.
   b. Further treatment is based on type of poison ingested (see Table 18-3).
2. Decreasing absorption.
   a. Gastric emesis.
      (1) Ipecac is the agent of choice to induce vomiting in the home. It should never be given prior to identification of specifically ingested substance. It is not generally recommended in the hospital because it delays the initiation of activated charcoal due to prolonged vomiting.
      (2) Ipecac is a gastric irritant and stimulates the vomiting center in the reticular formation.
      (3) Ipecac is contraindicated in infants and children:
         (a) Less than 6 months of age.
         (b) With neurologic impairment.
         (c) Who have ingested strong acids, alkali, or hydrocarbons.
         (d) Who have lost their gag reflex.
         (e) Who have ingested agents likely to cause rapid onset of CNS depression or seizures (Longo & Dickenson, 1996).
   b. Gastric lavage.
      (1) Empties the stomach and enhances decontamination of residual toxins.
      (2) Normally flushed through a large bore nasogastric tube with room temperature normal saline until the solution is clear.
      (3) Limited effectiveness when instituted more than 30 minutes after the ingestion.
      (4) Endotracheal intubation is necessary before this procedure is instituted in patients with an impaired gag reflex or in those patients with a potential for vomiting and subsequent aspiration.
3. Increasing elimination.
   a. Activated charcoal.
      (1) Decreases absorption and increases excretion of the toxin by binding with it in the gastrointestinal tract.
      (2) Usually administered by nasogastric tube; its unpleasant taste makes it difficult to drink.
      (3) Usual dose is 1 g/kg to a maximum of 50 g which should be given within 2 hours of the ingestion, following emesis and lavage (Woolf, Berkowitz, Liebelt, & Rogers, 1996).
      (4) The first dose is most effective when given with a cathartic such as sorbital. Sorbital binds with the charcoal and moves the toxin rapidly through the gastrointestinal tract.
      (5) Subsequent doses (0.5 g/kg every 4 hours) (Longo & Dickenson, 1996):
         (a) Stop recirculation into the liver.
         (b) Adsorb toxin secreted into the bowel lumen.
         (c) Continue adsorption throughout the gastrointestinal tract.
         (d) Given without a cathartic to prevent severe diarrhea and electrolyte abnormalities.
      (6) Activated charcoal should be mixed with water to decease its viscosity and prevent tube obstruction.
      (7) Patient's response varies.
         (a) Usually produces vomiting, especially if ipecac was given.
         (b) May need airway protection to decrease risk of aspiration.
      (8) Nursing priorities.
         (a) Position patient on right side with head of bed elevated.
         (b) Ensure suction is immediately available.
         (c) Maintain patency of the IV and gastric tube.
   b. Extracorporeal drug removal (Woolf et al., 1996).
      (1) Forced diuresis: when combined with alkalinization of the urine, traps the toxin in the tubular lumen, decreases reabsorption, and promotes elimination.
      (2) Dialysis: removes toxins by moving solutes across a semipermeable membrane across a concentration gradient.
      (3) Hemoperfusion: removes toxin from blood which is passed through a charcoal or resin filter.
      (4) Plasmapheresis: removes toxins from the plasma by continuous centrifugation.
4. When the toxin in unknown.
   a. Child is treated as though a harmful substance was ingested.
   b. Assessment includes evaluation for potential traumatic injuries and signs of ingestion, such as altered mental status.
   c. Airway is established (if necessary) and maintained.
   d. Patient is monitored and has intravenous access established.
   e. Appropriate specimens (serum, gastric, urine) are obtained.
   f. Supportive care given until definitive care prescribed.

Table 18-3
Selected Poisonings in Children

Type of Poison	Clinical Manifestations	Treatment

Corrosives
  Drain, toilet,
    oven cleaners
  Electric dishwasher
    detergent
  Mildew remover
  Batteries
  Denture cleaners
	Severe burning pain in mouth, throat, and stomach
	White, swollen mucous membranes, edema of lips, tongue, and pharynx
	Violent vomiting
	Drooling and inability to clear secretions
	Signs of shock
	Anxiety and agitation
		Inducing vomiting is contraindicated (vomiting redamages the mucosa).
		Dilute corrosive with water (usually no more than 120 ml [4 oz]), not milk (coats membranes, making assessment difficult) unless vomiting occurs.
		Provide patent airway if needed.
		Administer analgesics.
		Do not allow oral intake.
		Esophageal stricture may require repeated dilatations and/or surgery.

Hydrocarbons
  Gasoline
  Kerosene
  Lamp oil
  Lighter fluid
  Turpentine
  Paint thinner and remover
	Gagging, choking, coughing
	Nausea
	Vomiting
	Alterations in sensorium, such as lethargy
	Weakness
	Respiratory symptoms of pulmonary involvement: tachynea, cyanosis, retractions, grunting
		Treatment options are controversial.
		Inducing emesis is generally contraindicated.
		Gastric lavage may be used.
		Symptomatic treatment of chemical pneumonia includes high humidity, oxygen, hydration, and antidotes for secondary infection.

Acetaminophen	Occurs in four stages
	1. Initial period (2 to 4 hours after ingestion):
	    Nausea, vomiting, sweating, pallor
	2. Latent period (24 to 36 hours):
	    Patient improves
	3. Hepatic involvement (may last seven days and be permanent):
	    Pain in upper right quadrant, jaundice, confusion, stupor, coagulation abnormalities
	4. Patients who do not die in hepatic stage generally recover.
		Remove using induced vomiting; lavage, activated charcoal.
		Antidote *N*-acetylcysteine (NAC) is given, usually by nasogastric tube (smells like rotten eggs).
		NAC is given as one loading dose and usually 17 maintenance doses.
		NAC may be given intravenously, but use is investigational.

Aspirin (ASA)	Acute poisoning
	  Nausea
	  Disorientation
	  Vomiting
	  Dehydration
	  Diaphoresis
	  Hyperpnea
	  Hyperpyrexia
	  Oliguria
	  Tinnitus
	  Coma
	  Convulsions
	Chronic poisoning
	  Same as above but subtle onset (often confused with illness being treated)
	Dehydration, coma, and seizures may be more severe.
	Bleeding tendencies
		Use ipecac at home for moderate toxicity.
		Hospitalization is used for severe toxicity.
		Emesis, lavage, activated charcoal, and/or cathartics used.
		Activated charcoal is important early in ASA toxicity.
		Sodium bicarbonate transfusions to correct metabolic acidosis and urinary alkalinization is effective in enhancing elimination.
		Apply external cooling for hyperpyrexia.
		Administer diazepam for seizures.
		Administer oxygen and ventilation for respiratory depression.
		Administer vitamin K for bleeding.
		In extreme cases, hemodialysis (not peritoneal dialysis) may be used.

Table continues on next page

Table 18-3 (continued from previous page)
Selected Poisonings in Children

Type of Poison	Clinical Manifestations	Treatment

Barbiturates
Short-acting
  Hexobarbital
  Methohexital sodium
  Thiopental sodium
Short to Intermediate
  Amobarbital
  Butabarbital sodium
  Pentobarbital sodium
  Secobarbital
Long-acting
  Phenobarbital
  Mephobarbital
  Metharbital
	Mild sedation to deep coma with loss of deep tendon reflexes
	Miosis (early); dilated pupils unresponsive to light (late)
	Hypothermia
	Slow-to-rapid, shallow respirations
	May progress to Cheyne-Stokes respirations
	Hypoxemia
	Hypercarbia
	Depressed cough reflex
	Laryngospasm may occur
	Hypotension; Bradycardia
	Decreased urine output
		Gastric aspiration followed by lavage
		Endotracheal intubation if child is unconscious and overdose is suspected or is child exhibits respiratory depression
		Mechanical ventilation
		Fluid resuscitation, if in shock
		Vasopressor support if fluid does not correct hypotension
		Furosemide, if renal dysfunction occurs
		Urinary alkalinization for phenobarbital overdose
		Hemodialysis or hemoperfusion for severe barbiturate overdose not responsive to conventional therapies

Carbamazepine (Tegretol)	Neurologic status fluctuates with stage of absorption; increased absorption occurs in Stage 4 with resumption of normal peristalsis)
	1. Stage I (serum level >25 mcg/ml)
	  Stupor or coma
	  Abnormal pupillary reaction to light
	  Respiratory depression
	2. Stage II (serum level 15-25 mcg/ml)
	  Irritability
	  Combativeness
	  Choreiform movements
	  Hallucinations
	3. Stage III (serum level 11-15 mcg/ml)
	  Nystagmus, drowsiness, ataxia
	4. Stage IV (serum level <11 mcg/ml)
	  Normal mental examination
	  Mild ataxia
	  May relapse to earlier stages
	Cardiac conduction delays
	Hypotension
	Dysrhythmias
	May see acute hepatic dysfunction, hyponatremia, SIADH
		Lavage, activated charcoal
		If concretion has occurred, surgical gastrostomy may be necessary.
		Endotracheal intubation and mechanical ventilation if respiratory depression develops.
		Treat seizures if they occur.
		Seizures from hyponatremia require treatment with IV sodium replacement.
		Patients in status epilepticus or with dysrhythmias may require charcoal hemoperfusion.
		Conventional therapy for hypotension and altered hepatic function
		Water restriction and sodium supplementation for SIADH

Clonidine	Miosis Coma Respiratory depression Apnea Depressed level of consciousness to coma Hypothermia Hypotonia may be present Serum levels >10 to 15 mg/ml cause transient hypertension which is followed by hypotension. Serum levels <10 mg/ml may cause hypotension or patient may be normotensive. Bradycardia 1st degree heart block or PACs may be noted.	Lavage, activated charcoal Fluids for hypotension and shock if present; if no response, vasopressor support may be necessary. Passive warming to treat hypothermia Endotracheal intubation and mechanical ventilation if respiratory depression is present Atropine for bradycardia Sodium nitroprusside for hypertension; anticipate hypotensive phase Naloxone for any child with CNS, cardiovascular or respiratory depression

Table continues on next page

Table 18-3 *(continued from previous page)*
Selected Poisonings in Children

Type of Poison	Clinical Manifestations	Treatment
Cocaine	Sinus tachycardia Hypertension Ventricular ectopy Peripheral vasoconstriction With toxic dose, bradycardia and hypotension develop and ventricular dysrhythmias become more frequent. As toxicity progresses ventricular fibrillation, circulatory collapse, and ashen color appears. Emotional lability Overalertness Mydriasis Nausea Vomiting Hyperthermia Hyperreflexia May have seizures. CNS hyperexcitability progresses to coma and flaccid paralysis. Tachypnea, deep respirations progresses to dypsnea and respiratory failure.	Cannot decrease cocaine's absorption or increase excretion because of rapid absorption. Severe hypertension and seizures require treatment with sedatives such as diazepam or lorazepam. Sodium nitroprusside if sedatives not effective for hypertension Fluid resuscitation, if hypotensive Labetelol to treat tachycardia and ventricular dysrhythmias Lidocaine may be necessary to treat ventricular dysrhythmias. Cooling measures for hyperthermia Endotracheal intubation and mechanical ventilation for respiratory depression
Theophylline	Dysrhythmias Hypokalemia Hypophosphatemia Hyperglycemia Acidemia Hypotension Agitation Hyperreflexia Seizures Vomiting	Lavage, activated charcoal, sedatives for seizures Propanolol for dysrhythmias Administration of potassium, phosphate, sodium bicarbonate Metoclopramide or ranitidine may be given for vomiting.
Tricyclic antidepressants	Agitation and restlessness followed by sedation progressing to seizures or coma Some patients demonstrate myoclonus, tremors, chorea, choreoathetosis. Hypotension Decreased cardiac conduction rate Metabolic acidosis Signs of parasympathetic overstimulation: dry skin, axilla, mouth; mydriasis, flushed skin, agitation, hyperpyrexia	Lavage, activated charcoal Endotracheal intubation and mechanical ventilation for respiratory depression Fluids to treat hypotension; if no response vasopressor support Sodium bicarbonate for metabolic acidosis Sedatives for seizures

Table continues on next page

Table 18-3 *(continued from previous page)*
Selected Poisonings in Children

Type of Poison	Clinical Manifestations	Treatment
Iron Mineral supplement or vitamin containing iron	Occurs in 5 stages 1. Initial period ($\frac{1}{2}$ to 6 hours after ingestion). If child does not develop gastrointestinal symptom in 6 hours, toxicity is unlikely. 　Vomiting 　Hematemesis 　Diarrhea 　Bloody stools 　Gastric pain 2. Latency (2 to 12 hours) 　Patient improves 3. Systemic toxicity (4 to 24 hours after ingestion) 　Metabolic acidosis 　Fever 　Hyperglycemia 　Bleeding 　Shock 　Death (may occur) 4. Hepatic injury 　Seizures 　Coma 5. Although rare, pyloric stenosis may develop in 2 to 5 weeks	Emesis or lavage Lavage for all chewable tablets or liquids if spontaneous vomiting has not occurred. Chelation therapy with deferoxamine in severe intoxication (turns urine a red to orange color) If intravenous deferoxamine is given too rapidly, hypotension, facial flushing, rash, urticaria, tachycardia, and shock may occur; stop the infusion, maintain the intravenous line with normal saline, and notify the practitioner immediately.
Plants	Depends on type of plant ingested May cause local irritation of oropharynx and entire gastrointestinal tract May cause respiratory, renal, and central nervous system symptoms Topical contact with plants can cause dermatitis.	Remove plant parts (emesis) Wash from skin or eyes Supportive care as necessary

Adapted from Wong, D. (1995). *Whaley & Wong's nursing care of infants and children* (5th ed.). St. Louis: Mosby.

g. Antidotes to have available: nalaxone, glucose, oxygen, diphenhydramine, physostigmine, flumazenil, digoxin immune Fab, methylene blue, deferoxamine, acetylcysteine, calcium glucanate, glucagon.

D. Common nursing diagnoses, outcomes, and interventions.

1. Potential for injury related to ingestion of toxic substance.
   a. Outcome: Patient will not experience complications of toxic ingestion.
   b. Nursing interventions.
      (1) Monitor respiratory status and assist respirations as necessary.
      (2) Monitor for and treat signs of shock that may occur due to ingestion.
      (3) Obtain information about the time of ingestion, the substance and amount ingested, and any interventions that were initiated before coming to hospital.
      (4) Save any evidence of substance ingested to determine if a poisoning did occur.
      (5) If toxic substance is still present, remove from mouth, skin, eyes to decrease exposure to the poison.
      (6) Administer ipecac, if indicated, to induce vomiting.
      (7) Do not induce vomiting if:
         (a) Child is at risk for aspiration.
            [1] Comatose.
            [2] Severe shock.
            [3] Loss of gag reflex.
            [4] Seizures.
            [5] Substance is a low-viscosity hydrocarbon.

    (b) Substance is corrosive (vomiting produces further damage to the esophagus and mucosa).

  (8) Ensure that child is side-lying, sitting, or in knee-chest position to prevent aspiration during vomiting.

  (9) Administer charcoal, if indicated. If ipecac has been given, administer charcoal after vomiting has finished.

  (10) Administer cathartics, if indicated.

  (11) Perform gastric lavage.

  (12) Have antidotes available and administer, if indicated.

  (13) Assist with additional measure to eliminate toxins (forced diuresis, peritoneal dialysis, hemodialysis, hemoperfusion, plasmapheresis).

E. Home care considerations.

1. Educate family about poison prevention: safe storage of toxic substances, keeping medications out of the reach of children.
2. Advise parents against putting toxic substances in alternative containers, especially those that are similar to everyday food or drink containers.
3. Instruct parents to have syrup of ipecac available in home. Two doses are recommended for each child in family. Instruct parents on correct administration of ipecac.
4. Instruct parents to keep phone number of local poison control center posted by the telephone.
5. Assess need for referral to home health agency to evaluate home for injury prevention measures.

VI. FIREARM INJURY

A. Overview. Firearm injury has become a leading cause of mortality and morbidity in children. This violence affects children of every age, ethnic group, geographic area, and socioeconomic level in the United States. Firearm deaths include homicide, suicide, and unintentional injuries.

1. Pathophysiology.
  a. Two wounding mechanisms result from a bullet.
    (1) Crushing of tissues in the bullet's path which produces a permanent cavity. Destruction of tissue occurs due to:
      (a) Yaw: the deviation of a bullet from a straight path. If the bullet strikes the body at an angle, yaw angle is increased causing the bullet to slow and release more energy to the tissues, which will produce greater injury.
      (b) Tumbling: the somersault action of a bullet that also increases the area of the bullet as it strikes its target, causing a more severe wound.
      (c) Bullet deformation and fragmentation.
        [1] Soft-point and hollow-point bullets mushroom on impact which increases surface area and wound severity.
        [2] Bullets that fragment increase the surface area and volume of tissue crushed.
        [3] Bone fragments, produced by the bullet, can create secondary missiles increasing the severity of the wound.
    (2) The cavity created by the transfer of kinetic energy from the bullet to the tissue (temporary cavity).
      (a) As the bullet penetrates the tissue, kinetic energy is released which causes stretching, tearing, and displacement of tissue, causing a temporary cavity.
      (b) The maximum size of the cavity (can be many times the size of the bullet) is reached within milliseconds of penetration. The pressure exerted on cavity walls can be as much as 100 times atmospheric pressure.
      (c) The negative pressure created behind the missile can draw outside contaminants into the cavity and along the entire wound tract.
      (d) Bullet velocity defines the extent of cavitation and tissue destruction.
        [1] Low velocity bullets travel at less than 1000 feet/second; injury is confined to the area around the center of the tract and there is little cavitation.
        [2] High velocity bullets travel at 3000 feet/second, can cause a cavity with a diameter greater than 30 to 40 times greater than the diameter of the bullet.
          [a] Dense tissue with little elastic property, such as bone, brain, liver, and spleen, and fluid-filled organs, such as the heart and gastrointestinal tract, can be severely damaged by a temporary cavity because of the greater amount of energy imparted.

    [b] Low-density elastic tissue such as the lungs are less affected by the formation of a temporary cavity because less energy is transferred to the tissues.

b. Severe injury can also result from muzzle blast, which is the combustion of gas and powder that occurs when the gun is held to or in close contact with the victim.
    (1) Gas and powder enter the cavity after the shotgun pellet and cause an internal explosion, creating a burn.
    (2) Cavitation results from the combustion of powder and expansion of gases.
    (3) Muzzle blasts are common with shotgun wounds where gas enters the victim.
      (a) An explosive force is produced.
      (b) The elastic properties of the tissues are overwhelmed, causing severe stretching, tearing, and fragmentation.
      (c) Handguns produce this less because less gas is released and the wound is too small for gas to enter.

2. Incidence.
a. Over the past decade, childhood death from firearms have more than doubled.
b. Death rates from motor vehicle accidents have declined steadily; however, firearm fatalities have continued to increase.
c. Cost per firearm fatality is higher than for any other type of fatal injury.
d. Most children are shot in a familiar location by someone close to their own age or by an adult family member (Laraque et al., 1995).
e. Handguns account for the majority of firearm deaths and injuries in the United States.
f. Firearms are the weapons of choice in the majority of all completed teenage suicides.

3. Considerations across the life span.
a. Firearm deaths occur beginning in infancy, increase in frequency during childhood, and occur in large numbers into late adolescence.
b. Most unintentional injuries occur in children and adolescents less than 15 years of age. Most homicides occur in adolescents 15–19 years of age (Czerwinski & Moloney-Harmon, 1997).
c. The proportion of homicides committed with firearms increases with age, regardless of race or sex.

B. Assessment.
1. History and physical exam.
a. Determine the mechanism of injury, if possible. The characteristics and severity of the wound will depend upon the design of the weapon, the caliber and type of bullet, the bullet's velocity, the trajectory of the bullet, the distance of the victim from the weapon.
b. Bones that are struck by bullets may fragment, causing secondary paths.
c. Assessment of airway, breathing, and circulation is the first priority. The wound assessment is secondary unless extensive bleeding is present, which requires application of direct pressure.
d. A head, neck, or face wound requires careful assessment of airway patency and immediate intervention if an airway cannot be secured.
e. If the child experiences a firearm injury to the head, assessment for increased intracranial pressure and/or seizures should take place.
f. Assessment for life-threatening complications should also occur.
    (1) Hemopneumothoraces.
    (2) Pericardial tamponade.
    (3) Airway compromise.
    (4) Intraabdominal bleeding.
g. Firearm injury in the vicinity of major vessels requires frequent neurovascular checks and assessment for hematoma formation, which may compromise the upper airway.
h. Determine entrance and exit wounds. However, these wounds do not necessarily mark the beginning or the end of the wound. Bullets may take multiple paths causing injury to multiple organs. Entrance and exit wounds should be examined carefully and the appearance documented:
    (1) Description of powder soot and burns.
    (2) Scorching of wound edges.
    (3) Tearing of the skin around the wound.
    (4) Bruising and the presence of a muzzle imprint on the skin.
    (5) Location of unexited but palpable bullets.

2. Diagnostic tests.
a. Radiographic studies.
b. CT scan.
c. Angiogram.

C. Therapeutic management.
1. Surgical treatment may or may not be necessary.
2. Head injury.
a. The patient is stabilized and a CT scan obtained, if time permits.
b. Specific treatment depends upon the location of the wound.
3. Thoracic injury.
a. The first priority is pulmonary reexpansion, replacement of the circulating blood volume,

and relief of cardiac tamponade.
  b. Indications for surgical intervention:
    (1) Massive hemothorax (initial return of 20% of the child's estimated blood volume).
    (2) Continued bleeding (1 to 2 ml/kg/hr from the chest tube).
    (3) Persistent air leaks.
    (4) Esophageal injury.
4. Cardiac injury requires surgical repair and has a very high mortality rate.
5. Abdominal injury.
  a. Approximately 80% of gunshot wounds to the abdomen involve multiple organs and require surgical repair (Knudson, 1993).
  b. Indications for surgery.
    (1) Presence of peritoneal irritation on physical examination.
    (2) Hypovolemia.
    (3) Free air in the abdomen on x-ray.
    (4) Positive paracentesis.
6. Major vessel injury requires debridement and anastomosis.
7. Bone injury is treated as a compound fracture with surgical exploration, debridement, and antibiotics.

D. Common nursing diagnosis, outcomes, and interventions.
1. Potential for injury related to firearms.
  a. Outcome: Patient will not experience complications of injury.
  b. Nursing interventions.
    (1) Assess patient's ability to maintain airway and provide artificial airway as necessary.
    (2) Monitor respiratory status and assist respirations as necessary.
    (3) Monitor for and treat signs of shock that may occur due to bleeding.
    (4) Monitor for and treat increased intracranial pressure.
2. Alteration in physical regulation: infection.
  a. Outcome: Patient will have minimal potential for development of infection.
  b. Nursing interventions.
    (1) Use aseptic technique for all invasive lines, wound care, and dressing changes.
    (2) Administer antibiotics only if infection has been confirmed.
    (3) Provide good pulmonary toilet to prevent development of pulmonary infection.
    (4) Provide nutritional support as soon as possible.
3. Alteration in physical integrity.
  a. Patient will not experience skin breakdown or other complications of immobility.

  b. Nursing interventions.
    (1) Provide skin care and turn patient as much as possible.
    (2) Maintain mobility by range of motion exercises and placing limbs in position of function.
4. Alteration in comfort: pain.
  a. Outcome: Patient will experience minimal/reduced pain.
  b. Nursing interventions.
    (1) Begin standard analgesic therapy immediately.
    (2) Consider use of nonpharmacologic pain interventions appropriate to child's developmental level.
5. Potential for injury related to posttraumatic stress disorder.
  a. Outcome: Patient will not experience effects of posttraumatic stress disorder.
  b. Nursing interventions.
    (1) Provide time for child to discuss perception of events.
    (2) If child begins to exhibit signs of posttraumatic stress disorder, begin treatment for child and family as soon as possible.
    (3) Consider referral to mental health practitioner.

E. Home care considerations.
1. Assess for the presence of guns in the home.
2. If guns are present in the home, educate families about creating a gun-safe home environment.
3. If the child has been identified at risk for violence, consider family counseling and referral for support services.

BIBLIOGRAPHY

Campbell, L.S., & Campbell, J.D. (1991). Musculoskeletal trauma in children. *Critical Care Nursing Clinics of North America, 3*(3), 445–456.

Cusson, R.M. (1992). Rice-based oral rehydration fluid in the treatment of infant diarrhea. *Journal of Pediatric Nursing, 7*(6), 1–2.

Czerwinski, S.J., & Moloney-Harmon, P.A. (1997). Caught in the crossfire — Children, guns, and trauma: An update. *Critical Care Nursing Clinics of North America, 9*(2), 201–210.

Eagan, J.O. (1995). The child with cerebral dysfunction. In D.L. Wong (Ed.), *Whaley & Wong's Nursing care of infants and children* (5th ed.) (pp. 667–717). St. Louis: Mosby.

Knudson, M.M. (1993). Penetrating injuries. In M.R. Eichelberger (Ed.), *Pediatric trauma — Prevention, acute care, rehabilitation* (pp. 332–344). St. Louis: Mosby-Year Book.

Laraque, D., Barlow, B., Durkin, M., Howell, J., Cladis, F., Freidman, D., DiScala, C., Ivatury, R. & Stahl, W. (1995). Children who are shot: A 30-year experience. *Journal of Pediatric Surgery, 30*(7), 1072–1076.

Longo, C.B., & Dickenson, C.M. (1996). Toxic ingestions. In M.A.Q. Curley, J.B. Smith, & P.A. Moloney-Harmon (Eds.), *Critical care nursing of infants and children* (pp. 940–962). Philadelphia: Saunders.

Moloney-Harmon, P.A., Srnec, P., & Muir, R. (1996). Trauma. In M.A.Q. Curley, J.B. Smith, & P.A. Moloney-Harmon (Eds.), *Critical care nursing of infants and children* (pp. 893–923). Philadelphia: Saunders.

Thomas, M.D. (1993). Musculoskeletal injury. In M.R. Eichelberger (Ed.), *Pediatric trauma: Prevention, acute care, rehabilitation* (pp. 533–554). St. Louis: Mosby – Year Book.

Wong, D. (1995). *Whaley and Wong's nursing care of infants and children* (5th ed.). St. Louis: Mosby.

Wong, D. (1996). *Wong and Whaley's clinical manual of pediatric nursing* (4th ed.). Mosby: St. Louis.

Wong, D., & Mattis, L. (1995). Conditions that produce fluid and electrolyte imbalance. In D.L. Wong (Ed.), *Whaley and Wong's nursing care of infants and children* (5th ed., pp. 1233–1281). St. Louis: Mosby.

Woolf, A.D., Berkowitz, I.D., Liebelt, E., & Rogers, M. (1996). Poisoning and the critically ill child. In M.C. Rogers (Ed.), *Textbook of pediatric intensive care* (pp. 1315–1396). Baltimore: Williams & Wilkins.

Study Questions

Tanesha, a 2-month old female, presents to the emergency department with a 3-day history of vomiting and diarrhea. Upon physical examination, you note an irritable infant with a heart rate of 180, RR of 40, blood pressure of 78/40. Her skin remains tented when you pinch it, her fontanel is slightly sunken, and her eyeballs also appear to be sunken. She has a capillary refill time of 3 seconds, her peripheral pulses are present, and she is slightly pale. She has a large, watery stool in her diaper.

1. You are concerned about the possibility of dehydration. What laboratory tests would you obtain to confirm this finding?
   a. Blood cultures, bleeding time, and urine specific gravity
   b. Arterial blood gases, hematocrit, CBC, serum electrolytes
   c. Hemoglobin, BUN, and hematocrit
   d. Urine specific gravity, CBC, serum electrolytes, BUN

2. The appropriate treatment for Tanesha is:
   a. fluid resuscitation at 20 ml/kg.
   b. oral rehydrating solution.
   c. vasopressors.
   d. no treatment is necessary.

Jamie, a 14-month-old male, has a 2-day history of irritability and pulling at his left ear. He recently had a cold, and now has a temperature of 39°C. Examination of his left ear reveals inflammation of the middle ear with a collection of fluid in the middle ear space.

3. Jamie has:
   a. otitis media with effusion.
   b. subacute otitis media.
   c. chronic otitis media.
   d. otorrhea.

4. The initial treatment for Jamie is:
   a. myringotomy.
   b. steroids.
   c. antibiotics.
   d. placement of tympanostomy tubes.

Jessica, an 8-year old female, has been admitted to the pediatric unit following placement of an external fixation device for a compound fracture of her left femur. While assessing her affected extremity, you note that she cries out when you touch her leg, and that she is complaining of tingling. Her left leg seems to be pale and capillary refill time is 4 seconds. She does have a strong pulse in her left foot.

5. You suspect:
   a. infection.
   b. compartment syndrome.
   c. refracture of the bone.
   d. shock.

A few days later, Jessica is complaining of pain in her left leg. Your assessment reveals that all other parameters are stable.

6. You consider that she may need:
   a. fluid therapy.
   b. antibiotics.
   c. pain medication.
   d. distraction.

Michael, a 3-year old male, presents to the emergency department, with a 3 day history of fever, coughing, and irritability. On examination, you note a pale boy who is lethargic. He has a temperature of 41°C, heart rate of 130, and a blood pressure of 98/60. He has a positive Brudzinski's sign.

7. What are the appropriate laboratory tests to confirm a diagnosis in Michael?
   a. CBC, serum, and urine electrolytes
   b. Lumbar puncture, CSF culture and gram stain
   c. Arterial blood gases, lumbar puncture, and CBC
   d. Throat culture, serum glucose, and urine electrolytes

8. The initial intervention for Michael is:
   a. broad-spectrum antibiotics.
   b. corticosteroids.
   c. fluid resuscitation.
   d. antipyretics.

Serena, a 10-year old female, comes into the emergency department following the ingestion of 20 acetaminophen tablets.

9. The initial treatment is administration of:
   a. activated charcoal.
   b. fluids.
   c. N-acetylcysteine.
   d. dopamine.

10. The antidote for acetaminophen ingestion is:
    a. activated charcoal.
    b. sorbital.
    c. N-acetylcysteine.
    d. aspirin.

Richard, an 11-year old male, comes into the emergency department following a low-caliber gunshot wound to the face.

11. Your initial intervention is to:
    a. call the plastic surgeon.
    b. apply direct pressure to the face.
    c. assess airway, breathing, circulation.
    d. call the operating room.

12. Which type of firearm accounts for the majority of firearm injuries and deaths?
    a. Shotguns
    b. Handguns
    c. Semiautomatic weapons
    d. Pellet guns

Answers

1.d 2.b 3.a 4.c 5.b 6.c 7.b 8.a 9.a 10.c 11.c 12.b

Chapter 19

Chronic Conditions: Effects on the Child

Judith A. Vessey, PhD, RN, CRNP, FAAN
Maureen C. Maguire, MSN, RN, PNP

Concept

◆◆◆◆◆◆◆◆◆◆◆◆◆◆◆◆◆◆◆◆◆◆◆◆◆

◆ Children with a chronic condition, disability, or special health need and their families

Objectives

◆◆◆◆◆◆◆◆◆◆◆◆◆◆◆◆◆◆◆◆◆◆◆◆◆

At the completion of this chapter, the reader will be able to:

◆ Discuss the noncategorical approach to chronic conditions.

◆ Describe the effects of chronic conditions on physical growth.

◆ Identify the effect that chronic conditions have on development.

◆ Discuss the stressors a child with a chronic condition may experience.

◆ State the risk factors for children with chronic conditions.

◆ Describe the special heath care needs that might be required for a child with a chronic condition.

◆ Identify coping mechanisms that family members may display.

◆ Identify factors that influence the child's ability to cope with his/her chronic condition.

◆ Discuss techniques to normalize the health care routine of children with a chronic condition.

◆ Identify resources available for children with chronic conditions and their families.

Key Points

◆◆◆◆◆◆◆◆◆◆◆◆◆◆◆◆◆◆◆◆◆◆◆◆◆

◆ Chronic conditions need to be examined from a noncategorical approach as there are greater similarities than differences in responses to chronic health conditions.

◆ Chronic conditions require holistic health care that addresses a variety of health care needs.

◆ Children with chronic conditions can be affected physically, mentally, and developmentally.

◆ Nurses need to be aware of resources that are available for children with chronic conditions.

19

Chronic Conditions: Effects on the Child

I. OVERVIEW: NONCATEGORICAL APPROACH

In caring for children with chronic conditions, it is important to remember that they are more alike their unaffected peers than different from them (Patterson & Gerber, 1991). It is also critical to focus on the fact that the concerns and problems faced by children with differing chronic conditions are similar, regardless of the condition.

A. Definition: a long-term condition that is either not curable or has residual features that result in limitations in daily living requiring special assistance or adaptation in function (Jessop & Stein, 1988).

B. Sequelae associated with chronic conditions.
1. Limitation of function.
    a. Disruption in meeting developmental tasks.
    b. Dependency on parents or other family members beyond the usual developmental stage.
    c. Dependency on society if parents are unable to care for them.
2. Disfigurement.
3. Dependency on medication, diet, or treatments needed to maintain normal functioning or control condition.
4. Dependency on medical technology for optimal functioning.
5. Ongoing need for health care for management of the condition.

C. Major classifications of chronic conditions.
1. Chronic illnesses (e.g., asthma, rheumatoid arthritis).
2. Developmental disabilities (e.g., mental retardation, autism).
3. Mental health problems (e.g., depression, conduct disorder).

D. Incidence/prevalence (Newacheck & Taylor, 1992).
1. Incidence and prevalence are increasing.

a. Previously fatal childhood diseases are no longer fatal (e.g., HIV/AIDS, cystic fibrosis).
b. Improved survival rates for very low birth infants.
c. Improved survival rates for trauma victims.
d. Better case finding.
2. Rates.
    a. Estimated that 31% (20 million) of all children 0–18 years old have one or more chronic conditions.
    b. 17% have a developmental disability.
    c. Overall survival rate until adulthood now over 90%.
3. Disease severity in affected children.
    a. 66% have mild conditions with little or no limitations.
    b. 29% have conditions with limited limitations.
    c. 5% have conditions with constant limitations.
4. Distribution.
    a. Children from low socioeconomic backgrounds disproportionately affected.
    b. Minority children disproportionately affected.

II. EFFECTS ON PHYSICAL GROWTH

A. General growth retardation.
1. Generally grow slower.
2. Heights and weights are at the lower percentiles on growth charts.
3. Specific physiologic mechanisms affect growth (e.g., chronic hypoxemia, malabsorption).
4. Delayed growth is seen with some conditions more than with others (e.g., cystic fibrosis, end-stage renal disease).
5. Treatments and drugs either can hinder growth (e.g., chemotherapeutic agents, methylamphenidate) or improve growth.

B. Delayed puberty.
1. Generally enter puberty later than nonaffected peers.
2. Ultimate growth potential may or may not be affected, depending on the condition, its severity, and the child's therapeutic adherence.

III. EFFECTS ON DEVELOPMENT

A. Potential for slow development.
1. Delayed development: children advance through the normal sequence of milestones but at a slower rate (e.g., congenital heart disease).
2. Deviant development: children experience a disruption of the normal developmental sequences (e.g., cerebral palsy, infantile autism).
3. Parents, teachers, and others who are fearful of consequences of a child's symptomatology may unduly restrict a child's opportunities for interaction and subsequently hinder development (e.g., the child with asthma who is not allowed outside to play).

B. Effects of the condition's severity and pathophysiology.
1. Specific pathophysiologic mechanisms can alter development (e.g., hypoxemia, neurotransmitter deficits).
2. A correlation exists between the condition severity and developmental consequences.
   a. Many children with severe conditions have virtually normal development and vice versa.
   b. Children with developmental delays and other neurologic conditions are the most affected.
3. Children with mild conditions, no visible signs or symptoms, or only occasional exacerbations may have their condition unrecognized by families or providers; treatment is often delayed or overlooked.
4. Some families deny that the child has a chronic condition; this then places limitations on the child's potential development (e.g., parents who deny that their child has mental retardation).

C. Effects of treatment protocols.
1. Amelioration of symptoms by treatment results in better developmental outcomes (e.g., good pain management).
2. Improved case finding and an increase in early intervention programs have improved the developmental outcomes for many children.
3. Some developmental limitations can occur as a result of treatment because children have less time to interact with peers and their families.
   a. Time spent on treatments (e.g., pulmonary percussion).
   b. Energy needed to cope with disease.
   c. Physical constraints (e.g., ventilators).
4. More developmental sequelae are occurring as treatments improve life expectancy (e.g., developmental lag in children with HIV/AIDS; learning problems in cancer survivors).

D. Effects of prognosis.
1. If the prognosis is poor, children can lose developmental progression as their disease progresses (e.g., Tay-Sachs disease).
2. With a stable condition, greater developmental lags can be seen as the child matures and developmental expectations are increased (e.g., child with Down syndrome).
3. If the child's future is uncertain, family members and others may not help the child strive toward future goals.
4. If the condition is potentially fatal, parents may stop setting any limits; the child may experience increased anxiety and poorer developmental outcomes.

E. Effects of iatrogenic insults.
1. Some treatments can cause temporary or permanent developmental changes (e.g., effects of intrathecal chemotherapy on learning; aminoglycosides and hearing loss).
2. Some classes of drugs can affect cognitive performance and behavior (e.g., anticonvulsants).

F. Effects of age (see Table 19-1).
1. Chronic conditions have specific implications for each age group.
2. Children need to master developmental tasks of one age before moving on to the next (e.g., babbling prior to speech).
3. Achieving a developmental task for the first time is very different than relearning one (e.g., child who is born blind compared to one who loses vision during adolescence).

G. Effects of individualism and personality.
1. Characteristics that effect developmental attainment.
   a. Inborn temperament (e.g., "easy" baby, "slow to warmup," baby).
   b. Motivation; both intrinsic and extrinsic factors influence.
   c. Hardiness and resilience versus vulnerability.
   d. Intelligence.
   e. Attitudinal qualities (e.g., optimism versus pessimism).
   f. Interpersonal skills.
2. Children with chronic conditions have the same range of traits as their nonaffected peers.
3. Children with chronic conditions are at higher risk for developing vulnerable personalities.
   a. Fears may inhibit the child from taking part in activities that foster development (e.g., sports).
   b. Parental overprotectiveness may restrict independence.

Table 19-1
Developmental Aspects of Chronic Conditions

Developmental Tasks	Potential Effects of Chronic Conditions
INFANCY Develop a sense of trust.	• Multiple caregivers and frequent separations, especially if hospitalized. • Deprived of consistent nurturing.
Attach to parent.	• Delayed because of separation, parental grief for loss of "dream" child, parental inability to accept the condition, especially a visible defect.
Learn through sensorimotor experiences.	• Increased exposure to painful experiences over pleasurable ones. • Limited contact with environment from restricted movement or confinement.
Begin to develop a sense of separateness from parent.	• Increased dependency on parent for care. • Overinvolvement of parent in care.
TODDLERHOOD Develop autonomy.	• Increased dependency on parent.
Master locomotor and language skills.	• Limited opportunity to test on own abilities and limits.
Learn through sensorimotor experience, beginning preoperational thought.	• Increased exposure to painful experiences.
PRESCHOOL Develop initiative and purpose. Master self-care skills.	• Increased exposure to painful experiences. • Limited opportunities for success in accomplishing simple tasks or mastering self-care skills.
Begin to develop peer relationships.	• Limited opportunities for socialization with peers; may appear "like a baby" to age-mates. Protection within tolerant and secure family may cause child to fear criticism and withdraw.
Develop sense of body image.	• Awareness of body may center on pain, anxiety, and failure and sexual identification. • Sex role identification focused primarily on mothering skills.
Learn through preoperational thought (magical thinking).	• Guilt (thinking he or she caused the illness/disability or is being punished for wrongdoing).
SCHOOL AGE Develop a sense of accomplishment.	• Limited opportunities to achieve and compete, e.g., many school absences or inability to join regular athletic activities.
Form peer relationships.	• Limited opportunities for socialization.
Learn through concrete operations.	• Incomplete comprehension of the imposed physical limitations or treatment of the disorder.
ADOLESCENCE Develop personal and sexual identity.	• Increased sense of feeling different from peers and less able to complete with peers in appearance, abilities, special skills.
Achieve independence from family.	• Increased dependency on family; limited job/career opportunities.
Form heterosexual relationships.	• Limited opportunities for heterosexual friendships; less opportunity to discuss sexual concerns with peers.
Learn through abstract thinking.	• Increased concern with issues such as: Why did he or she get the disorder? Can he or she marry and have a family. • Decreased opportunity for earlier stages of cognition may impede achieving of abstract thinking.

Used with permission from Wong, D. L. (1995). *Whaley & Wong's nursing care of infants and children* (5th ed.). St. Louis: Mosby.

H. Effects of social networks.
1. Characteristics of the family. *See Chapter 7: Home and Family.*
2. Cultural orientation.
   a. Differences in perceived cause(s) of chronic conditions.
   b. Differences in expectations of survival.
   c. Differences in views of the child's ultimate potential.
3. Social class.
   a. Educational level of parents.
   b. Economic resources.
4. Educational resources.
   a. Availability of appropriate educational programs (see Table 19-2 on legislation).
   b. School reentry program.
   c. Adjunct supports.
      (1) Trained personnel to administer medications and treatments.
      (2) Symptom management protocols in place.
      (3) Policies supporting integration into student student activities.
   d. Increased absenteeism is associated with poorer outcomes.
5. Characteristics of the environment.
   a. Available support groups.
   b. Vocational supports (see Table 19-2).
   c. Community planning (e.g., handicap accessible playgrounds, camps, scouts, athletic programs, and after-school activities for children with chronic conditions).
   d. Availability of respite care.
   e. Potential for discrimination.

I. Internet services: use with care; no guarantee as to the accuracy of content.

J. Other risk factors.
1. Multiple chronic conditions.
   a. Certain factors increase the child's risk for poor outcomes.
   b. Poor self-concept (see section IV.A.).
   c. Dysfunctional family.
   d. Low socioeconomic status.
   e. Living in an isolated area.
2. The more risk factors, the greater the comorbidity.

IV. CHILD STRESSORS

A. Self-concept and body image.
1. A good self-concept is developed by mastering a variety of physical, emotional, cognitive, and social tasks.
   a. Good self-concept enables one to conquer most of life's challenges.

   b. These children educate those around them about the condition.
2. A poor self-concept can lead to a vulnerable personality.
   a. Poor self-concept is linked to poorer physical and socioemotional health.
   b. Children from dysfunctional families are at higher risk.

B. General mental health.
1. Children with chronic conditions experience higher rates of mental health problems.
2. Influencing factors.
   a. Age at which the chronic condition is diagnosed.
   b. Family and community receptiveness to the diagnosis.
   c. Child's personality.
   d. Medical and educational supports.
3. Mental health services remain limited; many insurance plans have limitations.

V. SPECIAL HEALTH CARE NEEDS

A. Coordinated, multidisciplinary comprehensive management facilitates optimal care. *See Chapter 17: Acute Illness: The Continuum of Care.*
1. Needs assessment.
   a. Physical needs (e.g., nutrition, elimination).
   b. Functional status needs (e.g., mobility, ability to perform activities of daily living).
   c. Socioeconomic needs (e.g., ability to afford necessary care).
   d. Educational needs (e.g., appropriate academic placements).
   e. Family members' needs (e.g., parents, siblings, extended family).
2. Service planning: coordination among agencies.
   a. Hospitals and clinics.
   b. Home health agencies.
   c. Schools.
   d. Respite care.
3. Access to needed services.
   a. Financial access.
      (1) Some well-coordinated programs are very effective but very expensive (e.g., Hemophilia Centers).
      (2) Some programs are tied into state and federal support (e.g., cystic fibrosis centers).
   b. Environmental access (e.g., ability to travel to treatment sites).
4. Facilitates:
   a. Monitoring service delivery.
   b. Advocating for the child and family.
   c. Evaluating service outcomes.

Table 19-2
An Overview Relevant of Legislation

Civil Rights Act of 1968	The protections afforded specific groups were later applied to persons with disabilities through the Americans with Disabilities Act, 1990 and the Rehabilitation Act of 1973.
Rehabilitation Act of 1973, Section 504	Applies to state, local, private, and religious schools receiving federal funds. The mandate for private and religious schools are somewhat minimized compared to those applied to public. This federal law mandate antidiscriminatory practices against individuals with disabilities. Requires schools to provide children with disabilities a free appropriate education.
Public Law 94-142, Education for All Handicapped Children Act, 1975.	Sweeping legislation relevant to education of children with disabilities.
Public Law 99-457, Education of the Handicapped Act Amendments of 1986	Extended the provisions of Public Law 94-142, to allow for of the early intervention for children from birth to 2 years of age. Also, expanded transitional and secondary education provisions.
The Carl D. Perkins Vocational Act of 1984	This Act addressed the post high school graduation needs of those children diagnosed as learning disabled.
Americans with Disabilities Act, 1990	Applies to state, local, and private schools with the exception of religious schools. Incorporated the ideology and federal protections previously outlined in the Civil Rights Act of 1968 and applied them to the public education and children with disabilities. Generally mirrors the protections afforded through Section 504.
Public Law 101-476, Individuals with Disabilities Education Act, 1990	Applies only to state and local schools except in the instance that the public school system places and funds a student in a private school. New title given the Education for the Handicapped Act. Some protections offered to children with disabilities are similar to Section 504 of the Rehabilitation Act, 1973.

Used with permission from Vessey, J.A. (1997). *The child with a learning disorder or ADHD: A manual for school nurses.* Scarborough, ME: Maine School Nurses Association.

B. Transition of adolescents to adult care.
1. Coordination and access more difficult.
2. Adult providers not knowledgeable about "pediatric" disease.
3. Management should build on prior experience.
4. Goals.
   a. Independence to the highest possible developmental level.
   b. Stabilizing the disease process/condition.
   c. Appropriate educational and vocational training.
   d. Maintenance of appropriate health insurance.

VI. ASSESSMENT STRATEGIES
◆ ◆ ◆ ◆ ◆ ◆ ◆ ◆ ◆ ◆ ◆ ◆ ◆ ◆ ◆ ◆ ◆ ◆
A. Need comprehensive assessment for diagnosis.
1. Use of valid instruments and tests to ascertain appropriate diagnoses.
2. Identification of risk factors for comorbidities.

B. Parent(s)' reaction to diagnosis is influenced by:
1. Sibling reaction.
2. Stage of family development at diagnosis.
3. Family resiliency (see Table 19-3).

Table 19-3
Traits of the Resilient Family System

- Balancing the illness with other family needs•
- Maintaining clear family boundaries
- Developing communication competence
- Attributing positive meaning to the experience
- Maintaining flexibility
- Maintaining a commitment to the family as a unit
- Engaging in active coping efforts
- Maintaining social integration
- Developing collaborative relationships with professionals

Used with permission from Patterson, J. M. (1991). Family resilience to the challenge of a child's disability. *Pediatric Annals, 20* (9),491–499.

VII. TREATMENT OPTIONS

◆ ◆ ◆ ◆ ◆ ◆ ◆ ◆ ◆ ◆ ◆ ◆ ◆ ◆ ◆ ◆ ◆ ◆ ◆

A. Collaboration with family in planning.
See Chapter 20: Chronic Conditions: Effects on the Child's Family and Chapter 28: Family-Centered Care.
1. Obtain family's perspective (see Table 19-4).
2. Work with family to plan care (see Table 19-5).
3. Negotiation when goals of the family and those of the health care team differ.

B. Management of the chronic condition.
1. Consistent monitoring of condition critical.
2. Appropriate therapeutics and other interventions.
   a. Medications.
   b. Surgical interventions.
   c. Dietary interventions.
      (1) Appropriate nutrient and caloric needs.
      (2) Dietary restrictions.
      (3) Modified route (e.g., gastrostomy tube).
   d. Symptom management.
      (1) Pain.
      (2) Nausea.
      (3) Fatigue.
      (4) Other symptoms.
   e. Adaptive devices.
      (1) Braces, crutches, walkers, wheelchairs.
      (2) Orthotics.
      (3) Oxygen, humidity, air purification.
      (4) Glasses, hearing aids.
      (5) Other adaptive aids to assist with activities of daily living.
   f. Training in activities of daily living (as needed).
3. Management of acute episodes or exacerbation.
   a. Need appropriate ongoing assessment.

Table 19-4
Information Families Can Be Asked to Provide as Part of the Assessment
© Elizabeth Ahmann, 1990, 1991

Observations regarding child's development
- overall development
- specific strengths
- problem areas (explicit observations)
   motor – gross and fine
   cognitive
   feeding
   speech/communication
   social/emotional

Observations regarding developmental impact of child's condition
- environmental limitations
- tolerance for activity
- recovery postactivity

Suggestions for intervention plan
- specific activity ideas
- priorities
- desired outcomes
- extent of desire to participate in interventions
- scheduling suggestions
- equipment needs

Other family concerns
- information needs
- long-term concerns
- concerns regarding sibling effects.

Preferred methods of sharing information.

Used with permission from Ahmann, E., & Lipsi, K. (1992). Developmental assessment of the technology dependent infant and young child. *Pediatric Nursing, 18*(3), 303.

   b. Decision as to whether the primary care or specialty care provider should manage acute episode.
4. Child and family education.
   a. Teach family the information and skills necessary to provide optimum care to the child.
   b. Information must be developmentally, experientially, and age-appropriate (see Table 19-6).
      (1) Reinforce correct information.
      (2) Clarify misconceptions.
      (3) Repeat information as often as necessary.
      (4) Encourage questions.
      (5) Always give a written or audiotaped copy of the information.
   c. Provide information about:
      (1) General anatomy and physiology.
      (2) The condition's pathophysiology.
      (3) Treatment protocols.

Table 19-5
Encouraging Collaboration with Family Members

Professionals can encourage collaboration with family members in the following ways:

- Meeting with family members at the family's convenience
- Sharing complete and unbiased information with families
- Developing good communication skills
- Reinforcing family members' observational skills
- Concentrating on family's priorities and goals
- Building trust by being constructive and positive
- Promoting tolerance by agreeing to disagree
- Avoiding punitive statements and actions
- Developing systems for conflict resolution
- Affording parental views appropriate weight in decision-making

Used with permission from Ahmann, E., & Lipsi, K. (1992). Developmental assessment of the technology dependent infant and young child. *Pediatric Nursing, 18*(3), 304.

Table 19-6
Possible Family Information Needs
Regarding Growth and Development

- ◆ How the condition affects child's physical growth and development
- ◆ How to provide for child's emotional needs
- ◆ How to improve communication among all the people caring for the child
- ◆ Behavior management/discipline
- ◆ How to plan for the child's future
- ◆ Services available in the community

Used with permission from Ahmann, E., & Lierman, C. (1992). Promoting normal development in technology dependent children: An introduction to the issues. *Pediatric Nursing, 18*(2), 147.

    (4) Signs and symptoms needing intervention.
    (5) Information about skill attainment needed for independence.
    (6) Genetic counseling.
  d. Suggest family maintain their own home health record.
 5. Primary care management.
  a. Same needs as unaffected children.
  b. Health care maintenance/disease prevention.
    (1) Monitor growth and development.
    (2) Nutrition counseling.
    (3) Safety counseling.
    (4) Immunizations.
    (5) Routine well-child screening.
    (6) Screening specific for family risk factors (e.g., cholesterol).
    (7) Condition-specific screening: varies according to condition (e.g., glycosolated hemoglobin in children with diabetes).
  c. Guidance around developmental issues.
    (1) Safety issues.
    (2) Sleep patterns.
    (3) Toileting.
    (4) Discipline.
    (5) Child care/schooling.
    (6) Sexuality.
 6. Counseling to address specific family concerns.
  a. Goal: normalization of life for parents, child, siblings, extended family.
  b. Family assessment: explore the family's reaction to the disorder and the child.
  c. Provide support at diagnosis.

  d. Accept family's emotions.
  e. Encourage expression of feelings and concerns.
  f. Be honest.
  g. Encourage family members, the child, and others to ask questions.
  h. Emphasize the positive aspects of the child's attributes and abilities.
  i. Help family gain confidence in their ability to cope and meet the child's needs.
  j. Help family to foster the child's development by stimulating the child to participate in age-appropriate activities.
  k. Provide support and be available.
  l. Help family to understand that anger and frustration are normal reactions.
  m. Assist family in problem solving.
  n. Refer to community organizations and support groups.
  o. Assist family to obtain needed equipment, supplies, and drugs.
  p. Arrange for consults and follow-up care.
  q. Provide family with phone numbers for seeking additional information or dealing with a crisis.
  r. Identify sources of child and family stress. *See Chapter 7: Home and Family.*
  s. Explore options for respite care.
 7. Promote self-care as appropriate.

VIII. COPING MECHANISMS USED BY FAMILY MEMBERS

◆ ◆ ◆ ◆ ◆ ◆ ◆ ◆ ◆ ◆ ◆ ◆ ◆ ◆ ◆ ◆ ◆ ◆ ◆ ◆

Also see Chapter 20: Chronic Conditions: Effects on the Child's Family.

A. Avoidance behaviors.
 1. Deny seriousness of problems.

2. Have unrealistic goals for child.
3. Continually look for new cures.
4. Avoid child and/or staff.
5. Act hostile toward staff without provocation.
6. Blame themselves.
7. Use alcohol, drugs excessively.
8. Withdraw from outside world.
9. Refuse to admit child's understanding of the problem.
10. Refuse reasonable treatment plans.

B. Approach behaviors.
1. Ask for information about child's condition.
2. Seek help and support.
3. Plan realistically for child's future.
4. Express feelings.
5. Share burden with others.
6. Acknowledge child's understanding of the problem.

C. Degree of adaptation needed.

D. Degree of adaptation/maladaption.

E. Factors affecting adjustment by family.
1. Family's sense of coherence.
   a. Ability to comprehend information.
   b. Ability to meet demands.
   c. Ability to find meaning in situation.
2. Intrafamily communication.
3. Social support systems.
4. Previous experience in dealing with crises.
5. Available resources.
6. Necessary lifestyle changes.
7. Blaming among family members.
8. Other concurrent stresses.
9. Religious/philosophic beliefs.

IX. COPING MECHANISMS USED BY CHILD
◆ ◆ ◆ ◆ ◆ ◆ ◆ ◆ ◆ ◆ ◆ ◆ ◆ ◆ ◆ ◆ ◆ ◆

A. Factors influencing child's ability to cope.
1. Gender.
2. Age at diagnosis.
3. Temperament.
4. Self-concept.
5. Intelligence.
6. Social skills.
7. Family's reaction.
   a. Denial.
   b. Overprotection.
      (1) Hover.
      (2) Assist child when not necessary.
      (3) Try to protect child from everything.
      (4) Are permissive or inconsistent with discipline.

(5) Restrict play and out of home activities.
(6) Sacrifice the needs/desires of other family members.
   c. Rejection.
   d. Acceptance.
8. Degree of support available.

B. Factors promoting normalization.
1. Prepare child for treatments, side effects.
2. Allow child to participate in decision making.
3. Give child some situational control whenever possible.
4. Foster intrafamily communication.
5. Apply the same rules for child with chronic conditions as for other children.

C. Interventions supportive of child's development (Wong, 1995).
1. Infancy.
   a. Encourage parents to be with child as much as possible.
   b. Provide consistent caregivers.
   c. Teach family members child's special care needs.
   d. Provide positive, multisensory experiences.
2. Toddler years.
   a. Encourage independence in areas where possible.
   b. Modify toys, equipment to increase gross motor activity.
   c. Give child choices when possible.
   d. Provide sensory experience.
3. Preschool years.
   a. Provide devices to assist in self-help skills.
   b. Encourage socialization.
   c. Help child deal with others' reactions to him or her.
   d. Reassure child that the condition/disability is not his fault.
4. School years.
   a. Encourage school attendance.
   b. Teach child about his or her condition.
   c. Educate teachers and classmates about child's abilities and special needs.
   d. Encourage participation in organizations, clubs, sports as possible.
   e. Encourage creative activities.
5. Adolescence.
   a. Provide instruction on interpersonal and coping skills, and decisions-making.
   b. Encourage socialization with peers, with and without disabilities.
   c. Give increased responsibility for self-management of condition/disability.
   d. Encourage age-appropriate activities.
   e. Modify equipment/environment to allow for

activities such as driving a car.
  f. Discuss how condition/disability may affect future choices.
  g. Discuss how condition/disability may affect sexual behavior and reproductive ability.

X. COMMUNITY RESOURCES

A. Hospital.
  1. Department of Social Work.
  2. Special programs for transition into community.

B. Governmental.
  1. State: Programs for Children with Special Needs.
  2. Medicaid.
  3. Supplemental Security Income.
  4. Services provided through Maternal and Child Health Block Grants.
  5. Federal laws specific to disability (see Table 19-2).

C. Disease/disorder specific organizations.
  1. Many chronic conditions have specific organizations (e.g., Juvenile Diabetes Association, Muscular Dystrophy Association, American Association of Mental Retardation).
  2. Services provided for affected child, family, siblings.
    a. Newsletters, lay materials.
    b. Audiovisual materials.
    c. Money for research.
    d. Child advocacy.
    e. Speakers' bureaus.
    f. Support groups.

D. Sources of information.
  1. Medic-Alert Bracelet
     P.O. Box 1009
     Turlock, CA 95381
     800-ID-ALERT
  2. Federation for Children with Special Needs
     95 Berkeley Street, Suite 104
     Boston, MA 02116
     617-482-2915
  3. Automotive Safety for Children Program
     (Auto restraints for children with special needs)
     Riley Hospital for Children
     534 N. Clinical Drive, Room 118
     Indianapolis, IN 46202
     317-274-2977
  4. National Information Center for Children and Youth with Disabilities
     P.O. Box 1492
     Washington, DC 20013
     202-884-8200

  5. National Easter Seal Society
     23 W. Monroe Street, Suite 1800
     Chicago, IL 60606
     312-726-6200
  6. Association for the Care of Children's Health
     19 Mantua Road
     Mount Royal, NJ 08061
     609-224-1742
  7. National Self-Help Clearinghouse
     CUNY Graduate Center
     25 W. 43rd Street
     New York, NY 10036
     212-642-2944
  8. Sibling Information Network
     The Information Network
     The A.J. Pappanikou Center
     A-VAP
     62 Washington Street
     Middleton, CT 06457
     203-344-7500
  9. The President's Committee on Employment of People with Disabilities
     1331 F. Street, N.W
     Washington, DC 20004
     202-376-6200
  10. Local libraries.
  11. School services: federal law mandates a free and appropriate education for children with disabilities (see Table 19-2).

BIBLIOGRAPHY

Ahmann, E., & Lipsi, K. (1992). Developmental assessment of the technology dependent infant and young children. *Pediatric Nursing, 18*(3), 299–305.

Boyle, C.A., Decoufle, P., & Yeargin-Allsopp, M. (1994). Prevalence and health impact of developmental disabilities in U.S. children. *Pediatrics, 93*(3), 399–403.

Committee on Children with Disabilities: Pediatric services for infants and children with special health care needs. (1993). *Pediatrics, 92*(1), 163–165.

Gortmaker, S.L., Walker, D.K., Weitzman, M., & Sobol, A.M. (1990). Chronic conditions, socioeconomic risks, and behavioral problems in children and adolescents. *Pediatrics, 85*(3), 267–276.

Graff, J.C., & Ault, M.M. (1993). Guidelines for working with students having special health care needs. *Journal of School Health, 63*(8), 335–338.

Groce, N.E., & Zola, I.K. (1993). Multiculturalism, chronic illness, and disability. *Pediatrics, 91*(5), 1048–1055.

Jackson, P.L., & Vessey, J.A. (1996). *Primary care of the children with a chronic condition* (2nd ed.). St. Louis: Mosby-Yearbook.

Jessop, D.J., & Stein, R.E.K. (1994). Providing comprehensive health care to children with chronic illness. *Pediatrics, 93*(4), 602–607.

Luthar, S.S., & Zigler, E. (1991). Vulnerability and competence: A review of research on resilience in childhood. *American Journal of Orthopsychiatry, 61,* 6–22.

McCabe, M.A. (1996). Involving children and adolescents in medical decision making: Developmental and clinical considerations. *Journal of Pediatric Psychology, 21*(4), 505–516.

McCubbin, H.I., Thompson, E.A., Thompson, A.I., McCubbin, M.A., & Kaston, A.J. (1993). Culture, ethnicity, and the family: Critical factors in childhood chronic illnesses and disabilities. *Pediatrics, 91*(5), 1063–1070.

Newacheck, P.W., Stoddard, J.J., & McManus, M. (1993). Ethnocultural variations in the prevalence and impact of childhood chronic conditions. *Pediatrics, 91*(5), 1031–1039.

Newacheck, J., & Taylor, W. (1992). Childhood chronic illness: Prevalence, severity and impact. *American Journal of Public Health, 82,* 364–371.

Passarelli, C. (1992). Case management of chronic health conditions of school-age youth. In H. M. Wallace, K. Patrick, G.S. Parcel, & J.B. Igoe (Eds.), *Principles and practices of student health: School health* (Vol. 2, pp. 350–389). Oakland, CA: Third Party Publishing Co.

Patterson, J.M., & Gerber, M. (1991). Family resilience to the challenge of a child's disability. *Pediatric Annals, 20*(9), 491–499.

Perrin, E.C., Newacheck, P., Pless, I.B., Drotar, D., Gortmaker, S.L., Leventhal, J., Perrin, J.M., Stein, R.E.K., Walker, D.K., & Weitzman, M. (1993). Issues involved in the definition and classification of chronic health conditions. *Pediatrics, 91*(4), 787–793.

Rabin, N.B. (1994). School reentry and the child with a chronic illness: The role of the pediatric nurse practitioner. *Journal of Pediatric Health Care, 8*(5), 227–232.

Stein, R.E. (1992). Chronic physical disorders. *Pediatric Review, 13,* 224-229.

Turner-Henson, A., Holaday, B., Corser, N., Ogletree, G., & Swan, J.H. (1994). The experiences of discrimination: Challenges for chronically ill children. *Pediatric Nursing, 20*(6), 571–577.

Vessey, J.A. (1997). *The child with a learning disorder or ADHD: A manual for school nurses.* Scarborough, ME: Maine School Nurses Association.

Wolman, C., Resnick, M.D., Harris, L.J., & Blum, R.W. (1994). Emotional well-being among adolescents with and without chronic conditions. *Journal of Adolescent Health, 15*(3), 199–204.

Wong, D.L. (1995). *Whaley & Wong's nursing care of infants and children* (5th ed.). St. Louis: Mosby.

STUDY QUESTIONS

1. Which of the following is a true statement about the noncategorical approach to the health care of children with chronic conditions?
   a. Adaptations imposed by each chronic illness/condition make the usual well child care standards nonapplicable.
   b. Designations such as "handicapped" or "disabled" are never to be used.
   c. Children with chronic conditions must be regarded as different from children without such problems in order to ensure availability of services.
   d. Children with differing chronic conditions are more alike than different.

2. The definition of a chronic condition is "a long-term condition that:
   a. includes some degree of mental retardation."
   b. is not curable or has residual features."
   c. is potentially fatal."
   d. has genetic or congenital origins."

3. One of the reasons that the incidence and prevalence of chronic conditions are increasing is:
   a. higher survivor rates of children with conditions that were previously fatal.
   b. fewer very low birth weight infants are being born.
   c. prenatal genetic counseling is rarely available in a managed care environment.
   d. the federal government's classification of chronic diseases was expanded.

4. The degree of limitation for more than half of the estimated 20 million children with one or more chronic conditions is:
   a. severe/constant.
   b. moderate/intermittent.
   c. mild or none.
   d. unknown due to data collection problems.

5. For which of the following children would you expect to have long-term growth retardation?
   a. 3-year-old with cystic fibrosis.
   b. 9-year-old receiving radiation for a bone tumor.
   c. 7-year-old asthmatic on inhaler treatment only.
   d. 10-month-old born at 38 weeks gestation.

6. Which of the following would be a true statement about the correlation between the severity of the chronic condition and the developmental consequences?
   a. A child with any severe chronic illness will have significant developmental delay.
   b. The correlation between severity and developmental outcome is NOT very robust.
   c. A child with only periodic exacerbations of the chronic condition will NOT have developmental consequences.
   d. Condition severity has a direct linear correlation with developmental outcome with a magnitude of r=.96.

7. Which of the following is a true statement about routine well child care and children with chronic conditions?
   a. These children need the same care as children without a chronic disease but there may be some modification of the vaccines used for immunization.
   b. These children are seen regularly by a health care provider for the chronic disease so routine screening is not needed.
   c. Children with chronic diseases should not receive any immunizations until right before starting first grade.
   d. Since these children will be developmentally delayed, monitoring growth and development is not necessary.

8. Lowanda, 11 years old, has Cerebral Palsy (CP). She has normal intelligence. She wears leg braces and uses crutches to ambulate. Which of the following statements is correct regarding anticipatory guidance for her in the area of sexuality?
   a. Because she will not be able to participate in intercourse, it is unnecessary to discuss sexual issues with her.
   b. Sexual counseling should be delayed until she is 16 years old because menarche is very late in girls with CP.
   c. Girls with CP cannot get pregnant, but she still needs information about sexually transmitted diseases.
   d. She needs the same basic information about sexuality as other children but might have some additional questions because of her CP.

9. Barbara, 22 months old, has mild mental retardation. Her mother refuses to discuss any special stimulation/education options and insists Barbara will "grow out of this problem." Your assessment?
   a. These are avoidance behaviors the mother is using in trying to cope with the diagnosis.
   b. The mother is probably retarded also and cannot understand the explanations being given to her.
   c. The child should be reevaluated to determine if the mother's assessment is correct.
   d. The mother's hostility to the staff is injuring her child so the situation should be referred to Child Protective Services.

10. Which of the following would be a good strategy to promote normalization for 16-year-old Carlos who has cancer? Allowing him to:
    a. decide when and if he will take his medication.
    b. refuse any household chores he does not like.
    c. stay home from school when he does not feel like going.
    d. order in pizza when he does not like what is being served for dinner.

ANSWERS

1.d 2.b 3.a 4.c 5.a 6.b 7.a 8.d 9.a 10.d

Chapter 20

Chronic Conditions: Effects on the Child's Family

Carolyn L. Walker, PhD, RN, CPON

Concept

◆◆◆◆◆◆◆◆◆◆◆◆◆◆◆◆◆◆◆◆◆◆◆◆◆◆◆◆

- ◆ Children with chronic condition, disability, or special health need and their families

Objectives

◆◆◆◆◆◆◆◆◆◆◆◆◆◆◆◆◆◆◆◆◆◆◆◆◆◆◆◆

At the completion of this chapter, the reader will be able to:

- ◆ Identify stressors common to parents of children with chronic conditions.

- ◆ Describe coping strategies used by parents of children with chronic conditions.

- ◆ Identify stressors common to siblings of children with chronic conditions.

- ◆ Describe coping strategies used by siblings of children with chronic conditions.

- ◆ Conduct an assessment of stressors, coping resources, coping restraints, and coping strategies of families of children with a chronic conditions.

Key Points

◆◆◆◆◆◆◆◆◆◆◆◆◆◆◆◆◆◆◆◆◆◆◆◆◆◆◆◆

- ◆ All families are unique, but they will experience some stressors related to the diagnosis and treatment of a chronic condition in their child.

- ◆ Although families will experience stress, the majority of them will cope with the stress and adapt to the demands of the chronic condition.

- ◆ Family-centered care includes assessing and intervening with the siblings as well as the parents and the child with the chronic condition.

20

Chronic Conditions: Effects on the Child's Family

◆ ◆

I. OVERVIEW

A. Definition of chronic illness.
1. An illness with a protracted course, frequently with periods of acute exacerbations, that may be progressive and/or fatal.
2. A disorder associated with a relatively normal life span despite physical or mental impairment.

B. Incidence of chronic illness: The overall incidence of children with chronic conditions has increased due to:
1. Improved medical and nursing treatment that has extended life expectancy.
2. Improved medical and nursing treatment of premature neonates has increased their survival rate, but many survive with chronic conditions.
3. The advent of new medical conditions of a chronic nature such as drug and alcohol exposed infants and Acquired Immune Deficiency Syndrome (AIDS).

II. FAMILY RESPONSE TO CHRONIC ILLNESS

A. Theoretical perspectives in chronic illness and family.
1. Theoretical frameworks are important as they direct nursing interventions.
2. Systems Theory: assists the nurse in viewing the family as dynamic and interactive. What happens to one member (a chronic illness) affects all the members.
3. Stress, Appraisal and Coping Theory (Lazarus & Folkman, 1984): assists the nurse in assessing and intervening in stressful situations to influence adaptation and minimize or eliminate maladaptation to a chronic illness.

B. Impact of chronic illness on the greater community.
1. Increased use of health care services.
2. Increased use of special education services.
3. Possible increased use of legal services.
4. Possible decrease in lifetime work productivity (parents and child).
5. Possible loss of societal contribution due to limited attainment of individual potential.

C. Six dimensions have been found to have implications for service delivery and public policy when distinguishing among classes of chronic illnesses.
1. Prevalence: with the exception of asthma and allergies, most chronic illnesses in childhood are rare.
2. Age of onset: coping with a condition from birth is different from coping with a later onset after a period of normal development.
3. Mobility: the degree of limitation on mobility affects participation in sports and other activities. Greater frustration and psychologic distress is found in children with moderate limitations rather than those severely affected.
4. Course of the illness: whether the condition is static or dynamic appears to have an effect on the child's and family's distress.
5. Cognitive and/or sensory functioning: impairment of cognitive functioning or sensory communication (hearing, language, vision) influences adjustment.
6. Visibility: the visibility of the child's illness may affect social relations with some evidence that "normal appearing" children (e.g., cyanotic heart disease) have poorer adjustment than those with visible conditions.

III. EFFECTS OF A CHRONIC CONDITION ON PARENTS

Research over the past 30 years has examined the impact of a specific chronic illness (e.g., cancer, asthma, diabetes) on the mother, with less attention to the father. A broader, more inclusive focus for research is needed to study the impact on the family system, soci-

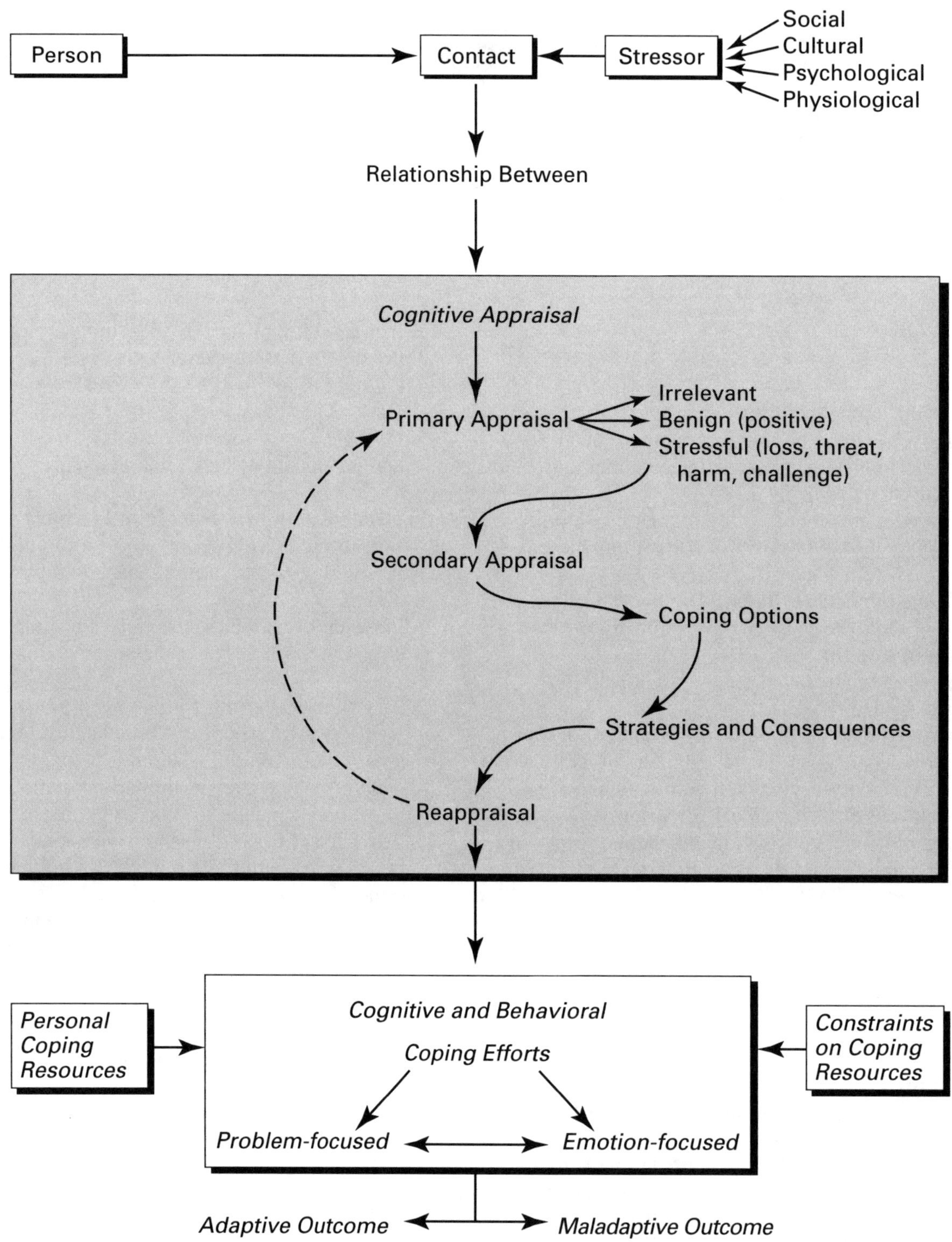

Figure 20-1
Model of Lazarus' stress, appraisal, and coping theory.

Used with permission from Walker, C.L. (1986). *Stress and coping in the siblings of children with cancer.* Doctoral Dissertation. Salt Lake City, UT: University of Utah.

ety, and culture, and on the broader concept of chronic illness, rather than specific diseases. Furthermore, although studies show that parents are at an increased risk for distress, most effectively cope with the demands of raising a child with a chronic condition, indicating a need for more research on resiliency.

A. Stress, Appraisal, and Coping Theory.
1. Stress is not inherent in the diagnosis of a chronic condition but results from the interaction of the individual (and hence family) and the environment.
2. Individuals and families may cognitively appraise or perceive the condition with varying degrees of threat, harm, loss, or challenge.
3. Once the stressor is cognitively judged to be stressful, the individual performs a secondary appraisal where a determination of what can or might be done is made (see Figure 20-1).
4. Once the stressor is appraised, some type of cognitive and/or behavioral coping effort will be used.
5. "Coping is the process through which the individual manages the demands of the person-environment that are appraised as stressful and the emotions they generate" (Lazarus & Folkman, 1984, p. 19).
6. Results of coping efforts may be either an adaptive or maladaptive outcome.

B. Stressors affecting parents.
1. Developmental and situational stressors.
    a. Developmental stressors are an expected part of life, such as birth of a child, toilet training, or beginning school. They are an inherent part of parenting.
    b. Situational stressors are not universal. Although all families will experience some stressors, not all families experience the same stressors. Having a child with a chronic illness, losing a job, and divorce are examples of situational stressors.
2. Role strain.
    a. Parents often assume new roles related to the child's illness including:
       (1) Case management.
       (2) Delivering nursing care.
       (3) Learning medical terminology, acquiring medical knowledge, and navigating health care system.
    b. Role confusion: husbands and wives frequently must overlap their roles and assist their spouse with a role that the spouse sees as primarily his or hers (e.g., wage earner, care giver, homemaker).
3. Financial stressors.

    a. Inadequate insurance coverage.
    b. Costs of care not covered by insurance.
    c. Concerns about changing or losing employment with loss of insurance.
    d. Lifestyle changes due to nonreimbursed medical care expenses.
4. Time constraints: in addition to the normal time demands of raising a child, parents may have to perform many routine nursing or medical care activities.
    a. Time demands increase in times of acute exacerbation or with progressive disease.
    b. Time demands of other family members continue during illness.
5. Energy demands: activities may be requested/required by the spouse, ill child, or other well children.
6. Psychosocial stressors.
    a. The emotional impact of the disease and the physical burden of care falls primarily on the mother.
    b. Mothers of chronically ill children experience more distress, frequently reflected in depressive symptoms, than mothers of healthy children.
    c. There is a relationship between the functional limitations of the child and the mother's distress.

C. Illness trajectory and parental stress.
1. Crisis Phase begins with prediagnosis concerns that something is wrong, through initial diagnosis and treatment when parents learn about the condition and begin to adjust.
2. Chronic Phase begins when parents learn to live with the condition on a daily basis.
3. Terminal Phase begins when the inevitability of death is apparent through death, bereavement, and life beyond the loss.
4. Sustained uncertainty has emerged as a major stressor for virtually all parents of children with potentially fatal chronic illnesses.

IV. COPING CONSTRAINTS AND RESOURCES FOR PARENTS

◆ ◆ ◆ ◆ ◆ ◆ ◆ ◆ ◆ ◆ ◆ ◆ ◆ ◆ ◆ ◆ ◆ ◆ ◆

The choice of a coping effort is influenced by individual constraints and resources. It must be noted that something that may be a "resource" for one family (e.g., relationship with the child's grandparents) may be a "constraint" for another family.

◆ ◆ ◆ ◆ ◆ ◆ ◆ ◆ ◆ ◆ ◆ ◆ ◆ ◆ ◆ ◆ ◆ ◆ ◆

A. Coping constraints.
1. Limited intellectual abilities.

2. Limited knowledge about the chronic condition.
3. Limited ability to perform required psychomotor skills.
4. Limited life experience with the chronic condition.
5. Perceived social stigma attached to condition.
6. Limited financial resources.
7. Limited social support system.
8. Concurrent demands from other life stressors.
9. Limited range of personal coping strategies.

B. Coping resources.
1. Adequate intellectual abilities.
2. Prior knowledge about the chronic condition.
3. Ability to perform psychomotor skills required.
4. Positive life experience with the chronic condition.
5. Lack of perceived social stigma attached to condition.
6. Adequate financial resources.
7. Extensive social support system.
8. Minimal demands from other life stressors.
9. Broad range of personal coping strategies.

V. COPING STRATEGIES

Coping efforts or strategies should not be evaluated as "good-bad," "positive-negative," or "adaptive-maladaptive." The outcome is evaluated as adaptive or maladaptive, not the individual coping effort.

A. Every coping method employed by each parent must be viewed from both the short-term and long-term effects on adaptation.

B. The choice of a specific coping strategy is also influenced by culture and ethnicity. Common strategies include:
1. Seeking out information.
2. Using social support resources.
3. Maintaining a sense of personal and family balance in life.
4. Maintaining hope.
5. Maintaining communication (with health care providers, spouse, children, extended family, friends).
6. Setting priorities.
7. Taking care of self (e.g., exercise, nutrition, rest, recreation, emotional needs).
8. Forgiving self (and others) when performance does not measure up to expectations.
9. Using support groups. For example, many specific chronic conditions have parent organizations that offer support groups that some parents find helpful.

10. Finding a personal sense of meaning in the experience.
11. Identifying positive aspects of living with a child who is chronically ill or disabled.
12. Identifying what can be controlled.
13. Keeping a sense of humor.
14. Living one day at a time.
15. Finding joy in life.
16. Utilizing spiritual supports.

VI. EFFECTS OF A CHRONIC CONDITION ON THE SIBLINGS

A. Findings of research on adjustment problems in siblings have yielded some contradictory results. Earlier studies tended to show greater adjustment problems than later studies.
1. The effects of stress on the siblings of chronic illness appear to be less than previously thought.
2. Each child will perceive stressors differently and there are significant differences in stressors at different ages, according to birth order, and gender.

B. Stressors affecting siblings.
1. Less attention from parents.
2. Emotional realignments within the family.
3. Physical and emotional separation from parents and/or ill sibling.
4. Lack of information or information that is understandable at their developmental level.
5. Disrupted family communication.
6. Perceived sense of guilt over causing the illness.
7. Negativity between how the ill child and siblings are disciplined.
8. Assumption of more household responsibilities and chores, often including care giving functions for the ill child.
9. Fear of the unknown (e.g., fears of what the treatments/hospitalizations are like, fear of death, fears of self or other family members becoming ill).
10. Changes in family routines.
11. Changes in recreation activities.

C. Coping constraints and resources for siblings.
1. Coping constraints.
   a. Developmental level may limit intellectual understanding.
   b. Limited repertoire of coping strategies.
   c. Limited knowledge about and experience with chronic illnesses.
   d. Lack of exposure to other siblings of chronically ill children for social support.

e. Limited language skills to express feelings.
2. Coping resources.
   a. Being born after or being very young when the chronic condition is diagnosed in sibling (never knowing a different family life).
   b. Having other well siblings to share feelings, concerns, and household tasks with.
   c. Extensive social support network available to provide physical and emotional care when needed.
   d. Open communication within family that promotes expression of feelings.

D. Coping strategies.
1. Seeking out information (see Table 20-1).
2. Using social support resources.
3. Having an outlet separate from the ill child and family as a means of distraction and source of esteem (e.g., school, recreation activities, clubs, friends).
4. Expressing emotions.
5. Thought stopping: the forced substitution of positive thoughts for negative ones.
6. Developing empathy: ability to assume the perspective of another.

VII. FAMILY ASSESSMENT
◆ ◆ ◆ ◆ ◆ ◆ ◆ ◆ ◆ ◆ ◆ ◆ ◆ ◆ ◆ ◆ ◆ ◆

Assessment of the family of a child who is chronically ill begins with a health assessment interview coupled with observations of family interactions.

A. Theoretical models: There are a number of theoretical models for assessing families
1. Systems theories.
   a. Social-Ecological Systems Theory.
      (1) Bronfenbrenner's (1979) ecological model proposes a series of concentric circles that have bidirectional influences on the child who is at the center.
      (2) Reciprocity: environments affect the child and the child affects the environment.
      (3) Interconnections between the setting and the child's development, and transitions across the life span influence achievement of developmental milestones.
   b. Family systems theories. The circumplex model of family systems (Olson, Sprenkle, & Russell, 1979) suggests that a balance of cohesion and adaptability are the central dimensions that are conductive to individual and family adjustment.
2. Cognitive-behavioral-social learning theories:
   a. The disability-stress-coping model (Wallander & Varni, 1992) is based on a risk-resistance framework. Risk factors engender stress, while resistance factors foster adaptation.
   b. The transactional stress and coping model. Thompson & Gustafson (1996) view adaptation as a function of the transaction of chronic illness and demographic parameters and how one processes stress.

B. Assessment strategies.
1. Assess what each family member knows about the condition and any previous experience with the same or similar condition including:
   a. Fears regarding prognosis.
   b. Concerns over etiology.
   c. Concerns over ability to manage care.
   d. Concerns over impact of chronic condition on personal and family life.
2. Assess coping resources and constraints such as:
   a. Family communication style.
   b. Social support systems.
   c. Need for financial assistance.
   d. Concurrent situational or developmental stressors in the family.
   e. Feelings about and emotional impact of the diagnosis.
3. Assess coping strategies previously used with other stressors. Ask parents:
   a. Do they think they will work now?
   b. Do they think the coping strategy was effective? If not, why?
4. Observe family interaction pattern. Ask the following questions:
   a. Are there special alliances? Relationships?
   b. Are there consistent dyads or triads?
   c. What roles does each member have within the family? Are they rigid or flexible?
   d. Who has power? What kind? How is power maintained?
   e. What are the family strengths and limitations?
   f. What is the family management style? Knafl, Breitmayer, Gallo, and Zoeller (1996) identified five styles in families with chronically ill children.
      (1) Thriving.
      (2) Accommodating.
      (3) Enduring.
      (4) Struggling.
      (5) Floundering.

C. Positive effects of childhood chronic conditions on the family.
1. The majority of families do cope with and adapt to the stressors associated with a chronic condition.

Table 20-1
National Resource List for Parents

Alexander Graham Bell Association for the Deaf 3417 Volta Place, NW Washington, DC 20007 202-337-5220	Association for Parents of the Visually Impaired 2180 Linway Dr Beloit, WI 53511 800-562-6265	Juvenile Diabetes Foundation International 432 Park Ave, S New York, NY 10016 800-223-1138	National Head Injury Foundation 1140 Connecticut Ave, NW Suite 812 Washington, DC 20036 800-444-6443 or 202-296-6443
American Burn Association New York-Cornell Medical Center 525 E 68th St, Room L-706 New York, NY 10021 800-548- BURN	Association of Birth Defect Children 827 Irma Ave Orlando, FL 32803 800-313-ABDC	March of Dimes -Birth Defects Foundation 1275 Mamaroneck Ave White Plains, NY 10605 914-428-7100	National Hemophilia Foundation 110 Green St, Room 303 New York, NY 10012 800-42HANDI or 212-219-8180
American Cancer Society 1599 Clifton Road, NE Atlanta, GA 30329 800-ACS-2345	Asthma & Allergy Foundation of America 1125 15th St, NW Washington, DC 20005 202-466-7643	Muscular Dystrophy Association of America 10 E. 40th St, Room 4105 New York, NY 10019 212-679-6215 or 212-689-9040	National Hospice Organization 1901 N Moore St Arlington, VA 22209 800-658-8898
American Celiac Society Dept. N 83 45 Gifford Ave Jersey City, NJ 07304	Autism Society of America 7910 Woodmont Ave, Suite 650 Bethesda, MD 20814	National Association for Sickle Cell Disease 3345 Wilshire Blvd, Suite 1106 Los Angeles, CA 90010-1880 800-421-8453	National Information Center for Children & Youth with Disabilities P.O. Box 1492 Washington, DC 20013 800-695-0285 or 202-884-8200
American Cleft Palate Association 1218 Grandview Avenue Pittsburgh, PA 15211 800-24-CLEFT or 412-418-1376	Candlelighters Childhood Cancer Foundation 7910 Woodmont Ave, Suite 460 Bethesda, MD 20814 800-366-2223 or 301-657-8401	National Association for Visually Handicapped 22 W. 21st St New York, NY 10010 212-889-3141	National Information Clearing-house for Infants with Disabilities and Life-Threatening Conditions Center for Developmental Disabilities University of South Carolina Benson Building Columbia, SC 29208 800-922-9234 ext 201
American Council of the Blind 1155 15th St, NW Washington, DC 20005 800-424-8666 or 202-467-5081	Children's Hospice International 901 N Washington St, 7th floor Alexandria, VA 22314 800-24-CHILD	National Center for Children with Chronic Illness & Disability Box 721-UMHC Harvard St. at East River Rd Minneapolis, MN 55455 612-626-4032	
American Diabetes Association 1660 Duke St Alexandria, VA 22314 800-232-3472	Children's Liver Foundation 76 S. Orange Ave, Suite 202 South Orange, NJ 07079		National Kidney Foundation 30 E. 33rd St. New York, NY 10016 800-622-9010 or 212-889-2210
American Foundation for the Blind 11 Penn Plaza, Suite 300 New York, NY 10001 212-502-7600	Cooley's Anemia Foundation 129-09 26th Ave Flushing, NY 11354 800-522-7222 or 718-321-2873	National Clearinghouse for Alcohol & Drug Information P.O. Box 2345 Rockville, MD 20847-2345 800-729-6686	National Pediatric HIV Resource Center 15 S 9th St. Newark, NJ 07107 800-362-0071 or 201-268-8251
American Juvenile Arthritis Foundation 1314 Spring St, NW Atlanta, GA 30309 800-283-7800 or 404-872-7100	Crohn's & Colitis Foundation of America 44 Park Ave, South New York, NY 10016 212-679-1570	National Diabetes Information Clearinghouse Box NDIC 9000 Rockville Pike Bethesda, MD 20892	Osteogenesis Imperfecta Foundation 5005 W. Laurel St. Tampa, FL 33607 813-282-1161
American Lung Association 1740 Broadway New York, NY 10019 212-315-8700	Cystic Fibrosis Foundation 6931 Arlington Road Bethesda, MD 20814-3205 800-FIGHT CF or 310-951-4422	National Downs Syndrome Society 666 Broadway New York, NY 10012 800-221-4602 or 212-460-9330	Sibling Information Network 991 Main St, Suite 3A East Hartford, CT 06108
American Lupus Society P.O. Box 9610 Marina Del Rey, CA 90215 310-390-6888	Family Resource Coalition (for aid to families of premature infants) 230 N. Michigan Ave, Suite 1625 Chicago, IL 60601	National Easter Seal Society 70 E. Lake St. Chicago, IL 60601 800-221-6827 or 312-726-6200	Special Olympics 1350 New York Ave, NW Suite 500 Washington, DC 20005-4709 202-628-3630
Aplastic Anemia Foundation of America P.O. Box 22689 Baltimore, MD 21203 800-747-2820	Federation for Children with Special Needs 95 Berkeley St, Suite 104 Boston, MA 02116 617-482-2915	National Federation of the Blind 1800 Johnson St Baltimore, MD 21230 410-659-9314	United Cerebral Palsy Association 710 Penn Plaza, Suite 804 New York, NY 10001 800-USA-IUCP

2. Individual or family psychopathology is not the inevitable outcome of a chronic childhood condition when nurses build upon the strengths of the family (Brett, 1988).
3. Family coping strategies used to successfully navigate the demands of the illness.
   a. Social support: Parents and siblings appear to cope when they can share their burdens with others (family, friends, professionals).
   b. Normalization: Families adjust best to the chronic illness when they can integrate the child into society, maintain their "normal" family interactions and routines, to some degree minimize the child's illness.
   c. Mastery: When families can master the specific demands of the illness, they tend to decrease anxiety and increase self-confidence and a sense of control.
   d. Assigning meaning: When family members see a meaning to life, there tends to be a transformation that leads to an affirmation of life. Family members experience a sense of pride, self-confidence, and a real life purpose that appears to mitigate the stressors.
   e. Open communication: Supportive, open communication skills appear to assist families in avoiding long-term emotional maladjustment.
4. Adaptation as a family process,
   a. Adaptation is viewed developmentally, is seen as a continual process, and sees the family as health-oriented, rather than from a pathologic perspective.
   b. Adaptive tasks of chronic illness.
      (1) Accepting the condition.
      (2) Daily management of the condition
      (3) Meeting the normal developmental needs of the child who is chronically ill.
      (4) Meeting the normal developmental needs of other family members.
      (5) Coping with ongoing stressors and periodic crisis.
      (6) Helping family members manage feelings.
      (7) Educating others about the chronic condition.
      (8) Establishing a support system.

BIBLIOGRAPHY

Brett, K.M. (1988). Sibling response to chronic childhood disorders: Research perspectives and practice implications. *Issues in Comprehensive Pediatric Nursing, 11,* 43–57.

Bronfenbrenner, U. (1979). *The ecology of human development.* Cambridge, MA: Harvard University Press.

Clawson, J.A. (1996). A child with chronic illness and the process of family adaptation. *Journal of Pediatric Nursing, 11,* 52–61.

Cohen, M.H. (1989). *Living under conditions of sustained uncertainty.* Doctoral dissertation. University of California, San Francisco.

Faux, S. A. (1993). Siblings of children with chronic physical and cognitive disabilities. *Journal of Pediatric Nursing, 8,* 305–317.

Gibson, C.H. (1995). The process of empowerment in mothers of chronically ill children. *Journal of Advanced Nursing, 21,* 1201–1210.

Knafl, K., Breitmayer, B., Gallo, A., & Zoeller, L. (1996). Family response to childhood chronic illness: Description of management styles. *Journal of Pediatric Nursing, 11,* 315–326.

Lazarus, R.S. & Folkman, S. (1984). *Stress, appraisal, and coping.* New York: Springer.

Olsen, D.H., Sprenkle, D., & Russell, C.S. (1979). Circumplex model of marital and family systems: I. Cohesion and adaptability dimensions, family types, and clinical applications. *Family Process, 18,* 3–28.

Pless, I.B., & Nolan, T. (1991). Revision, replication, and neglect – research on maladjustment in chronic illness. *Journal of Child Psychology and Psychiatry and applied Discipline, 32,* 347–365.

Thompson, R.J., & Gustafson, K.E. (1996). *Adaptation to chronic childhood illness.* Washington DC: American Psychological Association.

Walker, C.L. (1986). Stress and coping in the siblings of children with cancer. Doctoral dissertation. Salt Lake City, UT: University of Utah.

Walker, C.L. (1988). Stress and coping in siblings of childhood cancer patients. *Nursing Research, 37,* 208–212.

Wallander, J.L., & Varni, J.W. (1992). Adjustment in children with chronic physical disorders: Programmatic research on a disability-stress-coping model. In A.M. LaGreca, L. Siegal, J.L. Wallander, & C.E. Walker, (Eds.), *Stress and coping with pediatric conditions* (pp. 279–298). New York: Guilford Press.

STUDY QUESTIONS

1. The overall increased incidence in the number of children with chronic conditions is attributed to:
   a. improved treatment that extends life expectancy.
   b. improved survival rates of premature infants.
   c. several new chronic conditions.
   d. all of the above.
   e. none of the above; it is due to better reporting.

2. Although each type of chronic illness will impact community resources in different ways, every chronic illness will:
   a. require special education programs in schools.
   b. require legal services.
   c. increase use of health care services.
   d. decrease the parent's work productivity.
   e. decrease the individual's contribution to society.

3. Research has predominantly examined the impact of:
   a. specific chronic illness.
   b. chronic illness on society.
   c. chronic illness on the family system.
   d. cultural factors on chronic illness.

4. Parents must adapt to a variety of stressors related to their child's chronic illness. The financial stressor that reflects the hidden costs of care is:
   a. cost of insurance policy.
   b. nonreimbursed expenses.
   c. prescription costs.
   d. loss of insurance coverage with change of employment.
   e. limitations on insurance coverage.

5. An assessment of the family of a chronically ill child would include:
   a. concerns about etiology of condition.
   b. fears regarding prognosis.
   c. concerns about ability to manage care.
   d. concerns over impact of illness on family and personal life.
   e. concerns about being involved in clinical research.

The following situation pertains to questions 5 through 10:

Robert is a 5-year-old who was recently diagnosed with severe asthma requiring daily inhaled albuterol treatments. Robert's father and paternal grandfather both have asthma. Robert's mother, 9-year-old brother, and 3-year-old sister do not have any chronic illnesses. Both parents work in middle management positions and have excellent insurance coverage.

6. The family history of asthma most likely would be an example of:
   a. the cause of Robert's asthma.
   b. a coping constraint.
   c. a coping resource.
   d. a coping strategy.

7. Based on the situation presented, which of the following would NOT be a coping resource?
   a. Financial resources
   b. Life experiences with chronic illnesses
   c. Knowledge about chronic condition
   d. Concurrent demands from other life stressors
   e. Intellectual abilities

8. Robert's asthma treatment is different than his father's. Since his diagnosis, Robert's parents have done all of the following. Which is an example of an emotion-focused coping strategy as opposed to problem-focused coping strategies?
   a. Sought out information about asthma treatment in young children
   b. Maintained their own exercise programs despite his illness
   c. Altered housekeeping routines to reduce environmental antigens
   d. Changed each child's household chores to accommodate to Robert's limitations
   e. Kept a record of circumstances surrounding Robert's asthma attacks

9. Over the next 5 years, Robert experienced three hospitalizations for severe, life-threatening asthma attacks. During this time period, the family has altered the type of recreational activities they engage in, limited the amount and type of household chores Robert is responsible for, spent more time with Robert for his medical treatments, and assisted Robert with his schooling due to absences from school. His siblings (now ages 8 and 14) react differently to these family changes with the older sibling acting out and rebelling over extra chores assigned to him. Which is the most likely explanation for his behavior?
   a. Perceived sense of guilt over causing Robert's illness
   b. Resentment toward Robert for causing the changes
   c. Fears that he will also become ill or possibly die
   d. Lack of developmentally appropriate information
   e. Normal adolescent rebellious behavior not related to illness

10. Based on all of the above information about Robert's family, how would you describe the parents' management style?
    a. Thriving
    b. Accommodating
    c. Enduring
    d. Struggling
    e. Floundering

ANSWERS

1.d 2.c 3.a 4.b 5.e 6.c 7.d 8.b 9.b 10.b

Chapter 21

Chronic Conditions: Care Technologies

Judy Benka, MS, RN, PNP

Concept

◆◆◆◆◆◆◆◆◆◆◆◆◆◆◆◆◆◆◆◆◆◆◆◆◆◆

◆ Children with a chronic condition, disability, or special health need and their families

Objectives

◆◆◆◆◆◆◆◆◆◆◆◆◆◆◆◆◆◆◆◆◆◆◆◆◆◆

At the completion of this chapter, the reader will be able to:

◆ Identify nursing interventions used to care for children with chronic conditions requiring various venous access devices.

◆ Review the indications for parenteral/enteral therapy and appropriate nursing interventions.

◆ Discuss therapies that use home infusion pumps.

◆ Describe the equipment and the nurse's role in assisting the caregiver/child to use the equipment to monitor physical care.

◆ Review the specific needs of children receiving home peritoneal dialysis and mechanical ventilation.

Key Points

◆◆◆◆◆◆◆◆◆◆◆◆◆◆◆◆◆◆◆◆◆◆◆◆

◆ The technology-dependent child's and family's need for normalcy is extremely important.

◆ Establishing a safe environment in which the child's chronic care needs can be met minimizes the risk of injury.

◆ Continuing assessment of physical, emotional (family/child), and technologic needs is essential.

Chronic Conditions: Care Technologies

I. OVERVIEW: CONCEPTS RELATED TO HOME CARE EQUIPMENT

With the emphasis on early discharge from acute care hospitals and the increasing complexity of health care needs, more patients are relying on home medical equipment (HME) to meet their health needs in their own home. Previously, HME was known as durable medical equipment (DME); that is, it was not disposable and was medical in nature. HME is now an essential component of home health care. For each treatment attempted in the child's home, the nurse must be aware of the following (Birmingham & Jeffries, 1993):

A. Types of equipment.

B. Equipment features and general uses.

C. Nursing care related to incorporating the equipment into the plan of care.

D. Safety considerations and troubleshooting.

E. Developmental considerations of the child and family.

F. Infection control.

G. Documentation regarding medical necessity and patient response.

H. Reimbursement considerations.

II. HOME INFUSION THERAPY

A. Advantages of home infusion therapy.
1. Children are able to leave the hospital earlier or to avoid an admission to the hospital entirely.
2. Home-based infusion therapy is less expensive than traditional hospital-based therapy.
3. Treatment of child in the home environment leads to a happier, more relaxed, and comfortable patient.

4. Child and family are active participants in the delivery of care.
5. Continued parental employment may be possible.
6. Greater normalization and less disruption in the child and family's life are possible.

B. Patient selection criteria. Prior to initiating home infusion therapy, children must be carefully screened and specific criteria for some infusion therapy met (see Table 21-1) (Sheldon & Bender, 1994). These criteria include:
1. Appropriate diagnosis and treatment.
2. Child medically stable.
3. Reasonable plan for initiation and maintenance of venous access.
4. Best method of delivery for identified need.
5. Drug stability.
6. Safe and appropriate home environment (physical layout, cleanliness, functioning phone, electricity).
7. Patient and/or caregiver capable of learning and willing to perform prescribed care.
8. Financial resources to cover scope of home care verified.
9. Developmental considerations of child/family assessed.

Table 21-1
Common Uses of Home Infusion Therapies

Antibiotics (antibacterial)*	Antiviral
Hydration*	Antifungals
Pain management*	Antiemetics
Chemotherapies	Tocolytics
Total parenteral nutrition	Immunotherapy
Cardiovascular drugs	Hematopoietics
Blood products	Steroids
*Traditional therapies	

Adapted from Sheldon, P., & Bender, M. (1994). High technology in home care: An overview of intravenous therapy. *Nursing Clinics of North America, 29*(3), 507–519.

C. Evaluation criteria for home infusion therapy.
1. Child's physical response to therapy.
2. Ease of administration.
3. Parental and child feedback regarding infusion therapy.
4. Cost-effectiveness of therapy.

D. Concerns related to home infusion pumps.
1. Pump too cumbersome; makes mobility difficult.
2. Reliance on electricity poses restrictions.
3. Difficulty in reading pump.
4. Solutions (TPN) do not fit well into pump's carrying case.
5. Noisy pumps make sleeping difficult.
6. Inaccurate infusion rates.

III. INTRAVENOUS ACCESS DEVICES

A. Device selection based on:
1. Child diagnosis.
2. Type of prescribed therapy.
3. Expected length of treatment and dosing schedule.
4. Condition of child's anatomy.
5. Prior surgeries or illness.
6. Parent/child preference.
7. Developmental considerations.
8. Family competency and resources.

B. Short-term peripheral venous access.
1. Placed by nurse trained in proper insertion technique.
2. Considerations for site selection.
   a. Child's condition.
   b. Age.
   c. Diagnosis.
   d. Vein condition, size, location.
   e. Type and duration of therapy.
   f. Other therapies in progress.
3. Types and equipment features.
   a. Catheter material: Teflon, Aquavein (which softens and expands), and Vialon (which softens with body temperature). All are radiopaque.
   b. Over the needle catheter.
      (1) Needle within sheath.
      (2) Length ¾-inch to 2-inch and gauges of even numbers ranging from 12 to 24.
   c. Objective is to use the smallest gauge and length that will accommodate the therapy.

C. Nursing care.
1. Dressing: sterile, occlusive; may be tape and gauze or transparent semipermeable membrane (TSM) material.
2. Dressing change and site rotation per agency protocol.
3. Site assessment.
4. Flushing: controversies regarding use of heparin-flushing protocols and the use of saline flushes for maintaining patency of peripheral lines.
   a. Maintain patency according to agency policies.
   b. Flush with saline between medications.
5. Prevention of complications. Good venipuncture technique main factor in prevention of local complications (see Table 21-2).

IV. CENTRAL VENOUS ACCESS DEVICES

A. Types.
1. Nontunneled.
   a. Placed by specially trained nurse or physician.
   b. Peripheral inserted central catheter (PICC) and midline catheters (MLC) may be inserted in the home (with portable radiograph for confirmation of PICC placement).
   c. Appropriate for short-term or long-term therapy (several weeks to months).
   d. Indications.
      (1) Lack of peripheral access.
      (2) Infusion of vesicant or irritant drugs.
      (3) Infusion of hyperosmolar drugs and TPN.
      (4) Infusion of antineoplastic agents, blood, or blood components.
      (5) Patient/family/clinician preference.
   e. Advantages of PICC.
      (1) Inexpensive placement.
      (2) No surgical placement required; catheter inserted in antecubital fossa through basilic or cephalic vein into superior vena cava.
      (3) Preservation of peripheral venous system.
      (4) Decrease in discomfort.
      (5) Reliability.
      (6) Ease of discontinuation of catheter.
      (7) Diverse utilization of line.
      (8) Potential reduction in catheter sepsis.
   f. Disadvantages of PICC.
      (1) Daily care requirements.
      (2) Impact on activity and body image (line exits at antecubital space).
      (3) Occlusive dressing over exit site required because line not tunneled or sutured in place.
      (4) Risk of dislodgement because not sutured in place.
      (5) Requires radiographic verification.
      (6) Increased financial costs of caring for catheter.

Table 21-2
Complications, Prevention, and Treatment of Intravenous Therapy

Type	Etiology	Description	Prevention	Treatment
Hematoma	Venipuncture technique Large cannulas used in patients who bruise easily Discontinuing IV cannula without adequate pressure held over site after removal of needle	Discoloration of skin surrounding venipuncture Site swelling and discoloration	Use proper venipuncture technique Apply tourniquet just before venipuncture Use smallest gauge needle and catheter whenever possible	Apply direct pressure with sterile 2 x 2 gauze over site after catheter is removed Patient elevates extremity over head or on pillow
Thrombosis	Blood back up Low flow rate Cannula location Obstruction of flow rate Trauma to wall of vein	Site may appear healthy IV solution drips slowly Line does not flush well Resistance noted when flushing	Use infusion devices Avoid flexion areas for placement of IV cannulas	Discontinue cannula and restart in other site Apply cold compress to site to decrease flow of blood and increase further platelet adherence to formed clot Notify physician and assess for circulatory impairment
Phlebitis	Insertion technique Condition of patient Vein condition Inappropriate cannula selection Compatibility of medication/infusion	Redness at site Site warm to touch Local swelling Palpable cord along the vein Sluggish infusion rate Increase in basal temperature	Use larger veins for hypertonic solutions Long-term hypertonic solutions use central lines or long-arm catheters Insert smallest cannula appropriate for infusion Use in-line filter Rotate site every 72 hours Stabilize catheter Use good venipuncture technique	Apply hot or cold compress to affected site (cold decreases intradermal skin toxicity) for 45 minutes Notify physician >3+ (pain at site, erythema, or edema streak formation
Thrombophlebitis	Painful, inflamed vein develops from point of thrombosis	Sluggish flow rate Edema in limb Tender and cordlike vein Site warm to touch Visible red line above venipuncture site	Use veins in forearm preferably Do not use veins in joint flexion areas Assess infusion site every hour for signs and symptoms of redness, swelling, or pain at the site Anchor catheter securely Use smallest catheter as feasible Dilute irritating medications	Remove catheter and restart in opposite extremity Notify physician Apply warm, moist compress for 20 minutes to provide comfort
Infiltration	Seepage of nonvesicant solution or medication into surrounding tissues, due to dislodgement of cannula from vein Phlebitis	Coolness of skin around site Taut skin Dependent edema Backflow of blood absent Slowing infusion rate	Avoid flexor areas and multiple venipuncture attempts Secure catheter Apply armboard to avoid excessive movement Verify patency Assess site frequently	Discontinue infusion Elevate extremity Apply warm compresses

Table continues on next page

Table 21-2 (continued from page 271)
Complications, Prevention, and Treatment of Intravenous Therapy

Type	Etiology	Description	Prevention	Treatment
Extravasation	Infiltration of vesicant medication	Sloughing of tissues due to tissue necrosis Complaints of burning or pain Skin tightness at venipuncture site Blanching and coolness of skin Slow or stopped infusion Dependent enema affected extremity	In addition to prevention strategies for infiltration, avoid high-pressure infusion pumps when infusing vesicant drugs Educate patient to report any feelings of burning	Stop infusion and leave cannula in place If possible, aspirate any residual medication/blood and provide prescribed antidote after notifying physician Apply warm or cold compresses as indicated for agent extravasated Elevate arm
Local infection	Most commonly due to cannula contamination	Redness and swelling at site Possible purulent exudate Increased WBCs Elevated temperature	Inspect all solution containers for cracks and leaks before handling Change solution containers every 24 hours Maintain aseptic technique during cannula insertion, IV therapy, and catheter removal	Reevaluate dressing technique Stop infusion and discontinue cannula Culture site Notify physician Start topical/systemic antibiotics
Venous spasm	Can occur suddenly Usually results from administration of cold infusate, an irritating solution, or a too-rapid administration of IV solution or viscous solution (i.e., blood product)	Sharp pain at IV site traveling up arm Slowing of infusion	Dilute medication additive adequately Keep or let IV solution warm to room temperature Wrap extremity with warm compresses during infusion Administer solution at prescribed rate	Apply warm compresses Decrease flow rate until spasm subsides Restart IV if venospasm continues

Adapted with permission from Phillips, L.D. (1997). Complications of intravenous therapy. *Manual of IV therapeutics* (2nd ed.). Philadelphia: F.A. Davis Co.

(7) Small lumen may prohibit blood sampling due to risk of catheter collapse upon aspiration.

g. Equipment features.
   (1) Material: radiopaque silicone or polyurethane; 23 to 16 gauge.
   (2) Midline catheters (MLC): catheter is inserted in the antecubital fossa through the basilic or cephallic vein and threaded to level of subclavian vein or midaxilla area.
      (a) Does not require radiograph verification.
      (b) Common infusions via MLC: antibiotics, fluids for hydration, low osmolality TPN, pain management.
   (3) May be sutured in place or anchored by dressing only.

h. Nursing care.
   (1) Do not take blood pressure or draw blood from arm where PICC or MLC is inserted.
   (2) Dressing: policy varies by agency (3 to 7 days for transparent dressings, every 48 hours for dry sterile).
   (3) Flushing: flushing procedure varies by agency – see protocol.

i. Troubleshooting. See Table 21-3 regarding management of complications of all central venous access devices.

2. Tunneled catheters (i.e., Broviac, Hickman, Groshong) (see Figure 21-1).
   a. Appropriate for long-term therapy (months to years).
   b. Placed by a physician.
   c. Placement verified by radiograph prior to

Table 21-3
Venous Access Device Complications

Complication	Assessment	Prevention	Intervention
Catheter damage, breakage	1. Observe for pinholes, leaks, tears, every shift. 2. Assess for drainage after flushing.	1. Follow proper clamping procedure. 2. Avoid sharp objects near the catheter. 3. Avoid using >1″ needles through the injection cap. 4. Avoid larger than 21-gauge needles through injection cap.	1. Use a catheter stylet to temporarily repair. 2. Use permanent repair kit. 3. Remove catheter.
Occlusion: thrombus, precipitation, malposition	1. Assess for blood return. 2. Note inability to infuse. 3. Assess for drainage. 4. If port, reaccess to verify needle placement. 5. Assess with syringe directly on catheter. 6. Note discomfort or pain in shoulder, neck, or arm at insertion site. 7. Assess sutures to ensure no restriction.	1. Follow routine flushing with positive pressure. 2. Avoid tugging on line. 3. Use low-dose oral or intravenous anticoagulant therapy. 4. Avoid excessive force. 5. Flush between drugs. 6. Flush vigorously after viscous solutions. 7. Avoid mixing incompatible drugs. 8. Avoid kinking catheter.	1. Reposition patient. 2. Encourage patient to cough and deep breathe. 3. Raise patient's arm. 4. Obtain venogram 5. Administer thrombolytic agent. 6. Remove catheter. 7. Gentle push-pull technique with NS. 8. Obtain x-ray. 9. If precipitate, try hydrochloric acid or ethanol solution.
Infection: exit site, tunnel, thrombus, port pocket	1. Assess exit site for redness, drainage, edema, or tenderness. 2. Assess vital signs. 3. Monitor labs.	1. Use strict hand-washing. 2. Use aseptic technique. 3. Adhere to dressing change technique. 4. Apply dressing over exit site. 5. Apply antibiotic or antimicrobial ointment at exit site.	1. Administer antibiotic therapy. 2. Remove catheter. 3. Administer thrombolytic agent. 4. Replace catheter. 5. Obtain blood cultures, peripheral and from venous access devices (VAD)
Dislodgement, Twiddler's syndrome	1. Assess length of catheter daily. 2. Inform patient/parent of possible catheter dislodgement. 3. Note edema at exit site or drainage. 4. Palpate exit site and tunnel for coiling.	1. Loop and tape the catheter securely. 2. Use occlusive dressing. 3. Use athletic sock for PICC. 4. Avoid pulling on VAD. 5. Handle with care. 6. Avoid manipulating catheter (port) by hand.	1. Reinsert catheter. 2. Secure catheter with sutures. 3. Teach patient not to manipulate sutures.
Catheter migration, pinch-off syndrome, port separation	1. Patient complains of gurgling sounds. 2. Change in capability of catheter. 3. Obtain x-ray. 4. Assess edema of arm and hand on side of insertion. 5. Assess neck veins for distention. 6. Unable to infuse fluids. 7. Assess length of catheter daily.	1. Avoid trauma. 2. Avoid placement near site of local disease.	1. Reposition under fluoroscopy. 2. Remove catheter. 3. Stop all fluid administration.
Skin erosions, hematomas, cuff extrusion scar	1. Loss of viable tissue over implantation. 2. Separation of exit site edges. 3. Drainage at exit site. 4. Redness. 5. Edema, contusions. 6. Tunnelled catheter exposed.	1. Maintain nutritional status. 2. Minimize edema with cold packs. 3. Avoid pressure or trauma. 4. Rotate site with each port access.	1. Remove VAD. 2. Improve nutrition. 3. Provide appropriate skin care.
Infiltration, extravasation	1. Erythema. 2. Edema. 3. Spongy feeling. 4. Labored breathing. 5. No blood return. 6. Complaints of pain. 7. No free-flow IV drip.	1. Do not administer vesicants. 2. Use own judgment to use without a blood return. 3. Develop astute assessment skills. 4. Administer medications according to drug literature.	1. Apply warm compress. 2. Provide emotional support. 3. Obtain x-ray. 4. Use antidotes. 5. Discontinue IV fluids.

Used with permission from Camp-Sorrell, D. (1990). Advanced central venous access: Selection, catheter devices and nursing management. *Journal of Intravenous Nursing, 13*(6), 361–370. Original source: Carter, P., Engelking, C.H., Fiscus, J.A., Harvey, C., Hayes, N., Rostad, M., Vincent, B., Whedon, M. (1989). *Access device guidelines: Module I (pp. 2–3) and Module II (pp. 3–4)*. Pittsburgh: Oncology Nursing Society.

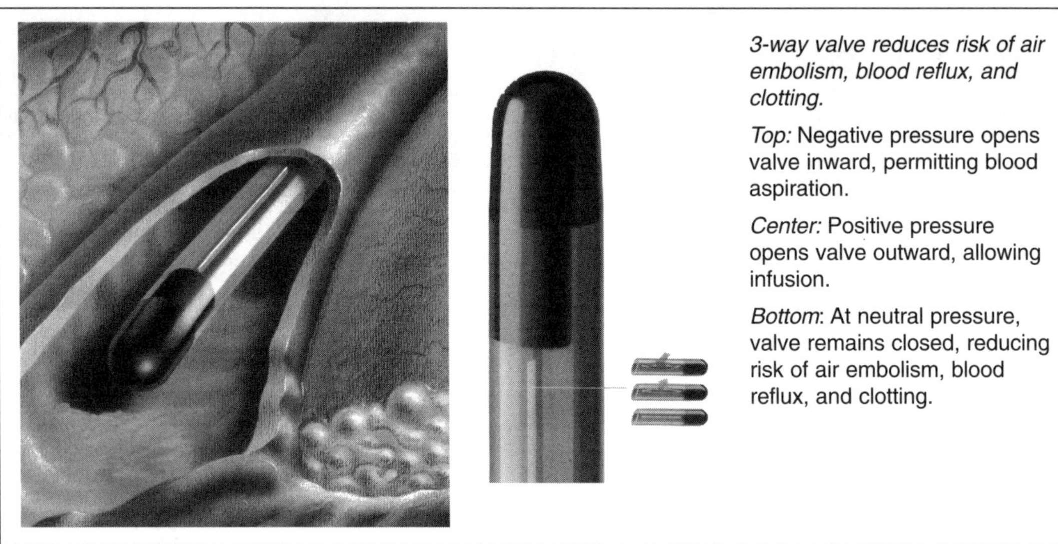

Figure 21-1
Valved Groshong® catheter.

Used with permission from Bard Access Systems, Salt Lake City, UT.

infusion; tip of catheter in superior vena cava.
d. Indications.
  (1) Refer to indications for PICC above.
  (2) Frequent blood withdrawal.
e. Advantages.
  (1) Multipurpose: blood sampling, drug administration, TPN administration, monitoring central venous pressure.
  (2) Can be repaired if it breaks or tears.
  (3) Useful for patients with long-term IV therapy needs.
f. Disadvantages.
  (1) Daily to weekly site care.
  (2) Costly maintenance supplies (i.e., dressing materials, frequency of flushing and cap changing).
  (3) Surgical placement required.
  (4) Impact on body image.
g. Equipment features.
  (1) Single, double, or triple lumen catheters.
  (2) Dacron/Vita-cuff anchors catheter in place subcutaneously and provides mechanical and chemical barrier against organisms.
h. Nursing care.
  (1) Dressing is same as for nontunneled catheter.
  (2) Never use metal clamps on catheter; use attached catheter clamp only.
  (3) Blood draws and flushing. Follow laboratory and/or agency policy.
i. Troubleshooting (see Table 21-3).

3. Implanted ports.
  a. Appropriate for long-term periodic therapy.
  b. Physician places catheter in subclavian vein and threads tip into the superior vena cava; may also be placed within hepatic vascular system (arterial port), peritoneal cavity, or epidural space.
  c. Indications: refer to nontunneled catheter indications.
  d. Contraindications.
    (1) Presence of known infection.
    (2) Inadequate body tissue to support the device.
    (3) Caregiver with severe emotional, psychiatric, or neurologic problems.
  e. Advantages.
    (1) Less impact on body image; apparatus not visible externally.
    (2) Less risk of dislodgement and infection.
    (3) Less interference with daily activities.
    (4) Decreased costs.
    (5) Fewer supplies needed and less frequent care needs.
  f. Disadvantages.
    (1) Discomfort associated with needle stick.
    (2) Expensive surgical fee for placement of port.
    (3) Minor surgical procedure required for removal.
  g. Equipment features.
    (1) Basic port design consists of a portal body, a central septum, a reservoir, and a catheter (see Figure 21-2).

(2) Self-sealing silicone septum in middle or side of portal body can withstand 1000 to 2000 needle punctures.
h. General uses.
(1) Venous access for blood withdrawal.
(2) IV solution infusion.
(3) Blood transfusions.
(4) Chemotherapy.
i. Nursing care.
(1) Follow agency protocol.
(2) Use only a noncoring needle to access port septum.
(3) Apply a dressing to stabilize the needle.
j. Troubleshooting (see Table 21-3).

V. Nutritional Support Enteral/Parenteral Therapy

A. Parenteral therapy: special considerations in children (Holden & Kelcey, 1997).
1. Body composition. Infants and children have limited energy reserves; therefore, they are particularly at risk for malnutrition.
2. Brain growth and injury. Rapidly growing brain extremely sensitive to periods of malnutrition as well as to metabolic insult; infant malnutrition is associated with intellectual impairment.
3. Nutritional requirements. Children's nutritional requirements vary with growth and increase during periods of nutritional stress.
4. Organ immaturity. Amino acid requirements differ in early infancy and deemed essential; excess administration of nutrients can lead to coma and brain damage.
5. Sepsis. Major concern for children and adults receiving parenteral nutrition.

B. Indications for parenteral therapy. Child unable to maintain nutritional status via the oral or enteral route due to gastrointestinal malabsorption, dysfunction, or hypermetabolic demands.

C. Assessment.
1. Nutritional assessment to determine degree of malnutrition and recommended daily intake of calories and protein.
a. Anthropometric. Weight, length/height, head circumference, growth percentiles.
b. Laboratory. Hemoglobin, hematocrit, albumin, total protein, total lymphocyte count, blood urea nitrogen.
c. Dietary. Typical intake pattern including vitamin and mineral supplement use (food history).
2. Ongoing assessment of growth parameters rec-

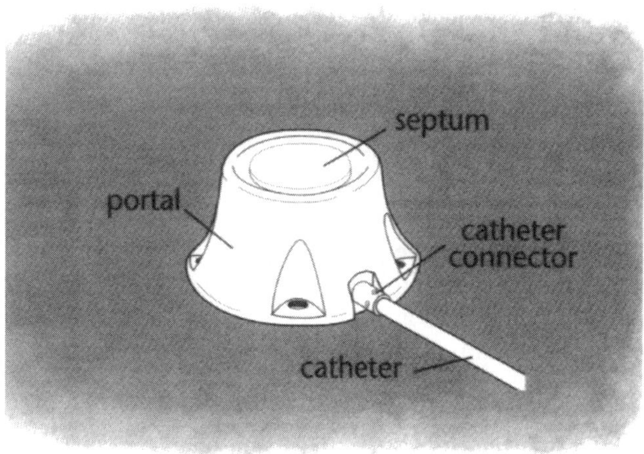

Figure 21-2
PORT-A-CATHETER® implantable venous access system.
Used with permission from SIMS Deltec, Inc., St. Paul, MN

ommended to determine whether calorie provision is adequate; energy needs may increase or decrease as clinical status changes.

D. Nutritional requirements.
1. Caloric requirement. *See Tables 13-1, 13-2, and 13-3 from Chapter 13: Acute Illness: Care Technologies.*
2. Calories are derived from dextrose and lipid (fat) sources; protein is derived from amino acids.
a. 1 g of dextrose = 4 cal.
b. 1 g of lipids = 9 cal.
c. Lipids 10% 500 cc = 550 cal.
d. Lipids 20% 1000 cc = 1000 cal.
e. Avoid lipid doses greater than 3g/kg/day.
3. Lipids are used in pediatric parenteral support as an additional source of calories and to prevent essential fatty acid deficiency.
4. Protein requirements to promote growth.
a. Term infants: 2.5 to 3.0 g/kg/day.
b. Older children: 1 to 2 g/kg/day (may increase or decrease on basis of clinical status of patient).

E. Fluid requirements.
1. Requirements increase in presence of respiratory distress, elevated body temperature, diuretic therapy, diarrhea, intravenous alimentation, fistulas/stomas.
2. TPN formulations may be concentrated to decrease fluid volume.
3. *Also see Chapter 13: Acute Illness: Care Technologies.*

F. Peripheral parenteral nutrition (PPN).
1. Provides partial or total nutrition for patients

who are unable to ingest adequate calories enterally or orally, or when central-vein parenteral nutrition is not feasible.

2. Can only provide short-term nutritional support (up to 2 weeks) due to limited peripheral vein access.
3. Nutritional replacement or aggressive nutritional support may be possible via PPN in older infants and children, but not those requiring fluid restriction.
4. Maximum dextrose concentration of infusion is 12%.

G. Central parenteral nutrition.
1. Can provide nutrients at greater concentrations and smaller fluid volumes than is possible with PPN.
2. Indications.
   a. Enteral support not tolerated.
   b. Limited peripheral access.
   c. Parenteral support is required for longer than 2 weeks.
   d. Nutrient needs not met by PPN.
   e. Fluid restriction is required.
3. Cyclic administration (8 to 16 hours/day, most of infusion at night) preferred over continuous infusion.

H. Nursing care of child receiving parenteral therapy.
1. Initiation of home TPN should be under close nursing supervision.
   a. Nurse must be present for initial hookup, first several hours of infusion, and disconnection.
   b. Monitor for hyperglycemia (>250 mg/dl) via home glucose monitor — every 6 hours at initiation of TPN, q.d. thereafter or as ordered.
2. Lipids may be piggy-packed into the TPN Y-site, past the filter.
3. Daily weights as ordered.
4. Laboratory testing (chemistry and hematology). Twice a week initially; decrease frequency as patient becomes stable on TPN.
5. Long-term TPN recipients require blood sampling for vitamin and trace element levels drawn every 6 months with periodic monitoring of liver function tests.
6. Monitor for metabolic bone disease (bone pain, decrease in bone density).
7. Assess tolerance and quantity of oral intake, if applicable.

I. Child/family teaching.
1. Instruct child/caregiver in injecting vitamins and/or insulin daily into TPN as ordered.
2. Instruct child/caregiver to keep TPN refrigerat-

ed and to remove at least 2 hours before administering; do not allow TPN to hang at room temperature for more than 24 hours.
3. Teach child/caregiver how to handle potential complications.

J. Potential complications.
1. Mechanical or technical. Involving catheters, pumps, and other apparatus for administration.
2. Infectious. Complicated by underlying health condition, risk of sepsis with parenteral nutrition.
3. Metabolic. Fluid, electrolyte, acid-base, and organ dysfunction.
4. Nutritional. Deficiency and/or excess of nutrients, electrolytes, minerals, vitamins, and trace elements.

K. Prevention of complications or adverse effects.
1. Strict aseptic care and maintenance of access site (catheter).
2. Proper preparation and storage of solutions.
3. Proper administration of parenteral nutrition.
4. Routine laboratory monitoring according to patient's individual status.

VI. ENTERAL NUTRITION

A. General information. *Also see Chapter 13: Acute Illness: Care Technologies.*
1. Appropriate for short-term or long-term therapy.
2. Preferred method of nutritional support when gastrointestinal tract can be used.

B. Advantages over parenteral therapy.
1. Maintains structure and function of gastrointestinal tract.
2. Decreased potential for bacterial translocation.
3. Enhanced use of nutrients.
4. Greater ease and safety of use.
5. Fewer hepatobiliary complications than associated with TPN.
6. Lower cost.

C. Indications.
1. Suck-swallow difficulties.
2. Esophageal abnormalities.
3. Hypermetabolism.
4. Failure to thrive.
5. Cystic fibrosis.
6. Renal disease.
7. Congenital heart disease.
8. Crohn's disease.
9. Short-bowel syndrome.
10. Chronic liver disease.

Table 21-4
Advantages and Disadvantages of the Button-Replacement Gastrostomy Device

Advantages	Disadvantages
Cosmetic: small, skin level device.	Small, easily lost parts.
Less obtrusive than a catheter and is well concealed under clothing	Feeding, giving medications, or venting requires an additional step not required with catheter tubes.
Durable: lasts 8-12 months or longer	Feeding extension setup or decompression tube must be attached to administer feeding.
Minimal site leakage.	Small internal diameter of venting or decompression.
Biocompatible (less irritation).	Limited sizes (18, 24, 28, Fr).
Decreased migration.	Requires MD placement for most patients.
Increased comfort between feedings.	Stomach tube limits expulsion of gas and emesis.

Adapted from Steele, N.F. (1991). The button: Replacement gastrostomy device. *Journal of Pediatric Nursing, 6*(6), 421–424.

D. Contraindications.
1. Peritonitis.
2. Intestinal obstruction or ileus that prohibits use of bowel.
3. Intractable vomiting and diarrhea.
4. Fistula.
5. Severe gastroesophageal reflux.

E. Types of enteral access devices.
1. Device selection depends on the anticipated duration of feeding, condition of the gastrointestinal tract, and potential for aspiration.
2. Orogastric rarely used and least safe at home.
3. Nasogastric (NG).
   a. Traditionally relied on for intermittent or short-term feeding, but now gaining acceptance for long-term use.
   b. Maximal patient comfort and acceptance due to tube texture and diameter.
   c. Easy insertion and reinsertion.
   d. Smaller tube lumen produces less discomfort and slower infusion of formula.
4. Gastrostomy tubes (G-tube).
   a. Long-term enteral access device.
   b. If gastroesophageal reflux is present, surgical placement of G-tube is performed with an antireflux procedure (Nissen fundoplication).
   c. If antireflux procedure has been performed, capacity of stomach has been altered.
   d. Malecot.
      (1) Tube has a basket-type end for securing placement.
      (2) Used as initial feeding tube after surgery when opened. Placement procedure performed (abdominal midline surgical incision).
   d. Foley.
      (1) Internal anchoring balloon has antimigration disk that prevents tube from moving inward and causing outlet obstruction.
      (2) Secures tube without need for tape.
   e. MIC (Medical Innovations Corporation).
      (1) Shorter, more aesthetically appealing.
      (2) Internal balloon and external anchoring device.
   f. PEG tube: Gastrostomy tube placed percutaneously via endoscopy rather than surgical placement.
   g. Skin surface devices (commonly referred to as gastrostomy "buttons").
      (1) Malecot-type button: requires an obturator for placement.
      (2) Balloon-type button.
      (3) Advantages and disadvantages (see Table 21-4).
5. Jejunal feeding tubes.
   a. Long-term nutritional support required (e.g., condition where medical management is not working and surgical intervention not possible.
   b. Placement.
      (1) Nasojejunal (NJ): placement through the nose.
      (2) Gastrojejunal (GJ): placement through an existing gastrostomy stoma.

(3) Jejunal (J-tube): surgical creation of jejunostomy.

F. Nursing care of child with enteral feedings
 1. Continuous feeding.
   a. Better tolerated by children with compromised GI function, delayed gastric emptying, or when feeding directly into small bowel.
   b. Position child during feeding: sitting, head elevated, or right side lying.
   c. Flush feeding through pump tubing and then attach to enteral feeding device.
   d. Interrupt feeding every 4 hours to infuse water into the line to clear the tubing and hydrate the patient.
   e. Instill no more than 4 hours of formula into feeding bag to avoid spoilage.
   f. Periodically check for residual.
 2. Bolus feeding.
   a. Positioning same as continuous.
   b. Height of prefilled feeding syringe affects the rate of of flow; observe infusion closely.
   c. Shorter delivery time, thereby has less impact on immobility and daily activities.
   d. Check for residual prior to initiation of next feeding.
   e. J-tube feedings seldomly given in bolus form due to risk of dumping syndrome.
 3. Oral-motor stimulation.
   a. Provides stimulation during real or simulated feeding.
   b. Allows infant to associate oral gratification and feelings of fullness with feeding.
   c. Promotes development of suck/swallow abilities.
 4. Safety concerns.
   a. Verify placement of tube by auscultation of air and/or aspiration of stomach contents; verification not required for jejunostomy feedings.
   b. Properly and brightly label all continuous feeding tubing and bags to distinguish from tubing of parenteral solutions to avoid potential for infusion of enteral formula parenterally.
   c. Secure tube to avoid dislodgement.
 5. Nursing care/care issues.
   a. Daily oral/nares care.
   b. Flush tube with water (2 to 5 cc/infant; 5 to 30 cc/child), both before and after giving each medication and immediately after completing a feeding.
   c. Dilute viscous medications with water prior to administration.
   d. Prevent aspiration of feeding.
     (1) Head of bed elevated during and after feeding.

(2) If gastric distention occurs, decrease flow rate.
   e. If diarrhea/dumping syndrome occurs.
     (1) Be certain formula and administration devices are not contaminated.
     (2) Alter flow rate, may need to move to slower continuous rate of flow via pump.
     (3) Request change in formula.
   f. If constipation occurs.
     (1) Increase water intake if not contraindicated.
     (2) Change formula as necessary.
     (3) Increase bulk in diet.
   g. If vomiting occurs.
     (1) Slow infusion rate.
     (2) Verify placement of tube.
     (3) Take aspiration precautions.
   h. Skin care around tube via agency protocol.
   i. Slight overgrowth of tissue and/or a small amount of fluid draining around feeding tube/button not uncommon

G. Troubleshooting.
 1. Clogged tube (Gebus, 1996).
   a. Changing tube (NG or G-tube) usually best option.
   b. Discuss methods for unclogging J-tube with physician.
   c. Use of carbonated beverages, cranberry juice, or fresh pineapple juice more effective than water.
 2. Skin breakdown: apply a stoma adhesive powder or a skin barrier.
 3. Skin overgrowth: overgrowth tissue causing excessive amounts of drainage or stomal erosion; apply silver nitrate as prescribed (Huddleston & Palmer, 1990).

H. Parental responses to feeding tubes (Micheals, Warzak, & VanRiper, 1992).
 1. Have difficulty in finding qualified babysitter who will tube feed child.
 2. Concerns regarding general public's ignorance about tube feeding.
 3. Social life revolves around child's tube feeding schedule.
 4. Sadness/depression regarding child's lack of participation in social activities that involve eating.
 5. Child's stools loose and messy.
 6. Burden of taking all feeding supplies along when traveling.
 7. Skin irritation around tube.
 8. Caring for child leaves little time for spouse/family/friends.

VII. EQUIPMENT FOR LONG-TERM/ HOME CARE

◆ ◆ ◆ ◆ ◆ ◆ ◆ ◆ ◆ ◆ ◆ ◆ ◆ ◆ ◆ ◆ ◆ ◆ ◆

A. Infusion pumps.
1. Guidelines for use of infusion pumps.
    a. Child/caregiver should:
        (1) Be provided written and verbal instructions regarding proper use of pump.
        (2) Be able to return demonstration prior to being allowed independence in performing the tasks.
        (3) Be able to effectively troubleshoot problems with the pump and be able to implement the established emergency medical plan.
        (4) Have 24-hour availability to the home infusion company and home care agency.
        (5) Be aware of battery capacity of pump.
    b. Nurse must document ongoing competency with the agency policy and equipment.
    c. Informed consent should be obtained prior to initiation of infusion pump.
    d. Blood and body fluid precautions must always be maintained.
2. Therapies using infusion pumps include:
    a. Enteral nutrition.
    b. Parenteral nutrition.
    c. Hydration.
        (1) Advanced dehydration requires intensive monitoring and care within an acute care setting.
        (2) Home nursing care.
            (a) Administer solution as ordered.
            (b) Assess urine output and need for electrolyte supplementation to IV solution.
            (c) Child's cardiac and renal status must be considered.
            (d) Instruct patient/family regarding signs/symptoms of dehydration and ongoing management plan.
            (e) Evaluation/ongoing monitoring.
                [1] Evaluate response to rehydration therapy.
                [2] Assess for reversal of dehydration.
                [3] Obtain laboratory tests as ordered.
                [4] If dehydration persists, evaluate efficacy of prescribed therapy & assess nutritional deficits.
                [5] Evaluate comfort level of family and home care agency in continuing hydration therapy at home.
    d. Antibiotics.
        (1) Document source of infection.
        (2) Document child's allergy history.
        (3) Assess adequacy of venous access or potential access site.
        (4) Administer drug according to prescribed treatment plan.
        (5) Instruct caregiver about:
            (a) Refrigeration of antibiotic-removal 1 hour prior to administration.
            (b) Drug side effects, adverse effects, and action if side effect/adverse effect occur.
            (c) Clarity of drug and particulate matter in drug.
            (d) Drug compatibilities/incompatibilities, photosensitivity, dilutional requirements.
        (6) Evaluation/monitoring.
            (a) Take evening temperatures daily; use consistent technique.
            (b) Note response to therapy (e.g., cessation of purulent drainage, afebrile) or presence of side/adverse effects.
    e. Pain management. *See Chapter 14: Acute Illness: Symptom Management.*
        (1) Use age-appropriate pain assessment tools.
        (2) Involve family in need for additional pain medication.
        (3) Provide home care pain management (see Table 21-5).
        (4) Review how to manage potential side effects with child/family.
        (5) Develop titration schedule and breakthrough pain management plan.
        (6) Consider patient-controlled analgesia pump (PCA).
        (7) Obtain order for narcotic antagonist; instruct family regarding indications for usage.
        (8) Evaluation/monitoring.
            (a) Evaluate patient's pain rating and compare to rating prior to administration of medication.
            (b) Evaluate patient/family competency in appropriately managing pain.
            (c) Assess child's/family's ability to appropriately use PCA (consider child's developmental level).
    f. Chemotherapy.
        (1) Prior to administration of chemotherapy, review patient's laboratory results (i.e., complete blood count) and overall treatment plan.
        (2) Explain potential side effects to patient and family; premedicate for symptom control as indicated (i.e., nausea and vomiting).

Table 21-5
Issues to Consider in Home Pain Management

- Thoroughly assess pain at every visit using assessment tool.

- Distinguish or define if this is a new pain or an increase in chronic pain.

- Assess what pain medications are in the home.

- Speak with physician regarding recommendations for pain medication and/or dosing schedule.

- Determine whether:
  - patient needs prescription refilled before the weekend
  - the patient's family has the money to buy the medication needed
  - the pharmacy stocks the prescription drug
  - the family has transportation resources available to pick up the prescription from the physician's office or pharmacy.

Adapted with permission from Bentzen, C. Magrum, L., & Weist, P. (1992, April). Unpublished observations. Source: Magrum, L.C., Bentzen, C., & Landmark, S. (1996). Pain management in home care. *Seminars in Oncology Nursing, 12*(3), 202–218.

Monitor responses to premedication and/or development of drug side effects.

(3) Prior to administration, venous access must be confirmed by obtaining blood return; instruct child/parent and observe for any signs of burning and pain during infusion.

(4) Antidote for chemotherapeutic agent should be accessible.

(5) Gown/apron, mask, latex gloves, and mask with face shield must be worn during administration.

(6) Reconfirm dosage of drug prior to administration.

(7) Dispose of all chemotherapy waste or spills in biohazardous container; home infusion company responsible for disposal.

(8) For accidental exposure: remove gloves and wash hands with soap and water; flood an exposed eye with water or isotonic eyewash for at least 5 minutes; seek medical evaluation as soon as possible; complete incident report.

(9) Each chemotherapy agent has a specific nadir; usually occurs 10 to 14 days after administration; susceptibility to infection is greatest during this time.

(10) Provide dietary consulting/interventions as needed.

(11) Instruct family to use care when handling vomitus or excreta for 48 hours after administration.

(12) Do follow-up within 24 to 48 hours after administration.

g. Blood components.

(1) Patients with myelosuppression and chronic blood loss are candidates for home infusion.

(2) Initial transfusion of blood products should be given in an acute care setting; if history of transfusion reactions, do not transfuse at home.

(3) Assess current health states (i.e., cardiac, renal, and hydration).

(4) Blood components appropriate for home transfusion: packed cells, platelets, immunoglobulins, coagulation factors.

(5) Recent laboratory results must be available prior to blood administration: complete blood count, platelets, coagulation studies, type and crossmatch.

(6) Informed consent must be obtained prior to administration of blood products.

(7) Family member must be present with RN during transfusion and must be available for 24 hours after transfusion.

(8) Follow blood bank and agency procedures for identification and transport of ordered blood components.

(9) Instruct family regarding signs/symptoms of reaction; blood transfusion reaction kit to be available.

(10) Follow agency protocol regarding patient and blood identification, timing of vital signs, specific observations, documentation, and follow-up lab work.

(11) Dispose of blood containers, tubing, etc. in biohazardous containers.

B. Blood glucose monitoring.
1. Indications.
    a. Diabetes mellitus.
    b. Patients at risk for hyper/hypoglycemia due to underlying illness or risks from infusion therapy (i.e., TPN).
2. Advantages.
    a. Provides immediate data to detect hypoglycemia or hyperglycemia.
    b. Data provides ability to evaluate effectiveness of therapeutic regimen.
3. Disadvantages.
    a. Cost, particularly if insurance reimbursement not available.
    b. Complexity of maintaining equipment accuracy.
    c. Possible malfunction of the meter.
    d. Discomfort when finger improperly lanced.
4. Equipment features and general uses.
    a. Machines require batteries and use test strips designed for each device.
    b. Validation of equipment accuracy must be done periodically.
5. Nursing care.
    a. If results of test are in question, nurse should observe the child/caregiver performing the test.
    b. Instruct the patient/caregiver to record all readings and to report abnormal results to the health care provider immediately.
6. Safety considerations.
    a. Store the meter and lancets in a safe place.
    b. If symptoms indicate that blood sugar is high and reading on the device is low, assess proper function of the meter and then repeat the test. If results are still low, verify glucose levels by laboratory blood test.
7. Infection control.
    a. Child should wash hands prior to finger stick.
    b. Discard sharps used to obtain specimen in a sharps container.
    c. Discard all materials contaminated with blood in appropriate containers.
8. Documentation.
    a. Child/caregiver should document all blood glucose results, insulin dosage, and any clinical symptoms in a patient log.
    b. All log entries should be reviewed regularly with the child and health care provider.
    c. Child/caregiver competency in use of the device should be documented.

C. Apnea monitoring.
1. Apnea: cessation of respiratory air flow.
    a. Causes of respiratory pauses may be central or diaphragmatic (i.e., no respiratory effort), obstructive, or mixed (National Institute of Health Consensus Development Conference Statement, 1986).
    b. Respiratory pauses of 15 seconds or longer are cause for concern in infants due to higher oxygen consumption needs, smaller lung volume, and lower oxygen stores than adults (Whitaker, 1995).
    c. Apparent life-threatening event (ALTE).
        (1) Characterized by apnea, cyanosis, altered muscle tone, choking, or gagging.
        (2) Cause may be multifactorial or may never be identified.
        (3) When cause cannot be identified, the infant may be at increased risk for for dying of SIDS (Steinschneider, Weinstein, & Diamond, 1982).
2. Home apnea monitoring: use of apnea monitoring equipment to detect apnea events.
    a. If monitor detects a symptom of possible apnea event, alarm alerts the caregiver.
    b. False alarms may occur; check equipment.
3. Indications for use of home apnea monitoring.
    a. A survivor of ALTE.
    b. A newborn in a family with previous SIDS. infants.
    c. Premature infant with symptoms of idiopathic apnea otherwise ready for hospital discharge.
    d. Child with a tracheostomy.
    e. Child with a sleep apnea syndrome caused by a neurologic disorder, periodic breathing, upper airway abnormality, or idiopathic syndromes (Hanley, 1992).
4. Equipment and supplies.
    a. Monitor, lead wires (two sets minimum), disposable patches (four sets minimum), belt and permanent electrodes (optional), monitor manual with troubleshooting guide, and battery pack (optional).
    b. Monitor plugged directly into grounded outlet.
    c. Keep monitor out of the reach of children.
    d. Monitor alarms should be heard throughout the home; if they cannot, an inexpensive intercom system is recommended.
    e. Keep monitor 3–4 feet away from sources of electrical interference, such as radios, remote telephones, and television sets. Signals may interfere with monitor's ability to detect apneic episode.
    f. Monitor should be placed on a hard surface with 8″ of ventilating space above or behind it.
    g. Periodically verify proper functioning of monitor by performing self-test according to manufacturer's directions.
5. Nursing care.

a Electrode placement.
  (1) Place symmetrically.
  (2) Replace every 2 days to ensure adequate monitoring to prevent skin breakdown.
  (3) An electrode belt should not be used until the infant weighs more than 8–10 lbs.
  (4) Proper skin care to prevent skin breakdown and infection.
b. Teach caregiver responses to alarms.
  (1) Apnea alarm: observe and feel the infant for respiratory movement.
    (a) If respiratory movement not noted, or infant appears lethargic, stimulate breathing by calling loudly, then touch the baby.
    (b) If no response, proceed with bag-mask ventilation and CPR if necessary. Notify emergency services (i.e., call 911).
  (2) Bradycardia alarm: stimulating infant may be sufficient; if alarm continues or infant is pale, cyanotic and/or lethargic:
    (a) Stimulate infant.
    (b) Verify a clear and patent airway, suctioning airway as necessary.
    (c) Initiate oxygen therapy, or if infant is already receiving oxygen, increase flow.
    (d) Increase stimulation from gentle to vigorous.
    (e) If response remains absent, initiate CPR, using bag-mask ventilation.
    (f) Notify emergency services (i.e., call 911).
  (3) Loose-lead or machine alarms: continuous alarm many indicate a loose electrode patch or belt, dirty electrode, or detachment/malfunction of wires from the electrode or cable.
c. Documentation: maintain cardiorespiratory event log.
6. Safety considerations.
a. Caregivers and babysitters must be knowledgeable about equipment use and care of child.
b. No one should sleep in the same bed with monitored infant due to the risk that the cables might become disconnected or choke the infant.
c. Electric company and community emergency services must be notified regarding the presence of the infant requiring home apnea monitoring.
d. Prior to leaving the hospital, all caregivers must be trained in infant CPR.

D. Pulse oximetry.
1. Indications: children with:
  a. Oxygen-dependency.
  b. Tracheostomies.
  c. Congenital heart disease.
  d. Disorders of airway, chest wall, and spine.
  e. Chronic lung disease.
  f. Neuromuscular disorders with subsequent abnormalities in breathing.
2. Equipment features.
  a. Pulse oximetry evidences oxygen availability or delivery to vital organs.
  b. Oximetry reading is assessed by placing a oximeter probe-detector on the fingertip or toe and attaching it securely.
    (1) Refer to manufacturer's recommendations regarding proper application of oximeter probe.
    (2) At least two additional probes should be available in home.
3. Nursing care.
  a. Periodically rotate the site of application of the probe.
  b. Assess and document integrity of skin prior to and after application.
  c. Review alarm limits periodically; after turning off monitor the limits need to be reset.
  d. Child/family teaching.
    (1) Teach child/family how to troubleshoot false alarms/malfunction and assess accuracy of O_2 saturation value.
    (2) Remove oximeter probe prior to bathing patient.
    (3) Administer oxygen as prescribed for desaturations. Document desaturation value, action taken, and patient response.

E. Home peak expiratory flow rate monitoring (PEFR).
1. Recommended for many patients with asthma to assist in:
  a. Assessment of severity of asthma.
  b. Determine when emergency medical care is needed.
  c. Recognize diurnal variations of PEFR (Li, 1995).
2. Advantages of home use of PEFR.
  a. Closer monitoring so child often experiences fewer: symptoms, days absent from school, emergency room visits, hospitalizations, and associated fatalities.
  b. Generally inexpensive ($23 to $45) and durable enough to last a year or more.
3. Disadvantage: when measured by a peak flow meter, the PEFR depends on patient effort and the strength of expiratory muscles.
4. Nursing care.
  a. Evaluate subjective data regarding impact of

disease on child's/family's normal daily activities.

  b. Child/family teaching.

    (1) Review proper peak flow technique.

    (2) Review management plan when patient's peak flow results are: 80–100% of personal best, 60–80% of personal best, <60% of personal best.

  c. Direct child/family to establish and maintain a peak flow diary.

  d. Patients with chronic, stable, and generally well-controlled asthma should monitor PEFR twice daily, or two or three times weekly.

F. Home continuous peritoneal dialysis (CPD).

  1. Indications: end-stage renal failure and children awaiting transplantation.

  2. Contraindications.

    a. Absence of an adequate or intact peritoneal cavity.

    b. Excessive intraabdominal adhesions may prevent successful peritoneal dialysis in some patients.

    c. Presence of ventriculoperitoneal shunt in hydrocephalic children.

  3. Equipment features and general uses.

    a. Permanent catheters (i.e., Tenckhoff – straight or curled); material: Silastic rubber with Dacron "cuff," which is used to fix the catheter into the subcutaneous tissue.

    b. Automated cyclers.

      (1) Computerized machine that provides dialysis exchanges with volumes as small as 100 cc.

      (2) Preferable schedule dialysis during evening and nighttime hours to minimize disruption of child's daily activities.

    c. Dialysate: must always be warmed to body temperature before it is instilled into peritoneal cavity.

      (1) Cool dialysate in an infant can rapidly lower core body temperature and result in an acute hypotensive episode.

      (2) Cycler machine has warming unit that warms fresh dialysate.

  4. Nursing care.

    a. Assessment: complete physical examination including daily weights, vital signs, and hydration status.

    b. Review intake and outtake log and cycler's historical data.

    c. Initiate connection to cycler via manufacturer's recommendations; sterile technique is essential.

      (1) Monitor exchange outcome of cycle; standard goal is 80% of input.

      (2) Observe and document characteristics of effluent: color, presence of fibrin, blood, or fecal material (rare).

      (3) Observe ease of inflow and outflow of dialysate.

      (4) Child must always be weighed at the end of the drain cycle.

    d. Dressing.

      (1) Follow agency policy regarding peritoneal catheter dressing change.

      (2) Assess for signs/symptoms of infection at exit site.

    e. Ongoing psychosocial assessment and support to patient/family.

  5. Child/family teaching: prior to hospital discharge patient/family demonstrates knowledge in:

    a. Initiating/discontinuing dialysis.

    b. Tenckhoff catheter care.

    c. Troubleshooting malfunctions/alarms from cycler.

    d. Identifying signs of hypo/hypervolemia, peritonitis, and dietary and infection control issues.

  6. Complications of CPD.

    a. Peritonitis.

      (1) Assess for:

        (a) Appearance of peritoneal dialysis effluent-cloudy/discolored.

        (b) Febrile child.

        (c) Complaints of abdominal pain and tenderness.

      (2) Intervention.

        (a) Notify health care provider to discuss plan.

        (b) Use sterile technique to obtain complete blood count with differential.

        (c) Culture effluent specimens.

        (d) Intraperitoneal antibiotic therapy is begun and continued for 7–10 days (may require hospitalization).

      (3) Prevention.

        (a) Consistent use of hand-washing and sterile technique when connecting or disconnecting cycler tubing and during dressing changes.

        (b) Minimize interruptions into cycler tubing.

    b. Fluid and electrolyte abnormalities.

      (1) Hypovolemia: can occur due too aggressive ultrafiltration and is most often seen with prolonged use of 4.25% solution.

        (a) Observe signs of advancing dehydration, monitor exchange balance and tube potency of cycler, review of intake and output, daily weights, complete physical exam and vital signs.

(b) Identify underlying etiology of dehydration (e.g., diarrhea, 4.25% dialysate used).

(c) Interventions: notify physician, notify emergency services if medically unstable, adjust dialysis regimen as ordered.

(d) Prevention: monitor amount of fluid removed with each exchange, frequent weighing, and frequent physical assessment.

(2) Hypervolemia: results from inadequate ultrafiltration. Most commonly result of mechanical factors interfering with complete drainage of the peritoneal cavity. Usually self-corrected with large drain volume with next exchange.

(a) Assessment: advancing signs of fluid overload, review exchange balance on cycler, review intake and output, daily weights, complete physical exam and vital signs, identify underlying etiology of fluid retention (e.g., mechanical problems with catheter, patient absorbing dialysate due to prolonged dwell times).

(b) Intervention: same as for hypovolemia.

(c) Prevention: same as for hypovolemia, and monitor patency of cycler tubing.

(3) Hyponatremia: inadequate dietary intake to replace peritoneal sodium losses caused by ultrafiltration.

(4) Hypernatremia: rarely a direct consequence of peritoneal dialysis; can occur due to frequent exchanges.

c. Hyperglycemia: frequently seen during first few days of dialysis when rapid exchange rates and high dialysate dextrose concentrations combine to deliver large amounts of dextrose to the infant/child.

d. Hypoproteinemia: commonly seen in patients on prolonged peritoneal dialysis; caused by the steady loss of protein into the dialysate.

e. Hypophosphatemia: phosphate removal by peritoneal dialysis is relatively inefficient, (late complication); temporary discontinuation of antacids may be sufficient enough to correct mild hypophosphatemia; little supplementation needed to correct levels.

7. Complications.

a. Dialysate leakage: reflux of small amounts of hypertonic dialysate into the subcutaneous tissue around the catheter tunnel.

(1) Can result in large accumulations of subcutaneous fluid being drawn into the hypertonic dialysate by osmosis; notify physician if observed.

(2) Small leaks may seal within a few days if dialysis can be suspended for 24 hours and then large leaks necessitate catheter revision.

b. Catheter exit site infection: minor irritation at catheter exit site may lead to local cellulitis; notify physician for further orders and plan.

c. Poor catheter drainage.

(1) If fluid flows freely into the peritoneal cavity but drains slowly or not at all, catheter probably wrapped in omentum.

(2) Tip of long catheters in infants can migrate against the posterior wall of the peritoneum; observe for presence of fibrin clots.

(3) Intervention: notify physician; surgical revision is often indicated.

d. Painful dialysis: optimal dialysis is painless.

(1) Pain noted during inflow (may result from dialysate hitting same point in peritoneum – slow rate of infusion.

(2) Cramping pain during dwell cycle (may be due to intolerance to acid pH or temperature of the dialysate) – warm dialysate.

(3) Pain occurring near end of a drain cycle (probably due to peritoneal tissues being drawn into the catheter) – should resolve spontaneously with next infusion.

(4) Shoulder pain when sitting up (probably caused by diaphragmatic irritation probably due to air entering peritoneal cavity) – purge air from tubing; eventually will resolve. Notify physician if shoulder pain persists or changes characteristics.

(5) Abdominal pain. Painful dialysis may be first sign of peritonitis.

e. Bloody peritoneal fluid.

(1) Usually result of coagulopathies or minor trauma to peritoneal membrane.

(2) May be seen in menstruating females.

(3) Rarely due to intraperitoneal hemorrhage.

(4) Notify physician and/or seek emergency medical assistance.

f. Respiratory compromise: patients with underlying respiratory compromise may experience further compromise as exchange volume elevates the diaphragm.

(1) Intervention: notify physician.

(2) Decrease infusion volume and increase cycling frequency.

(3) Evaluate patient for changes in respiratory status.

G. Long-term home care-respiratory therapies.

1. Indications: infant and children with disorders of:
   a. Airway and/or respiratory control.
   b. Neuromuscular system with subsequent abnormalities in breathing.
   c. Structural/functional disorders of chest, heart, longs, spine.
2. Types of equipment. *See Chapter 13: Acute Illness: Care Technologies.*
   a. Oxygen systems: wide variety available, liquid and gaseous.
      (1) Oxygen concentrator: an electrical device, separates oxygen from room air concentrates oxygen, and delivers more concentrated oxygen to the child.
         (a) Delivers O_2 up to 5L/min.
         (b) Cost-effective, but bulky to use.
      (2) Liquid oxygen: compressed into a cold liquid form and maintained under pressure.
         (a) Can be used with nasal cannula, tracheotomy collar, or ventilator.
         (b) Cannot be used with Venturi mask or medication nebulizer.
         (c) Cost-effective, light weight.
      (3) Cylinder oxygen: wide variety of sizes.
         (a) Most cost-effective.
         (b) Some types portable but bulky.
         (c) Can be used with most delivery mechanisms.
   b. Humidification devices: jet nebulizer, cascade, bubbler, or other heated system. Jet nebulizers may stimulate hyperactive airways.
   c. Suction equipment: battery or electric.
   d. Oxygen delivery methods.
      (1) Tracheostomy collar preferred O_2 delivery source for children with tracheostomy.
      (2) Oxygen mask: bulky, restrictive, and generally inappropriate for use with infants.
      (3) Venturi mask.
      (4) Nasal cannula least restrictive delivery mode.
      (5) Oxygen tent: sometimes used with infants, most circumstances less desirable than nasal cannula because it restricts visual and auditory environments so drastically.
      (6) Ventilator.
         (a) Requires backup power source when used in home or school.
         (b) Oxygen will bleed directly into line if room air not sufficient for child.
   e. Ventilators: home models less complicated than in acute setting, portable due to external battery capabilities. *Also see Chapter 13: Acute Illness: Care Technologies.*
      (1) Types.
         (a) Portable volume-cycled ventilator.
            [1] Provides intermittent positive pressure ventilation via tracheostomy (IPPV).
            [2] Major disadvantages: associated with barotrauma pneumothorax atelectasis and problems with tracheostomies (e.g., infection, bleeding, aspirations, difficulties with communication).
         (b) Pressure ventilator: used primarily in acute care setting, occasionally in home care.
      (2) Choice of mechanical support depends upon several factors (Jerome-Ebel, 1996).
         (a) Child's underlying disease process.
         (b) Mode of ventilation/assistance required.
         (c) Need for positive end-expiratory pressure.
         (d) Need for oxygen.
         (e) Device capabilities, including ease of operation, portability, reliability, and functioning alarm system.
         (f) Community support and resources.
      (3) Advantages of home ventilation (Ferns, 1994).
         (a) Extended life.
         (b) Enhanced quality of life.
         (c) Environment that will enhance individual potential.
         (d) Reduced morbidity/mortality.
         (e) Improved physiologic function.
         (f) Cost-effectiveness.
      (4) Disadvantages of home ventilation (Fern, 1994).
         (a) Client safety (risk of accidental disconnection).
         (b) 24-hour family accountability to caring for patient.
         (c) Home alteration for equipment.
         (d) Equipment malfunctions.
         (e) Family's lifestyle changes.
         (f) Family's fear of inadequacy and lack of external supports.
         (g) Family difficulty in adjusting to "strangers" present in home providing care to child.
      (5) BiPAP (Bilevel Positive Airway Pressure).
         (a) Provides pressurized air to the infant/child.
         (b) Given via face/nose mask or a tracheostomy tube.
3. Nursing care.
   a. Perform pulmonary assessment.
   b. Observe for signs of respiratory distress.

c. Assess quality of secretions.

d. Complete child/family psychosocial assessment.

e. Assess proper functioning of supportive and monitoring equipment.

f. Assess home environment (i.e., accessibility, safety, and comfort).

4. Management of child receiving oxygen therapy.

a. Discuss with caregiver any deviation from the child's normal patterns; if indicated, contact physician.

b. Determine frequency, duration, and use of treatment modality.

c. Assess reliability of monitors and equipment.

d. Patient teaching.

  (1) Review caregiver's assessment skill.

  (2) Assess caregiver's knowledge regarding oxygen delivery system (i.e., assess functioning, troubleshooting).

  (3) Review patient/caregiver's understanding regarding the management plan .

  (4) Reinforce knowledge deficit areas and emphasize strengths.

  (5) Observe caregiver's participation in care and proper use of equipment.

  (6) Review emergency procedures and safety considerations.

e. Identify alternative caregiver trained to give oxygen therapy.

5. Management of child requiring mechanical ventilation. *See Chapter 13: Acute Illness: Care Technologies.*

a. Observe and teach caregivers to observe for (Jerome-Abel, 1996).

  (1) Chest wall moves with ventilator breath.

  (2) Low-pressure alarm goes off with tubing disconnection.

  (3) Dial demonstrates cycling with each ventilator breath.

  (4) Dial returns to zero or recommended PEEP setting.

  (5) High-pressure alarm goes off with circuit occlusion or lack of patent airway (e.g., excessive secretions) or airway resistance (e.g., patient cough).

  (6) Circuit temperature is at recommended range.

  (7) Exhaled volumes, using respirometer, are within recommended range.

  (8) Oxygen saturations values are appropriate.

  (9) Oxygen input is accurate.

b. Any detection of discrepancies from prescribed management plan should be reviewed with the child/caregivers, and as appropriate, with physician or respiratory therapist.

c. Tracheostomy care: follow care plan and agency policy.

d. Administer chest physiotherapy and postural drainage as ordered.

e. Promote participation in developmental activities as able.

f. Provide means of communication (i.e., communication board, deflation of cuff, sign language, or computers with voice synthesizers).

6. Safety considerations.

a. Oxygen safety precautions.

  (1) Post "no smoking" signs at entry to house and appropriate rooms.

  (2) Teach family normal precautions for presence of oxygen.

    (a) Avoid use of alcohol, petroleum jelly (Vaseline) or other petroleum-based products, and aerosols.

    (b) Keep oxygen in a well-ventilated area at all times.

  (3) If using an oxygen concentrator, do not use an extension cord, and do not plug into outlets being used for other appliances.

  (4) If oxygen concentrator is used, an audible alarm will alert caregiver regarding power failure; a backup oxygen source must be available.

b. CPR guidelines and emergency telephone numbers should be posted near the patient's bed for easy reference. All caregivers should be knowledgeable about CPR.

c. Notify telephone company, electric company, and local emergency services of the presence of an oxygen- or ventilatory-dependent child in the community.

BIBLIOGRAPHY

◆ ◆ ◆ ◆ ◆ ◆ ◆ ◆ ◆ ◆ ◆ ◆ ◆ ◆ ◆ ◆ ◆

Birmingham, J., & Jeffries, C. (1993). Home medical equipment. In K.J. Morgan & S.L. McClain (Eds.), *Core curriculum for home health care nursing* (pp. 60–76). Gaithersburg, MD: Aspen.

Camp-Sorrell, D. (1990). Advanced central venous access: Selection, catheter devices and nursing management. *Journal of IV Nursing, 13*(6), 361–369.

Camp-Sorrell, D. (1992). Implantable ports: Everything you always wanted to know. *Journal of Intravenous Nursing, 15*(5), 262–273.

Carter, P., Engelking, C.H., Fiscus, J.A., Harvey, C., Hayes, N., Rostad, M., Vincent, B., Whedon, M. (1989). *Access device guidelines: Module I (pp. 2–3) and Module II (pp. 3–4).* Pittsburgh: Oncology Nursing Society.

Farrar-Simpson, M. (1996). Home care of the infant on a cardiorespiratory monitor. In E. Ahmann (Ed.), *Home care for the high risk neonate* (2nd ed., pp. 135–144). Gaithersburg, MD: Aspen.

Fern, T. (1994). Home mechanical ventilation in a changing health service. *Nursing Times, 90*(40), 43–45.

Free, F., & Hennessey, K. (1993). Enteral/parenteral therapy. In K.L. Morgan & S.L. McClain (Eds.), *Core curriculum for home health care nursing* (pp. 270–288). Gaithersburg, MD: Aspen.

Fry, B. (1992). Intermittent flushing protocols: A standardization issue. *Journal of Intravenous Nursing, 15*(3), 160–163.

Gebus, V.C. (1996). Home care of the infant or child requiring tube feeding. In E. Ahmann (Ed.), *Home care for the high risk neonate* (2nd ed., pp. 135–144). Gaithersburg, MD: Aspen.

Gropper, E. (1992). Promoting health by promoting comfort. *Nursing Forum, 27,* 5–8.

Hanley, R. (1992). Mechanisms and management of central sleep apnea. *Lung, 170,* 1017.

Holden, C., & Kelcey, H. (1997). Fluid systems…parenteral nutrition…pediatric patients. *Nursing Times, 93*(8), 61–62, 64.

Huddleston, K.C., & Ferraro, A.R. (1991). Preparing families with children with gastrostomies. *Pediatric Nursing, 17*(2), 153–158.

Huth, M.M., & O'Brien, M.E. (1987). The gastrostomy feeding button. *Pediatric Nursing, 13,* 241–245.

Jerome-Ebel, A. (1996) Home care of the infant requiring mechanical ventilation. In E. Ahmann (Ed.), *Home care for the high risk neonate* (2nd ed., pp. 229–234). Gaithersburg, MD: Aspen.

Kerner, J.A. (1991). Parenteral nutrition. In A. Walker (Ed.) *Pediatric GI disease* (pp. 1645–1675). St. Louis: B.C. Decker.

Knoeppen, M.A., & Caspers, S.M. (1994). Problems identified with home infusion pumps. *Journal of Intravenous Nursing, 17*(3), 151–156.

Lerner, A., & Russi, T.M. (1986). Techniques of nutritional assessment and their application to patients receiving total parenteral nutrition. In E. Leventhal (Ed.), *Total parenteral nutrition: Indications, utilization, complications and pathophysiological considerations* (pp. 155–172). New York: Raven Press.

Li, J.T.C. (1995). Home peak expiratory flow rate monitoring in patients with asthma. *Mayo Clinic Proceedings, 70*(7), 649–656.

Magrum, L.C., Bentzen, C., & Landmark, S. (1996). Pain management in home care. *Seminars in Oncology Nursing, 12*(3), 202–218.

Micheals, C.A., Warzak, K. S., & Van Riper, C. (1992). Parenteral and professional perceptions of problems associated with long-term pediatric home tube feeding. *Journal of the American Diabetic Association, 92*(10), 1235–1238.

National Institutes of Health Consensus Development Conference Statement (1986). *Infantile apnea and home monitoring. 6*(6), 1–2.

Phillips, L.D. (1997). Complications of intravenous therapy. *Manual of I.V. therapeutics* (2nd ed.). Philadelphia: Davis.

Schlichtig, R., & Ayres, S.M. (1988). Modes of delivery, rationale, implementation, and mechanical complications. *Nutritional support of the critically ill* (pp. 143–168). Chicago: Year Book Medical Publishers.

Sheldon, P., & Bender, M. (1994). High technology in home care: An overview of intravenous therapy. *Nursing Clinics of North America, 29*(3), 507–519.

Steele, N.S. (1991). The button: Replacement gastrostomy device. *Journal of Pediatric Nursing, 6*(6), 421–424.

Steinschneider, A., Weinstein, S., & Diamond, E. (1982). The sudden infant death syndrome and apnea: Obstruction during neonatal sleep and feeding. *Pediatrics, 70,* 858–863.

Weinstein, S.M. (1996). Advanced vascular access. *Plumer's principles and practice of intravenous therapy* (6th ed., pp. 205–259). Philadelphia: Lippincott.

Whitaker, S. (1995). The art and science of home infant apnea monitoring in the 1990s. *Journal of Obstetric, Gynecologic, & Neonatal Nursing, 24*(1), 84–89.

STUDY QUESTIONS

1. When determining the appropriateness of home infusion therapy for a child, which of the factors should NOT influence the decision?
   a. Availability of competent caregiver
   b. Developmental considerations of the child
   c. Drug stability
   d. Patient diagnosed as terminally ill
   e. Availability of electrical backup system

2. Which of the following procedures is performed to monitor for infiltration of a peripheral venous access device?
   a. Avoid armboards due to their potential restriction of circulation.
   b. Elevate the extremity with the IV.
   c. Assess site frequently.
   d. If possible, attempt venous cannulation in flexor areas.
   e. Verify patency of catheter by observing for pain reaction during infusion.

3. All of the following are potential indications for enteral nutrition EXCEPT:
   a. congenital heart disease.
   b. cystic fibrosis.
   c. failure to thrive.
   d. nausea/vomiting associated with migraines.
   e. renal disease.

4. Gastrostomy tubes are placed only when a Nissen-Fundoplication has been performed.
   a. False
   b. True

5. What is the most common side effect of central total parenteral therapy?
   a. Anorexia
   b. Dehydration
   c. Hyperglycemia
   d. Syncope
   e. Tachycardia

6. What is the most appropriate response when an apnea alarm sounds?
   a. Assess infant for shallow breathing, call for help, and initiate bag-mask ventilation.
   b. Assess for respiratory movement, stimulate baby if no movement; if no response, proceed with bag-mask ventilation and initiate CPR if necessary.
   c. Call for help, wake up the family, and initiate bag-mask ventilation and CPR if necessary.
   d. Initiate CPR, wake up the family, and have family member call 911; call home care agency for assistance.
   e. Turn off the monitor and assess for a malfunctioning alarm, observe infant for apneic events.

7. What action(s) should the nurse take if a child expresses pain during dialysis?
   a. Increase rate of infusion.
   b. Appropriately warm dialysate.
   c. Completely purge air out of the tubing.
   d. Notify physician.
   e. b and c

8. How is proper ventilator function determined?
   a. Dial indicates cycles only with patient-initiated breaths.
   b. High pressure alarm goes off when patient coughs.
   c. Low-pressure alarm goes off with excessive patient secretions.
   d. Patient's chest moves with spontaneously initiated breaths.
   e. None of the above

9. Which of the following actions best promotes safe use of oxygen?
   a. Discouraging patient use of Vaseline and aerosol sprays
   b. Encouraging family members to smoke at least 10 feet away from the oxygen source
   c. Keeping oxygen tanks and patient's bed at least 3 feet away from radiator or heater
   d. Placing the patient's oxygen tank beneath the bed to avoid damage to the canister
   e. Storing backup oxygen supply in a warm, dry, enclosed space

10. You are making a home visit to a child receiving TPN via a nontunneled PICC line. Which one of these factors is MOST important?
    a. Assessing correct line placement does not require x-ray monitoring.
    b. Line replacement is relatively inexpensive.
    c. There is a high risk of line dislodgement.
    d. TPN is being administered during child's sleeping hours.
    e. The large lumen of the line allows the TPN solution to flow freely and rapidly.

ANSWERS

1.d 2.c 3.d 4.a 5.c 6.b 7.e 8.b 9.a 10.c

Chapter 22

Chronic Conditions: Symptom Management

Myra Martz Huth, MSN, RN
Maureen E. O'Brien, PhD, RN

Concept

◆◆◆◆◆◆◆◆◆◆◆◆◆◆◆◆◆◆◆◆◆◆◆◆◆◆

◆ Children with a chronic condition, disability, or special health need and their families

Objectives

◆◆◆◆◆◆◆◆◆◆◆◆◆◆◆◆◆◆◆◆◆◆◆◆◆◆

At the completion of this chapter, the reader will be able to:

◆ Discuss pharmacologic and nonpharmacologic interventions for the child experiencing chronic pain.

◆ Recognize energy conserving and enhancing nursing interventions.

◆ Describe developmentally appropriate teaching strategies for assisting a child with self-care management of chronic dyspnea.

◆ Formulate a plan of care for the child with constipation.

◆ Explain strategies to assist the child and family in achieving success in bowel and bladder training programs.

◆ Identify parameters of altered skin integrity and selected interventions to improve skin integrity.

Key Points

◆◆◆◆◆◆◆◆◆◆◆◆◆◆◆◆◆◆◆◆◆◆◆◆◆◆

◆ The child and parent should be taught to recognize and manage fatigue by alternating rest and activity periods and increasing exercise gradually.

◆ The goals of child/parent self-care management of dyspnea are to: adjust medication and treatments to symptoms of severity, use relaxation and/or breathing techniques, avoid precipitants, balance rest and activity, and initiate contact with the health care team.

◆ Treatment of chronic constipation involves a combination of pharmacologic, dietary, and behavioral interventions.

◆ The processes of bowel and bladder training are multifaceted developmental tasks requiring coordination of motor, cognitive, and language skills.

◆ The child/adolescent with altered skin integrity should undergo a complete integumentary assessment.

◆ Chronic pain must be managed proactively with the health care team, child, and family mutually planning goals and interventions.

22

Chronic Conditions: Symptom Management

◆◆◆◆◆◆◆◆◆◆◆◆◆◆◆◆◆◆◆◆◆◆◆◆◆◆◆◆◆◆◆◆◆◆◆

I. PAIN

◆◆◆◆◆◆◆◆◆◆◆◆◆◆◆◆◆◆

A. Overview.

1. Definition: chronic pain is pain that extends about a month beyond the usual course of an acute illness/ injury or a reasonable period of time for an injury to heal or the pain returns at different intervals for months or years.
2. Etiology. Chronic pain results from pathologic processes in somatic structures or viscera, prolonged dysfunction or injury to the peripheral and/or central nervous system, and psychologic and/or environmental factors.
3. Pathophysiology.
   a. Peripheral and/or central mechanisms.
      (1) Tissue damage inherent in disease or injury causes release of chemical substances (e.g., histamine and prostaglandins) that have excitatory and sensitization effects on nociceptors (a high-threshold nerve ending in skin).
      (2) Damaged nociceptors become sensitive to noradrenaline released from efferent sympathetic nervous system (SNS) neurons.
      (3) Loss of inhibition on nonpain fibers at the "gate" in the dorsal horn or loss of inhibition produced by the descending endogenous analgesic system will cause persistent pain.
   b. Psychologic and/or environmental mechanisms.
      (1) Emotional stress may produce skeletal muscle spasm, local vasoconstriction, visceral dysfunction, and release of endogenous chemical substances like histamine, which in turn sensitize peripheral nerve endings and sustain a circle of pain.
      (2) The child's initial injury provokes responses positively reinforced by someone significant to the child; chronic pain behavior continues while the consequences are favorable, even after the pain is gone.
4. Incidence.
   a. Common locations.

(1) Recurrent abdominal pain occurs in as many as 25% of school-age children.
(2) Headache ranges from 75% in adolescents to 2% in young children.
(3) Limb pain occurs in 10% of latency age children.
   b. Children with sickle cell disease have recurrent episodes of severe pain in multiple sites that include abdomen, chest, and extremities.
   c. Children and adolescents who have musculoskeletal disease, cystic fibrosis, or asthma may also have chest pain.
   d. Fifty percent of hospitalized children and adolescents with cancer experience pain at the time of assessment as a result of a tumor or from recurrent painful procedures.
5. Developmentally based considerations.
   a. Premature infants respond to noxious stimulation with both behavioral and physiologic signs of stress.
   b. Children's understanding and descriptions of pain become more complex and precise with increasing age, cognitive level, verbal ability, and pain experiences.
   c. Pain must be assessed and intervened at the child's developmental level.
   d. Chronic pain may result in poor school attendance and performance.
   e. Prompt intervention in children and adolescents may prevent adult chronic pain behavior and disability.

B. Assessment.

1. History and physical exam. *Also see Chapter 4: Health, Psychosocial, and Developmental Screening and Assessment.*
   a. A comprehensive pain history includes:
      (1) A complete assessment of pain.
      (2) Impact of pain on school, play, friends, family interactions, mood, and sleep.
      (3) The potential for secondary gain.
      (4) Cultural influences on the pain response.
      (5) The verbal child's concept of the cause of pain.

(6) Family history of chronic pain or disability.

(7) Effectiveness of past pain control measures.

(8) Coping strategies used for pain control and pain behaviors.

b. Children with chronic pain may have the following symptoms:

(1) Sleep dysfunction.

(2) Fatigue.

(3) Nausea.

(4) Dizziness.

(5) Bloating.

(6) Sore throat.

(7) Blurred vision.

(8) Apathy.

(9) Inability to concentrate.

2. Physiologic pain measures.

a. Physiologic signs may include tachycardia, elevated blood pressure, sweating, or involuntary muscle spasm when the painful area is touched; however, children may develop habituation of the sympathetic responses and remain physiologically stable for long periods of time.

b. Muscle atrophy, trigger points, or skin temperature changes indicate organic pathology underlying the child/adolescent's pain.

c. Decreased levels of serotonin and endorphins can cause a decrease in pain tolerance so that even minor injuries provoke major responses.

3. Self-report measures.

a. Since pain is a subjective phenomenon, self-report methods are considered the gold standard, but the age of the child and type of pain are factors to consider when choosing a measurement tool. *See Table 14-5: Self-Report Measures of Pain in Children in Chapter 14: Acute Illness: Symptom Management.*

b. Assess quality, location, and intensity of pain.

(1) Location of pain can be marked on a body outline or by asking the child to point to their hurt.

(2) Quality, location, and intensity of pain can be assessed by listening to the words the child uses to describe their pain, with a word list that is appropriate for children, with the Pediatric Pain Questionnaire (PPQ) or the Adolescent Pediatric Pain Tool (APPT).

c. Assess the onset and duration of pain.

4. Observational measures.

a. Preverbal children communicate pain through a cry (long, high-pitched, shrill, and tense) followed by breath holding, then a lower-pitched, more rhythmic cry in bursts.

b. Chronic pain behaviors include:

(1) Posturing.

(2) Restricted movement.

(3) Absence of developmentally appropriate behaviors.

(4) Depressed mood or inactivity.

(5) Difficulty sleeping.

c. Behavior observation tools, like the Children's Hospital of Eastern Ontario Pain Scale (CHEOPS) and the Procedure Behavior Rating Scale (PBRS) are used for assessing behavioral indicators of pain and anxiety and do not always correlate with self-report measures (Berde, Schechter, & Yaster, 1993).

C. Common therapeutic modalities.

1. Nonpharmacologic treatment.

a. Self-regulatory techniques include, but are not limited to, relaxation techniques, guided imagery, biofeedback, and self-hypnosis.

b. Cutaneous stimulation includes application of ice, heat, massage, and transcutaneous electrical nerve stimulation (TENS).

2. Pharmacologic treatment.

a. Nonopioid analgesics.

(1) Nonsteroidal antiinflammatory drugs (NSAIDs) are used for children with pain and inflammation and given as adjuvants to opioid analgesia.

(2) Acetaminophen for mild to moderate pain is the most common NSAID administered to infants and children.

(3) Aspirin is recommended specifically for arthritis (antiinflammatory effects) but not generally for pain management due to concern with Reye's syndrome in children with viral illness.

(4) Choline magnesium trisalicylate is a useful analgesic and antiinflammatory agent.

(5) Naproxen and tolmetin are approved for children 2 to 12 years, but ibuprofen is more commonly used.

b. Opioid analgesics (Berde et al., 1993)

(1) Slow-release morphine or long-acting methadone can be given for moderate to severe pain due to terminal cancer and sickle cell disease.

(2) Infants 3 months and under may have an increased sensitivity to respiratory depression and need monitoring.

(3) Addiction is rare in children and adolescents receiving narcotics for pain.

c. Adjunctive medications.

(1) Tricyclic antidepressants: given for pain of neuropathic origin; pain associated with significant sleep disturbance or with

mild vegetative signs of depression; and with severe, unremitting pain that has not responded to NSAIDs, TENS, or other measures.

    (2) Stimulants: given to counteract the sedation of narcotics, increase analgesia, and provide some euphoria.

    (3) Anticonvulsants: neuropathic pain appears to be connected with increased excitability of peripheral nerves.

3. Psychotherapeutic treatments
  a. Mild to moderate depression is common in children and adolescents with chronic pain.
  b. Disturbed family dynamics are common; thus, family therapy may help.

D. Nursing outcomes and interventions.

1. Outcomes. The child/adolescent and/or parent will:
  a. Report reduction of pain to a level of acceptable comfort.
  b. Report an increase in activity level.
  c. Use personal actions to control pain.
  d. Report decreased disruptive effects on emotions and behavior.

2. Nursing interventions.
  a. Perform a comprehensive pain history.
  b. Provide information about pain, the cause, duration, expected discomfort from procedures, and misconceptions regarding pain management.
  c. Instruct child/parents in use of a developmentally appropriate pain measurement tool.
  d. Instruct and encourage use of a home diary to monitor pain, activity, and mood.
  e. Encourage a gradual program of activity and exercise despite pain.
  f. With the health care team, select and implement developmentally appropriate nonpharmacologic and/or pharmacologic measures to prevent or alleviate pain; consider the type and source of pain and child's preference of coping styles and strategies when selecting strategies.
  g. Teach child/family nonpharmacologic (e.g., relaxation, guided imagery, hot/cold applications) or pharmacologic techniques to use before pain occurs or increases; or after painful activities.
  h. Evaluate the effectiveness of pain control measures through ongoing assessment and reintervention if pain or side effects are unacceptable.

E. Home care considerations. *See Chapter 21: Chronic Conditions: Care Technologies.*

1. A child-family-health team partnership is required for the successful symptom management of chronic pain.
2. Changes in strategies over time or in response to the child's sensory, psychologic, emotional, and behavioral responses are a requirement of the management process.

II. FATIGUE

◆ ◆ ◆ ◆ ◆ ◆ ◆ ◆ ◆ ◆ ◆ ◆ ◆ ◆ ◆ ◆ ◆ ◆

A. Overview.

1. Definition: an overwhelming and continuing sense of exhaustion that limits one's capacity for physical and mental work. Fatigue is a subjective drained feeling that cannot be eliminated by rest and differs from tiredness, a temporary state that can be caused by an imbalance in exercise, diet, or rest.

2. Etiology: usually multiple and additive causes involving a combination of physiologic, biochemical, and/or behavioral mechanisms secondary to definable underlying health problems.
  a. Acute fatigue has a rapid onset, lasts less than a month, and usually resolves quickly with proper treatment.
  b. Chronic fatigue lasts anywhere from 1 to 6 months or longer, has a gradual onset, and may not be easily resolved.
  c. Chronic fatigue may precede, accompany, or follow acute illness and chronic health problems.

3. Pathophysiology.
  a. Physiologic and pathophysiologic mechanisms.
    (1) Central and/or peripheral mechanisms operate independently or in unison to produce fatigue.
    (2) The accumulation or depletion of certain metabolites can impair muscle performance and cause fatigue.
    (3) Changes in neurohormone levels (e.g., melatonin) or fluid and electrolyte imbalances affect neurotransmission and muscle force thus producing fatigue.
  b. Psychologic or environmental mechanisms.
    (1) There is an increased incidence of depression and anxiety in children with fatigue.
    (2) Decreased energy and activity may contribute to a sense of "learned helplessness," thus increasing dependency on family and isolation from peers.
    (3) Emotional stress caused by life events and transitions may influence fatigue.

4. Incidence.
  a. The incidence and prevalence of fatigue are

unknown, but fatigue accounts for up to 15% of referrals to pediatric disease specialists.

  b. Fatigue is prevalent in clinical populations because it frequently precedes, accompanies, or follows illness and treatments.

5. Developmental considerations.

  a. Infants and young children are unable to verbally explain/describe their fatigue, thus a comprehensive fatigue history is needed from the parents/primary caregiver.

  b. Chronic fatigue may result in poor school performance and attendance, decreased social activities, and an adverse effect on peer relationships; therefore, prompt intervention may prevent psychologic, behavioral, and social difficulties.

  c. Premature infants are at risk for respiratory muscle fatigue due to age-related muscle differences.

B. Assessment.

1. History and physical exam. *Also see Chapter 4: Health, Psychosocial, and Developmental Screening and Assessment.*

  a. Obtain a comprehensive fatigue history including an assessment of fatigue in terms of:

    (1) Duration.
    (2) Onset.
    (3) Severity.
    (4) Relationship to activities like play or sports.
    (5) The response of fatigue to rest.
    (6) Academic performance.
    (7) School attendance.
    (8) Sleep patterns.
    (9) Nutritional status.
    (10) Previous infections.
    (11) Use of medication.
    (12) Exposure to illnesses and environmental toxins.

  b. Areas of psychosocial assessment include peer relationships, family dynamics, substance use, family history of chronic health problems, abuse (sexual, physical, or emotional), significant life changes or losses, self-esteem, coping skills, and relaxation techniques.

  c. Information about the intensity of fatigue can be sought directly by self-report from children with the use of a visual analog scale (VAS) (Berde et al., 1993).

  d. Complete a comprehensive physical assessment including:
    (1) Lymph nodes.
    (2) Thyroid.
    (3) Liver.
    (4) Spleen should be palpated for tenderness and enlargement.
    (5) The abdomen palpated for masses.
    (6) Assess for scleral icterus, petechiae, pallor, clubbing, and cyanosis.

2. Diagnostic tests.

  a. Laboratory studies may indicate decreased hematocrit, hemoglobin, thyroid, and oxygen saturation levels, or alterations in pH, electrolytes and lactate secondary to acute or chronic illness or a treatment regimen.

  b. The laboratory workup for chronic fatigue in the absence of acute or chronic illness and treatment may include a complete blood count with differential, erythrocyte sedimentation rate (ESR), blood glucose, thyroid function studies, lead screen, screen for Epstein-Barr virus (mono spot), culture for cytomegalovirus (CMV), liver function tests, urinalysis, urine culture, BUN, creatinine, immunoglobulins, and pregnancy test.

C. Common therapeutic modalities.

1. Management is based on the illness or treatment regimen.

2. Psychosocial interventions.

  a. If fatigue persists in the presence of a normal physical exam and laboratory findings, psychotherapy (individual, family or group) may be needed while the child is being followed medically.

  b. Coping skills training may be used to reduce stress.

  c. Cognitive behavior therapy may be needed to change behaviors that maintain fatigue patterns.

D. Nursing outcomes and interventions.

1. Outcomes. The child/adolescent and/or parent will:

  a. Report reduction of fatigue to a level of satisfaction.

  b. Report an increase in daily activity level.

  c. Recognize energy limitations.

  d. Use energy conservation and coping skills techniques.

  e. Report decreased disruptive effects on social and family life.

2. Nursing interventions.

  a. Perform a comprehensive fatigue/psychosocial history.

  b. Provide information about fatigue (cause and duration).

  c. Instruct child/parent in use of a developmentally appropriate tool to measure fatigue.

    d. Instruct, encourage, and review use of a home fatigue diary with child/parent to help modify lifestyle.

    e. Teach energy conserving and enhancing techniques: alternate rest and activity periods (e.g., scheduling a study hall after lunch to offer opportunity for rest without missing class time).

    f. Teach parents/child to recognize symptoms of fatigue that indicate a need for reduced activity, management of fatigue, and gradual increase in activity.

    g. Instruct and encourage use of developmentally appropriate coping skill techniques; consider child's preferred coping styles and strategies.

    h. If needed, provide nutritional support and referral.

    i. Evaluate effectiveness of fatigue control measures with ongoing assessment and reintervention if fatigue persists.

E. Home care considerations.

  1. Children with chronic fatigue need to be monitored closely with particular attention to the development of a fever, weight loss, or any change from assessment data, physical exam, or laboratory findings.

  2. A child-family-health team approach with coordinated services is required to avoid family frustration that could lead to "health care shopping" and fad therapy.

III. DYSPNEA

◆ ◆ ◆ ◆ ◆ ◆ ◆ ◆ ◆ ◆ ◆ ◆ ◆ ◆ ◆ ◆ ◆ ◆ ◆

A. Overview.

  1. Definition: a subjective sensation of difficult, uncomfortable breathing or breathlessness.

  2. Etiology.

    a. Situational and personal factors such as environmental conditions, obesity, and smoking/passive-smoke exposure may result in the development of chronic dyspnea.

    b. Dyspnea is frequently associated with fatigue and physical inactivity and can lead to physical and social isolation.

    c. Respiratory disorders (cystic fibrosis, bronchopulmonary dysplasia, or asthma) and cardiac disease (congenital heart disease) account for the majority of causes of chronic dyspnea in children. Other causes of chronic dyspnea are anemia, diabetes, and human immunodeficiency virus.

    d. Self-care management to decrease the frequency and intensity of chronic dyspnea involves education, skill attainment, and constant adjustment.

  3. Pathophysiology.

    a. Increased respiratory muscle effort may be mediated by stretching of muscle spindles and tendons in the intercostal respiratory muscle, which results in afferent signals to the central nervous system (CNS). The increased muscle effort may be due to increased resistance to airflow and changes in airway caliber (as in asthma, cystic fibrosis, and chronic bronchitis) or from weak respiratory muscles.

    b. Increased respiratory drive causes stimulation of central and peripheral chemoreceptors that respond to changes in arterial pH, oxygen, and carbon dioxide concentrations (e.g., anemia).

    c. Increased sensitivity to changes in ventilation perceived through CNS mechanisms (e.g., mood states) may increase or decrease dyspnea.

  4. Incidence.

    a. The exact incidence of dyspnea is unknown; prevalence can only be estimated from the prevalence of the health problems in which it occurs.

    b. The reported incidence of bronchopulmonary dysplasia (BPD) varies between 10% and 30%.

B. Developmental considerations.

  1. Age-related differences in the infant and child's respiratory and cardiovascular systems have an impact on illness and assessment. *See Chapter 4: Health, Psychosocial, and Developmental Screening and Assessment.*

  2. Treatments presented as games or play create a sense of fun, provide a sense of normalcy, and give the child a sense of control.

C. Assessment.

  1. History and physical exam. *See Chapter 4: Health, Psychosocial, and Developmental Screening and Assessment.*

    a. Obtain a complete history, including an assessment of dyspnea in terms of:

      (1) Duration.

      (2) Temporal patterns.

      (3) Position in which dyspnea occurs.

      (4) Presence during sleep.

      (5) Onset and relationship to activities like play or sports.

      (6) Effect on other body systems.

      (7) Effect on school and social relationships.

      (8) Duration of the current illness.

    b. Observed signs of dyspnea may include flaring of the nostrils, subcostal and intercostal retractions, tachypnea, anxious expression, use of accessory muscles of respiration, pursed-lip breathing, a weak cry, shortness of breath during feeding and rest, and an audible wheeze.

2. Diagnostic tests.
   a. Laboratory tests include a complete blood count (CBC), peripheral blood smear, and arterial blood gas.
   b. Arterial oxygen saturation by pulse oximetry, airway and lung x-rays, and pulmonary function tests (e.g., forced and expiratory volume) provide further evaluation of respiratory function.

3. Self-report measures.
   a. Dyspnea is a subjective symptom; therefore, self-report measures are considered the best way of measuring intensity and distress.
   b. The intensity of dyspnea can be rated on scales similar to those used to assess pain.
   c. Quality and distress of dyspnea can be measured with a word list describing feelings in response to breathing and with a word list of emotions about responses to episodes of dyspnea.

D. Common therapeutic modalities.
1. Medical treatment.
   a. Treatment is based on the diagnosis of a disease or modification of a treatment regimen that is causing the symptom.
   b. Cardiac deviations may require surgical intervention to alleviate dyspnea.
   c. Oxygen with or without continuous positive airway pressure reduces respiratory drive.

2. Nonpharmacologic treatment.
   a. Energy conserving strategies and graduated exercise can reduce respiratory muscle effort.
   b. Pursed lip breathing and diaphragmatic breathing may decrease the effort of breathing.
   c. Sitting next to an open window and moving fan may decrease the breathless feeling.
   d. A leaning forward position, either sitting or standing, is a typical position for relieving acute breathlessness.
   e. Self-monitoring of dyspnea using a home diary and physiologic information, such as peak expiratory flow rate, can increase children's understanding and management of their symptoms and increase the perception of control.

3. Pharmacologic treatment.
   a. Medications that reduce dyspnea include beta-adrenergic aerosol treatments (albuterol, terbutaline), cromolyn sodium, corticosteriods, and theophylline.

b. Sedative and narcotics in low doses can reduce the intensity of dyspnea in a child who is chronically ill.
c. Diuretics may help alleviate dyspnea in children with heart disease.

4. Psychosocial interventions.
   a. Relaxation techniques, simple guided imagery, and hypnosis have proven helpful in treating dyspnea.
   b. Peer support groups may minimize distress and promote adjustment (e.g., asthma camp).

E. Nursing outcomes and interventions.
1. Outcomes. The child/adolescent and/or parent will:
   a. Report reduction in frequency and intensity of dyspnea.
   b. Report an increase in daily activity level.
   c. Recognize energy limitations.
   d. Use self-care strategies to conserve energy.
   e. Perform pharmacologic, nonpharmacologic, and/or psychosocial strategies based on symptom monitoring.

2. Nursing interventions.
   a. Complete respiratory assessment.
   b. Provide information about dyspnea (cause, anticipated sensations, duration, avoidance of precipitants, both environmental and personal).
   c. Instruct child/parent in use of a developmentally appropriate tool to measure dyspnea.
   d. Instruct and encourage use of a home diary to monitor dyspnea, activity, emotional changes, and environmental patterns.
   e. Review the dyspnea diary with child/parent to help modify their lifestyle.
   f. Teach energy conserving and enhancing techniques.
      (1) Balance rest and activity periods.
      (2) Teach parents/child to correlate monitored symptoms of dyspnea with appropriate self-care management strategies (e.g., altering dose or frequency of medication and/or treatment).
      (3) Make environmental alterations, avoid precipitants, and use techniques (pharmacologic and nonpharmacologic) in the order that works best.
   g. Evaluate effectiveness of dyspnea control measures with ongoing assessment if dyspnea increases in intensity and frequency.

F. Home care considerations.
1. The goal of self-management is to have the child/parent adjust medication dosage and frequency, alter self-management practices, and

initiate contact with the health care team.

2. Setting goals with the child/parent can be used to involve them in the decision making about management strategies specific to the child's lifestyle and may increase adherence to the regimen for reducing chronic dyspnea.

IV. CONSTIPATION

◆ ◆ ◆ ◆ ◆ ◆ ◆ ◆ ◆ ◆ ◆ ◆ ◆ ◆ ◆ ◆ ◆ ◆ ◆ ◆

A. Overview.

1. Definition: the passage of dry, hard stools that can be accompanied by painful bowel movements. It involves an alteration in frequency, size, or consistency of stooling.
2. Etiology.
   a. Physiologic factors that can lead to constipation are:
      (1) Inadequate fluid intake.
      (2) Dehydration due to illness and fever.
      (3) Change in diet such as introduction of solids or increased carbohydrates.
      (4) Lack of exercise.
      (5) Prolonged bed rest and/or immobility.
      (6) Stool retention secondary to decreased bowel motility.
      (7) Painful bowel movements.
      (8) Use of medications that have the side effect of constipation (such as antacids, diuretics, anticonvulsants, narcotic analgesics, antihistamines, and iron supplements.
      (9) Inappropriate use of laxatives, suppositories, or enemas by parents or caregivers.
   b. Psychosocial influences.
      (1) Stressful family or life adjustments such as divorce, birth of a sibling, death of a family member.
      (2) Inconsistent or inappropriate toileting habits.
      (3) Change in daily routine, including traveling or uncomfortable lavatory environment.
      (4) Physical or sexual abuse or neglect.
3. Pathophysiology.
   a. Constipation can arise from defects in filling or in emptying the rectum.
   b. Defective rectal filling occurs when colonic peristalsis is ineffective, such as in cases of Hirschsprung disease, hypothyroidism, or opioid use.
   c. Emptying the rectum depends on a defecation reflex initiated by pressure receptors in the rectal muscles. Stool retention may result from neuromuscular disorders affecting the rectal or abdominal muscles.
   d. Constipation tends to be self-perpetuating.

Hard, large stools become difficult or painful to evacuate so child resists stooling, and more retention occurs. Also, distention of the rectum and colon lessens defecation reflex sensitivity and the effectiveness of peristalsis.

4. Incidence.
   a. Constipation occurs in about 17% of children between the ages of 1 and 3 years and in 1% of 4-year-olds.
   b. In most children, no organic cause for constipation can be detected.
   c. Chronic conditions that involve decreased mobility, or prolonged use of medications such as narcotics, antidepressants, or anticonvulsants, may often be associated with constipation.
5. Developmental considerations.
   a. The frequency of defecation changes with age. Young infants have an average of 5 to 7 stools per day. During the second half of the first year of life, stooling decreases to 1 to 3 per day.
   b. Constipation may occur while toilet training is being instituted due to the toddler's need for autonomy and control.
   c. Constipation in the school-age child may be the result of a new school environment, reluctance to use toilet facilities when peers are present, or as a consequence of ignoring the urge to defecate when engaged in play or other activities.

B. Assessment.

1. History and physical exam.
   a. The history of the child with constipation can include:
      (1) Stained underwear.
      (2) Constant crossing legs.
      (3) Grimacing or shifting from one foot to another.
      (4) A bloating sensation.
      (5) Abdominal pain.
      (6) Complaints of pain with defecation.
      (7) Blood-streaked bowel movements.
      (8) Diet history.
      (9) Use of over the counter and prescription medications.
      (10) Toileting history.
   b. When obtaining the history from the child or parents, it is important to obtain the individual's definition of constipation. Normal patterns of defecation may be misinterpreted by the child or parents as a result of personal, social, familial, or cultural expectations.
   c. The physical exam should assess for the following:

(1) Overflow soiling.
(2) Abdominal distention.
(3) Abdominal tenderness on palpation.
(4) Impaction felt on rectal examination.
2. Diagnostic tests.
a. An abdominal x-ray is obtained if structural anomalies are suspected.
b. If mechanical obstruction is suspected, other diagnostic tests may include anal manometry, barium enema, or rectal biopsy.

C. Common therapeutic modalities.

1. Dietary management.
a. High-fiber diet. The minimal daily dietary fiber intake (grams/day) recommended for children 2 years of age and older can be calculated by taking the chronologic age of the child and adding 5.
b. Increased fluid intake.
(1) Encourage water and juices, 16–24 ounces/day.
(2) Whole milk, which can be constipating, should be limited to 16–24 ounces in children over 12 months of age.
c. Limited intake of highly processed foods such as white bread, sugared cereals, sugared cookies, and processed meats in children over age 2.
2. Pharmacologic interventions.
a. Impaction, if present, needs to be removed with isotonic (normal saline) enemas administered twice a day until impaction is cleared, though enemas should not be given for more than 3 days.
b. Stool softeners or laxatives may be necessary in cases of prolonged constipation. Laxatives are prescribed according to age, body weight, and severity of constipation. A specific starting dose is ordered, but the dosage is then increased until appropriate defecation patterns and stool consistency are established.
(1) For infants, malt soup extract (Maltsupex) or corn (Karo) syrup may be mixed in formula, water, or fruit juice. Half-strength prune juice may also be helpful.
(2) Children over 6 months of age may be given mineral oil, milk of magnesia, or lactulose.
(3) Children over 1 year of age may be given senna syrup (Senokot), which is available over the counter in syrup, tablet, or granule form. Senokot should be given at the same time every day.
3. Behavioral interventions.
a. Establish a routine for toileting; for example, have child sit on the toilet after meals for 10 minutes twice a day if possible.
b. Provide incentives for success (e.g., stickers or other small rewards).

D. Nursing outcomes and interventions.

1. Outcomes. The child and/or parent will report:
a. An elimination pattern of 1 to 2 soft stools per day.
b. Reduction in straining and discomfort associated with defecation.
2. Nursing interventions.
a. Discuss parental attitudes and expectations regarding toilet habits.
b. Modify diet by increasing fluid intake and fiber content.
c. Increase child's physical activity, if appropriate.
d. Provide information about bowel function, causes of constipation, and rationale for interventions.
e. Establish regular times for elimination and provide privacy for toileting appropriate to the child's age and developmental status.
f. Administer, and evaluate the effectiveness of, prescribed stool softeners and laxatives.
g. Support and encourage parental and child efforts to manage constipation.

E. Home care considerations.

1. The management of constipation requires considerable time, effort, and patience on the part of the child and parents.
2. Parents need to be consistent with behavioral interventions, diet, and medication administration.
3. Medication dosage is adjusted as necessary to achieve passage of one to two soft bowel movements per day.
4. Children with neuromuscular conditions may need long-term pharmacologic management and/or manual removal of stool on a regular basis.

V. BOWEL AND BLADDER TRAINING

◆ ◆ ◆ ◆ ◆ ◆ ◆ ◆ ◆ ◆ ◆ ◆ ◆ ◆ ◆ ◆ ◆ ◆ ◆

A. Overview.

1. Definition: combinations of specific strategies developed for a child/adolescent to support optimal bowel and bladder function and minimize incontinence. Most children, even those with chronic conditions, are toilet-trained by age 4 years.
2. Etiology: neurologic disorders such as myelomeningocele and spinal cord injury account for the majority of bowel and bladder

dysfunction in the children. Other causes of chronic bowel and/or bladder dysfunction are cerebral palsy, developmental disabilities, Hirschsprung disease, imperforate anus, and genitourinary system anomalies.

3. Pathophysiology.
   a. Neurogenic bowel, or bowel paralysis, can be caused by an absence of peristalsis (as in Hirschsprung disease) or interruption of the spinal cord nerves that innervate the bowel (e.g., meningomyelocele, spinal cord trauma). Deficits in innervation result in varying symptoms, depending on the location of the lesion.
      (1) Lesions occurring above the T12-L1 level (upper motor neuron lesions) result in loss of cortical and voluntary control of the bowel as well as sensory input from the perineal area, rectum, and anus.
         (a) Reflex arcs below the spinal cord lesion remain intact, however, and reflex contraction of the external anal sphincter still occurs.
         (b) Reflex emptying of the rectum occurs every 2 to 3 days.
      (2) Lower motor neuron lesions (at or below T12) generally result in an areflexive bowel.
         (a) The reflex arc is impaired, sphincter tone is flaccid, and there is sensory loss in the perineal and rectal areas.
         (b) If continence is to be maintained, daily emptying of stool is required.
   b. Neurogenic bladder occurs when the nerves that normally allow an individual to sense a full bladder and voluntarily control urination are impaired.
      (1) Urinary retention can ensue, which can result in bladder distention, infection, reflux, and permanent renal damage.
      (2) Neurogenic bladder may also result in urinary incontinence, ranging from constant dribbling of urine to incontinence of larger amounts of urine.
      (3) Incomplete bladder emptying is common.
4. Incidence: the specific incidence of bowel and bladder dysfunction can only be estimated from the prevalence of the health problems in which they occur.
5. Developmental considerations.
   a. A bowel or bladder training program must be individualized for the child/adolescent, taking into account his or her developmental level, emotional needs, family, and cultural background.
   b. Toddlers and preschoolers can take responsi-

bility for specific, developmentally appropriate aspects of a bowel/bladder training program (e.g., gather supplies, wash hands, cooperate with procedures).
   c. Rewards of praise or stickers may be helpful in increasing cooperation in young children.
   d. School-agers and adolescents can participate in all aspects of their bowel or bladder management program. It is important that bowel/bladder difficulties do not interfere with the child's school attendance.

B. Assessment.
1. History and physical exam.
   a. Components of a comprehensive assessment of bowel and bladder function include:
      (1) History and course of child's chronic condition.
      (2) Child's developmental level (cognitive, motor, language, and social/emotional).
      (3) Parental perceptions and feelings.
      (4) Past toilet training experiences.
      (5) Diet and fluid intake.
      (6) Stool consistency, quantity, and frequency.
      (7) Voiding patterns.
      (8) Past history of urinary tract infections.
      (9) Medication use.
      (10) Past problems with constipation, diarrhea, incontinence of stool or urine.
   b. The physical exam should assess for the following:
      (1) Overflow soiling.
      (2) Abdominal distention.
      (3) Abdominal tenderness on palpation.
      (4) Impaction felt on rectal examination, usually at midline in the suprapubic area.
      (5) Rectal tone.
      (6) Dribbling of urine.
      (7) Bladder fullness on palpation.
   c. Parents or caregivers should keep a diary of bowel movements and voiding patterns for 7–14 days to determine if there is any predisposition for regular toileting times.
2. Diagnostic tests.
   a. An abdominal x-ray can indicate accumulation of stool in the colon.
   b. A bladder scan may be used to determine the capacity of the bladder.
   c. If mechanical obstruction or other anomalies are suspected, additional diagnostic tests may include anal manometry, barium enema, rectal biopsy, voiding cystourethrogram (VCUG), or cystoscopy.

C. Common therapeutic modalities.
1. Mastery of bowel and bladder continence is of

major importance for social acceptance, self-esteem, and optimal functioning.

2. Bowel and bladder management programs include the use of exercise; fluids; dietary modifications; timing; medications; creation of a colostomy, ileostomy, or urostomy; and clean intermittent catheterization (CIC).
   a. The purpose of a bowel control program is to produce a complete evacuation of stool at regular, planned intervals with minimal or no leakage of stool at other times.
   b. The goals of a bladder program are a stable, healthy urinary tract and for the child to be dry and odor free.
3. Nonpharmacologic interventions.
   a. Reflex evacuation in the child with an upper motor neuron lesion can be enhanced by:
      (1) Timing elimination for 30 minutes after eating when the gastrocolic reflex is the strongest
      (2) Ingestion of warm fluid to stimulate evacuation.
      (3) Digital rectal stimulation.
   b. Digital evacuation may be necessary to prevent chronic distention of the rectum in the child with a lower motor neuron lesion.
   c. In the child with a neurogenic bladder, CIC is the most commonly used method to help achieve urinary continence. An external catheter may be used in males at times when CIC is not feasible.
   d. Diet should be well-balanced and high in fiber, with a large intake of fluids.
   e. Fluid intake may be restricted during the evening in the child with bladder dysfunction to decrease the frequency of CIC during the night.
   f. Biofeedback via bowel and/or bladder stimulation may be a helpful adjunctive therapy.
4. Pharmacologic interventions.
   a. Medications used in bowel management.
      (1) Bulk-forming agents.
      (2) Stool softeners.
      (3) Bowel stimulants (laxatives, glycerin suppositories).
      (4) Enemas.
   b. Medications for bladder management are generally used in conjunction with CIC and include anticholinergics and sympathomimetics.
5. Surgical interventions.
   a. Urinary continence may be successfully achieved through:
      (1) Bladder augmentation.
      (2) Bladder neck reconstruction.
      (3) Creation of continent stomas or artificial urinary sphincters.
   b. In some cases, bowel management may involve creation of a temporary or permanent ileostomy or colostomy.
6. Psychosocial interventions.
   a. Peer support groups may promote adjustment and increase self-esteem through sharing experiences and verbalizing emotions.
   b. Parent support groups enable verbalization of attitudes and expectations regarding toileting and exchange of management strategies, and assist in adaptation to childhood chronic illness.

D. Nursing outcomes and interventions.
1. Outcomes. The child and/or parent will:
   a. Report an elimination pattern of regular, complete evacuation of stool at a scheduled time each day.
   b. Establish a regular schedule for urinary elimination.
   c. Report minimal or no leakage of stool or urine.
   d. State signs and symptoms of urinary tract infection and/or impaction.
   e. Perform pharmacologic, nonpharmacologic, and/or psychosocial strategies to maintain optimal bowel and bladder function.
2. Nursing interventions.
   a. Perform a comprehensive history.
   b. Discuss parental attitudes and expectations regarding toilet habits.
   c. Modify diet by increasing fluid intake and fiber content.
   d. Provide information about bowel and bladder physiology and function, causes of child's bowel and/or bladder dysfunction, and rationale for interventions.
   e. Establish regular times for elimination and provide privacy for toileting appropriate to the child's age and developmental status.
   f. Administer and evaluate the effectiveness of prescribed medications.
   g. Initiate and evaluate measures to maintain skin integrity.
   h. Support and encourage parental and child efforts to implement successful bowel/bladder management regimens.

E. Home care considerations.
1. The management of bowel and bladder control requires time, effort, and patience on the part of the child and parents.
2. Parents need to be consistent with behavioral interventions, diet, medications, and other components of the bowel or bladder management program.

3. Child/adolescent participation in bowel/bladder management will foster self-care abilities, promote independence, and increase self-esteem.

VI. SKIN INTEGRITY

◆ ◆ ◆ ◆ ◆ ◆ ◆ ◆ ◆ ◆ ◆ ◆ ◆ ◆ ◆ ◆ ◆ ◆ ◆

A. Overview.
1. Definition: impaired skin integrity is a state in which the neonate's or child's skin is unfavorably altered. The problem is considered to be chronic when the alteration extends beyond the usual time for healing or becomes a recurrent problem.
2. Etiology: the problem may arise from multiple causes.
   a. Environmental factors such as radiation therapy, thermal injury, toxins, mechanical forces, moisture and immobilization may result in disruption of skin surface or destruction of skin layers.
   b. Internal factors like medications, immature organ system functioning, systemic disease, and alteration in nutritional, immunologic, metabolic, circulatory, and sensory states contribute to chronic alterations in the skin.
3. Pathophysiology.
   a. Reduced blood volume results in low tissue oxygenation, and wound healing is altered when circulating volume is decreased.
   b. Pressure produces toxic metabolites at the cellular level, leading to acidosis, increased capillary permeability, edema and cell death, thereby resulting in a pressure sore.
   c. Soft tissue injury can be caused by either high pressure maintained for a short period of time or low pressure for a long period of time.
   d. Emotional stress produces increased production of glucocorticoids, which inhibits the formation of collagen and predisposes tissue to breakdown.
   e. When energy is transferred from a heat source to the body, a burn will occur if heat absorption exceeds heat dissipation, thus causing cellular temperature to rise and varying degrees of cellular destruction to occur.
   f. Skin lesions involve a sequence of inflammatory changes in the skin that arise from a variety of causes.
      (1) Acute responses include intracellular and intercellular edema as well as infiltration of inflammatory cells in both the epidermis and the dermis, the formation of intradermal vesicles and vascular dilation in the dermal layer.
      (2) In chronic conditions, these responses are not reversible, and permanent changes are seen that vary according to the specific disorder, the overall health of the child, and the treatment regimen.
   g. Immune system dysfunction can lead to chronic alterations in skin integrity. For example, atopic dermatitis is characterized by two immunologic abnormalities, an increase in immunoglobulin E (IgE) and a decrease in T suppressor cells.
4. Incidence.
   a. Acne affects approximately 85% of adolescents, with boys affected more frequently and severely than girls.
   b. The prevalence of atopic dermatitis in the United States increased from 3% in the 1960s to 10% in the 1980s.
   c. Thermal injuries annually affect about 1 million children in the U.S.A.
   d. The incidence of pressure ulcers in the pediatric population is unknown; however, a 43% incidence of pressure ulcers in children with myelomeningocele has been reported.
5. Developmental considerations.
   a. The premature infant has a thin, poorly keratinized epidermis leading to decreased resilience, impaired barrier function, and increased insensible water losses.
   b. Neonatal immune system defense mechanisms are immature and incompetent and skin pH is more alkaline, thus making the neonate more susceptible to infection.
   c. Very low birth weight (VLBW) infants have poor nutritional stores, predisposing them to delayed wound healing.
   d. The sites of greatest pressure change with increasing age from the occiput, in infants and toddlers, to the sacral area in children.
   e. The pattern of burn injury is related to the child's age and developmental status, with infants and toddlers injured most frequently by scald burns, and flame burns most common in children 5 to 18 years.
   f. Increased sebaceous gland activity in response to hormone activity predisposes adolescents to acne.

B. Assessment.
1. History and physical exam.
   a. Components of a comprehensive integumentary history.
      (1) Onset of symptoms and course of illness.
      (2) Family history of integumentary disorders or allergies.
      (3) Health conditions, past medical history.
      (4) Nutritional and fluid intake.

(5) Activity level.

(6) Incontinence.

(7) Allergies.

(8) Medication use (e.g., low-dose steroids, photosensitizing drugs).

(9) Recent changes in environment.

(10) Use of skin care products.

b. Areas of psychosocial assessment.

(1) Stress levels.

(2) School and social relationships.

(3) Body image issues.

(4) Economic status.

(5) Family living conditions.

c. Assessment of the child's self-concept is important, since this can be significantly altered when skin integrity disruptions are visible.

d. Physical examination should include the following:

(1) Assessment of skin, hair, and nails.

(2) Skin temperature, color, consistency, and turgor.

(3) Appearance and characteristics of skin alteration (rash, lesion, or wound) including color, location, size in centimeters, whether raised or flat, and presence of exudate or odor.

(4) Staging (I-IV) may be used if a pressure ulcer is present.

e. Associated physical symptoms may include fever, pain, tenderness, lymphadenopathy, or pruritus.

f. The use of a body diagram provides a pictorial representation of the location and extent of pediatric skin disruptions.

g. Nurses can use a chart or scale to determine risk assessment (e.g., modified Braden Q scale for use in pediatric skin ulcer assessment. *See Table 14-3. Modified Braden Q Scale in Chapter 14: Acute Illness: Symptom Management.*

2. Diagnostic tests.

a. Laboratory tests may include a complete blood count (CBC), erythrocyte sedimentation rate (ESR), culture of the altered skin surface, and/or allergy testing.

b. Skin biopsy, scraping, or visual inspection may be useful in diagnosis.

C. Common therapeutic modalities.

1. Pressure ulcers and burns may need surgical intervention (e.g., grafting or debridement).

2. Nonpharmacologic treatment.

a. Provision of adequate oxygen, calories, and protein to tissues will promote medical and surgical wound healing.

b. The use of various types of dressings (e.g., transparent film dressing, hydrocolloid dressing, moisture barrier skin wafers) may help in preventing infection, providing protection for the skin, and promoting tissue regeneration.

c. The use of heat lamps is contraindicated, since small increases in skin temperature (1°C) cause a 10% increase in tissue metabolism and oxygen demand.

d. Pressure relief devices (water or air filled mattress overlay) may be applied.

e. Skin inspection every 1–2 hours and frequent turning may be needed.

f. Minimal use of abrasive or skin drying products such as adhesive tape, alcohol, and betadine is recommended, especially in neonates.

g. The child/adolescent should be encouraged to shift body weight frequently.

h. The head of the bed should be elevated no more than 30° for a maximum of 2 hours at a time to prevent shear injury to the sacral area.

3. Pharmacologic treatment.

a. Pharmacologic management is based on the specific skin alteration present, and may include topical and systemic medications.

b. Commonly used medications for dermatologic conditions.

(1) Antibiotics.

(2) Antipruritics.

(3) Topical anesthetics.

(4) Vitamins and minerals.

(5) Antifungals.

(6) Moisture barrier ointments or powders.

(7) Anti-acne agents.

(8) Corticosteroid preparations.

4. Psychosocial treatment.

a. Peer support groups may address body image concerns and promote adjustment through verbalizing emotions.

b. Counseling (individual or family) may be indicated for the child and family affected by visible cosmetic defects such as burns or congenital skin disorders.

D. Nursing outcomes and interventions.

1. Outcomes. The child and/or parent will:

a. Report a reduction in the amount and severity of skin disruption.

b. Express satisfaction with control of pain and/or itching.

c. Use pharmacologic and nonpharmacologic modalities to maintain or restore skin integrity.

d. Verbalize feelings and concerns related to alteration in body image or appearance.

2. Nursing interventions.
   a. Perform a comprehensive integumentary history and physical examination.
   b. Provide information about the cause and duration of skin disruption and rationale for interventions.
   c. With the health care team, select and implement appropriate nonpharmacologic and pharmacologic measures to promote skin integrity and healing.
   d. Teach self-care techniques (e.g., skin hygiene, prevention of infection, application of topical creams, avoidance of scratching, avoidance of exposure to sunlight) to maintain or improve skin integrity.
   e. Teach side effects of pharmacologic treatment.
   f. If needed, provide nutritional support and referral.
   g. Encourage child and family to express feelings about personal appearance and perceived reactions of others.
   h. Evaluate the effectiveness of skin integrity enhancement measures with ongoing assessment and reintervention if skin disruption persists.

E. Home care considerations.
1. Most childhood thermal injuries occur in the child's home, and approximately 80–90% of these injuries are potentially preventable.
2. Parents and caregivers need to safety-proof their homes and educate themselves about potential hazards that could lead to burn injury.
3. Treatments such as dressing changes may be easier for parents or caregivers if distraction techniques are used with infants and toddlers. Older children and adolescents will benefit if they can participate in the treatment process.

BIBLIOGRAPHY

Berde, C.B., Schechter, N.I., & Yaster, M. (Eds.). (1993). *Pain in infants, children, and adolescents.* Baltimore: Williams & Wilkins.

Edwards-Beckett, J., & King, H. (1996). The impact of spinal pathology on bowel control in children. *Rehabilitation Nursing, 21,* 292–297.

Fox, J.A. (1997). *Primary health care of children.* St. Louis: Mosby.

Frauman, A.C., & Brandon, D.H. (1996). Toilet training for the child with chronic illness. *Pediatric Nursing, 22,* 469–472.

Hoekelman, R.A., Friedman, S.B., Nelson, N.M., Seidel, H.M., & Weitzman, M.L. (Eds.). (1997). *Primary pediatric care* (3rd ed.). St. Louis: Mosby.

Keller, V.E. (1995). Management of nausea and vomiting in children. *Journal of Pediatric Nursing, 10,* 280–286.

Loening-Baucke, V. (1994). Assessment, diagnosis, and treatment of constipation in childhood. *Journal of WOCN, 21*(2), 49–58.

Quigley, S.M., & Curley, M.A.Q. (1996). Skin integrity in the pediatric population: Preventing and managing pressure ulcers. *Journal of the Society of Pediatric Nurses, 1,* 7–18.

STUDY QUESTIONS

1. An acute illness or injury that usually heals in 2 weeks would be considered chronic if pain is still present for what period of time after the illness or injury?
   a. 1 week
   b. 2 weeks
   c. 6 weeks
   d. 6 months
   e. 12 months

2. What is the best way to assess the severity of pain in children between 4 and 12 years of age?
   a. Measure physiologic responses to the pain experience.
   b. Ask the doctor what he/she has assessed.
   c. Ask the child to indicate on a self-rating scale such as the "Oucher" how much hurt they have.
   d. Determine the appropriate amount of analgesia necessary to bring an acceptable level of comfort.
   e. Observe the child's behavioral responses to pain.

3. Fifteen-year-old Meaghan tells the nurse she feels "exhausted" all the time, even after a good night's sleep. Which statement by Meaghan indicates a psychosocial concern that is characteristic of chronic fatigue?
   a. "I have an A average in school."
   b. "My mother is mad because my room is such a mess."
   c. "My friends don't call me anymore because I can't keep up with them at the mall."
   d. "I have had a sore throat for over a month."
   e. "On Sunday I stayed in bed all day."

4. Which of the following activities indicates that the nurse's teaching to 15-year-old Meaghan about energy conservation strategies has been successful?
   a. Schedules classes in the morning so she can rest in the afternoon
   b. Joins the swim team
   c. Signs up for extra credits so she won't get bored
   d. Takes a summer job as a camp counselor
   e. Takes classes located in several different buildings

5. When teaching a school-age child breathing techniques to help chronic dyspnea and encourage self-care management, it is most important that the nurse:
   a. explain to the child how this might help.
   b. medicate the child before starting the breathing technique.
   c. obtain the physician's permission before teaching the technique.
   d. teach the parents the technique before teaching the child.
   e. give the child a book to read on dyspnea before teaching.

6. Which of the following is a characteristic symptom of chronic dyspnea in a child?
   a. Hoarse voice
   b. Prolonged inspiration
   c. Cyanosis
   d. Nasal flaring
   e. Abdominal breathing.

7. Constipation has recently become a problem for Adam, age 10. He is healthy except for seasonal allergies, which are currently being successfully treated with decongestants and antihistamines. The nurse should suspect that Adam's constipation is most likely caused by which of the following?
   a. Diet
   b. Allergies
   c. Allergy medications
   d. Emotional factors
   e. Hirschsprung disease

8. Which of the following is a high-fiber food that the nurse could recommend as a snack for the child with chronic constipation?
   a. Cookies
   b. Popcorn
   c. Ripe bananas
   d. Grape jelly and white bread sandwich
   e. Crackers

9. A successful self-catheterization program for the child with spina bifida requires all of the following EXCEPT:
   a. ability of the child to perceive the sensation of bladder fullness.
   b. fine motor skills necessary to insert and remove the catheter.
   c. emotional support from the child's family.
   d. remembering the equipment necessary for catheterization.
   e. appropriate hygiene measures before and after catheterization.

10. Which of the following factors promotes restoration of skin integrity?
   a. Heat lamp treatments
   b. Emotional stress
   c. Liberal use of alcohol and betadine
   d. Restricted protein intake
   e. Adequate tissue oxygenation

ANSWERS

1.c 2.c 3.c 4.a 5.a 6.d 7.c 8.b 9.a 10.e

Chapter 23

Chronic Conditions: Intervention Strategies

Sandra R. Mott, PhD(c), MS, RN,C

Concept

◆◆◆◆◆◆◆◆◆◆◆◆◆◆◆◆◆◆◆◆◆◆◆◆◆◆◆◆◆

- ◆ Children with a chronic condition, disability, or special health need and their families

Objectives

◆◆◆◆◆◆◆◆◆◆◆◆◆◆◆◆◆◆◆◆◆◆◆◆◆◆◆◆◆

At the completion of this chapter, the reader will be able to:

- ◆ Describe the principles of nursing interventions that guide a nurse's care of a child with a chronic illness/condition.

- ◆ Describe key considerations that must be examined when planning interventions for the family living with a childhood chronic illness/condition.

- ◆ Develop a plan for a continuum of care that reflects collaboration between the child, caregiver(s), and health care provider(s).

- ◆ Discuss nursing interventions directed toward developmental changes/transitions experienced by the child who is chronically ill and family.

- ◆ Identify and discuss nursing interventions and strategies available to assist the child and family to cope with the uncertainty and multiple demands of living with the chronic illness/condition of a child.

Key Points

◆◆◆◆◆◆◆◆◆◆◆◆◆◆◆◆◆◆◆◆◆◆◆◆◆◆◆◆◆

- ◆ Nursing interventions must be modified according to the family's perception of the chronic illness/condition.

- ◆ Perception of chronic illness is influenced by cultural and ethnic heritage, religious beliefs and values, family traditions, and past experiences.

- ◆ All family members should be as involved as possible in planning care for the child with a chronic illness/condition, including the child and siblings.

- ◆ Interventions for the child with a chronic illness/condition need to be family-centered so that family functioning can be maintained.

- ◆ Nurses need to plan both short-term and long-term interventions that provide continuity of care, participation of child and family members, and resources for crisis events.

◆ 23 ◆

Chronic Conditions: Intervention Strategies

◆ ◆

I. GENERAL PRINCIPLES FOR PLANNING INTERVENTION STRATEGIES

A. Recognize the family as the constant in the child's life. *See Chapter 28: Family-Centered Care.*

B. Focus on the child's developmental age, rather than chronologic age.

C. Emphasize family and child strengths, instead of weaknesses.

D. Collaborate with parents in planning strategies.

E. Respect individuality in adaptive coping methods.

F. Collaborate with social workers and community and governmental resources to prevent depletion of financial resources.

G. Refer family to peer support groups.

H. Work with the family as a whole unit to facilitate the process of growth and understanding.
1. Create opportunities for all family members to display their present abilities and competencies while developing new ones.
2. Support families to maintain a sense of control and participation in decision making related to caregiving.
3. Encourage mutual participation in care by the child and parent to facilitate better communication and alleviate parental feelings of inadequacy and child inferiority.

II. INTERVENTION STRATEGIES
(Nursing Intervention Classifications [NIC], McCloskey & Bulechek, 1996)

◆ ◆

A. Negotiating care outcomes with families. There is no universal strategy that is effective for every family. Each family is unique and for any plan of care to be implemented, it must fit the beliefs, schedules, abilities, and goals of that family; the plan cannot be imposed.
1. Input from the family should be elicited and the plan modified to fit each family's situation.
2. Communication enhancement: interventions to facilitate the giving and receiving of verbal and nonverbal messages that can be used as a guide to support family functioning and facilitate life style changes. *See Chapter 30: Communication.*
   a. Active listening: attend closely to and attach significance to verbal and nonverbal messages from family members as well as the chronically ill child.
      (1) Display interest in the family unit.
      (2) Encourage expression of feelings.
      (3) Listen for unexpressed message and feeling, as well as content, of the conversation.
      (4) Clarify the message through the use of questions and feedback to learn the meaning attached to concerns expressed by the family members.
      (5) Verify understanding of message.
   b. Art therapy: facilitation of communication through drawings or other art forms; some parents and children may be better able to express their thoughts, feelings, and concerns using a neutral medium that facilitates interaction through verbal sharing. The goal of art therapy is to enhance communication, not probe for psychologic or emotional factors or determine self-concept or family dysfunction.
      (1) Provide art supplies (paper, pencil, crayons, clay) appropriate for developmental level and goals for therapy.
      (2) Discuss description of drawing or artistic creation with family member; use created medium as stimulus for interaction and communication.
      (3) Note any expression that relates to stressful events, especially fears, misconceptions, or concerns associated with illness, hospitalization, disability.

(4) Avoid reading meaning into art work; let creator tell story of drawing or artistic endeavor.

c. Bibliotherapy: use of literature to enhance the expression of feelings and the gaining of insight.
  (1) Select books that reflect the situation or feelings the child and/or family is experiencing.
  (2) Make selections appropriate for cognitive level and reading level for older child and adult.
  (3) Use pictures and illustrations.
  (4) Talk about the situation and feelings expressed by the story characters.

B. Collaboration for individualizing outcomes: importance of communication and cooperation between the health care team and the family to ensure both adherence to treatment and satisfaction.
1. Values clarification: assisting another to clarify her/his own values in order to facilitate effective decision making.
2. Culture brokerage: bridging, negotiating, or linking the orthodox health care system with a patient and family of a different culture. *See Chapter 29: Cultural Influences.*
3. Family process maintenance: minimization of family process disruptions or major role changes.
4. Mutual goal setting: collaborating with child and/or family to identify and prioritize care goals, then developing a plan for achieving those goals through the construction and use of goal attainment scaling.
5. Patient (family) contracting: negotiating an agreement with a patient (family) that reinforces a specific behavior change. When a child is the ill member, it usually involves taking on additional tasks as well as substantial changes in family roles and functioning.

C. Teaching disease process: assisting the child and family to understand information related to a specific disease process.
1. Provide general information to family members about the condition, etiology, signs and symptoms, and prognosis, as appropriate.
2. Assist family members in learning more specifics about the child's disease by providing clearly communicated, appropriately detailed information about its manifestations and usual course.
3. Provide family members with progress reports; be honest and avoid any empty reassurances.

4. Instruct family members on which signs and symptoms are significant indicators of the child's status, which need to be reported immediately to the health care provider, and which ones can wait .
5. Instruct family members on measures to prevent/minimize side effects of the disease.
6. Promote hope by informing families about recent advances and treatment as appropriate including any known limits or risks.
7. Reinforce information provided by other health care team members.

D. Learning facilitation: promoting the ability to process and comprehend information.
1. Adjust instruction to family members' level of knowledge and understanding by tailoring the content to fit their cognitive, psychomotor, and/or affective abilities.
2. Provide an environment conducive to learning: one that is quiet, away from the concerns of the child, and unhurried.
3. Arrange information logically, from simple to complex, known to unknown, concrete to abstract.
4. Adapt information so it is consistent with family's values and beliefs and meshes with their lifestyle and routines whenever possible.
5. Use familiar (nontechnical) language, encourage questions, and repeat or rephrase information not understood or found confusing.
6. Work with other health care members to ensure that information provided is consistent across disciplines.
7. Use pictures, diagrams, and models as teaching aids to enhance their understanding of the disease and its effects.
8. Provide written materials to reinforce and complement what was explained verbally and to serve as a quick reference when questions arise.
9. Introduce the family to other families who have a child with a similar diagnosis or who have had similar treatment-related experiences.
10. Provide frequent feedback during learning process, reinforce information, and include question/answer or discussion time with each session.

E. Decision-making support: provide information and support for a family who is making a decision regarding health care for their child with a chronic condition.
1. Presence: being with another during times of need.
  a. Establish trust and positive regard by demonstrating an accepting attitude and verbally

communicating empathy and understanding of the situation.

   b. Be physically present as appropriate to reassure, assist, explain, calm fears, and support.

2. Emotional support: provision of reassurance, acceptance, and encouragement during times of stress.

   a. Help family members recognize feelings such as disbelief, anxiety, anger, or sadness, and to express them.

   b. Provide support during shock, denial, anger, bargaining, and acceptance phases of grieving the lost "perfect child."

   c. Help family members to identify function of emotions, importance of dealing with them, and potential consequences if ignored.

   d. Encourage talking or crying as means to decrease the emotional response and free energy for decision making.

3. Family support: promotion of family values, interests, and goals.

   a. Promote trusting relationship with the family by actively listening to their concerns, feelings, and questions.

   b. Provide assistance in meeting basic needs for family such as shelter, food, and clothing.

   c. Identify congruence between family members and health professional's expectations.

   d. Counsel family members on effective coping skills.

   e. Include family members in decision making, especially when making long-term plans for the child's care that affect family structure and finances.

   f. Support the family in redefining their situation, planning new arrangements to provide for the health care needs of the child, and in deriving comfort and strength from their values and beliefs in determining priorities and task allocation.

   g. Assist family to acquire necessary knowledge, skills, and equipment to sustain their decision about providing for the child's care.

   h. Advocate for the family by fostering family assertiveness to meet caretaking needs and initiating referrals as appropriate.

   i. Arrange for peer support and/or respite care.

4. Spiritual support: assisting the family to feel balance and connection with a greater power.

   a. Be open to and supportive of family members' expressions of loneliness and powerlessness, and attentive to expression of feelings about illness and death.

   b. Encourage use of spiritual resources, offer referrals, or contact spiritual advisor of family's choice.

F. Teach new interventions related to the child's care. The acquisition of new skills and behaviors is a critical process in adjusting to the diagnosis and long-term care demands for the child who is chronically ill.

1. Teaching – individual (family members): planning, implementation, and evaluation of a teaching program designed to foster learning required to meet needs of the child.

   a. Discuss knowledge base, family decision about ongoing care; determine the learning needs of the family members.

   b. Present material in well organized, logical sequence that builds on the knowledge and competencies of the learner.

   c. Tailor instruction according to the educational level, cognitive, psychomotor, and affective abilities of the family members.

   d. Periodically evaluate learning, reinforce behaviors, or adjust instruction as needed; clarify misconceptions, answer questions, and discuss concerns.

2. Learning readiness enhancement (child): improving the ability and willingness to receive information; relates particularly to the child's maturity and participation in the daily management and caregiving.

   a. Establish rapport; provide nonthreatening environment.

   b. Apply principles of growth and development to assist the child to accept and learn about her/his condition and related care.

   c. Encourage verbalization of feelings, perceptions, and concerns.

   d. Provide time for questions; explain relationship between adherence to treatment and future goals as appropriate, and assist child in gaining confidence in her/his abilities.

3. Teaching – prescribed activity/exercise: preparing a child to achieve and/or maintain a prescribed level of activity and family members to assist and/or facilitate such achievement.

   a. Inform child and family of the purpose for, and the benefits of, the prescribed activity/exercise.

   b. Instruct the child and family, either verbally or via demonstration and return, how to perform the activity/exercise.

   c. Instruct the child and family to keep an exercise diary, to monitor tolerance, and how to safely progress.

   d. Discuss with family members the least disruptive way to incorporate the activity/exercise into the family's daily lifestyle.

   e. Provide information on available community resources that offer assistance or group activities for the child.

4. Teaching – prescribed diet: preparing the child and family to correctly follow a prescribed diet.
   a. Determine child and family members' knowledge of and attitude toward the prescribed diet.
   b. Instruct child and family on the purpose, rationale, and benefits of the diet.
   c. Provide written instructions of foods allowed and prohibited; recommended daily amount of calories, protein, carbohydrate, fat, and specific vitamins and minerals.
   d. Inform family how long the diet must be followed and any possible drug/food interactions.
   e. Assist the child and family to accommodate food preferences into the prescribed diet.
   f. Discuss with family the importance of reading labels, especially when buying prepared food.
   g. Provide family members with specific parameters that indicate the benefits of following the prescribed diet; suggest they maintain a written record of intake, weight gain or loss, presence or absence of disease manifestations.
   h. Refer family to dietitian/nutritionist as appropriate.
5. Teaching – procedure/treatment: preparing child and family to understand and mentally prepare for a prescribed procedure or treatment that is a necessary ingredient in the management plan for the child who is chronically ill.
   a. Determine family members' prior experiences and level of knowledge related to procedure/treatment.
   b. Discuss the purpose and goals of the procedure/treatment in terms of the child's health and long-term goals.
   c. Discuss family lifestyle routine and how best to integrate prescribed procedure/treatment to ensure cooperation without adding stress.
   d. Review with family members the availability of resources, both personnel and equipment.
   e. Discuss ways to incorporate developmental principles to gain child's cooperation, such as use of distraction, fantasy, imagery, relaxation.
   f. Provide time for questions, concerns, or ideas of alternative approaches based on child's temperament.
6. Teaching – psychomotor skill: prepare family members to perform psychomotor skills that are part of the child's health management plan.
7. Medication management: facilitation of safe and effective use of prescription and over-the-counter drugs.
8. Technology management: use of technical equipment and devices to monitor the child or sustain life while receiving care in the home.

See Chapter 21: Chronic Conditions: Care Technologies.

G. Enhancing self-efficacy within the family by strengthening family functioning. When families confront a stressor of the magnitude of a child's chronic illness, the potential exists for growth or disintegration. *See Chapter 28: Family-Centered Care.*
1. Focus on the family as a unit.
   a. Family integrity promotion: promotion of family cohesion and unity.
   b. Family involvement: facilitating family participation in the emotional and physical care of the child.
   c. Family mobilization: use of family strengths to influence child's health in a positive direction.
   d. Normalization promotion: assisting parents and other family members of children with chronic illnesses or disabilities in providing normal life experiences for their children and families. *See Chapter 20: Chronic Conditions: Effects on the Child's Family.*
      (1) Promote integration of the child into the family system without letting the child become the central focus.
      (2) Assist the family to interact with the child according to the child's developmental level, not according to the illness or disability.
      (3) Provide opportunities for the child to have normal childhood experiences, such as peer interaction in play, school, clubs, sports, music.
      (4) Identify adaptations needed to accommodate child's limitations, so child can participate in normal activities.
      (5) Communicate information about child's condition to those who need this information to provide safe supervision or appropriate educational opportunities for child.
      (6) Encourage parents to have same parenting expectations and to use the same techniques as they did, or would, if the child were not ill.
      (7) Include siblings in the care and activities of the child.
      (8) Encourage parents to balance involvement in special programs for the child's special needs and normal family and community activities.
      (9) Encourage the family to maintain their usual family habits, rituals, and routines including taking time to care for their personal needs as individuals.

e. Family therapy: assisting family members to move their family toward a more productive way of living.
   (1) Determine usual member roles within the family system and areas of dissatisfaction and/or conflict.
   (2) Incorporate therapeutic use of self as nurse change agent.
   (3) Help family members clarify what they need and expect from each other during times of increased stress as well as times of adaptation.
   (4) Refer to other health care professionals if needs require in-depth therapy.
2. Focus on the primary caregiver; important to verify who is the primary caregiver and not to assume it is the mother.
   a. Caregiver support: provision of the necessary information, advocacy, and support to facilitate care by someone other than a health care professional.
      (1) Determine primary caregiver's acceptance of role and associated responsibilities.
      (2) Explore with the caregiver perceived strengths and limitations.
      (3) Accept expression of negative emotion over dependency of child, and/or frustration about loss of freedom and time for self.
      (4) Encourage the acceptance of family members' offers of assistance.
      (5) Teach caregiver health maintenance strategies and stress management techniques to sustain own physical and mental health.
      (6) Identify health care and community resources and sources of respite care.
   b. Role enhancement: assisting the family to improve relationships by clarifying and supplementing specific role behaviors, especially in terms of adaptation to the new responsibilities related to the caregiver role.
      (1) Discuss behaviors of new or changed roles of each member necessitated by the caregiving needs of the child who is chronically ill.
      (2) Facilitate discussion about accepting new role responsibilities, expectations of each other, and potential barriers to fulfilling new role.
      (3) Facilitate interactions with groups of families with similar experiences.
   c. Assertiveness training: assistance with the effective expression of feelings, needs, and ideas while respecting the rights of others; to ward off caregiver 'burnout' it is important

that the caregiver learn to advocate for the child's well-being as well as for one's personal health.
   d. Energy management: regulating energy use to treat or prevent fatigue and optimize function.
      (1) Encourage verbalization of feelings about time demands and functional limitations.
      (2) Monitor nutritional intake to include intake of high-energy foods to ensure adequate energy resources.
      (3) Monitor sleep pattern and ensure adequate number of consecutive hours of sleep.
      (4) Discuss daily routine and possibility of including diversional activities that promote relaxation for both child and caregiver.
      (5) Discuss activity organization, prioritizing, and time management techniques to prevent fatigue.
      (6) Review goals of management plan to ascertain that they are realistic.
3. Focus on general interventions to facilitate development and meet the unique needs of the child who is chronically ill.
   a. Activity therapy: assistance with specific physical, cognitive, social, and spiritual activities to increase the range, frequency, or duration of the child's activity.
      (1) Collaborate with occupational, physical, and/or recreational therapists in planning and monitoring an activity program designed to support the developmental potential of the child.
      (2) Assist to choose activities consistent with physical, psychologic, and social capabilities.
      (3) Focus on what the child is capable of doing, rather than on the deficits.
      (4) Specify time periods for diversional activity into daily routine.
      (5) Provide gross motor activities that provide for learning needs and large muscle development.
      (6) Refer to community centers for activity programs.
      (7) Monitor emotional, physical, social, and spiritual response to activity.
   b. Play therapy: purposeful use of toys or other equipment to assist a child in communicating his/her perception of the world and to help in mastering the environment.
      (1) Provide developmentally-appropriate, safe play equipment that stimulates creative, expressive play.
      (2) Provide equipment that stimulates aggres-

sive or regressive play, expression of feelings about hospitalization, treatments, or illness.

(3) Provide a quiet environment that is free from interruptions.

(4) Communicate acceptance of feelings, both positive and negative, expressed through play.

(5) Discuss purpose and benefits of providing therapeutic play activities with family.

(6) Record observations made during play session.

(7) Encourage family to continue play sessions on a regular basis to foster sharing of feelings, knowledge, and perceptions.

c. Cognitive stimulation: promotion of awareness and comprehension of surroundings by use of planned stimuli.

(1) Use developmentally appropriate toys, games, and other activities to stimulate and support cognitive development.

(2) Keep learning sessions free from distractions.

(3) Concentrate on one skill at a time using repetition of information plus a variety of problem-solving tasks that require similar cognitive functioning.

(4) Present new information in small, concrete portions.

(5) Plan learning sessions at times when child is rested and alert.

(6) Provide feedback that praises the positive and constructively criticizes what needs improvement or correction.

d. Behavior modification – social skills: assisting the child to develop or improve interpersonal social skills.

(1) Discuss with family members potential and/or actual interpersonal problems resulting from the child's social skill deficits.

(2) Discuss strategies to promote the child's socialization and positive interactions with peers and adults.

(3) Arrange for child to participate in peer group activities with others.

(4) Discuss the disadvantages of treating the child who is chronically ill differently and advantage of expecting socially accepted, developmentally appropriate behavior from the child.

(5) Discuss with family any specific social skill or behavior that needs to be learned or behavior that needs to be changed.

(6) Identify goal for new or modified behavior and specific steps for achieving goal.

(7) Involve all family members in social skills training, use role play and modeling, and provide feedback via tangible and intangible rewards.

4. Focus on the environment in which the child and family interact.

a. Home Maintenance Assistance: helping the family to maintain the home as a clean, safe, and pleasant place to live.

(1) Involve family in deciding home maintenance requirements and if any structural changes are needed to accommodate care or equipment needs of the child who is chronically ill.

(2) Suggest services, such as homemaker, as alternatives to managing everything within the family, as appropriate.

b. Environmental management: manipulation of the surroundings for the therapeutic benefit of the child.

(1) Create a safe environment based on the child's physical and cognitive functioning.

(2) Place caregiving supplies together so they are easily accessible for respective treatments, procedures, or feedings.

(3) Arrange furniture in room(s) that best accommodates movement needs for the child and modify as child becomes more mobile (e.g., longer tubing for oxygen).

(4) Discuss use of special equipment back packs for children who need continuous feeds or intravenous therapy to increase mobility and developmentally appropriate behaviors.

(5) Individualize daily routine to meet child's needs and fit within other family responsibilities and routines.

H. Providing anticipatory guidance about developmental concerns and parenting issues. Teaching about normal developmental progression and issues is often forgotten or minimized when focus is on the child's chronic illness and related care.

1. Teaching – infant care: instruction on nurturing and physical care needed during the first year of life.

a. Provide verbal and written information about expected developmental progression during the first year of life.

b. Encourage family members to spend time holding, cuddling, and interacting with the infant at nontreatment times to foster attachment.

c. Encourage family members to spend time

playing with the infant and to talk and read to the infant thus providing pleasurable auditory and visual stimulation to promote growth and development.
   d. Give examples of safe toys or available things in home that can be used as toys.
   e. Provide verbal and written information about safety concerns (e.g., crib sides, type and size of toys, exposure to sun, cold, and environmental hazards such as stairs, cords, electrical outlets). *See Chapter 7: Home and Family.*
   f. Assist family members in describing infant's temperament and planning care and activities that complement infant's behavioral style.
2. Parent education – child-rearing family: helping the family understand and promote the physical, psychologic, and social growth and development of their toddler, preschool, or school-age child.
   a. Teach the physiologic, emotional, and behavioral characteristics of child according to that child's status given the chronic condition.
   b. Identify appropriate developmental tasks or goals for the child, emphasizing the areas of development that are not affected by the child's illness.
   c. Facilitate family members' discussion of different methods of discipline, selection, and results.
   d. Review nutritional requirements for specific age groups.
      (1) Teach the importance of a balanced diet and nutritious snacks.
      (2) Assist in modifying diet to accommodate special needs of child.
   e. Review dental hygiene and skin care; emphasize effects of long-term medication use on dental and dermatologic health, as appropriate.
   f. Discuss safety issues, such as talking to strangers and pedestrian, bike, wheelchair, passenger, and water safety.
3. Developmental enhancement: facilitating or teaching family members to facilitate the optimal gross motor, fine motor, language, cognitive, social, and emotional growth of preschool and school-age children.
   a. Build a trusting relationship with child and assist him/her to recognize his/her importance as an individual regardless of illness or disability.
   b. Discuss with the family the importance of providing activities that encourage interaction with other children to facilitate learning to share, take turns, cooperate, seek help when needed, and follow directions.
   c. Discuss helping the child learn self-help skills (feeding, toileting, brushing teeth, washing hands, and dressing) and ways to adapt to physical, cognitive, or psychosocial limitations.
   d. Discuss with the family the importance of providing opportunities for exercise, play, and cognitive developmental activities to the extent the child is capable.
4. Parent education – adolescent: assisting the family to understand and help their adolescent.
   a. Teach physiologic, emotional, and cognitive characteristics of adolescents, adapting the content to the unique characteristics of the adolescent with a chronic illness.
   b. Discuss necessity and legitimacy of limit setting for adolescents and explore some strategies to implement limits.
   c. Discuss concerns of family members; assist them to identify those over which they will accept compromise and those over which they cannot compromise, and ways to communicate this firmly and clearly to the adolescent.
5. General areas of family responsibility and strategies of discipline to promote the health and well-being of the child.
   a. Infection control: minimizing the acquisition and transmission of infectious agents.
      (1) Review with family members ways to prevent infections.
         (a) Hand-washing.
         (b) Proper dress for weather.
         (c) Avoiding crowds.
         (d) Restricting interactions with those who have colds or other illnesses.
         (e) Proper use of and disposal of tissue.
         (f) Covering mouth and nose when coughing or sneezing.
         (g) Good nutrition.
      (2) Teach family members about signs and symptoms of infection and when to report them to the health care provider.
   b. Environmental management – safety: monitoring and manipulation of the physical environment to promote safety.
      (1) Help family members identify the safety needs of the child based on level of physical and cognitive function.
      (2) Suggest ways to modify the environment to minimize hazards and risk.
      (3) Provide family with emergency phone numbers including poison control center.
   c. Distraction: purposeful focusing of attention away from undesirable sensation or unsafe area or behavior.

    (1) Describe the rationale for and the benefits, limits, and types of distraction techniques available.

    (2) Consider such distraction techniques as play, activity therapy, reading stories, singing songs, or rhythm activities for children.

    (3) Individualize the content of the distraction technique, based on those used successfully in the past and age or developmental level of the child.

    (4) Use distraction alone or in conjunction with other measures, as appropriate.

  d. Limit setting: establishing the parameters of desirable and acceptable behavior.

    (1) Clarify with family reasonable expectations for child's behavior, based on the situation and characteristics of the child.

    (2) Discuss strategies to communicate the established behavioral expectations and consequences to the child in language that is easily understood and nonpunitive.

    (3) Encourage the family to initiate the established consequences for the occurrence/nonoccurrence of the desired behaviors.

    (4) Suggest decreasing limit setting, as the child's behavior approximates the desired behaviors.

I. Preparing child and family for issues surrounding developmental transitions — as the child grows and matures, the child moves into new circumstances, new surroundings, and new expectations.

1. Body image enhancement: improve a child's conscious and unconscious perceptions and attitudes toward his/her body.

  a. Determine child's body image based on developmental stage.

    (1) Prepare the child for potential responses from strangers who are unfamiliar with the needs or appearance of a child with a chronic illness or disability.

    (2) Help the child to build a strong sense of self-confidence and self-knowledge.

  b. Assist child to discuss changes caused by illness, treatment, or surgery, as appropriate.

  c. Discuss the influence of peer group response on the child's perception of body image.

  d. Help the child to identify what stressors associated with his/her chronic condition most affect perception of body image.

  e. Identify the significance of the child's culture, religion, race, gender, and age on body image.

  f. Use self-drawing as a mechanism for understanding a child's body image.

  g. Identify coping strategies used by family members in response to changes in child's appearance and discuss with them the importance of their response to the child's future adjustment.

  h. Facilitate contact with individuals with similar changes in body image as well as encourage participation in support groups.

2. Self-responsibility – facilitation: encourage a child to assume more responsibility for own care and behavior by maximizing her/his level of independence.

3. Self-esteem – enhancement: assist a child/teen to increase her/his personal judgment of self-worth.

  a. Determine child's/teen's confidence in her/his own judgment.

  b. Reinforce the personal strengths that the child/teen identifies.

  c. Provide experiences that increase the child's/teen's autonomy.

  d. Convey confidence in the child's/teen's ability to handle situation.

  e. Explore previous achievements of success and encourage the child/teen to accept new challenges.

  f. Reward or praise child's/teen's progress toward reaching goals.

  g. Facilitate an environment and activities that will increase self-esteem.

  h. Discuss impact of peer group on feelings of self-worth.

  i. Discuss with family members the importance of their interest and support in the child's/teen's development of a positive self-concept.

  j. Encourage family members to value the child's/teen's ideas and to recognize all accomplishments and achievements.

4. Self-awareness – enhancement: assist a child/teen to explore and understand her/his thoughts, feelings, motivations, and behaviors.

  a. Encourage the child/teen to identify the values and factors that contribute to self-concept.

  b. Discuss with the child/teen usual feelings about self and assist her/him to realize that everyone is unique.

  c. Assist child/teen to identify the impact of chronic illness on self-concept and its role in her/his ambivalent, angry, guilty, or depressed feelings.

  d. Assist the child/teen to identify positive attributes of self and to focus on these, rather than any negative perceptions that exist.

  e. Explore with the child/teen the source of

motivation and facilitate opportunities for using it to elevate the self-concept.

f. Facilitate self-expression with peer group.

5. Behavior management – overactivity/inattention: provision of a therapeutic milieu that safely accommodates the child's attention deficit and/or overactivity while promoting optimal function.

a. Determine appropriate behavioral expectations and consequences, given the child's level of cognitive functioning and capacity for self-control.

b. Communicate rules, behavioral expectations, and consequences using simple language with visual cues, as necessary.

c. Use a calm, matter-of-fact, reassuring approach and praise desired behaviors and efforts at self-control.

d. Provide aides that will increase environmental structure, concentration, and attention to tasks to support effort and task completion.

e. Help child to maintain a routine schedule that includes a balance of structured time and quiet time.

f. Assist the family to set consistent limits on intrusive, interruptive behavior.

g. Teach social skills to facilitate child's acceptance by peers and his/her boost self-esteem.

III. CONCLUSION

Interventions related to the care of a chronically ill child are multidimensional and extensive because chronic illness affects the whole family. Although lengthy, the above list is not comprehensive; rather, it seeks to highlight the many facets of intervention that need to be considered when working with these families. Obviously, for each situation the list needs to be tailored to the circumstances and characteristics of the individuals involved.

The guiding source for all of the interventions and activities was McCloskey, J.C., & Bulechek, G.M. (1996). *Nursing interventions classification (NIC): Iowa intervention project.* St. Louis: Mosby–Year Book. The activities were either stated as suggested or modified to focus more accurately on the child and family members.

BIBLIOGRAPHY

Clements, D.B., Copeland, L.G., & Loftus, M. (1990). Critical times for families with a chronically ill child. *Pediatric Nursing, 16*(2), 157–161, 224.

Cohen, M.H. (1993). The unknown and the unknowable: Managing sustained uncertainty. *Western Journal of Nursing Research, 15*(1), 77–96.

Cohen, M.H. (1995a). The triggers of heightened parental uncertainty in chronic life-threatening childhood illness. *Qualitative Health Research, 5*(1), 63–77.

Cohen, M.H. (1995b). The stages of the prediagnostic period in chronic, life-threatening childhood illness: A process analysis. *Research in Nursing & Health, 18,* 39–48.

Gibson, C. (1995). The process of empowerment in mothers of chronically ill children. *Journal of Advanced Nursing, 21,* 1201–1210.

McCloskey, J.C. (1993) Caring for chronically ill children at home: Factors that influence parents' coping. *Journal of Pediatric Nursing, 8*(4), 217–225.

McCloskey, J.C. (1996). *Nursing interventions classification (NIC): Iowa intervention project.* St. Louis: Mosby–Year Book.

Sharkey, T. (1995). The effects of uncertainty in families with children who are chronically ill. *Home Healthcare Nurse, 13*(4), 37–42.

STUDY QUESTIONS

◆ ◆

1. Jason was diagnosed with a chronic illness a week ago. When his parents say, "We are doing fine. We don't need anything," a helpful response would be to:
   a. say, "I'm available if you feel like talking."
   b. grant his parents privacy and leave the room.
   c. add a note in the chart that Jason's parents have accepted the diagnosis.
   d. say, "You are coping so well. It doesn't seem like you need any extra help."
   e. say, "You will have good moments and difficult moments."

2. A nurse might provide anticipatory guidance for parents of a chronically ill child by explaining that as their child becomes an adolescent:
   a. negativism and defiance become common behavioral characteristics.
   b. issues around independence and dependence will arise.
   c. acceptance and adherence to treatment become normative behaviors.
   d. she/he will accept full responsibility for management of the condition.
   e. she/he will seek companionship within the family.

3. An important part of discharge planning for the child and family would be:
   a. making sure the child completely understands the chronic illness/condition.
   b. ascertaining that the parents understand the long-term complications of the illness.
   c. coordinating efforts of different health care providers to ensure a timely discharge and follow-up.
   d. doing all of the discharge teaching during the hour before discharge.
   e. making sure that the child and family has fully accepted the diagnosis.

4. The parent of a child with a newly diagnosed chronic illness is very upset and tearful. To facilitate the parent's coping skills, the nurse asks, "Whom do you talk to when something is worrying you?" This action is:
   a. appropriate because it builds on prior adaptive coping behaviors.
   b. a part of the general assessment of the number of available social supports.
   c. inappropriate because the parent is too upset to think about the past.
   d. appropriate because it serves as a diversion from the present stressor.
   e. inappropriate because the parent needs to learn a new coping strategy.

5. The nurse comes into the room of a child who was just diagnosed with a chronic disability. The child's family begin to yell at the nurse about a variety of issues. Which of the following is the nurse's best response?
   a. "What is really wrong?"
   b. "Being angry is only natural."
   c. "Yelling at me will not change things."
   d. "Calm down, you're only making matters worse."
   e. "I will come back when you settle down."

6. Pui, 10, is very quiet and seems to prefer to be by herself in her room than to interact with others in the playroom or to engage in conversation with others. Her nurse is concerned that Pui is afraid to express her concerns, perhaps thinking that her illness is punishment for some misdeed. Which of the following interventions might be most helpful?
   a. Select age-appropriate books that reflect the situation or feelings the child might be experiencing and read them with her.
   b. Discuss her withdrawal with her family and encourage them to seek counseling for her obvious depression.
   c. Provide her family with a referral to therapy so she can learn more adaptive coping instead of relying on maladaptive behavior.
   d. Support her preference to be alone as this is probably reflects some cultural, ethnic, or religious belief.
   e. All of the above

7. Nursing interventions to help the siblings of a chronically ill/disabled child cope include which of the following?
   a. Explain to the siblings that embarrassment is unhealthy and they should think of their sibling's feelings.
   b. Encourage the family not to ask the siblings to help in the care for the child with special needs.
   c. Provide information to the siblings about the child's condition only if or as they request it.
   d. Suggest to the family ways of showing gratitude to the siblings when they help care for the ill child.
   e. Discourage sibling participation in decision making as it would be too stressful for them.

8. In terms of promoting long-term family integrity and functioning, nursing interventions should be based on:
   a. the assumption that, over time, most families become maladaptive.
   b. the fact that most families comply with medical management plans.
   c. families do better if information about the child's condition is carefully screened.
   d. encouraging family members to change their lifestyle and priorities for the child.
   e. establishing a trusting, collaborative relationship with the family.

STUDY QUESTIONS

9. Karl's family is distrustful of the medical system and wants to use a spiritual healer. The best response would be:
   a. "We really can't support that option as it might interfere with his other treatments."
   b. "I suppose it would be all right but I have never seen anything like that work."
   c. "Let's talk about it. Maybe we can develop a plan using both systems of healing."
   d. "Sure, you can do whatever you think you need to, but only when he is home."
   e. "Why would you think a spiritual healer would know better how to treat Karl?"

10. During admission for an exacerbation of a child's chronic condition, the mother comments that her son feels safest under her care. In planning interventions, the nurse should say:
    a. "Don't worry, the nurses are proficient at all procedures and can do them while he is in the hospital."
    b. "Your nurses will collaborate with you so you can participate in as much of your son's care as you want."
    c. "Great! You can do all of his usual care just as if he were home and the nurses will do the additional treatments."
    d. "I wonder if this exacerbation might be related in some way to the manner in which his treatment regimen has been managed."
    e. "This will be a good time for him to learn to receive care from someone else so you can have a break."

ANSWERS

1.a 2.b 3.c 4.a 5.b 6.a 7.d 8.e 9.c 10.b

Chapter 24

Chronic Conditions: Outcomes of Care

Joan P. Totka, MSN, RN, CDE

Concept

◆◆◆◆◆◆◆◆◆◆◆◆◆◆◆◆◆◆◆◆◆◆◆◆◆◆◆◆◆◆◆◆◆◆◆

◆ Children with a chronic condition, disability, or special health need and their families

Objectives

◆◆◆◆◆◆◆◆◆◆◆◆◆◆◆◆◆◆◆◆◆◆◆◆◆◆◆◆◆◆◆◆◆◆◆

At the completion of this chapter, the reader will be able to:

◆ Identify examples of outcomes related to a family and child's short-term responses; physical and emotional, to an acute illness episode during the course of a chronic illness (care/clinical/critical pathway).

◆ Identify examples of outcomes related to a family and child's long-term responses; both physical and emotional, to a chronic illness (case management).

◆ Identify the difference between outcomes based on nursing interventions and medical therapies for the care of chronically ill children.

Key Points

◆◆◆◆◆◆◆◆◆◆◆◆◆◆◆◆◆◆◆◆◆◆◆◆◆◆◆◆◆◆◆◆◆◆◆

◆ Tracking of nursing outcomes related to care paths or critical pathway and case management plans is essential for quality improvement.

◆ Selection of outcomes that are developmentally based and family focused assures that the unique aspects of pediatric nursing care are not lost.

◆ An enhanced quality of life should be strived for in all physiologic and psychosocial aspects of care.

24

Chronic Conditions: Outcomes of Care

◆◆◆◆◆◆◆◆◆◆◆◆◆◆◆◆◆◆◆◆◆◆◆◆◆◆◆◆◆

I. OVERVIEW

◆◆◆◆◆◆◆◆◆◆◆◆◆◆◆◆◆◆

Tracking patient family outcomes for children with chronic illness and their families is essential for maintaining quality nursing care, changing practice, and justifying current care.

A. Health care practices must be quality based and cost effective .
1. Cares and interventions must be scrutinized on a regular basis.
2. Value is maintained through outcome-based quality improvement measures that reflect quality, process and resource use (Arford & Allred, 1995; Pierce, 1997).

B. Tracking outcomes related to nursing based interventions is the best method to systematically evaluate nursing care.
1. Historically outcome measures were variable.
2. It is difficult to compare one site to another (Grady & Wojner, 1996).
3. Nurses can develop systems to track outcomes that can be compared from site to site using taxonomies such as nursing outcomes classification (NOC) (Johnson & Maas, 1997).
4. Good outcome data can justify the need for professional nursing care.
5. Outcome data that is sensitive to nursing intervention can reflect effective nursing practice.

C. Outcomes that reflect child's growth and development during chronic illness (based on Green, 1994; Johnson & Maas, 1997).
1. Child development outcomes.
   a. Physical growth and development.
   b. Social growth and development.
   c. Development of verbalization.
   d. Development of mobilization.
   e. Development of eye hand coordination.
   f. Play.
   g. School performance and progression.
   h. Socially appropriate behavior and safety practices.
   i. Personal responsibility for behaviors.

   j. Transition to adulthood.
2. Grief resolution and coping related to chronic illness.
   a. Adjustment to actual or impending losses.
   b. Acceptance of health care regimen.
   c. Acceptance of health status.
3. Outcomes that reflect family cohesiveness, coping, and grief resolution.
   a. Caregiver/family emotional health.
   b. Caregiver/family home care readiness.
   c. Caregiver/family lifestyle disruption.
   d. Caregiver/family/child relationships.
   e. Caregiver/family performance: direct care.
   f. Caregiver/family performance: indirect care.
   g. Caregiver/family physical health.
   h. Caregiver/family stressors.
   i. Caregiver/family well-being.
   j. Caregiver/family endurance potential.
4. Physiologic outcome parameters.
   a. Bowel elimination.
   b. Circulation status.
   c. Electrolyte and acid/base balance and hydration.
   d. Endurance.
   e. Fluid balance.
   f. Immune status.
   g. Muscle function.
   h. Nutritional status.
   i. Oral health.
   j. Quality of life.
   k. Respiratory status: gas exchange and ventilation.
   l. Rest and sleep.
   m. Thermoregulation.
   n. Thermoregulation: neonate.
   o. Tissue integrity: skin and mucous membranes.
   p. Urinary elimination/continence.
   q. Ambulation: walking or wheelchair.
   r. Self-care: all activities of daily living (use those that apply).
   s. Joint movement: active and passive.
   t. Bone healing.
   u. Wound healing: primary and secondary intention.

II. CARE PATHS DURING AN ACUTE EXACERBATION OF CHRONIC ILLNESS: OUTCOMES OF CARE

◆ ◆ ◆ ◆ ◆ ◆ ◆ ◆ ◆ ◆ ◆ ◆ ◆ ◆ ◆ ◆ ◆ ◆ ◆

A. An outcome-based care path (clinical pathway or critical pathway) guides care.
   1. Invaluable for tracking variances and evaluating the care given during an acute illness.
   2. Day-to-day plan of care developed to achieve patient outcomes within a certain time frame.
   3. Outcomes associated with a care path are short-term; a resolution of an acute phase of an illness trajectory.
   4. Care paths must be developed within a multidisciplinary forum; these are often called collaborative practice teams (see Table 24-1)

B. Care path principles.
   1. A care path promotes standard level of care for child/ family.
      a. Collaborative practice protocols can be used concurrently with care path.
         (1) Collaborative practice protocols outline specific medical aspects of the care path: it is the delegation of medical care.
         (2) All parties must sign the protocol.
      b. Standard physician order sets should reflect care path/protocols.
         (1) Helps to avoid missed orders/consults on the path.
         (2) Reduces delays in care while waiting for orders.
   2. Quality of care demonstrated by tracking key outcomes.
      a. Must have systems in place to maintain and analyze data base.
         (1) Human resources assigned to the project.
         (2) Computer resources available.
            (a) Integrated with the hospital system (ideal).
            (b) Accessibility/availability of data reports to caregivers.
      b. Must have standard method to collect data.
         (1) Specific person assigned.
         (2) Data collection through a computer data base.
   3. Identify key outcomes to assess progress.
   4. Care path should guide care toward achieving outcomes.
      a. All documentation should reflect progression toward health/outcomes
      b. All documentation should reflect key aspects of care path.

C. Family response to diagnosis.
   1. Grief is an expected response to the diagnosis of chronic illness.
      a. Expression of grief may vary widely.
      b. Grief impacts extended family members strongly, especially grandparents and may strongly influence parents' response
   2. Denial is often an important coping mechanism.
      a. Parent may deny diagnosis but not withhold care.
      b. Child's response to care helps convince parents and child.
   3. Differences in the grief response of each parent is common.
      a. Parents may not be emotionally ready to support each other.
      b. Blame and guilt hamper their ability to support and be supported.

D. Knowledge outcomes: teaching a family newly diagnosed with a chronic illness (see Table 24-1).
   1. Give concrete information only during high stress times.
      a. When and how to provide immediate care are more important to the family than the details about pathophysiology and etiology.
      b. Skills and tasks should be taught first.
         (1) Parents are fearful of what they do not know.
         (2) Parents are empowered when they know how to do.
   2. Focus on information necessary to care for the child for the next 24 hours.
      a. Give them a schedule of cares for the next day: forever is overwhelming.
      b. Focus on only the "need to know" information at first.
         (1) Need to know includes information needed for the next days.
         (2) Any high level or theoretical information should be deferred.
   3. Give information in small doses and repeat as often as possible.
      a. Use as many ways as possible to provide information.
         (1) Verbal teaching.
         (2) Written information.
         (3) Videos and tapes.
         (4) Demonstration.
         (5) Analogies (e.g., the heart is like a pump).
      b. Use problem-solving examples to assess learning.
         (1) Assess the behaviors needed to achieve health.
         (2) Assess content related to daily health behaviors only at first.

Table 24-1
Clinical Pathway: Type 1 Diabetes

DRG: 295 Diabetic Ketoacidosis
Expected LOS: 1.5

Name:
DOB:
MR:
PMD:

Aspect of Care	1st Hour (First labs Drawn) EDTC Date: Time start:	Hour 2-24 Date: Time end:	Day 2 Date:
Physiologic Standards			
LABS	Blood: Glucose, pH, electrolytes, A1C BUN, creatinine Urine: Dip for ketones Critical DKA: pH<7.15 HCO3<10 Serious DKA: pH 7.15-7.25 HCO3 10-16 Mild DKA: pH 7.25-7.35 HCO3 16-18	Blood: Critical DKA: Glucose, pH, electrolytes q hour Serious DKA: Glucose, pH, electrolytes q 1hour until HCO3 > 15 then q 4 hours Mild DKA: Glucose pre-meal , HS, 2400, 0300, repeat electrolytes X 1 Urine: Ketones q void until neg.	Blood: Glucose pre-meal, HS, 2400, 0300 Urine: Ketones q void until negative
Outcomes	Identify level of DKA Admit if DKA present or any signs of concurrent illness	**Electrolyte & acid/base Balance achieved***	**Negative ketones*** Glucose 70-400
ASSESSMENT/ MONITORING (KEY SYSTEMS)	Respiratory: Fruity breath, Kussmaul breathing Hydration, neuro status Baseline vital signs Any signs of concurrent illness Accurate weight in kg.	Critical DKA: Neuro checks, cardiac monitor x 24 hours, VS q hr. Serious DKA: Neuro checks, VS q 1 hr. x 4 then q 4 hr. Mild DKA: VS q 4 hr. x 1 then q shift.	VS q shift Accurate weight in kg. Accurate height in cm.
Outcomes		No cerebral edema, no cardiac arrhythmias, arrest	Maintains/ regains weight
IV FLUIDS Maintenance = 100 x 1st 10 kg + 50 x 2nd 10 kg + 25 x > 20 kg	If Serious to Critical DKA or if Mild DKA & unable to tolerate PO then: Bolus: 20mo/kg LR or NS over first hour Repeat if in hypovolemic shock If Mild DKA & tol. PO then no IV	Serious to Critical DKA: 0.45NS 20 mEq Kphos 20 mEq Kacetate Rate: (85ml/kg + Maint.)- bolus(s) 23 Add D5 when glucose < 250 Add K+ if K+ drops < 3.0	DC IV if tolerates adequate PO fluids
Outcome	No shock	Neuro status maintained No cardiac arrhythmias/arrest	Hydration maintained
MEDICATIONS	If Serious to Critical DKA or if Mild DKA and unable to tolerate PO Insulin drip 0.1 u/kg Mannitol 1 gm/kg at bedside K+ PO/IV if K+ < 3.0 If Mild DKA and able to tol. PO then insulin SQ per MD order	Serious to Critical DKA: Insulin drip 0.1 u/kg until electrolytes WNL Mannitol 1 gm/kg at bedside until off insulin drip Glucose falls no more than 100 mg/dl/hr	Insulin SQ per MD order (give ½ hour before insulin drip turned off)
Outcome		No cerebral edema	Electrolyte & acid/base balance maintained
NUTRITION	Serious to Critical DKA: NPO Mild DKA and able to tolerate PO then push sugar free fluids: (Minimum per age) <1: 2 oz./hr x 16 hr. 1-3: 3 oz./hr x 16 hr. >4: 4 oz./hr. x 16 hr.	Critical DKA: NPO x 24 hr. Mild to Serious DKA: NPO until electrolytes corrected or per Endocrinology service order only. When able to drink: push sugar free fluids per age guideline.	Basic Meal Plan (In Safe at Home Book) per age Push sugar free fluids
Outcome		Neuro status maintained	Nutritional status/ hydration maintained
Behavioral/ Developmental			
TEACHING	Assess family knowledge/ experience with Type 1 diabetes Assess best way to learn and any barriers to learning (language, literacy, etc.) Begin teaching skills with 1st SQ Use Safe at Home with Diabetes book**	Once DKA at Mild level RN will: 1. Show Real Ins and Outs video** 2. Family to learn/do SQ dose 3. Family to learn/do blood sugar tests 4. Family to learn/do urine ketone test 5. Basic Meal Plan/ Schedule reviewed	On Day 2: 1. Show Balancing Highs and Lows video** 2. High and Low signs/ symptoms and treatment 3. Continue 2-5 from day 1 4. Family to draw mixed insulin
Outcomes	Identify factors that may affect learning	Family to learn/do all skills (2-4) Family has home schedule completed	Knowledge: Treatment regimen- daily cares

(Table 24-1 continues on next page)

Table 24-1
Clinical Pathway: Type 1 Diabetes (continued from previous page)

Family Centered			
FAMILY SUPPORT/ COPING	Prepare family for diagnosis of Type 1 diabetes Consult Diabetes MSW Consult Diabetes CNS	Usual coping methods assessed Developmentally appropriate methods for initiating invasive procedures presented to family	Family support systems assessed Plans for return to work and school assessed
Outcomes	Family grief acknowledged (ongoing)	**Child and family able to cope with procedures*** Home Nursing Care arranged for 1st injection after discharge	**Child and family plan to return to usual activities*** School Health Plan **given to the family
Health System			
PLACEMENT Discharge Criteria	Critical DKA- Intensive care unit Serious DKA- 7th floor (or 4th floor per Critical Care MD) Mild DKA- after electrolytes correct, no concurrent illness- may arrange for care outpatient Transition coordination to order blood sugar meter and home health nursing.	If all Day 1 outcomes achieved and no other concurrent illness, may finish plan outpatient Has blood sugar meter. Urine ketone strips ordered from pharmacy	All Day 2 Outcomes achieved or a plan to meet needs outpatient identified
CONSULTS	Pediatric Endocrine Case Manager Pediatric Social Worker Pediatric Dietitian ASR Finance	Home supplies prescription signed Discharge orders to reflect follow up care and plans faxed to Home Nursing Care agency **Follow up Diabetes Clinic appt. scheduled.***	Home Supplies prescription signed Discharge orders to reflect follow up care and plans faxed to Home Nursing Care agency Has blood sugar meter. **Follow up Diabetes Clinic appt. scheduled.***
Safety			
HEALTH AND SAFETY			Up to date in immunizations Wears well fitting shoes Wears helmet when appropriate Use of seatbelts/ pads Good oral hygiene Use of sharps container for disposal
Outcome			General health care maintained

* Tracked outcome   **Videos and teaching materials available through Maxishare 1-800-444-7747   © Totka, J. P., Children's Hospital of Wisconsin

E. Discharge planning: the key to maintaining outcomes through transition.
 1. Follow-up care should be scheduled before discharge.
 2. Follow-up care plan should be negotiated with family.
 3. Supplies needed should be assembled before discharge.
 4. Need for home health personnel should be assessed and scheduled.
   a. Example: home nurse to reinforce teaching.
   b. Example: home rehabilitation therapy.
 5. Need for home inspection assessed and done before discharge.
   a. Example: home checks for asthma triggers.
   b. Example: house able to receive special equipment.
 6. Schools able to accommodate cares.
   a. Information given to schools.
   b. Health care plan for schools.
     (1) Includes cares needed in the school.
     (2) Includes family and school responsibilities.
   c. Home schooling arranged if unable to safely treat at school.
     (1) Home schooling is least attractive option.
     (2) Incorporation back into school is long-term goal.
 7. Family aware of their resources and parameters to seek care.
   a. Discharge orders reflect when to call, whom to call.
   b. Family has access to phone or plan for maintaining communication.
   c. Discharge orders reflect an inpatient nurse's report to home care.

III. CASE MANAGEMENT PLAN TO TRACK LONG-TERM OUTCOMES

◆ ◆ ◆ ◆ ◆ ◆ ◆ ◆ ◆ ◆ ◆ ◆ ◆ ◆ ◆ ◆ ◆ ◆ ◆

A. Exacerbations and remissions reflected not only in physical parameters but emotional and coping parameters as well.
 1. Psychologic wellness and coping behaviors have impact on outcomes of health and quality of life as well as level of disability or impairment.
 2. Outcomes must not only reflect physiologic parameters, but psychosocial parameters as well.

3. Overall quality of life is the desired outcome for the children with chronic illness and their families.
4. Outcome quality is directly dependent on the knowledge, skills, abilities, efforts and motivations of the patient (Pierce, 1977, p. 6) See Table 24-2 for an example of an outcome-based case management plan.

B. Grief resolution in chronic illness: outcomes for parents and children.
1. Feelings of loss may be triggered at different times.
   a. Losses may be relived at ages of expected milestones.
      (1) Developmental milestones.
      (2) Social milestones.
   b. Losses may be impacted by date or time of year.
      (1) Anniversary date of diagnosis.
      (2) Holidays, birthdays, and special events.
2. Course of illness can impact grief response.
   a. Decline of health, complications.
   b. Resurgence of symptoms after remission.
3. Assessment of resolution includes the following (adapted from Johnson & Maas, 1997):
   a. Expressions of feelings.
   b. Verbalizations of acceptance.
   c. Describe personal meanings associated with illness.
   d. Describes personal feelings associated with illness.
   e. Discusses unresolved conflicts.
   f. Reports absence of sleep disturbance.
   g. Seeks social/peer support.
   h. Expresses positive expectations of the future.
      (1) Dreams.
      (2) Goals.
      (3) Hope.

C. Knowledge outcomes in ongoing care of chronic illness.
1. Ongoing knowledge and self-care needs include:
   a. Higher level self-management issues.
      (1) Family anticipation of needs and care.
         (a) Understanding when and whom to call.
         (b) Anticipating changes in health status.
      (2) Family adaptation of illness into life events.
         (a) Incorporating cares with family vacations/travel.
         (b) Incorporating cares on odd schedule days.
      (3) Family use of knowledge to promote optimum health.
         (a) Adjusting regimen to respond to other activities.
         (b) Adjusting regimen in response to body changes.
   b. Advocacy issues.
      (1) Accessing health care.
      (2) Accessing supplies needed for care.
      (3) Accessing health care support in schools.
      (4) Ensuring participation/nondiscrimination in schools.
   c. Transition of child to adulthood.
      (1) Transferring care from parent to child.
      (2) Promoting interdependence versus independence.
      (3) Accessing adult health care.
      (4) Planning for career.

D. Caregiver support and family cohesion.
1. Promotion of shared responsibility of cares.
   a. Primary caregiver support.
   b. Appropriate transitions of care.
2. Promotion of family communication related to chronic illness.
   a. Sharing of feelings.
   b. Sharing of challenges.
   c. Sharing of information related to cares.
   d. Sharing data related to medical outcomes without judgment.
3. Promotion of family communication outside of chronic illness.
   a. Relationship not defined by illness or cares.
   b. Family time spent in activities unrelated to illness.
   c. Communication not centered on illness.

IV. OUTCOMES RELATED TO NURSING INTERVENTIONS VERSUS MEDICAL OUTCOMES

◆ ◆ ◆ ◆ ◆ ◆ ◆ ◆ ◆ ◆ ◆ ◆ ◆ ◆ ◆ ◆ ◆ ◆ ◆

A. Medical outcomes.
1. Physiology based.
   a. Lab results.
   b. Physical assessment parameters.
2. Morbidity and mortality.

B. Nursing outcomes.
1. Measurements of functioning and well being.
   a. Functional status.
      (1) Ability to perform activities of daily living.
      (2) Movement and range of motion.
   b. Development.
      (1) School performance and behavior.
      (2) Peer interaction and play.
      (3) Age-appropriate activities and interests.

Table 24-2
Case Management Plan Type 1 Diabetes

Name:
DOB:
MR:

PMD:

Aspect of Care related to Quality of Life	Diagnosis to 1 year Date of dx __/__/__	Year 1- Adolescence Date: __/__/__	Year 5 - Transition to Adult Care Date: __/__/__
Physiologic Standards			
LABS / TESTS	Blood: T4, TSH, thyroid antibodies, cholesterol (lipid panel if random > 200) A1C q 3-4 mon.	Blood: A1C q 3-4 mon. T4, TSH- yearly if positive antibodies T4, TSH, lipid panel, celiac screen- frequency determined by initial screen, family history and symptoms Urine: Ketone check in clinic if A1C >10 Eye exam baseline and q 3 years	Blood: Same as previous Urine: Screen for micro albumin every year Dilated eye exam yearly
Outcomes	**A1C < 8.5*** Baseline abnormalities identified	**A1C < 8.5*** Other labs WNL	**A1C < 8.5*** Same as previous: Normal eye exam
ASSESSMENT/ MONITORING (KEY SYSTEMS)	BP/Pulse, accurate ht. & wt. Units of insulin per kg. Growth velocity, BMI, Injection sites, rotation Gross neuro status Tanner Stage ER visits/hospitalizations	Same as previous Contractures Feet	Same as previous Eyes
Outcomes	**Maintain growth curve*** No lypohypertrophy or atrophy No DKA	**Maintain growth curve*** Same as previous Maintain usual physical maturation No DKA	**Maintain growth curve*** Same as previous No DKA
MEDICATION	Insulin: 0.5-0.8 u/kg pre-pubertal 0.8-1.5 u/kg post pubertal (less during honeymoon) 2/3 in AM; 1/3 in PM 1/3 H 2/3 N in AM 1:1 ratio of H:N in PM Thyroid meds as directed if needed (Insulin type choice per MD preference)	Same as previous Insulin-Move to N at HS H/N + H/0 + 0/N if: AM Hyperglycemia and/or Hypoglycemia during sleep Move to multiple injection regimen for increased control and/or lifestyle flexibility (3 shot, 4 shot, insulin pump) Consider other insulins as needed.	Same as previous Consider insulin pump as an option for increased control and/or flexibility
Outcomes	Usual u/kg and split of dose **75% of blood sugars in target range*** **(Target range individually defined)**	Same as previous Regimen fits current lifestyle **75% of blood sugars in target range***	Same as previous Treatment options explored **75% of blood sugars in target range***
NUTRITION	Family given age appropriate meal plan that incorporates nutrition and carbohydrate guidelines	Family able to adjust meal plan related to hunger and lifestyle needs	Patient given age appropriate plan that incorporates nutrition and carbohydrate guidelines with lifestyle needs. Importance of fat intake in management of weight and lipid levels discussed.
Outcomes	Ht/Wt ratios maintained Knowledge related to carb goals	Ht/Wt ratios maintained Family able to adjust meal plan Family knows carb goals	Ht/Wt ratios maintained Patient able to adjust meal plan: carb goals: Serum lipids WNL
Behavioral/ Developmental			
TEACHING	**Class 1:** Label reading/ Meal plan adjustments Coping with injections and pokes **Class 2:** Hypoglycemia: anticipation, treatment, exercise, glucagon Coping with chronic illness **Class 3:** Insulin Adjustment: goals of care, odd days and schedules, flexibility **Class 4:** Sick day: red flags, insulin supplement, fluid guidelines, diabetic ketoacidosis	15 ADA Content Areas: Covered in teaching plan and curriculum Anticipatory guidance related to adolescence issues Safety behaviors: Helmets, shoes, pads, etc. Follow up 1:1 visits when appropriate with Dietitian, Clinical Nurse Specialist or Social Worker	Same as previous Driving issues Fat intake goals Risk taking behaviors: potential risks and consequences ■ Alcohol/Drug ■ Sexuality ■ Birth Control ■ Pregnancy ■ Cigarette use
Outcomes	Family knowledge: Care management Appropriate use of team and hospital resources	Same as previous and Family knowledge: Anticipatory care for changes in management	Knowledge: Self care management

(Table 24-2 continues on opposite page)

Table 24-2
Case Management Plan Type 1 Diabetes (continued from opposite page)

DEVELOPMENT: Cognitive and Psychosocial	Baseline assessments of milestones of cognitive and psychosocial progressions: School: Performance and behavior Peers: Play, interaction and identification Interests and activities	Assessment of progression through milestones of cognitive and psychosocial development: School adaptation and progression Peers: Play interaction, identification with same sex peers Anticipatory guidance related to adolescent changes	Same as previous: Peers: maintains relationships with peers of both genders Body image and self esteem: acceptance and acknowledgment of changes
Outcomes	Child development in expected range **Grade level appropriate for age and cognitive ability***	Child development in expected range **Grade level appropriate for age and cognitive ability***	Child development in expected range **Grade level appropriate for age and cognitive ability***
Family Centered			
FAMILY COHESION	Baseline assessment related to: Roles and responsibilities of family members Communication styles of family members Discipline styles and limit setting Family activities Feelings of grief and loss related to chronic illness Coping behaviors	Ongoing status of previous assessment and: Transitions of care from parent to child: maintenance of shared responsibility Caregiver support and feelings related to daily cares Parent's relationships as partners and family interactions outside of cares	Ongoing status of previous assessment and: Interdependence with daily cares of diabetes Mutual support of family members Independence and autonomy issues Conflict resolution skills
Outcomes	Assess base level of family cohesion Grief resolution: process **Age appropriate transitions of cares***	Same as previous Caregiver/family emotional health **Age appropriate transitions of cares***	Same as previous Family relationships maintained Appropriate conflict resolution **Age appropriate transitions of cares***
Health System/ Community			
LIFE TRANSITIONS	School Health Care Plan **filled out School video** request filled out Information to coaches, other activity leaders	Same as previous Anticipatory guidance and support related to changes in school structure and teachers	Same as previous Anticipatory guidance and support related to adult responsibilities (driving, work, parenting, etc.) and transition to adult care providers
Outcomes	Care maintained in school setting Care maintained with sports/activities Health Care Plan at school	Same as previous Care maintained with school, schedule changes Health Care Plan at school	Same as previous Plans for the future Care maintained through change of health providers Health Care Plan at School
Safety			
HEALTH AND SAFETY	Up to date in immunizations Wears well fitting shoes Wears helmet when appropriate Use of seatbelts/ pads Good oral hygiene Use of sharps containers for disposal	Same as previous Yearly check with PMD Dentist visit 2x/year	Same as previous Obstetric/gynecology consult if appropriate
Outcomes	General health care maintained	Same as previous	Same as previous

*** Tracked outcome **Videos and teaching materials available through Maxishare 1-800-444-7747   © Totka, J. P., Children's Hospital of Wisconsin**

    (4) Anticipatory guidance.
  c. Family cohesion.
    (1) Roles and responsibilities of family members.
      (a) Transitions of care.
      (b) Interdependence.
    (2) Communication styles of family members.
    (3) Discipline styles.
    (4) Caregiver grief and support.

    (5) Grief related to chronic illness.
    (6) Intrafamily relationships.
      (a) Parent/parent relationships.
      (b) Parent/child relationships.
      (c) Sibling relationships.
  d. Life transitions.
    (1) Beginning/changing schools.
    (2) Career goals/planning.
    (3) Move to adult health care.

BIBLIOGRAPHY

◆ ◆ ◆ ◆ ◆ ◆ ◆ ◆ ◆ ◆ ◆ ◆ ◆ ◆ ◆ ◆ ◆

Arford, P.H. & Allred, C.A. (1995) . Value = quality + cost. *Journal of Nursing Administration, 25,* 64–69.

Grady, G.F., & Wojner, A.W. (1996). Collaborative practice teams: The infrastructure of outcomes management. *AACN: Clinical Issues, 7,* 153–158.

Green, M. (1994). *Bright futures: Guidelines for health supervision of infants, children and adolescents.* Arlington, VA: National Center for Education in Maternal and Child Health.

Harris, M.R., & Warren, J.J. (1995). Patient outcomes: Assessment issues for the CNS. *Clinical Nurse Specialist, 9,* 82–86.

Johnson, M. & Maas, M. (Eds.). (1997). IOWA *Outcomes project: Nursing outcome classification (NOC).* St. Louis: Mosby–Year Book, Inc.

Mark, B.A., & Burleson, D.L. (1995). Measurement of patient outcomes: Data availability and consistency across hospitals. *Journal of Nursing Administration, 25,* 52–59.

Pierce, S.F. (1997). Nurse-Sensitive health care outcomes in acute care setting: Integrative analysis of the literature. *Journal of Nursing Care Quality, 11,* 60–72.

Pridham, K. (1995). *Standards and guidelines for pre-licensure and early professional education for the nursing care of children and their families.* Washington, DC: D.H.H.S. Bureau of Maternal-Child Health. Document No. H112.

Turley, K.M., & Higgins, S.S. (1996). When parents participate in critical pathway management following pediatric cardiovascular surgery. *MCN, 7,* 133–145.

STUDY QUESTIONS

◆ ◆

1. An example of a short-term outcome related to an acute illness is:
   a. grief resolution.
   b. transition back to work or school.
   c. maintenance of functional status.
   d. caregiver/family emotional health.
   e. frequent teaching by the caregiver.

2. The purpose of a care path in acute illness is to:
   a. provide a standard of care during the illness.
   b. provide documentation of care plan.
   c. delegate the medical management.
   d. provide a format for the day-to-day care.
   e. assist the patient in getting through their morning. cares.

3. When a diagnosis of chronic disease is initially made, what should the teaching be focused on?
   a. Medical causes of disease/pathophysiology
   b. Long-term health risks/complications
   c. Tasks needed for the next 24 hours
   d. Promoting self-care of the child
   e. Preventing further medical complications from the chronic condition

4. The primary outcome of using a care path is:
   a. resolution of acute illness.
   b. tracking of patient outcomes.
   c. decreased length of stay.
   d. increased patient satisfaction.
   e. preventing future acute exacerbations of chronic illness.

5. An example of a long-term outcome goal related to chronic illness is:
   a. maintenance of adequate hydration.
   b. knowledge: treatment regimen, daily cares.
   c. caregiver grief resolution.
   d. more focused individual learning needs.
   e. decreased ability to adapt to hospitalization.

6. What is the main purpose of a case management plan for a child who is chronically ill?
   a. To provide a format for day-to-day care
   b. To provide a format for documentation
   c. To provide a template for assessments over time
   d. To provide a protocol to delegate medical care
   e. To provide developmentally appropriate care

7. Ongoing teaching of families who have a child who is chronically ill:
   a. is focused on self-management only.
   b. is necessary only if rehospitalized.
   c. is an inefficient use of nursing time.
   d. must be individualized.
   e. is instituted initially, but not on subsequent hospitalizations.

8. The primary outcome of a case management plan is:
   a. justification of nursing interventions.
   b. promotion of quality of life.
   c. promotion of patient and health care provider relationships.
   d. increased patient satisfaction.
   e. increased professional staff ratio used in the hospital.

ANSWERS

◆ ◆

1.b 2.a 3.c 4.a 5.c 6.c 7.d 8.b

Chapter 25

Chronic Conditions:
The Continuum of Care

Wendy M. Nehring, PhD, RN, FAAMR

Concept

◆◆◆◆◆◆◆◆◆◆◆◆◆◆◆◆◆◆◆◆◆◆◆◆◆◆◆◆◆

◆ Children with a chronic condition, disability, or special health need and their families

Objectives

◆◆◆◆◆◆◆◆◆◆◆◆◆◆◆◆◆◆◆◆◆◆◆◆◆◆◆◆◆

At the completion of this chapter, the reader will be able to:

◆ List the elements of care that must be attained for the ideal continuum of care to occur.

◆ Differentiate between models of professional collaboration.

◆ Describe the process a child and his or her family follow once the point of entry is made to a system of care.

◆ Define the process of case management and the roles and responsibilities of the case manager.

◆ Discuss unique aspects of care to be considered during age periods of prenatal, infancy, toddler and preschool, school-age, and adolescence.

◆ Identify factors important for successful transition to adult systems of care.

Key Points

◆◆◆◆◆◆◆◆◆◆◆◆◆◆◆◆◆◆◆◆◆◆◆◆◆◆◆◆◆

◆ The continuum of care for children with chronic illness and/or developmental disabilities must be individualized and developed, implemented, and evaluated by the child, caregivers, and a team of professionals.

◆ The continuum of care exists across all levels of care and is family-centered, coordinated, community-based, comprehensive, and culturally competent.

◆ Collaboration between a team of professionals and the family is essential.

◆ It is important that family experiences at the point of entry to a care system are positive and that the family feels their needs and concerns are being heard.

◆ There are age-related considerations for comprehensive systems of care for children with chronic illness and or developmental disabilities.

25

Chronic Conditions: The Continuum of Care

◆◆◆◆◆◆◆◆◆◆◆◆◆◆◆◆◆◆◆◆◆◆◆◆◆◆◆◆◆◆◆◆◆◆◆◆

I. THE CONTINUUM OF CARE IN CHRONIC CONDITIONS

◆◆◆◆◆◆◆◆◆◆◆◆◆◆◆◆◆◆◆◆◆

The continuum of care includes chronic illness and developmental disabilities; exists across all levels of care; must be family-centered, coordinated, community-based, comprehensive, individualized and culturally competent (National Maternal and Child Health Resource Center, 1989).

A. Levels of care.

1. Primary or well-child care consists of basic health services for medical monitoring, care of routine health problems, immunizations, and anticipatory guidance in the clinic or office setting. Services include:
   a. Health promotion and prevention.
   b. Routine acute illnesses and injuries.
   c. Ongoing management/monitoring of non-routine problems.
   d. Child and family education and counseling.
   e. Family support and networking services.
   f. Case management.
2. Secondary care consists of direct services by members of an interdisciplinary team and specialized consultants, as needed, for complex and unusual health problems in a community hospital setting. Services include:
   a. Complex and specialized interdisciplinary services.
   b. Child and family education and counseling.
   c. Education and training for primary health care providers.
   d. Development of a service and education plan for community.
3. Tertiary or specialized care consists of direct services by highly specialized members of an interdisciplinary team and specialized consultants, as needed, for complex and unusual health problems in a medical center or university health science center setting. Services include:
   a. Highly complex and specialized services by interdisciplinary team.

b. Child and family education and counseling.
   c. Education and training for primary health care providers and other professionals.
   d. Development of individualized hospital discharge plans.
   e. Development of collaborative community service projects.
   f. Research.

B. Family-centered care (FCC).

1. Family-centered care is considered the best practice in the care of children with chronic illness and/or developmental disabilities.
2. FCC is specified in state Title V programs and Part H of the Individuals with Disabilities Act of 1991 (renewed in 1997). *See Chapter 28: Family-Centered Care.*

C. Coordinated services.

1. Interagency collaboration may include links between:
   a. Primary health care providers.
   b. Public health programs.
   c. Community and regional hospitals.
   d. Early intervention programs.
   e. Early childhood daycare or preschool programs.
   f. Public and private schools.
   g. Special education programs.
   h. Community and special recreational programs.
   i. Medical and university health science centers.
   j. Voluntary agencies and specialized social service agencies across various geographica areas.
2. Benefits of coordinated services for families.
   a. Increased empowerment.
   b. Increased acceptance and support for families' decisions.
   c. Increased family and professional collaboration.
   d. Better assistance from professionals to meet identified needs of family.
   e. Identification and use of resources help to decrease need for help.
   f. Increased independence of family in accessing needed support and services.

g. Decreased fragmentation and/or duplication of services.
3. Benefits of coordinated services for professionals.
   a. Increased sensitivity to clients' needs increase depth of professional skills.
   b. Improved communication skills.
   c. Improved ease in working with a diverse clientele.
   d. Greater satisfaction in family and professional collaboration.
   e. Increased clarification of role and satisfaction with job.
4. Barriers to coordinated services.
   a. Mindset that the program or professional must address each identified family need.
   b. Coordination takes time and planning.

D. Community-based services.
1. Must be accessible.
2. Contract for service can be time-limited or long-term.
3. Care is given across the lifespan.
4. Services rendered by a system may be general or highly specialized.

E. Comprehensive services.
1. Many children with chronic illness and/or developmental disabilities do not require significant coordination of their care on an ongoing basis. For other children, constant coordination of care is essential.
2. Although most children will not require all of these services, a comprehensive list of services for children with chronic illness and/or developmental disabilities include:
   a. Ongoing, comprehensive primary, well-child, and preventive care according to American Academy of Pediatrics (AAP) guidelines.
   b. Periodic primary care for common childhood illnesses and injuries.
   c. Specialty medical care, including education, training, and consultations as needed.
   d. Durable and nondurable medical supplies and equipment.
   e. Durable and nondurable adaptive devices and assistive technology, including equipment for fine and gross motor needs and home adaptation.
   f. Mental health and social support services for individuals and family.
   g. Case management.
   h. Nursing services, including home and school.
   i. Medications.
   j. Special education from birth through age 21 years.

k. Diagnostic services, including lab work and x-rays.
l. Personal assistance services to aid with activities of daily living.
m. Respite care.
n. Physical, speech, and occupational therapies, including speech, language, vision, and hearing devices.
o. Community recreational programs, including toy-lending libraries and camps.
p. Transportation, including automobile modifications.
q. Vocation, rehabilitation, and habilitation programs.
r. Emergency services.
s. Family planning and genetic counseling for child and other family members.
t. Dental services.
u. Dietary services.
v. 24-hour access to medical information.
w. Legal and financial support services.

F. Culturally competent.
See Chapter 29: Cultural Influences.
1. Must consider the cultural and ethnic diversity of children in this country.
   a. 1 in 6 children have a foreign born mother.
   b. 1 in 9 children is born into a family living at less than half the poverty level (1995).
   c. 1 in 12 children has a disability (Children's Defense Fund, 1997).
2. Current lack of culturally diverse service providers.
3. Need for better outreach programs and services.
4. Barriers to improved culturally competent programs and services.
   a. Lack of community ownership.
   b. Racism.
   c. Lack of knowledge of cultural mores and beliefs.
   d. Lack of money and time to create and maintain programs in culturally diverse areas.
   e. Scarcity of minority health care providers.
   f. Insensitivity and lack of support among politicians and policy makers.

II. PROFESSIONAL COLLABORATION

◆ ◆ ◆ ◆ ◆ ◆ ◆ ◆ ◆ ◆ ◆ ◆ ◆ ◆ ◆ ◆ ◆ ◆ ◆

Various models of professional collaboration have arisen in the last half of the 20th century. These models include multidisciplinary, interdisciplinary, and transdisciplinary.

A. Multidisciplinary care.
1. Definition: multiple disciplines provide independent assessments of a child. The information is usually shared with the child and family by a coordinating physician.
2. Used most often during the 1960s and early 1970s. Increased use today by some physicians operating under managed care.

B. Interdisciplinary care.
1. Definition: a collaborative plan of care by various disciplines and the family. A case manager is often identified.
2. Used in the majority of cases by early interventionists and professionals in the University Affiliated Programs (UAPs – programs servicing individuals with developmental disabilities and their families through education, programming, research, and service) since the early 1960s.
3. First mentioned in the Education of the Handicapped Act Amendments of 1986 (P.L. 99-457) as services were mandated to be interdisciplinary.
4. Characteristics of interdisciplinary teams (Ducanis & Golin, as cited in Robinson, 1997).
   a. A team of two or more disciplines.
   b. Interactions may or may not be face-to-face.
   c. A case manager is identified, but this individual may change depending on the child's needs.
   d. Teams may be comprised of disciplines that are within and across organizational systems.
   e. Roles among the disciplines are clearly delineated.
   f. Active collaboration exists between the professionals and the family.
   g. The team is child and family-centered.
   h. Individual and team tasks are identified.
   i. The team operates under specific rules of operation.
5. Composition of the interdisciplinary team may include:
   a. Child and family members.
   b. Family support members (e.g. extended family, friends, professional friends, clergy).
   c. Developmental pediatrician.
   d. Nurse.
   e. Physical therapist.
   f. Occupational therapist.
   g. Speech and language pathologist.
   h. Special educator.
   i. Social worker.
   j. Other pediatric subspecialists (e.g., orthopedists, ophthalmologists, geneticists, neurologists).

C. Transdisciplinary care.
1. Definition: a collaborative process whereby the roles of the professionals and family members are blurred.
2. Usually a case manager who serves as the primary interventionist is identified and directly works with the child and his or her family to carry out the activities/interventions recommended by the other team members.
3. This model has achieved much use in early intervention programs since the 1980s, but was first described by nurses several years earlier (Haynes, 1976; Hutchinson, 1974).

III. MANAGED CARE

Due to the rising health care costs, managed care programs have surfaced in the 1990s. These programs have been designed to coordinate health care services at a manageable cost while still providing quality to its customers. Many states have instituted state-supported Medicaid managed care programs for persons of low income and persons with disabilities. The efficacy of these programs is not yet known. Managed care for persons with long-term health concerns, such as children with chronic illness and developmental disabilities, must include health, educational, and social service systems in the managed care plan. Such comprehensive plans are only in the initial stages and have only begun to be evaluated, although not longitudinally (Smith & Ashbaugh, 1996). *See Chapter 9: Influences of Regulatory Mechanisms and Policies of Health Care.*

A. Types of managed care insurance plans.
1. HMO (Health Maintenance Organization): a type of insurance plan that emphasizes preventive services and is usually the employer of the service providers.
2. PPO (Preferred Provider Organization): a type of insurance plan that offers a list of contracted providers that the customer chooses from.
3. POS (Point of Service): a type of insurance plan where the amount of reimbursement is equal to the contracted provider charges.

B. Integrated delivery networks: a conglomeration of contracted providers, including professionals and hospitals, that offer a comprehensive variety of health care services.
1. All levels of care, inpatient, outpatient, and home health services are included.
2. Offers "one-stop shopping" and lowered costs.
3. Has also been referred to as a system of care.

4. Few such networks offer additional educational and social services as part of the package that would be helpful for children with chronic illness and/or developmental disabilities.

IV. CASE MANAGEMENT

A. Definition: the collaborative provision of coordinated care by professionals from multiple disciplines, in one or more settings, over a stated period of time, to achieve specific outcomes (Trachtenberg & Lewis, 1996, p. 203)**.**

B. The case manager is usually the professional who will have the most input into the care of the child. For example, a physical therapist may be the best case manager for a child with cerebral palsy, whereas a nurse may be the best case manager for a child with diabetes.

C. Models of case management (Trachtenberg & Lewis, 1996).
1. Client driven: the case manager, along with the team, develops and implements the plan of care around the goals identified by the child and his or her family. The client holds the primary power.
2. Funding-stream driven: the plan of care is developed and implemented by the case manager and the team based on the payor's priorities for cost containment.
   a. Services may be rationed.
   b. The case manager and the client have no power.
3. Provider-driven: the case manager adheres to the treatment plans based on functional outcomes that are developed by the service provider/agency. The case manager and client have little power.
4. Although it would be ideal to have one case manager, often a child has two or more case managers from different systems. For example, a case manager is identified from the health care system and another case manager is identified from the insurance agency, each safeguarding different interests.

D. Responsibilities of the case manager.
1. Provides leadership and consultation.
   a. Identifies and prioritizes goals and outcomes.
   b. Plans for interventions and resources for implementing the care plan.
2. Provides background information on the child and his or her diagnosis.

a. Current plan of care.
b. Strengths and gaps of the plan are discussed.
3. Documents the team process,
   a. Information shared and decisions made.
   b. Sources of referrals and the family's financial information are discussed.
4. Evaluates present plan for quality, access, and cost.
5. Evaluates present plan for:
   a. Achievement of goals according to estimated time given.
   b. Readjusts plan according to need to successfully meet the goals.
   c. New or additional education, therapy, or social supports might be arranged to meet goals.

E. Credentials for case manager.
1. Master's degree provides best preparation.
2. Certification exam.
3. Practice guidelines for case management (Coeur, 1996).

V. POINT OF ENTRY

The child and his or her family enters the care system at diagnosis. Many sensory deficits, learning disabilities, and chronic illnesses are discovered during the preschool and school-age years. Chronic illnesses and developmental disabilities continue throughout the child's lifetime.

A. The initial point of entry is diagnosis.
1. The setting for telling the diagnosis must be free of distractions.
   a. Both parents should be present.
   b. Time should not be limited.
   c. Professional(s) present themselves in a collaborative, empathetic, and hopeful manner.
   d. Define the diagnosis, prognosis, etiology, symptomatology, and short and long-term health and social service needs.
   e. Use first-person language.
2. Allow time for questions, comments, and emotional reactions.
3. Give ways of reaching the professional(s) to parents.
4. Focus on the present status of the child and the immediate treatment goals and decisions.
5. Realize and inform the parents that early decisions will not "feel good" as the idealization of the child has been altered.
6. Initial assessment.
   a. Health history and physical examination of

the child, including a neurologic examination if needed. *See Chapter 4: Health, Psychosocial, and Developmental Screening and Assessment.*

   b. Gestational and birth history.

   c. Past surgeries and hospitalizations.

   d. Developmental milestones.

   e. Dietary history and current nutritional status.

   f. Daily care needs, including infusion therapy if needed.

   g. Educational/school history, including results of most recent psychometric tests.

   h. Assessment of the family's coping style. *See Chapter 12: Acute Illness: Effects on the Child's Family.*

   i. History of the family's past medical use.

   j. Current informal and formal support systems.

   k. Home environment, especially if adaptations will be needed.

   l. Transportation needs.

   m. Safety precautions.

   n. Financial status, including present insurance.

   o. Current list of health care providers for child and family.

7. Documented assessment in a life care plan is kept by the family and shared with each service provider across time. Additional information would include:

   a. Architectural modifications to the home and alterations to the automobile.

   b. A list of goals, including services and supplies needed, a beginning and ending date and age of child, frequency of use of supplies or replacement needs of equipment, costs, vendor(s), recommending service provider, and additional comments.

   c. Activity of daily living needs, including supplies, equipment, and personnel needs.

   d. Financial information (DiLima & Niemeyer, 1997).

B. Locations for point of entry.

1. Primary provider.
2. Subspecialty clinic or program.
3. Public health clinic.
4. Provider referral system.
5. University-affiliated program.
6. Community hospital.
7. University health sciences center.
8. Emergency room or urgent care centers.

C. Duration of services by providers or agencies.

1. Immediate (1 to 2 visits).
2. Short-term (weeks or months).
3. Intermediate (1 to 5 years; e.g. physical, occu-

pational and/or speech therapy).

4. Long-term (greater than 5 years; e.g. pediatrician or subspeciality services).

D. Illustration of movement through a system once entered (see Figure 25-1).

VI. Developmental Aspects

The continuum of care for children with chronic illness and or developmental disabilities changes somewhat as the child grows. Different considerations for care, treatment, consultation, educational, and social services are made prior to the child's birth and as the child ages. *See:*

Chapter 4: Health, Psychosocial, and Developmental Screening and Assessment
Chapter 5: Health Behavior
Chapter 9: Influences of Regulatory Mechanisms and Policies of Health Care
Chapter 12: Acute Illness: Effects on the Child's Family
Chapter 18: Acute Illness: Selected Acute Illnesses and Injuries

At each developmental stage, a physical examination and systems review for secondary disabilities and dysmorphology is necessary. Additional and unique requirements for care for each developmental period are discussed below.

A. Prenatal.

1. Genetic counseling and diagnostic studies. May be determined by the mother's age, ethnic background, consanquinity, or personal request.
2. Information is given on the diagnosis and options for carrying the fetus to term are presented.

B. Birth of infant.

1. Newborn neurodevelopmental screening should be completed. This screening should include:

   a. Primitive reflexes.

   b. Posture.

   c. Muscle tone.

   d. Axial tone.

   e. Deep tendon reflexes.

   f. Cranial nerve assessment.

   g. Sensory and behavioral responses.

2. Discharge planning is completed and links to community agencies made for specific diagnosis.
3. Financial assistance as necessary (e.g.,managed care plan, Medicaid, SSI, AFDC, state Medicaid subsidies).

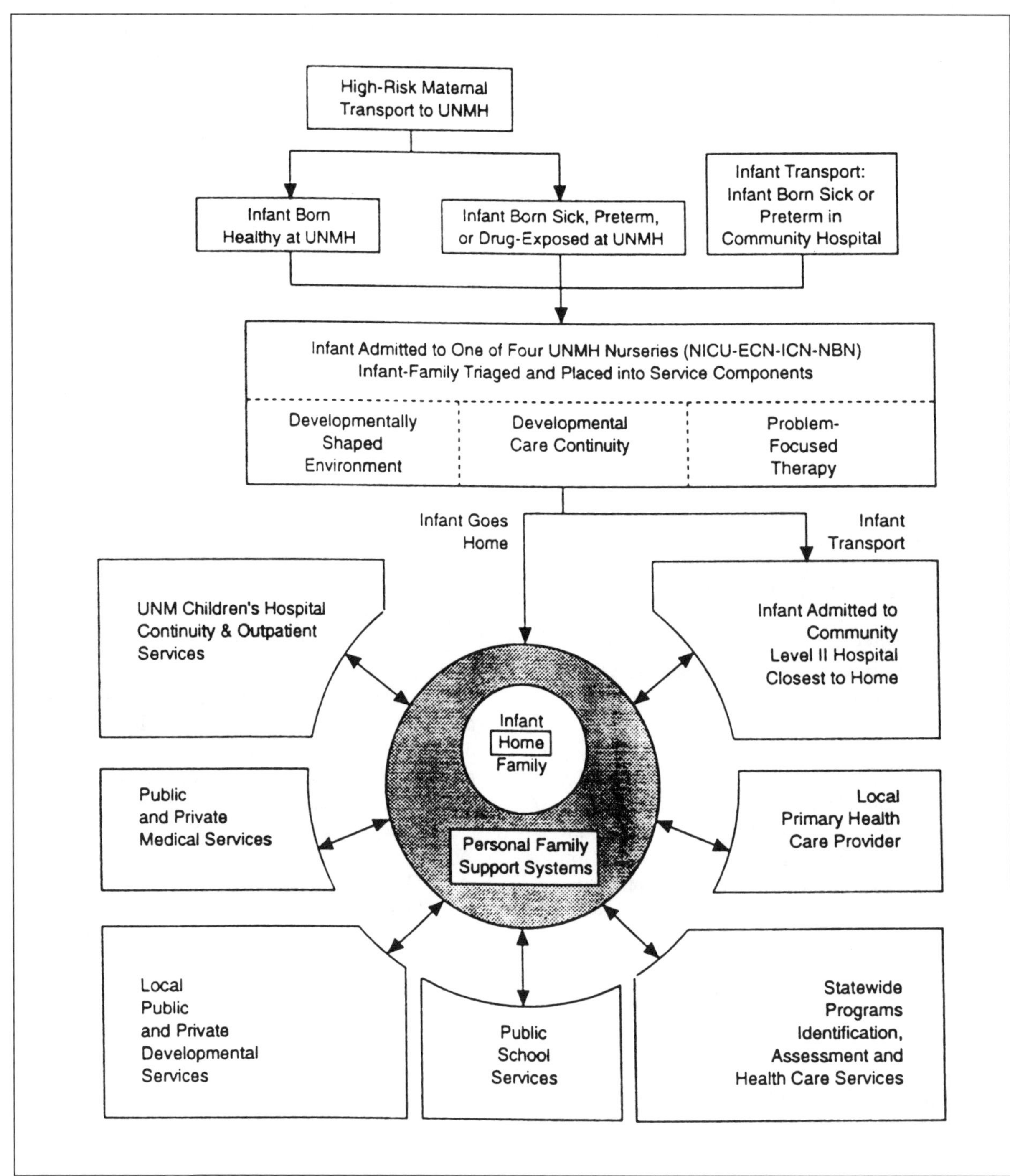

Figure 25-1. Infant-Family Care Continuum Between Hospital and Home/Community.

Reprinted with permission from Laadt-Bruno, G. (1993). Infant-family care continuum between hospital and home/community. Originally printed in Laadt-Bruno, G., Lilley, P.K., & Westby, C.E. (1993). A collaborative approach to developmental care continuity with infants born at-risk and their families. *Topics in Language Disorders, 14*(1), 15–28.

C. Infancy.

1. Infant neurodevelopmental screening should include primitive reflexes, posture, muscle tone, axial tone, deep tendon reflexes, cranial nerve assessment, and sensory and behavioral responses as described for the neonate above.
2. Developmental screening should be done at each primary care visit and referred for abnormal and at-risk results. Examples: Denver II Screening Exam (1 mo. to 6 yrs.), Ages and Stages Questionnaires (4 to 48 mos.), and the Batelle Developmental Inventory Screening Test (birth to 8 yrs) (Bricker et al., 1995; Drumwright & Frankenberg, 1973). *See Chapter 4: Health, Psychosocial, and Developmental Screening and Assessment.*
3. The infant should continue to be assessed for dysmorphology.
4. Growth parameters should be documented on a growth grid. Separate growth grids are available for children with Down syndrome.
5. Attendance in early intervention programs should be initiated if necessary. *See Chapter 9: Influences of Regulatory Mechanisms and Policies of Health Care.*
6. Case management needed when the child requires hospitalization. Provide prehospitalization preparation if possible, inpatient support, and discharge planning, including home health care and alterations in care plan.

D. Toddlers and preschoolers.

1. Continue to assess parent's knowledge of the diagnosis, treatment plans, medications, long-term prognosis, etc.
2. Developmental screening should be done at each primary care visit and referred for abnormal and at-risk results.
   a. Specific screening is done for sensory (e.g., hearing and vision) and language development.
   b. Examples of developmental screening tools include above plus the Early Language Milestone Scale (1 to 36 mos) and the Denver Articulation Screening Exam (2.5 to 6 yrs). *See Chapter 4: Health, Psychosocial, and Developmental Screening and Assessment.*
3. Child should continue to be assessed for dysmorphology.
4. Assess mobility needs: arrange for physical and or occupational therapy as needed.
5. Assess whether child knows his or her diagnosis and what care is necessary.

6. Begin to develop and implement age-appropriate goals for beginning self-management.
7. Assess for any behavioral issues and socialization experiences.
8. Case management needed when the child requires hospitalization. Provide prehospitalization preparation if possible, inpatient support, and discharge planning, including home health care and alterations in care plan.
9. Attendance in early childhood programs should be initiated if necessary. An Individualized Family Support Plan (IFSP) should be developed and implemented by the interdisciplinary team, which includes the family.

E. School-age.

1. Developmental screening done at each primary care visit; referred for abnormal and at-risk results. Specific screening is done for sensory, learning disabilities, and school-related problems. Screening must focus on cognitive, perceptual, and behavioral problems (Aylward, 1994). Examples of screening tools include the Goodenough-Harris Drawing Test (3 to 15 yrs), the Wide Range Achievement Test-revised (5 to 75 yrs) and the Conners Behavior Scales (3 to 17 yrs). *See Chapter 4: Health, Psychosocial, and Developmental Screening and Assessment.*
2. A functional assessment of the child's ability to carry out his or her activities of daily living. Example of a standardized measure is the WeeFIM (A Pediatric Functional Independence Measure for Neurodevelopmental Disabilities) (6 mos to 7 yrs) (WeeFIM, 1998).
3. School assessment for placement in specialized programs. Full inclusion currently recommended. Children with severe cognitive and behavioral problems often require specialized educational settings. An IEP (Individualized Education Plan) should be developed and implemented by the school's interdisciplinary team, which includes the family. For further discussion of the rights and rules governing the child with special needs in the classroom. *See Chapter 9: Influences of Regulatory Mechanisms and Policies of Health Care.*
4. Assess for family roles and responsibilities, focusing on whether the affected child performs chores and is treated similar to the other siblings.
5. Case management needed when the child requires hospitalization. Provide prehospitalization preparation if possible, inpatient support, and discharge planning, including home health care and alterations in care plan.

F. Adolescents.
  1. Gynecologic care begins for girls. Sexuality and concerns regarding sexuality specific to the diagnosis are discussed. *See Chapter 5: Health Behavior.*
  2. Assessment of school progress and placement done. An IEP plan should be developed.
     a. Vocational or higher education plans.
     b. Development and implementation of a prevocational program begins at age 14 years and no later than 16 years for students not planning on attending higher education settings.
     c. Contact Department of Rehabilitation Services (DORS) as needed.
  3. A functional assessment of the adolescent's ability to carry out his or her activities of daily living should be completed. The adolescent should be fully independent in carrying out these tasks.
  4. Assess driver's education opportunities and acquire adaptive equipment and automobile alterations, if necessary.
  5. Assess adolescent's knowledge of his or her diagnosis, medications, what care is necessary, and how to contact their primary health care provider. The adolescent should be self-managing his or her own care.
  6. Case management needed when the adolescent requires hospitalization. Provide prehospitalization preparation if possible, inpatient support, and discharge planning, including home health care and alterations in care plan.

G. Transition to adulthood and adult care. An Individualized Transition Plan is developed.
  1. Evaluate the adolescent's knowledge of the diagnosis, plan of care, medications, and health care and social service providers.
     a. Knows where to go for health care.
     b. Can verbalize health care concerns and needs.
     c. Knows where to get social support services.
     d. Knows where to purchase medications and medical supplies.
  2. Plan for and implement an independent living trial if needed. Plan in-home support services to assist with activities of daily living.
  3. Plan for career choices and assist with educational plans or vocational placement.
  4. Plan for independent financial status.
     a. Insurance.
     b. SSI and or Medicaid.
     c. Job income.
  5. Barriers to transition.
     a. Adult care provider knowledge and skills related to diagnosis and adult manifestations

of the diagnosis. Trend is toward pediatric health care providers continuing with care of child into adulthood.
     b. Economic issues: insurance coverage often decreased or eliminated at 21 years.
     c. Philosophic issues: adult care has been less developmentally oriented and family-centered.
     d. Readiness issues: attachment and trust in pediatric health care providers may interfere.
  6. Encourage the adolescent to become a self-advocate.
  7. Public policy.
     a. Rehabilitation Act of 1973 (PL 93-112) and Rehabilitation Act Amendments of 1992 (PL 102-569). *See Chapter 9: Influences of Regulatory Mechanisms and Policies of Health Care.*
     b. Americans with Disabilities Act (PL 101-336).

VII. ADDITIONAL CONSIDERATIONS

A number of additional aspects affect the continuum of care for children with chronic illness and/or developmental disabilities. These include disease progression, institutionalization, foster care, nonstandard therapies, and standards of care and care guidelines.

A. Disease progression.
  1. Frequent hospitalizations.
  2. Cyclic course of active treatment to period of no treatment during remissions.
  3. Terminal care and hospice. *See Chapter 6: Separation, Loss, and Bereavement.*

B. Institutionalization.
  1. Children with severe disabilities and/or behavioral problems may require residential placement.
  2. Comprehensive planning is needed between the interdisciplinary team and the parents. Assistance in the move from home to residential placement is also required.

C. Foster care.
  1. Specialized foster care for children with special health care needs, including developmental disabilities and some chronic illnesses.
  2. Accessing health and social service providers according to state and/or agency policies.

D. Nonstandard therapies.
  1. Identify nonstandard therapies for specific diagnosis (e.g., megavitamins for children with Down syndrome).

2. Assess research base for any claims.
3. Assist parents to understand benefits versus risks for acquiring the therapies for their child.

E. Standards of care and care guidelines.

1. Standards of Nursing Practice for the Care of Children and Adolescents with Special Health and Developmental Needs (1994).
2. National Health and Safety Performance Standards Guidelines for Out-of-Home Child Care Programs (1997).
3. Statement on the Scope and Standards for the Nurse Who Specializes in Developmental Disbilities and/or Mental Retardation (1998).

BIBLIOGRAPHY

◆ ◆

Aylward, G.P. (1994). *Practitioner's guide to developmental and psychological testing*. New York: Plenum.

Bricker, D., Squires, J., Mounts, L., Potter, L., Nickel, R., & Farrell, J. (1995). *Ages and stages questionnaires (ASQ)*. Baltimore: Brookes.

Children's Defense Fund. (1997). *The state of America's children yearbook*. Washington, DC: Author.

Coeur, M. (Ed.). (1996). *Case management practice guidelines*. St Louis: Mosby.

Consensus Committee and the Maternal and Child Health Bureau (1994). *Standards of nursing practice for the care of children and adolescents with special health and developmental needs*. Washington, DC: American Nurses Association.

DiLima, S.N., & Niemeyer, S. (Eds.). (1997). *Caregiver education guide for children with developmental disabilities*. Gaithersburg, MD: Aspen.

Drumwright A.F., & Frankenburg, W.K. (1973). *Denver articulation screening exam (DASE)*. Denver: Denver Developmental Materials, Inc.

Haynes, U. (1976). Highlights of the UCPA project. In Programming for atypical infants and their families. Monograph 2. New York: United Cerebral Palsy Associations, Inc.

Hutchison, D. (1974). A model for staff development: Transdisciplinary teams. In *The first three years: Programming for atypical infants and their families*. New York: United Cerebral Palsy Associations, Inc.

Krajicek, M., & the Maternal and Child Health Bureau (1997). *National health and safety performance standards guidelines for out-of-home child care programs*. Rockville, MD: Maternal and Child Health Bureau and the University of Colorado Health Sciences Center.

Laadt-Bruno, G., Lilley, P.K., & Westby, P.E. (1993). A collaborative approach to developmental care continuity with infants born at-risk and their families. *Topics in Language Disorders, 14*(1), *15–28*.

National Maternal and Child Health Resource Center (1989). *A national goal: Building service delivery systems for children with special health care needs and their families: Family centered, community-based, coordinated care*. Iowa City, IA: National Maternal and Child Health Resource Center.

Nehring, W.M., Roth. S., P., Natvig, D., Morse, J.S., Savage, T., & Krajicek, M. (1998). *Statement on the scope and standards for the nurse who specializes in developmental disabilities and/or mental retardation*. Washington, DC : American Nurses Association and the American Association on Mental Retardation.

Robinson, C. (1997). Team organization and function. In H.M. Wallace, J. C MacQueen, R.F. Biehl, & J.A. Blackman (Eds.), *Mosby's resource guide to children with disabilities and chronic illness* (pp. 268–280). St. Louis: Mosby.

Sheldon, T.L., & Stepanek, J.S. (1994). *Family-centered care for children needing specialized health and developmental services* (2nd ed.). Bethesda, MD: Association for the Care of Children's Health.

Smith, G., & Ashbaugh, J. (1996). *Managed care and people with developmental disabilities: A guidebook*. Alexandria, VA: National Association of State Directors of Developmental Disabilities Services, Inc., and Human Services Research Institute.

Trachtenberg, S.W., & Lewis, D.F. (1996). Case management. In L.A. Kurtz, P.W. Dowrick, S.E. Levy, & M.L. Batshaw (Eds.), *Handbook of developmental disabilities: Resources for interdisciplinary care* (pp. 203–208). Gaithersburg, MD: Aspen.

STUDY QUESTIONS

1. The model of professional collaboration that defines a group of professionals who work together, using their expertise, along with the family to develop and implement a plan of care is:
   a. an unidisciplinary team.
   b. a multidisciplinary team.
   c. an interdisciplinary team.
   d. a transdisciplinary team.

Situation: Timmy, is a 4-year-old boy with cerebral palsy who lives in a rural town. He and his family travel to a large, urban medical center once a year for an annual physical and developmental evaluation by a group of professionals who, along with his parents, have developed and revised his plan of care. Throughout the year, his case manager, a physical therapist, visits Timmy in his home to assist in carrying out the plan of care.

2. To make sure that Timmy receives the ideal continuum of care, it is important that his plan is:
   a. family-centered, coordinated, comprehensive, community-based, individualized, and culturally-competent.
   b. family-centered, inexpensive, accessible, and physician-centered.
   c. community-based, accessible, physician-centered, and affordable.
   d. community-based, integrated in one building, disease-specific, and age-appropriate.

3. The model of professional collaboration that Timmy is receiving is:
   a. unidisciplinary.
   b. multidisciplinary.
   c. interdisciplinary.
   d. transdisciplinary.

4. Which of the following does not represent care appropriate for Timmy's developmental age?
   a. Well-child care
   b. Dietary assessment
   c. Developmental screening
   d. Individualized Transition Plan

5. Which model of case management is being used in Timmy's case?
   a. Client driven
   b. Funding-stream driven
   c. Provider-driven
   d. Federally driven

6. The responsibilities of the case manager includes:
   a. providing leadership and consultation to the team.
   b. discussing strengths and gaps in the current plan in preparation for revision.
   c. evaluating the present plan of care.
   d. all of the above.

Situation: Laura is a 16-year-old with spina bifida and hydrocephaly. She has been shunted and is currently having no difficulties. She attends high school where she takes some classes for students with learning disabilities. She would like to be a secretary when she graduates.

7. At what age is it mandatory that Laura receive prevocational training and services as a result of her disability?
   a. 12 years
   b. 14 years
   c. 16 years
   d. 18 years

8. It is very important that Laura is able to:
   a. declare her college major.
   b. perform her activities of daily living and manage her health care independently with minimal assistance.
   c. seek out her parents for assistance with health care concerns.
   d. tell all of her friends about her diagnosis and health history.

9. Sid and Connie have just had their first child who was born with Down syndrome. They learned of the diagnosis after an amniocentesis during pregnancy. At that time, it was important for the professionals involved in the care of Connie and her child to:
   a. discuss the diagnosis in a hopeful, empathetic, and value-free manner.
   b. tell Connie immediately of the diagnosis after the child was born.
   c. arrange to talk to the parents about the diagnosis at the 2-week visit.
   d. tell the parents that everything will be all right.

10. When developing a plan of care for a child with a chronic illness or developmental disability, the team of professionals and family should use which of the following as a template for planning?
    a. Standards of care
    b. Old nursing care plan
    c. A treatment plan for someone with the same diagnosis
    d. Care guidelines used at another service agency

ANSWERS

1.c 2.a 3.d 4.d 5.a 6.d 7.c 8.b 9.a 10.a

Chapter 26

Chronic Conditions: Selected Chronic Conditions

Janice Selekman, DNSc, RN

Concept

◆◆◆◆◆◆◆◆◆◆◆◆◆◆◆◆◆◆◆◆◆◆◆◆◆◆◆◆◆◆

- ◆ Children with a chronic condition, disability, or special health need and their families

Objectives

◆◆◆◆◆◆◆◆◆◆◆◆◆◆◆◆◆◆◆◆◆◆◆◆◆◆◆◆◆◆

At the completion of this chapter, the reader will be able to:

- ◆ Select a framework in which they can organize the pediatric content on chronic conditions within their existing curriculum.

- ◆ Identify selected chronic conditions that fit that framework.

- ◆ Prepare content so that students can make assessments, plan strategies of care and intervene in ways that promote the growth and development of the child with a chronic condition or disability.

- ◆ Identify multiple and varied approaches to presenting content related to the needs of children with chronic conditions.

Key Points

◆◆◆◆◆◆◆◆◆◆◆◆◆◆◆◆◆◆◆◆◆◆◆◆◆◆◆◆◆◆

- ◆ There are multiple frameworks available to organize content on chronic pediatric conditions.

- ◆ The study of each condition should be based in social and health care sciences and should include some components of pathophysiology, pharmacology, medical and nursing assessments and the rationales for them, and medical and nursing interventions and the rationales for them.

- ◆ Content related to the needs of children with chronic conditions can be taught in multiple and varied modalities, depending on the resources available.

26

Chronic Conditions: Selected Chronic Conditions

◆◆◆◆◆◆◆◆◆◆◆◆◆◆◆◆◆◆◆◆◆◆◆◆◆◆◆◆◆◆◆◆◆◆

I. OVERVIEW

◆◆◆◆◆◆◆◆◆◆◆◆◆◆◆◆◆◆

"A chronic condition, disability, or special need in children is a long-term condition resulting in ongoing concerns/lifestyle changes. The chronic condition may involve episodes of exacerbations and remissions. A developmental disability is a lifelong condition that originates before the age of 22 years and affects one or more areas of development and self-care activities" (Pridham, 1995).

II. SELECTED PROTOTYPE CONDITIONS

◆◆◆◆◆◆◆◆◆◆◆◆◆◆◆◆◆◆◆◆◆◆

Prototypes can be chosen to fit into the organizing framework of the curriculum.

A. Body systems.
1. Hematologic.
   a. Hemolytic anemia (sickle cell).
   b. Clotting disorders (hemophilia, idiopathic thrombocytopenic purpura).
2. Immunologic.
   a. Human Immune Deficiency Syndrome.
   b. Allergies (respiratory, food, and contact).
   c. Autoimmune disorders (lupus erythematosus).
3. Central nervous system.
   a. Sensory alterations (blindness, deafness).
   b. Learning disorders (learning disabilities and Attention Deficit Hyperactivity Disorder).
   c. Cognitive impairment (mental retardation/ Down syndrome).
   d. Motor impairment (cerebral palsy).
   e. Seizure disorders.
   f. Brain tumors and neuroblastoma.
4. Respiratory.
   a. Bronchopulmonary dysplasia.
   b. Asthma.
   c. Cystic fibrosis.
5. Cardiac.
   a. Congenital heart anomalies.
   b. Acquired heart conditions (rheumatic fever).
6. Gastrointestinal.
   a. Congenital anomalies (cleft lip and palate, esophageal atresia/tracheoesophageal fistula).
   b. Inflammatory conditions (Inflammatory Bowel Disease [Crohn's] and ulcerative colitis).
   c. Sequelae to necrotizing enterocolitis (Short Bowel Syndrome).
7. Genitourinary.
   a. Autoimmune conditions (nephrotic syndrome, glomerulonephritis).
   b. Cancer (Wilm's tumor).
8. Musculoskeletal.
   a. Congenital orthopedic conditions (hip dysplasia, clubfoot).
   b. Scoliosis.
   c. Juvenile rheumatoid arthritis.
   d. Muscular dystrophy.
   e. Bone tumors (osteogenic sarcoma).
9. Endocrine.
   a. Diabetes (Type I).
   b. Growth hormone alterations.
   c. Thyroid deficiency.
10. Mental health disorders.
    a. Autism.
    b. Eating disorders.
    c. Conduct disorders.
    d. Drug-exposed babies (cocaine, heroin, and fetal alcohol syndrome).
    e. Drug and alcohol abuse.

B. Developmental approaches.
1. Neonatal.
   a. Congenital anomalies.
   b. Problems of prematurity.
2. Infant.
   a. Chronic respiratory problems.
   b. Developmental delay.
3. Toddler.
   a. Chronic problems related to safety concerns (burns/ingestions).
   b. Cerebral palsy.
4. Preschool.
   a. Mental retardation.
   b. Renal problems.
5. School-age.

    a. Learning disabilities and Attention Deficit Hyperactivity Disorder.
    b. Diabetes.
    c. Cancer.
  6. Adolescence.
    a. Scoliosis.
    b. Drug and alcohol abuse.

C. Nursing diagnoses categories.
  1. Altered nutrition.
  2. Ineffective breathing.
  3. Anxiety.
  4. Potential for infection.
  5. Gastrointestinal irritation.

D. Most common national and regional conditions.
  1. Learning disorders/Attention Deficit Hyperactivity Disorder.
  2. Asthma.
  3. Mental and emotional problems.
  4. Sensory deficits.
  5. Cerebral palsy.
  6. Allergies.
  7. Congenital anomalies.
  8. Drug and alcohol problems.
  9. Cancer.
 10. Diabetes.

E. Fully integrated curriculum.
  1. Pediatric nursing faculty should provide pediatric-related content for each topic taught.
  2. Clinical experiences related to providing health care and/or nursing care for children 0–18 years should be included in one or multiple courses.

F. Health continuum.
  1. Provide a breadth of chronic conditions that have exacerbations, remissions, and sequelae.
  2. Focus on chronic conditions that are both limited and nonprogressive as well as progressive and terminal.

G. It is ideal to choose conditions that:
  1. Span the pediatric age ranges.
  2. Cover multiple organ system groups.
  3. Cover the health continuum (well, acute, chronic; recoverable, terminal).
  4. Cover genetic, idiopathic, and environmentally-caused conditions.

III. Selected Conditions

(presented alphabetically)

A. Acquired Immune Deficiency Syndrome (HIV Disease)
  1. The science.
    a. Children acquire Human Immunodeficiency Virus from the uterine and vaginal environment before and/or during birth, infected breast milk, and sexual and other contact with infected blood and body secretions.
    b. HIV is an ribonucleic acid (RNA) retrovirus and attacks the helper T cells (CD4) and depletes them; there are then more suppressor T cells than helper cells and the immune system is inefficient in its protective role.
    c. There is an 8–30% risk of perinatal transmission if the mother is HIV positive.
  2. Assessment.
    a. All infants born to HIV positive mothers will also be HIV positive. Most are NOT infected, but have passive antibodies from the mother.
    b. Infected children may have no symptoms: blood and body secretions are infectious.
    c. Assess status of the immune system (T4 count; ability to mount an immune assault).
    d. Assess for the following manifestations:
      (1) Failure to thrive; developmental delay; loss of developmental milestones.
      (2) Recurrent diarrhea.
      (3) Hepatosplenomegaly; lymphadenopathy.
      (4) Recurrent opportunistic infections.
        (a) Lymphoid interstitial pneumonia.
        (b) *Pneumocystis carinii* pneumonia.
        (c) Recurrent fungal infections, usually in the mouth (thrush) or diaper area.
  3. Interventions.
    a. Initiate universal precautions.
    b. Zidovudine is administered to pregnant women from their second trimester through delivery and then to the newborn.
    c. Observe for opportunistic infections.
    d. Administer monthly IV immune globulin to provide immune protection.
    e. Immunize as scheduled, but use inactivated polio vaccine.
    f. Make additional plans for the child if the parent is ill with HIV and/or engages in high risk behaviors.
    g. For the older child, instruct on modes of transmission of the virus.
    h. Instruct the family about infection control measures in the home.

B. Allergies.
  1. The science.
    a. Immediate hypersensitivity (or Type I

Allergy) is the most common type.
(1) Mediated by IgE that is made during the initial contact with an allergen, attaches to mast cells, and on subsequent contact with the allergen, results in degranulation of the mast cells and release of products such as histamine.
(2) Can result in anaphylaxis; reactions occur within minutes.
(3) Examples include hayfever and reactions to bee stings.
b. Delayed hypersensitivity (or Type IV Allergy) is T cell mediated and does not involve immunoglobulins.
(1) The reaction can occur within 48–72 hours.
(2) Examples include contact dermatitis, such as poison ivy.
c. The most common manifestations of allergies in children are respiratory, gastrointestinal, and dermatologic.
2. Assessment.
a. For respiratory allergies.
(1) Identify pattern of symptoms: seasonal, location.
(2) Conduct allergy skin testing to identify the cause.
(3) Note the following symptoms:
(a) Persistent sneezing.
(b) Rhinorrhea and nasal congestion.
(c) Complaints of itchy eyes, throat, and ears.
(d) Allergic shiners (dark circles under the eyes from edema).
(e) Allergic salute (wiping the nose straight up to free the turbinates); this results in a crease across the bridge of the nose.
(f) Open mouth breathing.
b. For gastrointestinal allergies.
(1) Identify food allergies: most common are cow's milk, shellfish, nuts, wheat, citrus, egg whites, chocolate.
(2) Differentiate between food allergies and food intolerance.
(3) Note time between contact and development of symptoms.
(4) Symptoms include vomiting, colic, diarrhea, or immediate skin reactions at the point of contact with the mouth.
c. For dermatologic allergies.
(1) Note location of rash.
(2) Note level of discomfort (irritable, complaining of itching).
(3) Note type of skin reaction (macular, dry, etc).

(4) If eczema is suspected:
(a) Note its relationship to foods, contact, temperature changes, bathing, sweating, and emotional factors.
(b) Check for lesions on areas prone to moisture.
(5) Note secondary infection from scratching.
3. Interventions.
a. For Type I reactions, administer antihistamines.
b. Relieve itching with antipruritics; apply cool compresses to eyes.
c. Avoid contact with allergen.
(1) Keep indoors during high pollen counts or when grass is cut.
(2) Use damp dusting, frequently.
(3) Avoid smoking in the child's environment.
(4) Decrease use of products that collect dust (curtains, clutter).
(5) Discourage use of natural fibers (wool).
(6) Read food labels carefully.
d. Keep nails short to decrease scratching.
e. Keep affected skin areas covered with light cotton clothing.
f. Eczema.
(1) Keep the child dry.
(2) Avoid heat and sweating.
(3) Bathe only twice a week and without soap.
(4) Apply topical emolients after bathing and pat dry.
(5) Use a cortisone cream to decrease inflammation.
g. Administer allergy shots, if appropriate.

C. Asthma/reactive airway disease.
1. The science.
a. Characteristics include airway obstruction that may be reversed, airway inflammation, and hyperreactive airway responsiveness to stimuli.
b. Attacks can be caused by allergens, viral infections, exercise, and irritants, such as dust and cold air.
c. Bronchospasm occurs early, followed by inflammation of mucous membranes and increased mucus secretion; can lead to airway obstruction and air trapping.
2. Assessment.
a. Respiratory distress.
(1) Use of accessory muscles; prolonged expiratory effort.
(2) Unequal or decreased breath sounds.
(3) Wheezing may or may not be present; usually expiratory.

(4) Flat diaphragm on x-ray and barrel chest due to air trapping.
(5) Increased pCO_2 and decreased pO_2.
b. Nocturnal cough in the absence of infection.
c. Shortness of breath with exercise.
3. Interventions during an attack.
a. Provide oxygen.
b. Sit child upright or raise the head of the bed.
c. Administer bronchodilator and corticosteroid.
d. Administer fluids, intravenously if necessary.
e. Maintain a calm environment.
f. Be aware that failure to resolve the bronchospasm and inflammation results in status asthmaticus and can be fatal.
4. Interventions to prevent an attack.
a. Take environmental measures to avoid contact with the allergen or offending irritant.
b. Administer cromolyn sodium by inhalation to prevent mast cell degranulation.
c. Teach child breathing exercises to increase ventilatory capacity.
d. Forbid smoking in the child's environment.
e. Teach child to monitor his or her respiratory status with a peak flow meter.
f. Teach the child to use a metered dose inhaler and a spacer.
g. Initiate asthma education for the child and family.

D. Attention Deficit Hyperactivity Disorder (ADHD).
1. The science.
a. ADHD is defined as a persistent pattern of inattention and/or hyperactivity-impulsivity that is more frequent and severe than is typically observed in individuals at a comparable level of development.
b. Multiple causes including genetic predisposition and catecholamine deficiency.
c. There is significant comorbidity with learning disabilities, Tourette's syndrome, and conduct disorders.
2. Assessment.
a. Must have at least 6 symptoms from each category below that began before 7 years of age, persisted for at least 6 months to a degree that is maladaptive and inconsistent with developmental level and are evident across 2 or more settings.
b. Inattention.
(1) Has difficulty sustaining attention in tasks.
(2) Makes careless mistakes.
(3) Does not seem to listen when spoken to.
(4) Fails to follow through on instructions.
(5) Has difficulty organizing tasks.

(6) Avoids engaging in tasks that require sustained mental effort.
(7) Often loses things.
(8) Is easily distracted.
(9) Is often forgetful.
c. Hyperactivity.
(1) Fidgets or squirms.
(2) Leaves seat when expected to stay seated.
(3) Runs or climbs excessively.
(4) Has difficulty engaging in activities quietly.
(5) Is "on the go" as if "driven by a motor."
(6) Talks excessively.
d. Impulsivity.
(1) Blurts out answers before the question is completed.
(2) Has difficulty awaiting turn.
(3) Interrupts or intrudes on others.
3. Interventions.
a. Psychostimulants (e.g., methylpenidate hydrochloride [Ritalin]).
(1) Actions: increase attention span and short-term memory, reduce distractibility, reduce motor activity, and make children more ready for learning to occur.
(2) Adverse effects include anorexia, insomnia, weight loss, growth suppression, lowering of the seizure threshold, and the development or worsening of tics.
b. Other medications used include tricyclic antidepressants and clonidine.
c. Medication should never be the sole treatment initiated.
d. Mandatory access to services include continual testing, free and appropriate education in the least restrictive environment, and an Individualized Education Plan (IEP) outlined in the Individuals with Disabilities Education Act (IDEA – Public Law 101-476).
e. Ensure adequate nutrition.
f. Decrease distraction in the environment.
g. Provide consistency and routine.

E. Bronchopulmonary dysplasia.
1. The science.
a. This condition is the sequelae of positive pressure ventilation during the first weeks of life, usually following treatment for Respiratory Distress Syndrome.
b. It is commonly seen in infants born prematurely.
c. The damage to the lungs is thought to be due to barotrauma and oxygen stimuli that initiate the inflammatory process, cause cellular damage, fibrosis, and smooth muscle hypertrophy.
2. Assessment.
a. Signs of respiratory distress include tachyp-

nea, retractions, wheezing, rales, cyanosis, and decreased oxygen saturation.
  b. Assess for activity and handling intolerance.
  c. Decreased energy for growth and development; assess developmental parameters.
3. Interventions.
  a. Provide supplemental oxygen and adequate rest times.
  b. Diuretics are used to decrease pulmonary congestion.
  c. Bronchodilators and antiinflammatory medications are also administered.
  d. Avoid contact with children with respiratory infections.
  e. Teach sign language if child ventilated for a significant period of time.
  f. Total parenteral nutrition necessary if oral aversion or gastroesophageal reflux prevents adequate intake.

F. Cancer.
1. The science.
  a. Cancer is second to accidents as the cause of death in children.
  b. In children, it occurs most commonly in rapidly differentiating tissues, e.g., bone marrow and neurologic tissues.
  c. The most common types in children are leukemia, neurologic tumors, lymphomas, neuroblastomas, Wilm's and bone tumors.
  d. Childhood tumors are fast growing because their metabolism is normally at a higher rate than adults.
  e. The incidence of cancer increases with age.
  f. Causes may include genetic factors, ionizing radiation, viral infections, and chronic chemical exposure.
2. Leukemia: assessment.
  a. Anemia (pallor, fatigue, headache).
  b. Platelet deficiency (bruising, purpura).
  c. Immune suppression (fever, infection, organomegaly, poor wound healing).
  d. Bone pain due to hypertrophy of the bone marrow.
3. Brain tumors: assessment.
  a. Personality changes.
  b. Loss of developmental milestones.
  c. Decreased academic performance.
  d. Intermittent headaches.
  e. Difficulty with balance; vision.
  f. Seizures; hemiparesis.
4. Lymphomas: assessment.
  a. Mass may occur in lymph nodes, bone marrow, anterior mediastinum.
  b. Lymphadenopathy resulting in symptoms in that area (swelling of neck, abdominal pain,

bowel changes, dysphagia, dyspnea).
5. Neuroblastoma: assessment.
  a. Nodes most common near the adrenal gland, the thorax, or the neck.
  b. Presence of mass causes compression on other systems.
  c. Metastasis is present in 70% of cases at the time of diagnosis.
6. Cancer-related interventions.
  a. Surgical removal of the tumor, if possible.
  b. Radiation therapy.
  c. Combination chemotherapy.
  d. Bone marrow transplant, in some cases.
  e. Biologic response modifiers to stimulate the immune system.
  f. Other measures.
    (1) Avoid contact with infectious individuals.
    (2) Institute measures to decrease nausea, vomiting, and stomatitis related to chemotherapy and promote adequate nutrition.
    (3) Institute measures to decrease bruising (gentle handling, soft toys, toothettes) and conserve energy (passive stimulation, promote rest).
    (4) Immunizations should not be given while the child is still on immunosuppressive therapy; then inactivated vaccines may be given.
    (5) Anticipate late effects from these treatments, such as secondary cancers, learning disabilities, and altered functioning of specific organ systems.

G. Cardiac anomalies.
1. The science.
  a. Results from the abnormal development of the heart structures during embryonic development.
  b. In acyanotic heart conditions, the systemic circulation is not exposed to unoxygenated blood; eg. atrial septal defect, ventricular septal defect, patent ductus arteriosus, coarctation of the aorta.
  c. In cyanotic heart conditions, there is a mixing of oxygenated and unoxygenated blood into the systemic circulation; e.g., tetralogy of Fallot, transposition of the great arteries, hypoplastic left heart syndrome, pulmonary or tricuspid atresia.
  d. Heart defects can also occur due to failure of normal fetal heart structures to close.
  e. Because the pressure is higher on the left side of the heart, there is frequently a left to right shunting of blood.
2. Assessment.

a. Acyanotic conditions primarily manifest with signs of congestive heart failure including tachypnea, tachycardia, dyspnea, diaphoresis, hepatomegaly, persistent cough, easily fatigued, decreased energy to feed, failure to thrive, heart murmurs, and pale, cool skin.

b. Cyanotic conditions primarily manifest with:
   (1) Cyanosis, especially around the mouth, gums, and nailbeds.
   (2) Polycythemia and its sequelae (increased hematocrit).
   (3) Tachypnea and tachycardia.
   (4) Clubbing of digits.
   (5) Child assuming a squatting posture.
   (6) Fatigue and failure to thrive.
   (7) Heart murmurs.

3. Interventions.
   a. Decrease oxygen demands.
   b. Provide oxygen if necessary.
   c. Anticipate needs.
   d. Provide passive stimulation.
   e. Position infant in knee-chest position for comfort.
   f. Use a preemie nipple to decrease the energy needed for sucking.
   g. Give high calorie foods that are easy to digest.
   h. Provide good skin care.
   i. Administer digoxin and diuretics as ordered.
   j. Administer Prostaglandin E to keep the ductus arteriosus open, indomethacin to attempt pharmacologic closure.
   k. Prevent cold stress.
   l. Prepare child for cardiac catheterization if indicated; take measurements of pulse pressures, extremity temperatures, color, and movement in all extremities both before and after the procedure.

H. Cerebral palsy.
1. The science.
   a. Defined as a nonprogressive motor disorder of the central nervous system causing aberrant movement and posturing.
   b. Classified as spastic, dyskinesia, ataxia, and mixed.
   c. Caused by trauma/hemorrhage, anoxia, or infection before, during, or after birth.
   d. Approximately 33% of children with cerebral palsy have mental retardation.
2. Assessment. Assess for:
   a. Abnormal muscle tone and coordination.
   b. Altered speech, vision, and hearing.
   c. Delayed developmental milestones.
   d. The presence or absence of reflexes; dental anomalies.
   e. Seizures.

f. Spastic CP may be partial or involve the entire body; results in hypertonicity with poor posture control, leg scissoring, persistent primitive reflexes, and contractures.

g. Dyskinetic CP demonstrates as constant wormlike movements that increase with stress and disappear during sleep.

h. Ataxic CP results in poor equilibrium.

3. Interventions.
   a. Increase calorie intake due to increased motor function.
   b. Provide a safe environment (use protective headgear and environmental padding).
   c. Promote range of motion; maintain proper body alignment.
   d. Divide tasks into small steps.
   e. Promote age-appropriate mental activities.
   f. Use communication boards if speaking is difficult.
   g. Refer for speech, nutrition, occupational, and physical therapies.
   h. Promote good skin care, especially if orthotic devices are used.
   i. Attend to constipation, pain management, and dental care.

I. Cleft lip and palate.
1. The science.
   a. This congenital defect occurs due to failure of the median maxillary, premaxillary, and palatine processes to fuse early in gestation.
      (1) Failure of the lip/palate to fuse.
      (2) Deformed nasal bridge.
   b. The lip and/or the palate may be involved; it can be a partial or complete cleft; it can be unilateral or bilateral.
   c. Cause unknown, but suggested causes include genetic predisposition, folic acid deficiency, and phenytoin ingestion.
2. Assessment.
   a. Difficulty forming a seal around the nipple; results in feeding difficulties.
   b. Speech/cry sounds nasal.
   c. Possible respiratory distress.
3. Intervention.
   a. Teach parent to provide adequate nutrition to infant prior to surgery.
      (1) Use cleft palate nipple, large nipple, or a syringe with tubing attached to put formula into the side of the child's mouth.
      (2) Burp frequently to eliminate air that is swallowed.
      (3) Feed upright to decrease risk of aspiration.
      (4) Provide small frequent feedings.
   b. Cleft lip surgery is completed in early infancy to provide proper alignment for teeth.

c. Cleft palate surgery is completed during early toddlerhood in anticipation of speech development; child must be weaned from nipples/pacifiers/thumbs prior to surgery.

d. Follow-up therapies include dental/orthodontic, speech, and plastic surgery.

J. Cystic fibrosis.

1. The science.

   a. A multisystem disorder of the exocrine glands; appears to involve the chloride ion channel across epithelial cells.

   b. An autosomal recessive disorder passed on Chromosome 7.

   c. Average age of death usually young adulthood, with respiratory compromise being the primary cause. However, recent advances in care have extended the lifespan of many into middle adulthood.

2. Assessment.

   a. Respiratory system.

      (1) Persistent thick tenacious mucus.

      (2) Persistent congested cough.

      (3) Decreased exercise tolerance.

      (4) Air trapping, areas of atelectasis, barrel chest.

      (5) Crackles and wheezes.

      (6) Clubbing of digits.

      (7) Presence of nasal polyps.

   b. Sweat glands.

      (1) Normal amount of sweat but significantly increased sodium and chloride in the sweat.

      (2) High rate of salt loss, especially in hot weather.

   c. Pancreas.

      (1) Meconium ileus possible in newborns.

      (2) Decrease or absence of release of exocrine pancreatic enzymes to digest fats.

      (3) Malabsorption (fatty, foul smelling, frequent, foamy, and undigested food in stool); steatorrhea.

      (4) Fat soluble vitamin deficiency (A, D, E, and K).

      (5) Failure to gain weight.

   d. Reproductive tract.

      (1) Viscous secretions make fertility difficult for females.

      (2) Obliteration of the vas deferens in males may result in sterility.

   e. Other: may develop glucose intolerance, rectal prolapse, esophageal varices, cor pulmonale.

3. Interventions.

   a. Administer chest physiotherapy (percussion and postural drainage).

   b. Administer bronchodilators, DNase, and anti-inflammatories.

   c. Antibiotics may be required for infection.

   d. Increase dietary salt intake.

   e. Administer pancreatic enzymes with meals and snacks.

   f. Administer fat soluble vitamins (A, D, E, and K).

   g. Provide high calorie, high protein foods to enhance growth.

   h. Genetic counseling.

   i. Encourage physical activity.

   j. Avoid cough suppressants and antihistamines.

K. Diabetes (Type I).

1. The science.

   a. May be caused by an autoimmune process characterized by beta cell failure.

   b. Results in inability of the pancreas to make insulin.

   c. Glucose does not have enough insulin to get into the cells and builds up in the blood. Available insulin inadequate to transport glucose into cells.

   d. Glucose acts as an osmotic diuretic.

   e. Classified as Type I or Type II diabetes, based upon onset and treatment requirements.

2. Assessment.

   a. Polydipsia.

   b. Polyphagia.

   c. Polyuria.

   d. Hyperglycemia.

   e. Glucosuria and ketonuria.

   f. Dry, flushed skin.

   g. Note "fruity" odor to breath (ketones).

3. Interventions.

   a. Children are almost always insulin dependent.

   b. Insulin preparation.

      (1) Administer regular insulin for fast action (onset in 30 minutes; peaks 2–4 hours).

      (2) Administer intermediate insulin for more sustained duration (onset in 1 hour; peaks in 8 hours).

      (3) Provide a snack at the time insulin peaks.

   c. Give fluids without sugar.

   d. Observe for hypoglycemia symptoms including sweating, tremors, palpitations, and behavior changes.

   e. If hypoglycemia suspected, give fast acting carbohydrate, such as honey or orange juice, followed by a protein source.

   f. For insulin administration.

      (1) Teach child to administer own insulin as soon as developmentally capable (8+ years).

(2) When giving two types of insulin, draw up clear insulin first to prevent contamination.

(3) Do not shake vial; gently rotate it.

(4) Rotate injection sites to prevent lipodystrophy.

g. Insulin requirements will change with illness, activity, stress, and growth.

h. Prevent complications by managing insulin need.

(1) Balance activity, diet and insulin.

(2) Assess blood sugars using home glucose monitor 4–6 times per day. Teach child/family to manage this.

i. Provide consistent follow up to assess for the common complications of diabetes.

(1) Nephropathy.

(2) Premature atherosclerosis.

(3) Retinopathy.

(4) Poor wound healing.

L. Drug-exposed infants (cocaine, heroin, fetal alcohol syndrome).

1. The science.

a. Cocaine in the mother's system causes placental and uterine vasoconstriction; this results in fetal hypoxia and the development of CNS abnormalities.

b. Heroin in the mother's system is transferred to the fetus and soon after delivery, the child enters withdrawal.

c. Fetal alcohol syndrome results in malformations and CNS deficits; milder form is called fetal alcohol effects.

d. Many drug-abusing women use multiple substances.

2. Assessment.

a. Withdrawal from heroin and alcohol.

(1) Irritability.

(2) Tremors.

(3) Hypertonicity.

(4) Tachycardia and hypertension.

(5) Difficult to feed and soothe.

(6) Difficulty in maternal-infant interaction and bonding.

b. Fetal alcohol syndrome.

(1) Intrauterine growth retardation.

(2) Significant learning disabilities.

(3) Craniofacial abnormalities.

3. Interventions.

a. Assist infant through the withdrawal process.

(1) Swaddle.

(2) Decrease environmental stimuli.

b. Feed small frequent feedings every 2 hours.

c. Provide support services for the substance abusing mother.

d. Anticipate learning problems and developmental delay.

M. Eating disorders.

1. The science.

a. Common in adolescents.

b. Often a result of poor perception of physical self, poor parent-child interactional skills.

c. Anorexia nervosa is the refusal to eat accompanied by a loss of more than 25% of body weight without an organic cause.

d. Bulimia is referred to as the "binge-purge" syndrome; a huge intake is followed by forced vomiting.

2. Assessment.

a. Measure weight and muscle mass.

b. Assess for metabolic alkalosis related to vomiting.

c. Assess for electrolyte imbalance, especially potassium; observe for changes in cardiac status.

d. Note changes in menses or other signs of malnutrition.

e. Assess how the child/teen feels about the way they look.

f. Note dental deterioration, mouth/lip ulcerations related to gastric acid reflux during vomiting.

3. Interventions.

a. Refer for psychotherapy.

b. Provide nutritional assistance and monitoring to regain homeostasis and to enhance nutritional status.

c. Contract with the child to develop a plan of action.

d. Initiate behavior modification to achieve the above plan.

e. Caregivers usually involved in counseling along with child.

N. Failure to thrive (related to deficient parenting).

1. The science.

a. Defined as a child who remains below the third percentile; may be due to physical causes or deficient parenting.

b. Most commonly seen in infants; premature infants and those with special needs are at higher risk.

c. Physical causes must be ruled out before other causes are explored.

2. Assessment.

a. Compare height, weight, head and chest circumferences, and bone age on growth charts.

b. Compare cognitive and psychosocial development to chronologic age.

c. Note altered body posture (hypertonicity or hypotonicity).

d. Note quality and length of sleeping behaviors.

e. Note child's response to cuddling.

f. Note child's response to parents and interactions with caregivers.

g. Note child's intake, feeding techniques (e.g., bottle propping), burping.

h. Note amount of stimulation caregiver provides.

3. Interventions.

a. Work with caregiver to teach appropriate parenting behaviors (feeding, bathing, holding, stimulation, providing love).

b. Help caregiver learn to identify and respond to infant's cues.

c. Act as role model for the caregiver.

O. Hemophilia.

1. The science.

a. Involves a deficiency in one of the intrinsic clotting factors, usually Factor VIII (classical hemophilia or Hemophilia A) or Factor IX (Christmas disease or Hemophilia B); it is not a platelet deficiency.

b. Severity of the disease is determined by the degree of the clotting factor deficiency.

c. Inherited from the mother on the sex-linked chromosome.

d. Due to the opposition of healthy X chromosome in females, only males develop this disorder.

2. Assessment. Observe for:

a. Prolonged bleeding following circumcision, from the umbilical cord stump, following dental care, and after injections and heel sticks.

b. Excessive bruising.

c. Swollen, painful joints (due to hemarthrosis [bleeding into the joints]).

d. Elevated partial thromboplastin time.

e. Bleeding into areas of the central nervous system or other organ systems.

3. Interventions.

a. Pad objects in the child's environment; recommend helmets and soft tooth brushes if needed.

b. Replace deficient factor and initiate bleeding control measures; teach child and/or caregiver home administration of Factors.

c. If bleeding occurs, apply ice compresses and pressure, raise extremity in a slightly flexed position, and immobilize the site for 48 hours.

d. Avoid aspirin, sutures, and excessive handling.

e. Deal with caregiver tendency to overprotect child.

P. Inflammatory bowel disease.

1. The science.

a. Includes Crohn's disease and ulcerative colitis.

b. Crohn's disease involves asymmetric, patchy lesions of all layers of the GI track.

c. Ulcerative colitis involves symmetric and contiguous ulcers of the mucosa of the GI track.

d. The cause is unknown, but the conditions are exacerbated by stress.

e. More common in adolescents.

2. Assessment.

a. Diarrhea is common; constipation may also be seen.

b. Grossly bloody stools (pus and mucus are also in the stools in ulcerative colitis).

c. Skin breakdown around rectum.

d. Abdominal pain, cramping.

e. Anorexia, nausea, vomiting.

f. Weight loss.

g. Delayed growth and development, especially sexual development.

h. Anemia is possible related to the amount of blood loss.

3. Interventions.

a. Administer antiinflammatory, antispasmodic, antibiotic, steroids, and/or pain medications.

(1) Teach purpose for each drug or combination.

(2) Instruct concerning discontinuation of steroids.

b. Teach the use of the elemental diet or the use of parenteral hyperalimentation.

c. Foster stress reduction activities.

d. Surgery may be required to develop an ostomy or to resect sections of bowel.

Q. Learning disabilities.

1. The science.

a. The number one chronic, non-illness condition in children.

b. A heterogeneous group of disorders.

(1) Alteration in sensory-receptive processing.

(2) Alteration in integrative processing.

(3) Alterations in motor-expressive performance.

(4) Diffuse.

c. Individual has at least a normal Intelligence Quotient; may be above average.

d. Affects both academic and nonacademic life skills.

2. Assessment.

a. For sensory-receptive deficits.

(1) Dyslexia.

(2) Altered depth and distance perception.

(3) Difficulty with visual memory.
(4) Difficulty understanding directions.
(5) Difficulty interpreting tone of conversation.
(6) Difficulty differentiating similar sounds.
(7) Difficulty sensing onset of menses or need to void or defecate.
(8) Distracted by the sensation of certain materials on their skin.
  b. For integrative deficits.
    (1) Difficulty retrieving and using information that has been received.
    (2) Difficulty with sequencing events and planning activities.
    (3) Difficulty with analysis, understanding cause and effect, and abstract thought.
    (4) Difficulty with reading comprehension.
    (5) Difficulty setting priorities.
  c. For motor-expressive.
    (1) May appear clumsy.
    (2) Poor hand-eye coordination.
    (3) Motor skills may be affected (hand writing, speech, coordination).
  d. For all learning disabilities.
    (1) Multiple failures.
    (2) Poor self-esteem.
    (3) Multiple types of psychologic testing are required to make an accurate diagnosis.
3. Interventions.
  a. Develop teaching modalities based on the child's strengths.
  b. Teach the child to compensate for their deficit.
  c. Decrease distractions.
  d. Make tasks achievable.
  e. Build self-esteem.
  f. Develop an Individualized Education Plan.

R. Mental retardation/cognitive impairment (using Down syndrome as a prototype).
1. The science.
  a. Defined as significantly subaverage general intelligence that exists concurrently with deficits in adaptive behavior; is manifest during the developmental period.
  b. Differentiated as mild (IQ 54–69), moderate (IQ 36–53), and severe/profound (IQ<36).
  c. Due to hundreds of causes, including trauma, anoxia, genetic/chromosomal, congenital defects, and inborn errors of metabolism.
  d. Down syndrome is usually due to nondisjunction of chromosome 21 resulting in 47 chromosomes.
2. Assessment.
  a. Mild retardation: is educable to a mental age of 8–12 years and is capable of most activities of daily living.
  b. Moderate retardation: can function at mental ages of 3–7 and is trainable in self-care activities.
  c. Severe retardation: requires complete care with a mental age of toddlerhood or lower.
  d. Assess cognitive, growth, and developmental parameters.
  e. For Down syndrome.
    (1) Small head with upward slanting palpebral fissures (the opening between the lids), Brushfield's spots, a flat nose, a protruding tongue.
    (2) Short stature.
    (3) A single simian crease across palm and other dermatoglyphics.
    (4) Hypotonia.
    (5) Increased risk of congenital heart defects, myelogenous leukemia, and altered immune function.
    (6) Mild to moderate retardation.
3. Interventions.
  a. Initiate activities that promote the optimal development of the child.
  b. Set realistic goals; break activities into smaller components.
  c. Promote safety.
  d. Be consistent in presenting rules and expectations.
  e. Provide interventions and communication based on the child's mental age.
  f. Initiate early intervention programs for stimulation and family teaching; develop an Individualized Family Service Plan for those under age 3 and an Individualized Education Plan (IFSP) for those above 3 years old.

S. Myelomeningocele (spina bifida).
1. The science.
  a. This neural tube defect occurs during the first trimester of embryonic gestation.
  b. Also referred to as myelodysplasia.
  c. Can occur anywhere along the spinal canal.
  d. Cause is unknown but is thought to be related to folic acid deficiency in the mother.
  e. The degree of disability depends on the location of the sac and the amount of spinal nerves encased in it.
2. Assessment.
  a. Defect can be detected in utero by the high alpha-fetoprotein level in the amniotic fluid.
  b. Assess for leakage of spinal fluid from the sac; also assess for degree of skin integrity of the sac.
  c. Assess for loss of sensation at and below the level of the lesion (lack of movement of or sensation in the legs, neurogenic bladder, neurogenic bowel).

d. Assess for infection around sac, infection of the central nervous system or septicemia.

e. Measure head circumference due to the high risk of hydrocephalus.

3. Interventions.

a. Primary surgical repair occurs within 48 hours of birth.

b. Prior to surgery, prevent trauma to sac.

(1) Place child on abdomen or side, support sac if necessary.

(2) Keep sac free from infection; avoid contamination by urine and stool (use of diaper generally not possible).

(3) Keep sac moist with saline-soaked sterile dressings.

c. After surgery, note degree of sensation and movement at and below the level of the lesion.

d. Monitor head circumference, because scarring from surgery may result in noncommunicating hydrocephalus.

e. Be aware of the increased incidence of latex allergies in individuals with myelomeningocele, primarily from all of the intermittent catheterizations done to compensate for neurogenic bladder.

T. Nephrosis (nephrotic syndrome)/glomerulonephritis.

1. The science.

a. Both are due to autoimmune processes in the glomerulus of the kidney due to an initial immune insult; in glomerulonephritis, the cause is often infection with group A beta hemolytic streptococcus, although there is no infection at any time in the kidney.

b. Interferes with glomerular permeability.

(1) Nephrosis results in release of protein, especially albumin.

(2) Nephritis results in release of protein as well as red blood cells.

2. Assessment.

a. Check urine for protein and blood.

(1) Urine will be dark and foamy with a high specific gravity

(2) Test first void of the day.

b. Assess for signs of hypovolemia.

c. Closely monitor and record intake and output.

d. Assess for edema.

(1) Nephrosis results in dependent edema, which starts around the eyes in the morning and shifts to the perineum and ankles.

(2) Weigh child daily.

(3) Note diarrhea, anorexia, and malnutrition due to edema of intestines.

e. Assess for electrolyte imbalance.

f. Assess skin turgor and skin breakdown due to edema.

g. Note fatigue and lethargy.

h. For nephritis, note increased sedimentation rate and increased antistreptolysin-O titer; hypertension might also be present.

3. Interventions.

a. Avoid adhesives, injections, or trauma to edematous skin.

b. Provide supportive treatment for edematous areas.

(1) Elevate areas of edema.

(2) Provide scrotal supports if needed.

(3) Provide warm compresses to edematous eyes.

(4) Prevent irritation from edematous tissues rubbing together.

(5) Keep skin dry; prevent trauma.

c. Provide small frequent meals; sodium restriction may be implemented with hypertension or edema.

d. For nephritis, the child may be placed on prophylactic antibiotics to prevent a reattack of the kidneys.

U. Scoliosis.

1. The science.

a. A lateral curvature of the spine.

b. Structural scoliosis is progressive with an S curve.

c. Nonstructural functional scoliosis is nonprogressive and involves a C curve.

d. Usually identified during the growth spurt of puberty; progression of the curve ceases when bone growth stops.

e. Cause can be unknown or may be due to a congenital condition, muscle weakness, trauma, or nutritional problem.

2. Assessment for structural scoliosis.

a. When child bends forward with knees straight and arms hanging down, the spinal curve fails to straighten.

b. There is asymmetry in the heights of the shoulders, scapula, hips, and ribs.

c. X-rays assist in the diagnosis.

d. Altered structure of the rib cage may result in compression of other organ structures.

e. Seen most frequently in female adolescents.

3. Interventions.

a. Prolonged bracing requires teaching of skin care measures and correct bracing techniques (Boston brace and the Milwaukee brace).

b. External electrical stimulation of spinal muscles may be used.

c. Surgical instrumentation to stabilize the spine may be necessary, often including spinal fusion.

d. Assist the teen to deal with body image and compliance to wearing the brace.

e. Postoperatively, maintain proper body alignment to avoid twisting or bending of spine.

V. Seizure disorder (epilepsy).

1. The science.
   a. A sudden, episodic, involuntary alteration in consciousness, motor activity, behavior, sensation, or autonomic function.
   b. A convulsion is an involuntary muscular contraction and relaxation; terms *seizure* and *convulsion* may be used synonymously.
   c. Excessive neuronal discharges can be due to infection, lesions, pressure, chemical imbalances, and medications.
   d. Seizures are differentiated as simple or complex partial (localized to one area of the brain), convulsive or nonconvulsive generalized (involves both hemispheres), status epilepticus, or febrile.

2. Assessment.
   a. Note type of seizure by describing:
      (1) What parts of body move.
      (2) The quality of the movement (clonic/tonic).
      (3) The timing of the event.
      (4) The level of consciousness.
      (5) Whether or not incontinence is present.
   b. Note whether there are preictal symptoms (aura or particular sensations) and the degree of postictal symptoms (drowsy, orientation to person, place and time, and coordination).
   c. Serial electroencephalogram (EEG), sleep EEG, and multiple brain scans are helpful in diagnosis.
   d. Note impact on growth and development.

3. Interventions.
   a. During a seizure.
      (1) Promote an open airway as possible; never attempt to insert anything into mouth.
      (2) Maintain safe environment.
         (a) Place child on floor or bed with padded siderails raised.
         (b) Remove objects that may cause injury.
         (c) Place pad under head to prevent banging on the floor.
         (d) Do not restrain child.
      (3) Maintain a calm environment.
      (4) Place individual on side so that secretions can drain and tongue does not block airway.
      (5) Assist the child to regain orientation.
   b. Administer prophylactic seizure medications (dilantin, tegretol, depakene, phenobarbital); be aware of nursing interventions for these medications, especially the dental care needed due to the gingival hyperplasia of dilantin.
   c. Promote compliance with treatment regimen: reinforce need for long-term commitment to treatment regimen.
   d. Surgery may be indicated to correct the problem.
   e. The use of the ketogenic diet (high fat and low carbohydrate and protein) is sometimes used.

W. Sickle cell disease.

1. The science.
   a. An autosomal recessive disorder more common in African Americans and those of mediterranean origin.
   b. Due to a defective hemoglobin chain.
   c. Results in alteration of the oxygen carrying capacity of red blood cells (RBCs).
   d. RBC shape changes to shape of a sickle when vaso-occlusive episode (crisis) occurs.
   e. Altered shape results in hemolysis and subsequent anemia.
   f. The amount of the sickle cell hemoglobin determines the level of risk.
   g. Sickle cell crisis is initiated by dehydration, deoxygenation, or acidosis.

2. Assessment.
   a. Symptoms are rare before age 4 months because the infant still has fetal hemoglobin.
   b. Note degree and location of pain; crisis results in significant pain without overt signs.
   c. Note hand-foot syndrome in the infant due to infarction of small bones of hands and feet.
   d. Note enlarged spleen (due to its role in homeostasis); spleen may infarct and become nonfunctional.
   e. Assess degree of anemia.
   f. Assess for hypovolemia due to sequestering of RBCs in spleen.
   g. Assess for priapism and enuresis.
   h. Assess for cause (oxygen status, hydration status, acid/base status).
   i. Note if any developmental delay exists.

3. Interventions.
   a. During a crisis, provide:
      (1) Large amounts of fluids.
      (2) Adequate pain relief.
      (3) Oxygen and correct acid/base balance.
   b. Avoid tight clothing that can restrict circulation.
   c. Prevent infections with prophylactic antibiotics; assure that the child receives pneumococcal and influenza vaccines.
   d. Spleen may have to be surgically removed.
   e. Initiate genetic counseling.
   f. Initiate measures for anemia, related to diet and activity.

BIBLIOGRAPHY

Bowden, V., Dickey, S., & Greenberg, C. (1998). *Children and their families.* Philadelphia: Saunders.

Disabilities Among Children Aged ≤ 17 Years-United States, 1991-1992. (1995, August 25). *Morbidity and Mortality Weekly Report, 44*(33), 609–613.

Jackson, P. & Vessey, J. (1996). *Primary care of the child with a chronic condition.* St. Louis: Mosby–Year Book, Inc.

Oski, F., DeAngelis, C., Feigin, R., McMillan, J., & Warshaw, J. (1994). *Principles and practice of pediatrics.* Philadelphia: Lippincott.

Pridhum, K. (1995). *Standards and guidelines for prelicensure and early professional education for the nursing care of children and their families.* Washington, DC: DHHS, Maternal-Child Health Bureau: Document No. H112.

Selekman, J., & Saunders, A. (1997). *Pediatric nursing.* Springhouse, PA: Springhouse.

Wong, D. (1995). *Whaley & Wong's nursing care of infants and children.* St. Louis: Mosby–Year Book, Inc.

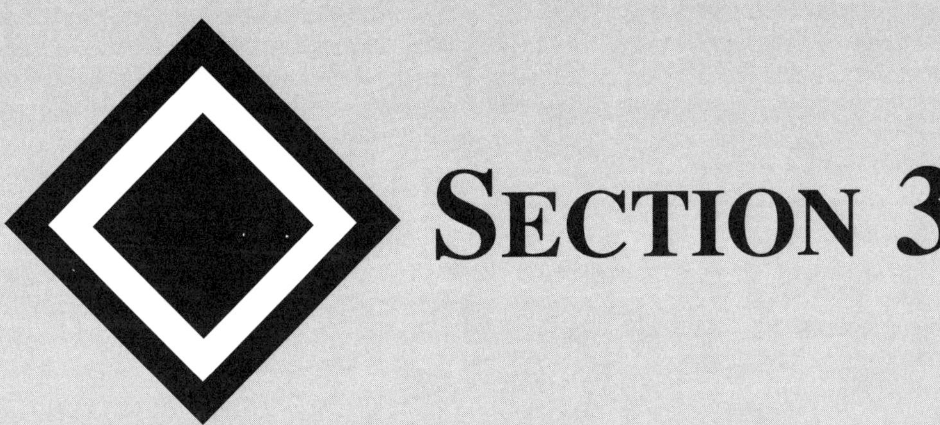

SECTION 3

Care Delivery

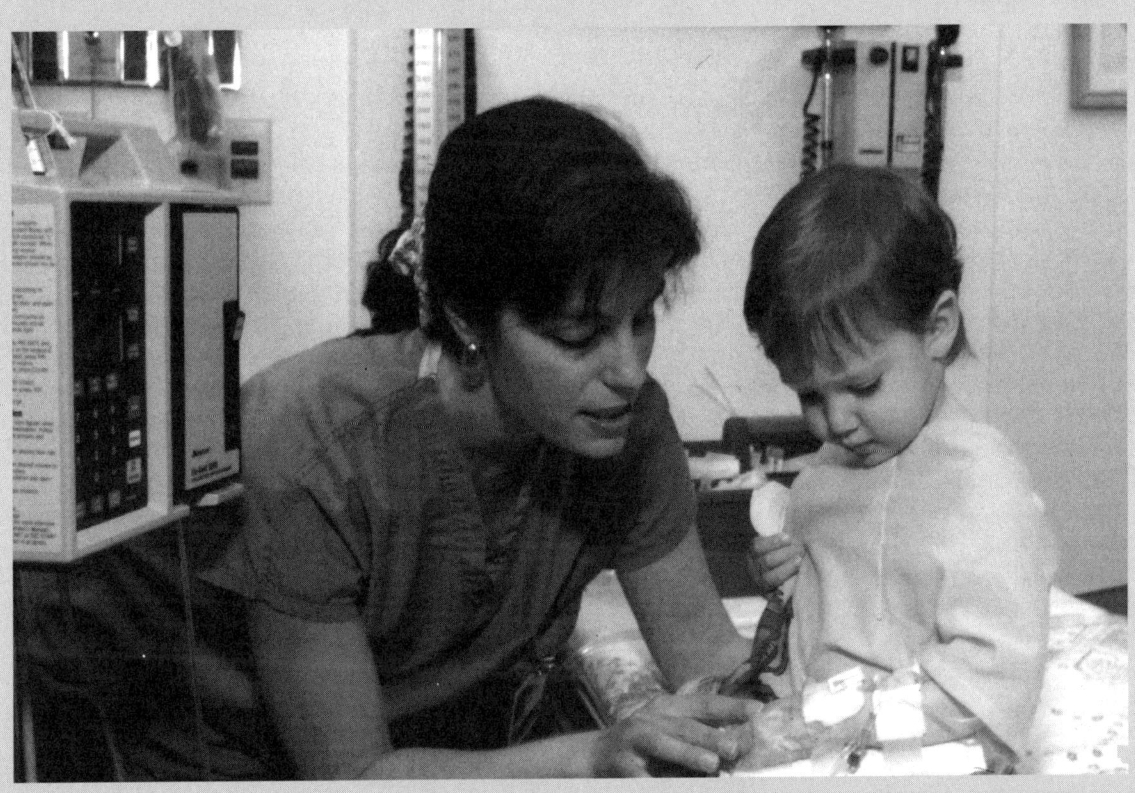

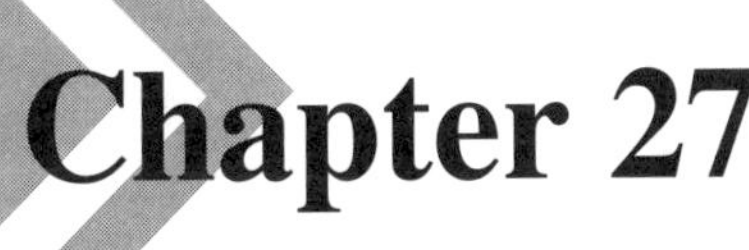

Chapter 27

Caring for the Child and Family Across the Continuum of Care

Carol C. Beausang, PhD, RN

Concept

◆◆◆◆◆◆◆◆◆◆◆◆◆◆◆◆◆◆◆◆◆◆◆◆

◆ Family-centered care

Objectives

◆◆◆◆◆◆◆◆◆◆◆◆◆◆◆◆◆◆◆◆◆◆◆◆

At the completion of this chapter, the reader will be able to:

◆ Identify three ways the nurse can care for the child and family across the continuum of care.

◆ Give examples of *community-based care* and *community health care.*

◆ Cite aspects of the home setting that are important to consider for discharge planning.

◆ Review developmentally appropriate ways to teach the child about health-related issues.

◆ Discuss the importance of anticipatory guidance for the child and family.

◆ Explain the relationships among supporting, teaching, counseling, and advocating for the child and family.

Key Points

◆◆◆◆◆◆◆◆◆◆◆◆◆◆◆◆◆◆◆◆◆◆

◆ The nurse needs to be knowledgeable about ways to care for the child and family beyond the more typical practice settings, i.e., the hospital, clinic, or physician's office.

◆ *Community-based care* refers to the community as the setting for care, whereas *community health care* means that the community as a whole is the unit of care.

◆ To promote health, the home needs to be safe and clean, with adequate utilities and nutritious food.

◆ Developmental characteristics are the basis for teaching the child effectively.

◆ Anticipatory guidance is used to prepare the child and family for developmental milestones and what to expect concerning other health-related experiences.

◆ Supporting, teaching, counseling, and advocating for the child and family are both distinct and interrelated; for example, providing information may be perceived as teaching but it may also provide support.

27

Caring for the Child and Family Across the Continuum of Care

◆◆◆◆◆◆◆◆◆◆◆◆◆◆◆◆◆◆◆◆◆◆◆◆◆◆◆◆◆◆◆◆◆

I. SUPPORTING THE CHILD AND FAMILY

◆◆◆◆◆◆◆◆◆◆◆◆◆◆◆◆◆◆◆◆

A mother brings her 2-year-old child to the clinic with vomiting and diarrhea. The nurse asks the mother about the onset, frequency, and severity of symptoms. She inquires whether or not any other family members are sick. Then she asks, "Has anything like this ever happened to you before?…What did you do?…How did that work?"

A. Assess the child and family's needs.

Also see Chapter 28: Family-Centered Care and Chapter 29: Cultural Influences.
1. For understanding.
   a. Of current situation.
   b. Of past experiences.
   c. Of future concerns.
2. For information.
   a. About who is doing what.
   b. About what is going to happen.
   c. About when something is going to happen.
   d. About where something is going to happen.
   e. About why something is being done.
3. For resources.
   a. Health care.
      (1) Primary care.
      (2) Acute care.
      (3) Emergency care.
      (4) Home care.
      (5) Respite care.
      (6) Hospice care.
   b. Child care.
   c. Early intervention programs.
   d. Rehabilitation services.
   e. Marital or family counseling.
   f. Financial resources.
   g. Health insurance.
      (1) Trends.
         (a) The percentage of children covered by employer-based health insurance is decreasing.
         (b) Responsibility for insuring children is shifting from the private to the public sector.
      (2) Issues.
         (a) Children who lack health insurance are disproportionately poor and Black or Hispanic.
         (b) In 1993-94, 13% of children younger than age 18 had no health insurance (Data from the National Health Interview Survey cited in Newacheck, Stoddard, Hughes, & Pearl, 1998).
         (c) Children without insurance typically receive inadequate health care.

A 14-year-old boy is admitted to the intensive care unit in critical condition following a bicycle accident. His anxious parents arrive. The nurse explains the purposes of the tubes and machines, and she encourages them to talk to their son even though he seems unresponsive. She listens carefully to the parents as they talk about arguing with their son about the need to wear a helmet and their feelings of helplessness when he refused to wear one.

B. Meet identified and potential needs.

1. Listen actively.
   a. Sit down, if possible.
   b. Minimize interruptions.
      (1) Close the door.
      (2) Pull the curtains.
      (3) Go to a quiet place.
   c. Facilitate expressions of feelings.
      (1) Be tolerant of silences.
      (2) Have tissues available.
      (3) Observe nonverbal expressions of feelings.
      (4) Provide appropriate play material for children.
      (5) Use appropriate touch.
   d. Clarify with the person what, if any, follow-up is needed.
2. Prepare the child and family for health care-related experiences. *Refer to the subsequent section on teaching the child and family; also see Chapter 28: Family-Centered Care.*
   a. Physical examination.

b. Immunizations.
c. Emergency department visit.
d. Pain management.
e. Hospital admission.
f. Intravenous fluids.
g. Medications.
h. Diagnostic tests.
i. Surgery.
  (1) Separation from parents.
  (2) Experience of anesthesia.
  (3) Recovery from surgery.
3. Plan for discharge, if hospitalized.
  a. Initiate discharge planning on admission to hospital.
  b. Continually involve the child and family in discharge planning.
  c. With child and family, identify goals for discharge.
  d. Use clinical pathways to monitor process toward discharge goals.
  e. If needed, arrange for car restraint device for trip home.
  f. Depending on child's needs, get as realistic a picture as possible of the home situation. *See Chapter 7: Home and Family* and *Caldwell and Bradley (1984)* and *Frankenburg and Coons (1986).*
    (1) What is the neighborhood like generally and child's home in particular?
    (2) Is the home basically safe?
      (a) Are smoke detectors working?
      (b) How would inhabitants escape in case of fire?
      (c) If firearms are kept in the home, are they locked?
      (d) Are drugs and other toxic substances locked and inaccessible to children?
      (e) Is there possible exposure to lead-based paint?
      (f) If there are stairs, where are they and are they solid and uncluttered?
      (g) Is there a safe place for children to play?
    (3) Are utilities available, dependable, and working correctly?
      (a) Water.
      (b) Heat.
      (c) Gas.
      (d) Electricity.
      (e) Telephone.
    (4) Who is living in the home?
      (a) Is a responsible adult able to stay at home?
      (b) Are there other children or adults who need care?
    (5) Is the home basically clean?
      (a) Is there at least one place to wash hands with soap?
      (b) How are clothes and linens laundered?
      (c) If animals are in the home, how are they managed?
      (d) How is garbage disposed of?
    (6) Are cooking facilities adequate?
      (a) Is there a working refrigerator?
      (b) Can food be stored safely?
      (c) Can food be cooked adequately?
    (7) Is there sufficient food for good nutrition?
    (8) What are sleeping arrangements for the child?
      (a) Does child need a special bed?
      (b) Where will the bed be placed?
      (c) If able, how will child communicate needs to others?
    (9) Are there adequate toilet facilities?
      (a) Does plumbing work reliably?
      (b) Are hand-washing facilities nearby?
    (10) What resources does the family have in emergencies?
      (a) 911.
      (b) Neighbors.
      (c) Other family members.
    (11) Is the home and/or child's room accessible?
      (a) Is there easy accessible entry to the house for a child with a disability (e.g., child who uses a wheelchair)?
      (b) Are door entries of adequate size to enable passage (e.g., child in large hip spica cast)?
  g. Consult resource people about unusual or complex situations.
    (1) Physicians.
    (2) Clinical nurse specialists.
    (3) Social workers.
    (4) Discharge planners.
    (5) Child life specialists.
    (6) Respiratory therapists.
    (7) Physical therapists.
    (8) Occupational therapists.
    (9) Speech therapists.
    (10) Home health nurses.
    (11) School nurses.
4. Use community-based resources.
  a. Local telephone books should list:
    (1) Government and official agencies in a separate section.
    (2) Specific resources in the white pages, e.g., the Kidney Foundation or parent stress hotlines.
    (3) General categories in the yellow pages, e.g., child care.

b. Public libraries.
  (1) May provide helpful books and periodicals (caution user about the need for current information and authoritative sources).
  (2) May offer special programs for children.
  (3) May provide computers for access to the Internet.
c. Health departments.
  (1) May provide well-child health supervision.
  (2) Will provide immunizations.
  (3) Can provide information on community health issues, e.g.,communicable diseases or food borne illnesses.
  (4) Has information about other resources, e.g., food stamps.
d. Public schools.
  (1) May provide early intervention programs.
  (2) Should provide special education.
  (3) May provide health screening for:
    (a) Vision.
    (b) Hearing.
    (c) Scoliosis.
  (4) May offer health education programs in:
    (a) Nutrition and health.
    (b) Physical activity and health.
    (c) Sexuality education.
    (d) Prevention of communicable diseases.
  (5) May have resource people available, such as a:
    (a) School nurse.
    (b) Social worker.
    (c) Counselor.
    (d) Psychologist.
    (e) Speech therapist.
e. Churches and synagogues.
  (1) May have services for children, such as:
    (a) Preschool education.
    (b) After-school programs.
    (c) Youth group activities.
    (d) Host of support groups, such as:
      [1] Coping with divorce.
      [2] Experiencing grief and bereavement.
      [3] Coping with alcoholism, e.g., Alateen.
  (2) May have services for parents, such as:
    (a) Peer group support.
    (b) Social networking.
    (c) Spiritual support.
    (d) Counseling services for issues such as:
      [1] Marital issues.
      [2] Divorce.
      [3] Bereavement.
    (e) Support groups for:
      [1] Bereavement, e.g., Compassionate Friends.
      [2] Alcoholism, e.g., Alcoholics Anonymous.
    (f) Time for self, e.g., babysitting cooperatives.
5. Use resources on the Internet.
  a. Newsgroups.
  b. Web sites. For example:
    (1) Creative Link and Graphics (1995): Foster Parent Home Page provides resources about foster parenting and parenting children with special health care needs: http://worldaccess.comFPHP.
    (2) Family Resource Center (1996): Parents Helping Parents is a national resource directory containing agencies, service providers, conference and workshop information concerning children with special needs, especially rare conditions: http://www.php.com.
    (3) Needleman and Cohen (1995): Parent's Place has regularly scheduled live chat sessions and information about parenting issues: http://parentsplace.com.
6. Be a critical consumer.
  a. Look for current resources.
  b. Gather resources from more than one place.
  c. Compare resources.
7. Continue to reach out for what is needed, e.g., a 3-year-old boy was a typical preschooler except for the fact that he did not talk, so his mother sought information and support from books, articles, pediatricians, nurses, teachers, therapists, and other parents before finally finding what she needed on the internet.

II. TEACHING THE CHILD AND FAMILY

◆ ◆ ◆ ◆ ◆ ◆ ◆ ◆ ◆ ◆ ◆ ◆ ◆ ◆ ◆ ◆ ◆ ◆ ◆

A. Theoretical foundations (scc Table 27-1).

B. Teaching needs. *See Chapter 15: Acute Care: Intervention Strategies.*
1. Situational needs.
  a. Planned events, e.g., elective surgery.
  b. Unplanned events, e.g., traumatic injury.
2. Child's needs.
  a. Developmental level.
    (1) The toddler.
      (a) Encourage parents' presence for support to child.
      (b) Have security object nearby, if child has one.
      (c) Tell child that something is going to happen.

Table 27-1
Theoretical Foundations

	Principles	Uses
Behavior Modification	1. Behavior that is rewarded will be repeated. 2. Punishment or fear of punishment will extinguish behavior. 3. To be effective, rewards and punishments need to be developmentally appropriate and meaningful.	1. To teach and maintain desired behavior, e.g., self-feeding 2. To decrease undesirable behavior, e.g., aggression
Health Belief Model	1. Various factors contribute to one's perceptions of health and illness. • Demographic variables, e.g. age and gender • Socioeconomic variables, e.g. education • Risk factors associated with disease • Past experiences with health care 2. Additional factors may motivate one to take action. • Exposure to advertising • Advice from others, including health professionals • Illness experiences of family members or friends 3. Health behavior may be the result of balancing perceived benefits of and barriers to taking preventive actions.	1. To analyze factors contributing to one's perceived state of health and susceptibility to illness 2. To assess the likelihood that one will take actions to promote health or prevent illness 3. To choose educational strategies based on clients' values and beliefs
Social Leaning Theory	1. Observational learning by modeling behavior is apt to occur when one identifies with the person modeling the behavior. 2. Reinforcement perpetuates learned behavior. 3. Adopting a behavior is the result of believing that the behavior will benefit health and that one is capable of behaving in the new way.	1. To design effective health education strategies, i.e., reflecting one's developmental level and past experiences 2. To analyze why people may not follow health education instructions or behave in ways they know to be healthy, e.g., an adolescent with diabetes who eats unhealthily

(d) If the child is going to encounter people with masks over their mouths and noses, prepare him or her for this. Bring the mask up and down from the face, so the child can see that people wearing masks have whole faces. Engage parents in this game that is like "peek-a-boo."

(e) Time preparation close to actual event.

(f) Model honesty, gentleness, and firmness, especially when separation from parents is necessary.

(g) Expect the toddler to protest health-related experiences.

(2) The preschooler.

(a) Encourage parents' presence for support to child.

(b) Tell child why something is going to happen, e.g., "This operation is to fix your ears."

(c) If possible, give child some time to think about it.

(d) Reassure child that he or she has not been "bad."

(e) Prepare child only for what he or she will actually experience.

(f) Use teaching dolls for explanation, then for child to play; using the child's own doll may be intrusive.

(g) Describe sensations child will experience, e.g., cool.

(h) Describe anesthesia as "a special sleep during your operation; then you wake up."

(i) If the child will have a mask put over his or her face, prepare the child for

this by gently bringing the mask up to the face from below and reassuring him or her that one can breathe through the mask.
(j) Be honest about possible separation from parents ("They will wait for you here.") and painful experiences ("We will do our best to make the pain go away.").
(k) Recognizing that the preschooler has permeable body boundaries, cover small wounds with band-aids and if the child sees some blood, reassure the child that he or she still has plenty of blood left inside.
(l) Offer the child coping techniques.
[1] "Say 'ouch.'"
[2] "Squeeze my hand."
[3] "Blow into the party blower."
[4] "Bring a favorite toy or blanket with you."
(m)Acknowledge the child's feelings and give him or her confidence, e.g., "I know this can be scary. I think you will do fine."
(n) Regardless how the child behaves, give him or her positive feedback, e.g., "You did a good job, you really tried."
(3) The school-ager.
(a) Encourage parents' presence for support to child.
(b) Teach the child how something is going to happen.
(c) Recognizing the child is learning how the inside of the body works, use simple pictures to explain relevant anatomy and physiology.
(d) If possible, use actual equipment in teaching.
(e) Though the school-age child may try to seem "grown up," be sensitive to needs for parents' presence, orientation to new surroundings, and preparation for health-related experiences.
(4) The adolescent.
(a) Similar to the school-age child, the adolescent may try to seem "grown up." Be sensitive to needs for parents' presence, orientation to new surroundings, and preparation for health-related experiences.
(b) If the adolescent's appearance will be altered, prepare him or her for this and provide suggestions for ways to manage it, e.g., cap or wig for hair loss.

(c) Acknowledge the adolescent's sexual maturation, e.g., provide needed menstrual supplies. Be sensitive to questions or other teaching needs.
b. Past history.
(1) Children usually enjoy talking about past experiences.
(2) Quiet or shy children may need more time and often respond well to watching other children in a group or being encouraged to draw pictures or play.
(3) Parents' memories may be similar or quite different from the child's; listen to the child and parents.
(4) Use memories of past experiences to reinforce or clarify the current situation.
c. Current readiness.
(1) Assess readiness to learn.
(a) Does the child seem somewhat anxious?
(b) Does the child seek information?
[1] Asks questions.
[2] Pursues resources, e.g., the library.
(2) Provide cues to stimulate learning.
(a) Books about subject matter, e.g., having surgery.
(b) Equipment to be used, e.g., mask for anesthesia.
(c) Others modeling behavior, e.g., breathing with mask.
(d) Tour of new surroundings, e.g., hospital unit, surgery.
(e) Therapeutic play equipment, e.g., dolls, syringes.
3. Family's needs.
a. Child.
(1) Determine role in family.
(2) Assess capabilities for learning.
(3) Identify reasonable expectations for responsibilities.
(4) Verify expectations with child and parents.
(5) Recognize that despite health problems the child needs to be held accountable for reasonable family responsibilities.
b. Parents.
(1) Determine how parents manage caregiving responsibilities.
(2) Assess what the current situation means to each parent.
(3) Recognize that parental responsibilities may shift between partners or one partner may experience health-related experiences as overwhelming.
(4) Provide parents with support for learning new skills, information, or behavior.

c. Siblings.
  (1) Assess siblings' roles in family.
  (2) Address legitimate feelings of jealousy, anger, resentment.
  (3) Involve siblings in ways appropriate to family situation.
  (4) Recognize that involvement may change over time.
d. Extended family members, e.g., grandparents.
  (1) Identify roles of extended family members.
    (a) Continually provide direct care.
    (b) Occasionally care for child.
    (c) Special support person to child.
    (d) Concerned but uninvolved.
  (2) Attend to their relationships with parents.
  (3) Involve extended family members in ways appropriate to their involvement in the family system.

C. Teaching strategies.
1. To learn a psychomotor skill.
  a. Observe skill, e.g., changing a central line dressing.
  b. Practice skill, e.g., on a doll.
  c. Return demonstrate skill, e.g., on a person.
2. To acquire information.
  a. Question-and-answer sessions.
  b. Printed information.
    (1) Books.
    (2) Pamphlets.
    (3) Posters.
  c. Audiovisual media.
    (1) Television.
    (2) Videotapes.
    (3) CD-ROMs.
  d. Web sites.
    (1) The American Academy of Pediatrics (1996) has health information for professionals and parents: http://www.aap.org.
    (2) KidsHealth (1996) has educational resources for parents and children: http://www.kidshealth.org/index2.html.
    (3) KidSource(1995) has health information for parents and children: http://www.kidsource.com.
    (4) Points of Pediatric Interest (1995) from Johns Hopkins University Department of Pediatrics includes patient education materials for parents and activities for children: http://www.med.jhu.edu/peds/neonatology/poi.html.
3. To change behavior.
  a. Provide models for behavior.

  (1) Support groups.
  (2) "Buddy" systems.
  (3) Personal stories.
  (4) Role play, e.g., to teach alternatives to violence.
b. Provide simulated experiences, e.g., special houses that fill with smoke to teach children about fire safety.

D. Special issues.
1. Low literacy skills.
  a. Be sensitive to cues suggesting difficulty reading.
    (1) Giving excuses, e.g., "I lost my glasses."
    (2) Difficulty telling time.
    (3) Mistakes giving medicines.
  b. Use verbal instructions and elicit feedback carefully.
  c. Provide pictures and illustrations.
2. Cultural differences. *See Chapter 29: Cultural Influences.*
  a. Be knowledgeable about cultural values.
    (1) Beliefs about health.
      (a) Illness.
      (b) Medicines.
      (c) Nutrition.
      (d) Sexuality.
    (2) Beliefs about gender roles.
      (a) Men may not relate well to female health professionals.
      (b) Women may be caregivers but have little power in the family system.
    (3) Patterns of communication.
  b. Discuss cultural adaptations to teaching with others involved.
3. Withholding information, i.e., parents refusing to have children taught.
  a. Try to identify underlying issues.
    (1) Parents may have had traumatic health-related experiences or are afraid themselves.
    (2) Parents may think that teaching and preparation will upset the child unnecessarily.
  b. Clarify misconceptions about current practices.
  c. Adapt teaching to meet identified needs.
4. Handicapping conditions.
  a. Sensory handicaps.
  b. Motor handicaps.
  c. Mental handicaps.
  d. Emotional handicaps.
5. Lack of time.
6. Lack of resources.
7. Lack of motivation.

III. COUNSELING THE CHILD AND FAMILY

◆ ◆

A. Principles of therapeutic relationships.

See Chapter 30: Communication.

1. Taking time to make introductions identifies who people are and clarifies roles.
2. Communication in a pediatric setting is usually triangular, involving the parent, child, and nurse.
3. Physical surroundings influence interactions, e.g., a private place usually promotes expressions of feelings.
4. A mutual exchange of ideas and opinions fosters understanding and problem solving.
5. Issues concerning confidentiality must be discussed honestly, i.e., most information will be shared with other health professionals.
6. Relationships need to be close enough to be meaningful yet separate enough for people to identify their own feelings and needs.
7. Ultimately, decisions made and actions taken are the child and family's.

B. Issues for counseling.

1. Anticipatory guidance.
   a. For the infant.
      (1) Meanings of infant crying.
      (2) Patterns of sleeping behavior.
      (3) Foods and feeding behavior.
      (4) Patterns of physical growth.
      (5) Ways to provide appropriate stimulation.
      (6) How to provide a safe environment.
      (7) Issues related to safe, reliable child care.
      (8) Appearance of temperament characteristics.
      (9) Need for health supervision visits.
      (10) Signs and symptoms of illness.
   b. For the toddler.
      (1) How to balance the child's need for independence with the need for safety.
      (2) Principles of giving the child choices.
         (a) Do not offer the child choices if he or she does not have options, e.g., taking medications.
         (b) Give no more than two or three options.
         (c) Each option must be a realistic possibility.
      (3) How to manage separation honestly.
      (4) The importance of routines in providing security.
      (5) How to manage temper tantrums.
      (6) Signs of readiness for toilet training.
   c. For the preschooler.
      (1) Reflections of the preschooler's vivid imagination.
         (a) Usually enjoys role playing, e.g., "house."
         (b) May have imaginary friends.
         (c) May have fears, e.g., of monsters, of the dark.
      (2) The importance of learning to share and cooperate.
      (3) How to respond to the preschooler's curiosity about gender differences: simply, naturally, and honestly.
      (4) Need for reasonable, consistent limit setting.
   d. For the school-ager.
      (1) Support for expanding social environment.
      (2) Need for safety precautions during activities.
      (3) The importance of acquiring basic academic skills, e.g., reading, writing, studying.
      (4) Need for acquiring basic knowledge about the world, e.g., history, science, sexuality, finances, sports.
   e. For the adolescent.
      (1) Seems to have a physiologic need to sleep later in the morning.
      (2) Increasingly takes responsibility for self.
      (3) Balance between maintaining ties with family and forming separate relationships.
      (4) Need to review personal safety practices, e.g., driving, drugs, sexual behavior.

Parents bring their 6-month-old daughter to the clinic for her routine check-up. The baby is sitting well without support and has begun to show indications of crawling behavior. Learning that the parents have little experience caring for young children, the nurse counsels them to start "childproofing" the house. She advises them to begin by continually inspecting the floors for small articles like coins and buttons that the baby could put in her mouth.

2. Specific problems.
   a. Related to the child's behavior.
   b. Related to health issues.

C. Strategies for counseling.

1. Face-to-face.
2. Telephone.
   a. Potential problems occur because advice is given without direct observation.
   b. Established protocols can help the clinician ask informative questions and dispense appropriate advice.

IV. ADVOCATING FOR THE CHILD AND FAMILY

A. Goals.

1. To assist the child and family to obtain what they are entitled to have:
   a. Access to basic primary care.
   b. Developmentally appropriate health care.
   c. Family-centered health care.
   d. Culturally sensitive health care.
   e. Special treatment if the child has disabilities.
   f. A safe and nurturing environment.
2. To attempt to make systems more responsive to the needs of the child and family.
   a. Broader insurance coverage for children.
   b. Data-based decisions regarding hospital practices.
   c. Increased community-based supports for the child and family.

B. Strategies.

1. Inform families of resources that might be helpful to them, e.g., hospital ombudsman.
2. If needed, help families articulate their needs to other health professionals.
3. Promote parental involvement on committees and boards.
4. Participate in professional organizations, e.g., Association for the Care of Children's Health, Society of Pediatric Nurses.
5. Become involved in local school programming.
6. Participate in community coalitions.
7. Lobby legislators.
8. Become involved in politics.

BIBLIOGRAPHY

Anticipatory Guidance for Children and Families. (1990). In S.R. Mott, S.R. James, & A.M Sperhac. *Nursing care of children and families* (2nd ed.) (Poster). Redwood City, CA: Addison-Wesley.

Barnes, L.P. (1997). Linking discharge planning and family teaching. *MCN, The American Journal of Maternal/ Child Nursing, 22,* 103.

Caldwell, B., & Bradley, R. (1984). *Home observation for measurement of the environment* (Rev. ed.). Little Rock, AR: University of Arkansas.

Chachkes, E., & Christ, G. (1996). Cross cultural issues in patient education. *Patient Education and Counseling, 27,* 13–21.

Edelman, C.L., & Mandle, C.L. (1994). *Health promotion throughout the lifespan* (3rd ed.). St. Louis: Mosby.

Frankenburg, W., & Coons, C. (1986). Home screening questionnaire: Its validity in assessing home environment. *Journal of Pediatrics, 108*(4), 624–626.

Havens, D.M.H., & Hannan, C. (1997). Children first: Expanding health insurance coverage for children. *Journal of Pediatric Health Care, 11*(2), 85–88.

Lobo, M.L. (1993). Listening to parents. *Journal of Pediatric Nursing, 8*(2), 68–69.

Mackenburg, M., & Hobbie, C. (1997). Patient education on the Web. *Journal of Pediatric Health Care, 11*(2), 89–91.

Nelms, B.C. (1992). Lessons to be learned. *Journal of Pediatric Health Care, 6*(5), 233–234.

Newacheck, P.W., Hughes, D.C., & Cisternas, M. (1995). Children and health insurance: An overview of recent trends. *Health Affairs, 14*(1), 244–254.

Newacheck, P.W., Hughes, D.C., & Stoddard, J.J. (1996). Children's access to primary care: Differences by race, income, and insurance status. *Pediatrics, 97*(1), 26–32.

Newacheck, P.W., Stoddard, J.J., Hughes, D.C., and Pearl, M. (1998). Health insurance and access to primary care for children. *The New England Journal of Medicine, 338*(8), 513–519.

Robinson, D., Anderson, M.M., & Erpenbeck, P.M. (1997). Telephone advice: New solutions for old problems. *The Nurse Practitioner, 22*(3), 179–192.

Shoultz, J., & Hatcher, P.A. (1997). Looking beyond primary care to primary health care: An approach to community-based action. *Nursing Outlook, 45*(1), 23–26.

Wandersman, A., Valois, R., Ochs, L., de la Cruz, D.S., Adkins, E., & Goodman, R.M. (1996). Toward a social ecology of community coalitions. A*merican Journal of Health Promotion, 10*(4), 299–307.

Wong, D.L. (1995). *Whaley & Wong's nursing care of infants and children* (5th ed.). St. Louis: Mosby.

Zink, K.A. (1996). Emotional support in pediatric trauma: Remembering children like Caleb. *Journal of Pediatric Nursing, 11*(6), 345–346.

Zotti, M.E., Brown, P., & Stotts, R.C. (1996). Community-based nursing versus community health nursing: What does it all mean? *Nursing Outlook, 44*(5), 211–217.

STUDY QUESTIONS

1. Which of the following is the best example of community health care?
   a. A comprehensive immunization program
   b. A parent stress hotline to prevent child abuse
   c. An ambulatory care clinic for well-children
   d. An early intervention program for children with special needs

2. Which of the following best describes a current trend in health care insurance coverage for children?
   a. Employer-based insurance is covering a greater percentage of children.
   b. Health insurance for children is shifting from the private to the public sector.
   c. More insurance providers are expanding coverage for children with special needs.
   d. The percentage of children without health insurance coverage is decreasing.

3. Discharge planning should begin when:
   a. discharge orders are written.
   b. home care instructions are complete.
   c. parents begin to ask questions.
   d. the child is admitted to the hospital.

4. Which of the following is the most important way to provide emotional support for the child?
   a. Advocate for greater access to comprehensive health care.
   b. Encourage the presence of parents for health-related experiences.
   c. Promote appropriate play activities in health care settings.
   d. Provide developmentally appropriate preparation for health-related experiences.

5. Which of the following two concepts are included in Social Learning Theory?
   a. Avoidance and restraint
   b. Empowerment and nurturing
   c. Modeling and reinforcement
   d. Risk-taking and saturation

6. During which developmental level does the child usually develop an understanding of the inside of the body?
   a. Adolescence
   b. Preschool
   c. School-age
   d. Toddler

7. Which of the following teaching strategies is most appropriate for helping a parent learn how to give an injection?
   a. Demonstrate and return-demonstrate
   b. Question-and-answer sessions
   c. Printed information in a notebook
   d. Role play in simulated situations

8. Which of the following best describes therapeutic relationships in pediatric settings?
   a. Confidentiality can always be promised to parents.
   b. Mutual exchanges of thoughts and feelings bias decisions.
   c. The nurse is responsible for decisions the family makes.
   d. Triangular communication involves the parent, child, and nurse.

9. The primary purpose of anticipatory guidance is to:
   a. advise the child and family how to change behavior.
   b. improve the recognition of developmentally-related problems.
   c. maximize the possibility of using community-based resources.
   d. prepare the child and family for expected developmental milestones.

10. The most important problem with giving advice over the telephone is:
    a. advice is given without direct observation.
    b. callers frequently disregard advice given.
    c. insurance companies will not provide reimbursement.
    d. professional practice laws do not include giving advice.

ANSWERS

◆ ◆

1.a   2.b   3.d   4.b   5.c   6.c   7.a   8.d   9.d   10.a

Chapter 28

Family-Centered Care

Elizabeth Ahmann, ScD, RN

Concept

◆◆◆◆◆◆◆◆◆◆◆◆◆◆◆◆◆◆◆◆◆◆◆◆◆

◆ Family-centered care

Objectives

◆◆◆◆◆◆◆◆◆◆◆◆◆◆◆◆◆◆◆◆◆◆◆◆◆

At the completion of this chapter, the reader will be able to:

◆ Recognize the significance of family-centered care.

◆ Identify the key elements of family-centered care and practice examples.

◆ Identify approaches to parent-professional collaboration.

◆ Describe a family-centered nursing process.

◆ Identify strategies for the application of family-centered care in various practice settings.

Key Points

◆◆◆◆◆◆◆◆◆◆◆◆◆◆◆◆◆◆◆◆◆◆◆◆

◆ Family-centered care is an evolving concept.

◆ Family/professional collaboration is essential for providing appropriate and optimal care.

◆ Family-centered care is not a blueprint, but a process that will differ based on variations in situations, families, cultures, health care settings, and providers.

◆ Family/professional collaboration should encompass assessment, planning care strategies, implementing care, and the evaluation of care and services.

◆ The principles and practice of family-centered care apply in all practice settings.

◆ Family-centered care requires learning new ways of relating to and working with families.

28

Family-Centered Care

I. FAMILY-CENTERED CARE

A. Overview.

"Family-centered care refers to nursing care that recognizes the central role of the family, however defined by its members, in the health of children. It is based on a partnership of health care professionals, other professionals, the child, and the family. Its goal is to support, respect, encourage, and enhance the strengths and participation of children and families in the child's health care" (Pridham, 1995) and provide for optimal care of the child. (See Table 28-1 for elements of family-centered care.)

B. Definition of family.

"Families are big, small, extended, nuclear, multigenerational, with one parent, two parents, and grandparents. We live under one roof or many. A family can be as temporary as a few weeks, as permanent as forever. We become part of a family by birth, adoption, marriage, or from a desire for mutual support. A family is a culture unto itself, with different values and unique ways of realizing its dreams; together, our families become the source of our rich cultural heritage and spiritual diversity" (House Memorial, 1990, p. 1).

II. SIGNIFICANCE OF FAMILY-CENTERED CARE

A. Family-centered care has an evolving history.

1. The term was used 30 years ago in relation to maternity nursing (Wiedenbach, 1967).
2. The consumer movement in the 1960s laid the groundwork for family-centered care (Beach Center, 1996), followed in the 1980s by family support programs, early intervention practices, and changing maternity care practices (Dunst, Johanson, Trivette, & Hamby, 1991, cited in Shelton & Stepanek, 1994).
3. Passage of PL 99-457 required Individual Family Service Plans for families of children having special needs, and mandated a family-centered approach and family/professional collaboration.
4. Supported by the federal Maternal and Child Health Bureau in response to the new directions mandated by PL 99-457, the Association for the Care of Children's Health articulated the elements of family care (Shelton, Jeppson, & Johnson, 1987).
5. Increasingly complex care, rising costs, and the movement toward home care in the late 1980s and early 1990s fueled the move toward viewing family-centered care as the best model of care in pediatrics; decreased costs and improved clinical outcomes were motivations.
6. Early application of family-centered care concepts included less restrictive visiting hours; rooming-in; developmentally-appropriate care; teaching parents aspects of complex medical care of the child before discharge; developing home care services; and ensuring transition to related services and follow-up in the community.
7. The recent evolution of family-centered care includes more focus on the family-professional interface and models of parent/professional collaboration.

B. Family-centered care is a new paradigm, distinguished from medical, child-centered, and family-focused models; the end result is development of mutually identified outcomes, not seen with other models.

1. Medical model.
   a. Professionals conduct assessment and develop plan.
   b. Orientation is to disease and disability.
   c. Family is expected to comply with treatment recommendations.
   d. Family access to information is often restricted.
2. Child-focused model.
   a. Concepts of child development influence provision of care (e.g., presurgical preparation).
   b. Professionals conduct assessment and develop plan based on perceived needs of the child.
   c. Family is expected to comply with treatment recommendations.
3. Family-focused model.
   a. Family members' needs are considered important.

Table 28-1
The Key Elements of Family-Centered Care

- Incorporating into policy and practice the recognition that the family is the constant in a child's life, while the service systems and support personnel within those systems fluctuate.

- Facilitating family/professional collaboration at all levels of hospital, home, and community care:
  - care of an individual child;
  - program development, implementation, evaluation, and evolution; and,
  - policy formation.

- Exchanging complete and unbiased information between families and professionals in a supportive manner at all times.

- Incorporating into policy and practice the recognition and honoring of cultural diversity, strengths, and individuality within and across all families, including ethnic, racial, spiritual, social, economic, educational, and geographic diversity.

- Recognizing and respecting different methods of coping and implementing comprehensive policies and programs that provide developmental, educational, emotional, environmental, and financial supports to meet the diverse needs of families.

- Encouraging and facilitating family-to-family support and networking.

- Ensuring that hospital, home, and community service and support systems for children needing specialized health and developmental care and their families are flexible, accessible, and comprehensive in responding to diverse family-identified needs.

- Appreciating families as families and children as children, recognizing that they possess a wide range of strengths, concerns, emotions, and aspirations beyond their need for specialized health and developmental services and support.

Reproduced with permission from the Association for the Care of Children's Health, 19 Mantua Road, Mount Royal, NJ 08061; 609-224-1742 from Shelton, T.L., & Stepanek, J.S. (1994). *Family-centered care for children needing specialized health and developmental services.* Bethesda, MD: ACCH.

b. In addition to assessing needs of the child, professionals assess family structure, functioning, problems, needs, and coping skills.
c. Intervention plans include recommendations related to family needs (e.g., social work referrals, parent group referrals).
4. Family-centered model.
   a. Professionals recognize central role of the family in the child's life.
   b. Family actively participates in assessment, planning, implementation, and evaluation of care, to the extent they choose; their concerns are addressed in the care plan.
   c. Information is shared openly between families and professionals.
   d. Family strengths and capabilities are recognized and valued in the planning and provision of care.
   e. Collaborative methods are the foundation of professional practice.

C. **Family-centered care has many demonstrated benefits not observed with other models, including improvements in the following** (Beach Center, 1996; Hanson, Jeppson, Johnson, & Thomas, 1997):
   1. Health and developmental outcomes.
   2. Parental skills and emotional well-being.
   3. Parental view of service effectiveness and sense

of control over their child's care.
   4. Problem solving.
   5. Ability of families to care for their child at home.
   6. Service delivery.
   7. Cost effectiveness.
   8. Efficient, effective use of resources.
   9. Family empowerment.
   10. Positive, proactive models of support.
   11. Professional satisfaction.
   12. Mutually respectful parent-professional interactions.

D. **Family-centered care is a philosophy of care that has implications for change in management, education, and clinical practice.**

III. ELEMENTS OF FAMILY-CENTERED CARE

A. **Family as the center.**
   1. Explanation: "Incorporating into policy and practice the recognition that the family is the constant in a child's life, while the service systems and support personnel within those systems fluctuate" (Shelton & Stepanek, 1994, p. 5).
   2. Rationale.
      a. Families care for their children's health,

developmental, educational, social, and emotional needs across settings and over a period of many years.
  b. Professionals and service-systems have specific and time-limited therapeutic interactions with the child and family.
  c. Research demonstrates that families of children with critical and chronic illnesses and disabilities prefer family-centered approaches to care (Diehl, Moffitt, & Wade, 1991; McNeil, 1992).
3. Practice examples.
  a. Providing comfortable places for family members to stay in health care settings.
  b. Supplying pagers for family members in acute care settings.
  c. Using collaborative care conferences.
  d. Showing respect for family choices and autonomy.
  e. Offering parents the opportunity to participate in care.
  f. Listening to parental observations and expertise.
  g. Providing interpreters as requested.
  h. Supporting home and community-based care.

B. Collaboration.
1. Explanation: "Facilitating family/professional collaboration at all levels of hospital, home and community care: care of an individual child; program development, implementation, evaluation, and evolution; and, policy formation" (Shelton & Stepanek, 1994, p. 14).
2. Rationale.
  a. Families know the child best and should be active participants in assessing needs, and in planning and implementing care.
  b. As consumers of care, families have an essential perspective to contribute on the program and policy levels.
3. Practice examples.
  a. Instituting and facilitating family presence and participation in collaborative care conferences.
  b. Facilitating family self-assessments.
  c. Negotiating of the plan of care.
  d. Assuring family advisory councils.
  e. Facilitating family evaluation of care.
  f. Providing for family representation in policy-making meetings and on institutional, state, and national committees.

C. Sharing information.
1. Explanation: "Exchanging complete and unbiased information between families and professionals in a supportive manner at all times"

(Shelton & Stepanek, 1994, p. 25).
2. Rationale.
  a. Families need complete information on diagnosis, prognosis, options, care strategies, services available, negotiating the system, and other details, to participate in decision making about their child's needs and care, to build skills and competence as caregivers (Hanson et al., 1997), and to cope with the challenges they face.
  b. Professionals need information on family values, cultural beliefs and practices, strengths, concerns, and preferences to collaborate with families in providing relevant and appropriate care for the child.
  c. Families have vital information about their child, including how the child responds to treatments and medications.
3. Practice examples.
  a. Meeting with families in a private, quiet place.
  b. Inviting questions and observations.
  c. Providing relevant handouts and references in a family's own language whenever possible.
  d. Repeating information as necessary.
  e. Explaining the reasons any personal questions are asked.

D. Respect for cultural diversity. *See Chapter 29: Cultural Influences.*
1. Explanation: "Incorporating into policy and practice the recognition and honoring of cultural diversity, strengths, and individuality within and across families, including ethnic, racial, spiritual, social, economic, educational, and geographic diversity" (Shelton & Stepanek, 1994, p. 37).
2. Rationale.
  a. Culture and ethnicity have an impact on access to care, use of services, perceived meaning of illness, health care practices and intervention plans, and communication (Ahmann, 1994a).
  b. Cultural traditions give families guidance, support, comfort, and meaning and can become more important in stressful or challenging circumstances.
  c. The health care system has its own cultural biases, as do individual practitioners; these may differ from those of families served.
3. Practice examples.
  a. Providing translators.
  b. Providing written information in a family's own language when possible.
  c. Examining one's own belief system and biases.
  d. Accepting alternative viewpoints as valid.

e. Learning about dominant cultures in a practice setting.
f. Inquiring about a family's cultural healing practices.
g. Explaining terminology.
h. Interpreting mainstream medical practices.
i. Providing for interreligious worship space in hospital settings.

E. Broad array of supports.
1. Explanation: "Recognizing and respecting different methods of coping and implementing comprehensive policies and programs that provide developmental, educational, emotional, environmental, and financial supports to meet the diverse needs of families" (Shelton & Stepanek, 1994, p. 51).
2. Rationale.
   a. While many issues are common to families having a child with special needs, family strengths, needs, and coping strategies will vary.
      (1) Often, several members of the same family may cope differently.
      (2) Families cope differently at different times in their lives.
   b. Supporting families requires the availability of traditional health services, but may also mean linking families with educational, emotional, and instructional support; financial support; environmental and material support; and emotional, recreational, and respite support (Shelton & Stepanek, 1994).
3. Practice examples.
   a. Respecting varied coping styles.
   b. Helping families build on their strengths.
   c. Acknowledging normalcy of family members coping differently.
   d. Valuing a father's perspective as different from a mother's.
   e. Providing information or offering referrals, as appropriate, to social work, developmental services, early intervention and special education, parent-to-parent support groups, and other community services.
   f. Providing all care in a developmentally-appropriate manner.
   g. Assisting families in mobilizing their own networks (Dokken & Sydnor-Greenberg, 1998).
   h. Welcoming siblings in the care environment.
   i. Assuring comfortable accommodations for families in hospital settings.
   j. Advocating for needed services and supports in the institution and community.

F. Family-to-family supports.
1. Explanation: "Encouraging and facilitating family-to-family support and networking" (Shelton & Stepanek, 1994, p. 66).
2. Rationale.
   a. Support provided by peers is unique, complements that provided by professionals, and may have an impact lasting beyond the initial reasons for contact. It can provide families with information, emotional support, a sense of being understood, friendship, mentoring, role modeling, assistance with problem solving, and a base for advocacy efforts.
   b. Peer support for fathers is less common than that for mothers, but men benefit from avenues for talking to other men in similar circumstances, in a group or one-to-one (May, 1996).
   c. Siblings and the child with special needs can benefit from peer support provided in a fun, engaging manner (Meyer & Vadasy, 1994).
   d. Extended family-members caring for the child (kinship care) have unique issues to face and may benefit from peer support (Ahmann, 1997).
3. Practice examples.
   a. Making referrals to parent-to-parent groups, if a family wishes.
   b. Facilitating meetings by arranging for meeting location, transportation, child care.
   c. Linking parents one-to-one when no formal support group is available.
   d. Providing referrals to national parent and peer support newsletters and organizations (see Table 28-2).
   e. Encouraging development of peer support for fathers, siblings, grandparents, and the child.
   f. Offering referrals to disability-specific camps.
   g. Developing peer support networks in the practice setting (Jarrett, 1996).

G. Flexible systems of care.
1. Explanation: "Ensuring that hospital, home and community service and support systems for children needing specialized health and developmental care and their families are flexible, accessible, and comprehensive in responding to diverse family-identified needs" (Shelton & Stepanek, 1994, p. 79).
2. Rationale.
   a. Families and children typically have many varied service and support needs that change over time.
   b. Optimal outcomes for the child and family are supported by allowing families to make choices about needed services and assuring

Table 28-2
Selected Organizations for Family Member Peer Support

Partners in Intensive Care 504 North Drive Tracy's Landing, MD 20779 301-681-2708	National Parent Network on Disabilities 1600 Prince St. Alexandria, VA 22314 703-684-6763
ROCKING, Inc. (Raising Our Children's Kids: An Intergenerational Network of Grandparenting, Inc.) PO Box 96 Niles, MI 49120 616-683-9038	National Father's Network Merrywood School 16120 NE Eighth St. Bellevue, WA 98008 206-747-4004 or 206-282-1334
National Parent to Parent Support and Information System (NPPSIS) PO Box 907 Blue Ridge, GA 30513 800-651-1151	Sibling Information Network The University of Connecticut AJ Pappanikou Center on Special Education and Rehabilitation 1776 Ellington Rd. South Windsor, CT 06084 860-648-1205 or 860-486-5035
Family Voices Box 769 Algodones, NM 87001 505-867-2368	

coordination of care when multiple providers or agencies are involved.

3. Practice examples.
   a. Offering flexible scheduling of clinic visits based on family transportation or other needs.
   b. Providing, and training families in, care coordination.
   c. Planning for smooth transitions between service providers.
   d. Advocating for sufficient and flexible financial supports.

H. Appreciating families.
1. Explanation: "Appreciating families as families and children as children, recognizing that they possess a wide range of strengths, concerns, emotions, and aspirations beyond their need for specialized health and developmental services and support" (Shelton & Stepanek, 1994, p. 92).
2. Rationale.
   a. Families are multidimensional and must balance a child's health care needs with other needs and interests of the child as well as needs and interests of other family members, in the short and long term.
   b. It is common for health care providers to focus on the immediate crisis and see the child and family only in that limited context.
3. Practice examples.
   a. Respecting family choices, even when fami-

lies would rather not share their reasons for the choice.
   b. Negotiating when there are differing points of view.
   c. Asking parents how they would like to be addressed.
   d. Calling parents by their names rather than "mom" or "dad."
   e. Being sensitive to the use of language (e.g., avoiding such terms as "crippled," "handicapped" or "defective").
   f. Encouraging opportunities for family times during hospital stays.
   g. In home care settings, maintaining therapeutic boundaries and respecting house rules (Klug, 1993).

IV. STAFF COMMITMENT TO FAMILY-CENTERED CARE

A. Value of commitment to family-centered care.
1. Care is more relevant to child as whole person.
2. Plans address family priorities and reflect family values.
3. Care is more likely to meet needs.
4. Greater professional satisfaction and growth occur.
5. Family and professionals are empowered.
6. Cost effectiveness improves.

Table 28-3
**Key Content for Family-Centered
Training Programs**

- Principles of family-centered care
- Cultural competence
- Child development
- Family systems
- Communication with children and families
- Building collaborative relationships with families
- Supporting and strengthening families in their caregiving roles
- The impact of hospitalization, illness, and injury on children and families, including the impact of health care costs on family resources
- Supporting the developmental and psychosocial needs of children and families through hospital policies and programs
- Function and expertise of each discipline in the medical setting
- Multidisciplinary collaboration and team building
- Ethical issues and decision making
- Community resources for children and families

Reproduced with permission from the Association for the Care of Children's Health, 19 Mantua Road, Mount Royal, NJ 08061; 609-224-1742 from Johnson, B.H., Jeppson, E.S., & Redburn, L. (1992). *Caring for children and families: Guidelines for hospitals.* Bethesda, MD: ACCH.

7. Improved clinical outcomes are seen.
8. Shortened hospital stays may be possible.

B. Strategies for promoting positive staff attitudes and behaviors related to family-centered care.
1. Cultivate the following:
   a. Respect for differences.
   b. Active listening.
   c. Exploring one's own values.
   d. Collaborative practice.
   e. Advocating for institution-wide support for family-centered care.
2. Avoid the following attitudes:
   a. Professionals know best.
   b. Family-centered care is too much trouble.
   c. Family-centered care doesn't apply to difficult families (e.g., assertive, poorly educated, culturally different from provider, "uncooperative").
3. Be aware of one's own attitudes, values, beliefs, and practices regarding family structures, lifestyle choices, cultural differences, economic differences, coping strategies, and other factors that may pose potential barriers to or limitations

in practicing family-centered care (Pridham, 1995).
4. Learn related concepts and skills, including child health, growth and development, interactions of child and family with health care environment, theories of family development and functioning, impact of illness, hospitalization, and disability on children and families, coping and management strategies, parenting styles and skills, communication strategies, team building skills, and community resources (Pridham, 1995).
5. Recognize the need for ongoing training. Growing in communication skills, collaboration, and the provision of family-centered care is a life-long process.
6. Use self-reflection, with or without a mentor or group of colleagues, as a way of assessing one's own attitudes and beliefs about families and family-centered practice (see evaluation section).

C. Advocacy for systemwide support for family-centered care.
1. Institutional mission statement, bill of rights, policies, and procedures should support family-centered care.
2. Nursing department and pediatric unit mission statements should address family-centered care; family-centered care should be an institutional standard of care.
3. Nursing leadership should be values driven, with family-centered care as a core value.
4. Nursing department and individual nurses should serve as change agents to better the institutional commitment to and practice of family centered care.
5. Staff should receive training for family-centered care (at orientation and in-services), including the following (see Table 28-3 for key training content):
   a. Presentations by families.
   b. Films about families.
   c. Skills laboratories (including mock family conferences).
   d. Information about community resources.
   e. An introduction to culturally competent care.
   f. Principles and practice of collaboration.
   g. Therapeutic relationships.
6. Staff should receive support, encouragement, and acknowledgment for family-centered efforts.
7. Institutional environment should welcome families and include (Johnson, Jeppson, & Redburn, 1992):
   a. Family-friendly spaces and furniture.
   b. Activities, opportunities for distraction and relaxation.

Table 28-4
Principles of Family/Professional Collaboration

Family/professional collaboration:

1. Promotes a relationship in which family members and professionals work together to ensure the best services for the child and family.

2. Recognizes and respects the knowledge, skills, and experience that families and professionals bring to the relationship.

3. Acknowledges that the development of trust is an integral part of a collaborative relationship.

4. Facilitates open communication so that families and professionals feel free to express themselves.

5. Creates an atmosphere in which the cultural traditions, values, and diversity of families are acknowledged and honored.

6. Recognizes that negotiation is essential in a collaborative relationship.

7. Brings to the relationship the mutual commitment of families, professionals, and communities to meet the needs of children with special health needs and their families.

Reprinted with permission from Bishop K.K., Woll J., & Arango P. (1993). *Family-professional collaboration for children with special health care needs and their families.* Burlington, VT: University of Vermont Department of Social Work, p. 15.

Table 28-5
Language that Facilitates Collaboration

"Do you prefer us to call you by your first name or your last name?"

"Here's what I'm thinking, but I'm wondering how this will work for you."

"Tell me how can I help you."

"Our institution usually does _______ this way. Would that work for you?"

"These are the things I plan to do for your child today. Would you like to do some of these activities?"

"What goals do you have for your child's care?"

"How does your child look to you today?"

"Do you have any questions or suggestions about your child's care?"

"This sounds important; help me understand your concern."

"Who would you like to have included in discussions about your child's care?"

"Let's talk about how much you want to be consulted."

Some of these examples are excerpted or modified from: Fialka, J. (1994). You can make a difference in our lives. *Early On Michigan, 3*(4), 6–7, 11; and Curley, M.A. (1988). Effects of the Nursing Mutual Participation Model of Care on parental stress in the pediatric intensive care unit. *Heart and Lung, 17*(6), 682–688; *Family Centered Care in Practice* (no date). British Columbia Children's Hospital.

---

   c. Opportunities for privacy.
   d. Transitional living-in facilities.
   e. Accessibility.
8. Family members should serve in advisory capacities to institutions and departments; options include (Jeppson & Thomas, no date).
   a. Surveys at discharge.
   b. Family presentations to staff.
   c. Family focus groups on specific issues.
   d. Family review of draft policies, procedures, and other written materials.
   e. Advisory board participation.
   f. Paid consultant positions.
   g. Family members on board of trustees.
9. Nursing should reach out to involve other disciplines in change activities.
10. Institutional policies should include consideration for the needs of staff and their families as well.

V. FAMILY/PROFESSIONAL COLLABORATION

A. Family/professional collaboration (see Table 28-4) is a process of working together that includes shared responsibility and shared success.

1. It may be easy or difficult, depending on the situation.
2. The process of family-professional collaboration promotes respect for families, empowers family members, and can result in optimal outcomes for the child and family (Bishop, Woll, & Arango, 1993).

B. Strategies that promote family/professional collaboration include:

1. Use active listening.
2. Choose collaborative language (see Table 28-5); avoid language such as "family should," "family needs to," "family must," "families always."
3. Have honest and clear communication, including use of the following: reading, writing, speaking, listening, teaching, and eliciting family stories (Pridham, 1995).
4. Respect family skills and knowledge.
5. Respect family choices and values, even if differing from one's own.
6. Share information readily, through discussions and written materials.
7. Help family members identify and evaluate options (Dokken, 1993).
8. Develop negotiation skills to use when disagree-

Table 28-6
Example of Negotiation

> **Family's goal:** Oral feeding for their 3-year-old child who is ventilator-dependent and currently tube fed.
>
> **Conflict with medical management:** Child is at high risk of aspiration and already has compromised respiratory status.
>
> **Nursing actions:**
>
> 1. Acknowledge the family's expressed goal.
>
> 2. State concern of health team – risk of aspiration, possible pneumonia, difficulties that can arise in treating pneumonia given child's other diagnoses.
>
> 3. Suggest smaller incremental steps – for example, obtaining an oral-motor assessment and/or having speech therapist provide oral motor therapy program.
>
> 4. Involve parents in the oral motor therapy so they can develop an understanding of child's progress or the unrealistic nature of their original goal.
>
> 5. Explore with parents the reason they desire oral feeding. Normalizing meal time and reducing parental burden of care in this case led to scheduling tube feeding during family meal times and teaching the child to assist in administration of tube feeding with the goal of eventually taking over the responsibility completely.

Copyright 1992, E. Ahmann and N. Bond. Used by permission.

ments arise (see example in Table 28-6). Strategies include the following (Ahmann & Bond, 1992, p. 402):
  a. Jointly identify the problem(s).
  b. Elicit family perspective.
  c. Share one's professional perspective.
  d. Explain the risks or drawbacks, if any, to the family's suggestions.
  e. Work with the family's priorities.
  f. Summarize the concern(s).
  g. Identify areas of agreement.
  h. Jointly brainstorm options.
  i. Agree on a plan.
  j. Jointly evaluate over time.
9. Evaluate progress together; avoid labeling and blame; celebrate success.

C. **Maintaining therapeutic boundaries supports effective help-giving and advocacy and promotes family-centered care** (Rushton, Armstrong, & McEnhill, 1996).
  1. Qualities of supportive help-giving relationships include (Dunst, Trivette, & Deal, 1988):
    a. Honesty.
    b. Confidentiality.
    c. Empathetic communication skills.
  2. Features of a therapeutic relationship include:
    a. Reciprocity.
    b. Mutual respect
    c. Trust.
    d. Empathy.
    e. Mutual goal setting.
    f. Empowerment (as opposed to dependency).

3. Behaviors indicating boundary problems include (Willis-Brandon, 1990):
    a. Exaggerated feelings of shame.
    b. Guilt.
    c. Inadequacy.
    d. Exaggerated sense of responsibility.
    e. Unrealistic expectations.
    f. Avoiding conflict and confrontation.
    g. Giving help that is not needed or requested.
    h. Putting the needs of others above personal needs.
    i. Burnout.
  4. Institutional promotion of therapeutic boundaries can include (Rushton et al., 1996):
    a. Recognition of the dilemmas of helping.
    b. Provision of forums for discussing the issue, self-assessment, team strategizing, and role-playing.
    c. Provision of values clarification discussions.
    d. Assignment of supportive, honest "accountability partners" or mentors.
    e. Establishment of standards for therapeutic relationships (Barnsteiner & Gillis-Donovan, 1990).
  5. For communication strategies that foster therapeutic relationships, *see Chapter 30: Communication.*

D. **Families may need support for the collaboration process; strategies to address this issue include:**
  1. Anticipate and accept the range of family member feelings, including anger, confusion, fear,

Table 28-7
Measures to Help Families Identify Concerns, Priorities, Resources, and Sources of Support

Measure	Author(s)	Source
1. Family Needs Survey, Revised Edition (1990)	D. Bailey & R. Simeonsson	Frank Porter Graham Child Development Center, CB#180, University of North Carolina, Chapel Hill, NC 27599
2. How Can We Help? (1988)	Child Development Resources	Child Development Resources, Post Office Box 299, Lightfoot, VA 230980
3. Parent Needs Survey (1988)	B. Darling	Seligman, M., & Darling, B. (1989). *Ordinary families, special children: A systems approach to childhood disability.* New York: Guilford Press.
4. Family Needs Scale (1988)	C. Dunst, C. Cooper, J. Weeldreyer, K. Snyder, & J. Chase	Dunst, D., Trivette, C., & Deal, A. (1988). *Enabling and empowering families: Principles and guidelines for practice.* Cambridge, MA: Brookline Books.
5. Family Support Scale (1984)	C. Dunst, V. Jenkins, & C. Trivette	Dunst, D., Trivette, C., & Deal, A. (1988). *Enabling and empowering families: Principles and guidelines for practice.* Cambridge, MA: Brookline Books.
6. Exercise: Social Support (1985)	J. Summers, A. Turnbull, & M. Brotherson	Summers, J., Turnbull, A., & Brotherson, M. (1985). *Coping strategies for families with disabled children.* Unpublished manuscript, University of Kansas, Kansas University Affiliated Facility at Lawrence.
7. Family Profile (1993)	B. McCord	The Coordinating Center for Home and Community Care, 8258 Veterans Highway, Suite 13, Millersville, MD 21108.

Note: Measures 1–6 may be found in Appendix D of McGonigel, M., Kaufmann, R., Johnson, B. (Eds.). (1991). *Guidelines and recommended practices for the Individualized Family Service Plan* (2nd ed.). Bethesda, MD: Association for the Care of Children's Health. ACCH is located at 19 Mantua Road, Mount Royal, NJ 08061; 609-224-1742. For more information regarding measure 7, contact The Coordinating Center for Home and Community Care, 8258 Veterans Highway, Suite 13, Millersville, MD 21108; 410-987-1048.

Source: Bond, N., Phillips, P., & Rollins, J. (1994). Family-centered care at home for families with children who are technology dependent. *Pediatric Nursing, 20*(2), p. 125. Reprinted by permission.

tears (Fialka, 1994); avoid personalizing feelings.
2. Recognize and validate family member skills, expertise, and experience.
3. Provide encouragement and recognition for all that family members do and have become (Fialka, 1994): a word of praise, a compassionate remark, a note or phone call.
4. Educate family members about collaboration, and model the collaborative approach.
5. Ensure time and opportunities for building trusting relationships between staff and families.
6. Provide a supportive presence for families during conferences and meetings.
7. Ensure that agency/institutional policies support collaboration.

VI. FAMILY-CENTERED NURSING PROCESS

◆ ◆ ◆ ◆ ◆ ◆ ◆ ◆ ◆ ◆ ◆ ◆ ◆ ◆ ◆ ◆ ◆ ◆ ◆

A. Application of a family-centered nursing process will vary in form and character based on the following factors:
1. Setting (e.g. acute inpatient, chronic outpatient, home care).
2. Situation.
3. Characteristics of the individual families and professionals involved (e.g., experience, personal strengths, cultural background).

B. A family-centered approach is not prescriptive; rather, it is a process, unique in each application.

C. Assessment.
1. Assessment of the child should include child and parental point of view about the symptoms or problems and their origin.
2. Reasons for questions and procedures should be explained in a manner understood by all, for example: "We are asking about this because…"
3. The following options for involvement in the assessment process can be offered to families:
   a. List observations or concerns in writing.
   b. Talk with one professional.
   c. Participate in interdisciplinary meetings.
4. Family identification of needs and resources can be facilitated by the use of open-ended questions and self-report tools (see Table 28-7).
5. A family "assessment" should be done by the family (see Table 28-7) or as a collaborative process; its purpose should be explained.
6. Assessment should focus on strengths as well as problems, needs, and concerns.
   a. Building on strengths is empowering.
   b. Examples of strengths (Dunst et al., 1988).
      (1) Commitment.
      (2) Close relationships within family.
      (3) Ability to communicate needs and support.
      (4) Coping strategies.
      (5) Problem solving skills.
      (6) Flexibility.
      (7) Strong network of friends and family.
      (8) Strong faith.
      (9) Loving manner.
      (10) Courage.
   c. Examples of family needs.
      (1) Information about the child's condition and prognosis.
      (2) Information about hospital or clinic facilities and services.
      (3) Training in skills related to care of the child.
      (4) Financial assistance.
      (5) Identification of community resources.
      (6) Access to a parent network.
      (7) Child care.
7. A collaborative assessment process (see discussion of collaboration above) results in the best set of data upon which to base a plan of care.

D. Planning strategies of care.
1. Family goals and priorities should be central in the plan of care.
2. Plan of care should reflect family values and the needs of all family members.
3. Normalization principles are central in planning family-centered care.
4. Developmental considerations are central in any care plan for a child.

5. Collaborative methods, including negotiation strategies when appropriate, should guide the process of developing the plan of care.
6. Outcome measures should be part of the plan of care.
7. Care plans should address transitions from one setting to another.
8. Coordination of care should be addressed whenever multiple providers or agencies are involved.

E. Providing care.
1. Families should have options, whenever possible, in regard to who provides care and when and how it is provided.
2. Defining roles and responsibilities can assure a smooth implementation of the plan of care.
3. Skill building education for families allows them to confidently care for their children in ways they choose.

F. Evaluating care.
1. Evaluating the plan of care is an ongoing process and occurs in formal and informal ways.
2. Mutually agreed upon goals and outcome criteria guide evaluation of the plan of care.
3. Care conferences can be used to encourage communication between the family and multiple professionals involved in care provision; families may benefit from the presence of a supportive professional or friend to help them articulate their concerns.
4. Evaluation can result in altering the plan of care and/or celebrating successes.
5. Family-centered care can be evaluated using informal surveys or formal tools (see evaluation section and Table 28-8).

VII. FAMILY-CENTERED CARE IN AND ACROSS CARE SETTINGS

A. Principles of family-centered care will have somewhat different interpretation and application in various care settings. For example:
1. In an acute crisis in the emergency department, communication with families, while no less complete, will have a different flavor and purpose than communication in the outpatient setting about management of a chronic illness or disability.
2. Similarly, parent-professional collaboration, while composed of the same features across settings, will play out differently in the hospital or home care setting.

Table 28-8
Tools for Evaluation of Family-Centered Care Practices

Tool	Use
McWilliam, P.J, & Winton, P. (1991). *Brass Tacks: A Self-Rating of Family-Centered Practices in Early Intervention. Part I: Program Policies and Practices.* Chapel Hill, NC: Frank Porter Graham Child Development Center, The University of North Carolina at Chapel Hill.	This scale is designed for early intervention programs to use in determining the extent to which their policies and practices are family-centered.
McWilliam, P.J, & Winton, P. (1991). *Brass Tacks: A Self-Rating of Family-Centered Practices in Early Intervention. Part II: Individual Interactions with Families.* Chapel Hill, NC: Frank Porter Graham Child Development Center, The University of North Carolina at Chapel Hill.	This scale is designed for staff members in early intervention programs to use in determining the extent to which their one-to-one interactions with families are family-centered. Many of the questions are applicable to nursing practice as well.
Murphy, D.L., Lee, I. M., Turbiville, V., Turnbull, A. P., & Summers, J.A. (1991). *Family-Centered Program Rating Scale: Parents' Scale.* Lawrence, KS: The Beach Center on Families and Disability, University of Kansas.	This scale is designed for use by parents whose children receive early intervention or special education services to evaluate how family-centered the practices of a program and its staff are. With few exceptions, the questions are applicable to nursing practice as well. *The Family-Centered Program Rating Scale: User's Manual, 2nd ed.* will augment the use of this scale.
Murphy, D.L., Lee, I. M., Turbiville, V., Turnbull, A. P., & Summers, J. A. (1991). *Family-Centered Program Rating Scale: Providers' Scale.* Lawrence, KS: The Beach Center on Families and Disability, University of Kansas.	This scale is designed for use by staff members in organizations that serve children and families to use in evaluation of how family-centered their practices are. Most questions are applicable to nursing practice. *The Family-Centered Program Rating Scale: User's Manual, 2nd ed.* will augment the use of this scale.
Jeppson, E.S., & Thomas, J. (no date). *Essential Allies: Families as Advisors.* Bethesda, MD: Institute for Family-Centered Care.	The Institute for Family Centered Care publishes this and a number of other publications that include checklists and inventories that can be used for formal or informal evaluation of family-centered care. Publications include *Hospitals Moving Forward with Family-Centered Care; Family-Centered Care: Changing Practice, Changing Attitudes; and Newborn Intensive Care: Resources for Family-Centered Practice.* The latter includes a tool that can be used by individual nurses for self-reflection.
Johnson, B.H., Jeppson, E.S., & Redburn, L. (1992). *Caring for Children and Families: Guidelines for Hospitals.* Bethesda, MD: Association for the Care of Children's Health.	This book includes numerous checklists that can be used by parents and professionals for informal evaluation of aspects of family-centered care.

B. Examples of best practice in family-centered care in varied settings form the basis for developing approaches to quality nursing care.

C. Types of health care settings.
1. Critical care settings.
    a. Description: "In critical care areas, children's medical needs are intense. They receive sophisticated, specialized care and treatments from highly skilled professionals. However, the technology that may save their lives has potentially dehumanizing effects. Therefore, children in these areas and their families have greater requirements for psychosocial care and increased needs for information, support and comfort" (Johnson, Jeppson, & Redburn, 1992, p. 371).
    b. Environmental considerations.
        (1) Welcome families 24 hours a day, even during rounds. Extend welcome to the family's natural support persons. Provide for sibling visitation.
        (2) Protect child and family from unnecessary noise, light, and distressing sights (Johnson, Jeppson, & Redburn, 1992).
        (3) Provide for family:
            (a) Space for family members and their siblings at the bedside.
            (b) Spaces for family privacy.
            (c) Comfortable, close-by waiting areas.
            (d) Rocking chairs, beds, and other comfortable furniture.
            (e) Telephone access.
            (f) Places to store coats.
            (g) Easy availability to meals, laundry, showers, and other resources to meet family needs.
        (4) Make beepers available to give family members freedom to leave the unit without concern they will miss important meetings or moments.
        (5) Encourage family members to make the child's area homelike (e.g., photos, favorite doll or stuffed animal, tape of family members' voices or favorite songs).
        (6) Advocate for institutional attention to design considerations reflecting attention to child and family needs.
    c. Practice considerations.
        (1) Recognize common stresses on child and family in critical care environment; respect varied coping mechanisms.
        (2) In conjunction with child life specialists, occupational and physical therapists, and the family, attend to the developmental needs of the child in critical care.

(3) Cluster treatments and care procedures to minimize disturbance of the child.
(4) Provide information to families, both verbally and in writing (in their language when possible), about the critical care environment, unit guidelines, family services, strategies for communication with staff, and answers to common questions.
(5) Prepare siblings, or arrange for others (e.g., child life specialists) to prepare them, for visits to the critical care setting.
(6) Share information in an honest, supportive, sensitive, and timely manner.
    (a) Provide family members with information about medical terms used.
    (b) In conjunction with medical team members, explain the child's medical status and review treatment options; repeat explanations as necessary.
    (c) Invite and, as necessary, facilitate articulation of questions and concerns.
    (d) Explain to family common emotional and behavioral reactions of children in critical care.
    (e) Ask about the child's previous responses in this or similar settings.
(7) Ask family members how they usually touch, hold, comfort the child and suggest adaptations appropriate to the setting, if necessary; offer options for appropriate involvement in the care of the child (e.g., wiping the brow, feeding the infant).
(8) Involve families in decision making to the extent they desire.
    (a) Establish collaborative relationships.
    (b) Learn about family member's values and goals.
    (c) Inquire about family preferences.
    (d) Ask family members how they would like to participate in decision making; offer options.
(9) Advocate for primary nursing care to provide stability for child and family and enhance coordination and communication (Curley, 1988). *Also see Chapter 17: Acute Illness: The Continuum of Care.*
(10) Assure continuity of care when infant/child and family transfer to another unit.
(11) Provide respectful, supportive care at the end of life. *Also see Chapter 6: Separation, Loss, and Bereavement* and *Chapter 30: Communication; Chapter 31: Legal, Moral, and Ethical Issues of Care.*
    (a) Recognize barriers to open communi-

cation: parental stress, overworked staff, staff attitudes (End of Life Care, 1997).

(b) Assure open communication by: allowing difficult discussions, using therapeutic communication, providing information (End of Life Care, 1997).

(c) Recognize parent's legal, moral and emotional responsibility to act on behalf of the child. Be aware of their value systems. Address ethical conflicts tactfully and collaboratively (End of Life Care, 1997).

(d) When death is imminent, explain what the family may see and hear.

(e) Respect families' grief, sadness, or silence.

(f) Offer to call other family members, clergy, or supportive friends.

(g) Provide the family with privacy; inform them if there is a chapel or quiet room nearby.

(h) Entrust their care to a staff member at shift change; make introductions.

(i) Recognize the lengthy bereavement process families experience; provide follow-up care/contact and/or a referral to a formal bereavement program (Stewart, 1995).

(j) Consider institution or agency development of a formal bereavement follow-up program (Stewart, 1995).

2. Other inpatient settings (see also critical care suggestions).

a. Description: " The family is the context in which quality pediatric care is planned and delivered. Therefore, support for the family is neither a discrete task nor an extra burden; it is fundamental to all hospital policies, programs, and practices" (Johnson, Jeppson, & Redburn, 1992, p. 174).

b. Environmental considerations.

(1) Advocate for signs that provide clear directions for children and families throughout the hospital.

(2) Assist families in finding affordable housing near the hospital if facing a prolonged stay.

c. Practice considerations.

(1) Promote primary nursing care to optimize communication and coordination.

(2) Offer choices for parental participation in the child's care.

(3) Encourage parent-professional collaboration.

(a) Assure that family members know names of all team members.

(b) Involve family in rounds and care conferences.

(4) Include family goals in Kardex and medical record.

(5) Strive for comfortable routine schedules for child and family during hospital stay.

(6) Provide information and activities to support family coping with hospitalization (e.g., preadmission programs, information booklets, patient education materials for children and adults).

(7) Recognize when policies may need to be altered to meet family needs (Johnson, Jeppson, & Redburn, 1992).

(8) Provide instruction to prepare child and family for discharge to home setting.

(9) Provide referrals to parent-to-parent support and sibling groups.

3. Ambulatory care.

a. Description: In ambulatory settings, the skilled practitioner will develop collaborative relationships that assure families' priorities are addressed and that care provided and home care plans agreed upon are relevant to the child and family in the context of their values, priorities, other commitments, and schedules.

b. Environmental considerations.

(1) Advocate for ambulatory care hours that are responsive to family schedules and needs (including evening and Saturday hours).

(2) Waiting areas should contain comfortable furniture, toys and books, and patient/family education materials.

(3) Parking should be convenient and affordable.

(4) Treatment areas should be comfortable, contain toys and books, and should be roomy enough to accommodate several family members.

(5) Siblings should be welcomed into treatment areas and/or child care should be provided.

c. Practice considerations.

(1) Be informed about common concerns of families in a primary or specialty care environment. (A family-centered approach to health supervision is provided in detail in Green, 1994.)

(2) Be informed about family adjustment to chronic illness and disability (e.g., family management styles, coping mechanisms, life cycle effects, changes in family needs over time).

(3) Actively involve the family in the process of assessment, developing the plan of care, intervention, and evaluation of the care plan.

(4) Provide distraction for the child undergoing tedious, lengthy or uncomfortable procedures.

(5) Assure appropriate pain management during painful procedures. *See Chapter 14: Acute Illness: Symptom Management.*

(6) Continue family support beyond the time of initial diagnosis of a chronic illness or disability as changes in family needs occur over time.

(7) In conjunction with child life specialists, occupational and physical therapists, and the family, incorporate the child's developmental needs into plans for outpatient or home care.

(8) Promote normalization as a goal of care by family and professionals.

(9) Provide information to families, verbally and in writing (in their language when possible), about the ambulatory care environment, strategies for communicating with staff, and answers to common questions related to the child's needs or diagnosis.

(10) Share information in an honest, supportive, sensitive, and timely manner.
 (a) Provide family members with information about medical terms used.
 (b) In conjunction with medical team members, explain the child's medical status and review treatment options; repeat explanations as necessary.
 (c) Invite and, as necessary, facilitate articulation of questions and concerns.
 (d) Provide information about various coping mechanisms or approaches to management of care needs, if appropriate.
 (e) Provide anticipatory guidance.

(11) Involve families in decision making to the extent they desire:
 (a) Establish collaborative relationships.
 (b) Learn about family member values and goals.
 (c) Inquire about family preferences.
 (d) Ask family members how they would like to participate in decision making; offer options.
 (e) Respect family decisions and choices; integrate them into the plan of care.

(12) With family, make plans for care coordination if more than one service is needed or desired.

(13) Assure continuity of care when child is seen in other settings, including health, developmental, and educational settings.

(14) Assure that family has information about community resources.

4. Emergency department care.
 a. Description: While the focus in emergency department care must be to stabilize the child's condition, it should always be remembered that the family is the child's key support. The nurse and other team members should make the family comfortable, and provide the family with information, support, and the opportunity to be involved in decision making to the extent they may desire.
 b. Environmental considerations.
  (1) Advocate for designs and decorations that are interesting, to provide distraction, yet are soothing.
  (2) Provide comfortable furniture in waiting areas and seats for family members in treatment areas.
  (3) Protect child and family from unnecessary noise, light, and distressing sights (Johnson, Jeppson, & Redburn, 1992).
  (4) Provide for privacy.
  (5) In conjunction with child life specialists (if available), provide spaces and activities (crayons, paper, toys) for siblings who may accompany family to the emergency visit.
 c. Practice considerations.
  (1) Recognize stresses on child and family in various emergency situations.
  (2) Share information in an honest, supportive, sensitive, and timely manner (see details in previous section on ambulatory care).
  (3) Permit family in treatment area if they wish to be present; prepare them for what they may see and hear.
  (4) Introduce family members to appropriate ways to touch, hold, comfort their child, and explain what they both can and should not do during evaluation and treatment.
  (5) Involve families in decision making to the extent they desire:
   (a) Explain treatment options.
   (b) Inquire about family preferences.
   (c) Ask family members how they would like to participate in decision making; offer options.
  (6) Encourage family members to consult their natural support systems.
  (7) Assure continuity of care if the child is admitted to the hospital or needs follow-

up care in the community. *See Chapter 17: Acute Illness: The Continuum of Care.*

   (8) Provide for distraction during long waits in the treatment area.

   (9) Assure appropriate pain management.

  (10) If appropriate, see section on end of life care in critical care section above.

5. Home care.

  a. Description: The home is the family's domain. Family values, choices, and priorities should drive the plan of care. Flexible, collaborative parent-professional relationships in the home setting promote family strengths, maintain therapeutic boundaries, and encourage normalization practices.

  b. Environmental considerations.

   (1) Recognize and respect that the home is the family's domain.

   (2) Negotiate "house rules" regarding the use of the telephone, refrigerator, and other details (see Klug, 1993).

  c. Practice considerations.

   (1) Develop collaborative relationships with family members.

   (2) Respect family choices and priorities; remain flexible (Ahmann & Bond, 1992; Klug, 1993).

   (3) Negotiate differences.

   (4) Maintain confidentiality.

    (a) Much of what is seen or heard in the home is not necessary to report in the record and should not be discussed with others.

    (b) Inform family, explain reasons, and obtain consent when information must be shared.

   (5) Assist family in assessing their own needs and strengths if they choose (see Table 28-7, noting that the Family Profile is designed specifically for use in the home care setting).

   (6) Provide information to families about community resources (e.g., developmental services, parent-to-parent support, special education services, Women, Infants, and Children (WIC), Medicaid, respite care, social work, counseling).

   (7) Maintain well-defined therapeutic boundaries.

   (8) Promote normalization.

    (a) Organize caregiving activities around family's schedule.

    (b) Encourage sibling relationships in the manner preferred by family.

    (c) In conjunction with other team members, instruct family in how to combine therapeutic activities with other activities (e.g., range of motion during dressing or diaper change, special feedings during family meal time, physical therapy as part of play between brothers and sisters).

    (d) Assist family in attending to normal developmental needs of child, despite medical or technologic needs (e.g., provide lengthy IV or oxygen tubing to promote mobility; provide tube-fed infant with opportunity to suck; provide portable oxygen and ventilation equipment). (For additional suggestions see Ahmann, 1994b.)

   (9) Prepare family for transition as home care services draw to a close.

  (10) Assure coordination of care.

  (11) If appropriate, see section on end of life care in critical care section above.

VIII. EVALUATION

◆ ◆ ◆ ◆ ◆ ◆ ◆ ◆ ◆ ◆ ◆ ◆ ◆ ◆ ◆ ◆ ◆ ◆ ◆ ◆

A. Rationale.

1. Research has demonstrated that the practices of nurses and other professionals are often not as family-centered as professionals might think.
2. Institutional or agency self-assessment, individual self-evaluation, and evaluation by families are important for encouraging family-centered policies, programs, and nursing practice (see Table 28-8 for evaluation tools).

B. Purposes of evaluation of family-centered care.

1. Evaluation is the ongoing process of assessment.
2. Evaluation is a part of problem identification.
3. Evaluation is a tool for planning and implementing change.
4. Evaluation is responsiveness to consumer needs and desires.

C. Barriers to evaluation of family-centered care.
(Johnson, Jeppson, & Redburn, 1992).

1. Assumption that services are family-centered.
2. Resistance to change; reluctance to challenge traditional models of practice.
3. Complexity of evaluation of process (as opposed to outcomes) of care.
4. Challenge of evaluating care that crosses departments.

D. Types of evaluations (Johnson, personal communication, July 22, 1997).

1. Family evaluation, which addresses:
  a. Satisfaction with care.

   b. Perceptions of care.
   c. Perceived control.
2. Staff evaluation, which addresses:
   a. Satisfaction with work environment.
   b. Professional self-evaluation of attitudes regarding families and family-centered care.
   c. Peer or supervisor evaluation of staff member's practice of family-centered care.
   d. Agency or institutional self-assessment of family-centered care.
3. Outcomes evaluation, which addresses:
   a. Health outcomes.
   b. Utilization of health care services.

E. Evaluation methods (Johnson, Jeppson, & Redburn, 1992).
1. Informal observations and discussions.
2. "Comments" or "Suggestions" forms and boxes.
3. Formal or informal surveys/questionnaires, both regarding satisfaction broadly and/or about specific policies and procedures (see Table 28-8).
4. Interviews (e.g., at or after discharge).
5. Focus groups.
6. Inclusion of psychosocial and family support indicators as part of quality improvement or quality assurance programs.

F. Strategies for implementing change.
1. Use evaluation information in planning change.
2. Take family feedback seriously.
3. Respond promptly to individual situations and concerns (risk management).

BIBLIOGRAPHY

◆ ◆ ◆ ◆ ◆ ◆ ◆ ◆ ◆ ◆ ◆ ◆ ◆ ◆ ◆ ◆ ◆ ◆ ◆

Ahmann, E. (1994a). "Chunky stew:" Appreciating cultural diversity while providing health care for children. *Pediatric Nursing, 20*(3), 320–324.

Ahmann, E. (1994b). An overview of issues in pediatric high-tech home care. In L. Gorski, (Ed.), *High-tech home care manual.* Gaithersburg, MD: Aspen.

Ahmann, E. (1997). Kinship care: An emerging issue. *Pediatric Nursing, 23*(6), 598–600.

Ahmann, E., & Bond, N. (1992). Promoting normal development in school-age children and adolescents who are technology-dependent: A family-centered model. *Pediatric Nursing, 18*(4), 399–401.

Barnsteiner, J.H., & Gillis-Donovan, J. (1990). Being related and separate: A standard for therapeutic relationships. *The Journal of Maternal-Child Nursing, 15*(4), 223–228.

Beach Center on Families and Disability. (1996). *What research says: Family-centered service delivery.* Lawrence, KS: The University of Kansas.

Bishop, K.K., Woll, J., & Arango, P. (1993). *Family/professional collaboration for children with special health care needs.* Burlington, VT: University of Vermont, Department of Social Work.

Bond, N., Phillips, P., & Rollins, J. (1994). Family-centered care at home for families with children who are technology dependent. *Pediatric Nursing, 20*(2), 123–130.

Curley, M.A. (1988). Effects of the Nursing Mutual Participation Model of Care on parental stress in the pediatric intensive care unit. *Heart and Lung, 17*(6), 682–688.

Diehl, S.F., Moffitt, K.A., & Wade, S.M. (1991). Focus group interview with parents of children with medically complex needs: An intimate look at their perceptions and feelings. *Children's Health Care, 20*(3), 170–178.

Dokken, D. (1993, summer). The physician as enabler. *Ethiscope.* Washington, DC: Children's National Medical Center, 3–4.

Dokken, D., & Sydnor-Greenberg, N. (1998). Helping families mobilize their personal resources. *Pediatric Nursing, 24*(1), 66–69.

Dunst, C.J., Trivette, C.M., & Deal, A.G. (1988). *Enabling and empowering families: Principles and guidelines for practice.* Cambridge, MA: Brookline Books.

End-of-life care for children and their families: Ethical dimensions. (1997, February). [Monograph]. Research Triangle, NC: Glaxo Wellcome, Inc.

Family Centered Care in Practice (pamphlet, no date). British Columbia Children's Hospital.

Fialka, J. (1994). You can make difference in our lives. *Early On: Michigan, 3*(4), 6–7, 11.

Green, M. (1994). *Bright futures: Guidelines for health supervision of infants, children and adolescents.* Arlington, VA: National Center for Education in Maternal and Child Health. (See also www.brightfutures.org/)

Hanson, J.L., Jeppson, E.S., Johnson, B.H., & Thomas, J. (1997). *Newborn intensive care: Resources for family-centered practice.* Bethesda, MD: Institute for Family-Centered Care.

House Memorial Task Force on Young Children and Families. (1990, November 6). *First steps to a community based, coordinated continuum of care for New Mexico children and families.* Available from Family Voices, PO Box 338, Algodones, NM 87001.

Jarrett, M.H. (1996). Parent Partners: A parent-to-parent support program in the NICU. Part I: Program development. *Pediatric Nursing, 22*(1), 60–63.

Jeppson, E.S., & Thomas, J. (no date). *Essential allies: Families as advisors.* Bethesda, MD: Institute for Family-Centered Care.

Johnson, B.H., Jeppson, E.S., & Redburn, L. (1992). *Caring for children and families: Guidelines for hospitals.* Bethesda, MD: The Association for the Care of Children's Health.

Klug, R.M. (1993). Clarifying roles and expectations in home care. *Pediatric Nursing, 19*(4), 374–376.

May, J. (1996). Fathers: The forgotten parent. *Pediatric Nursing, 22*(3), 243–246, 271.

McNeil, D. (1992, March). *Uncertainty, waiting and possibilities: Becoming a mother in the NICU.* Paper presented at the National Association of Neonatal Nurses' Preconference Research Symposium, Washington, DC.

Meyer, D.J., & Vadasy, P.F. (1994). *Sibshops: Workshops for siblings of children with special needs.* Baltimore: Paul H. Brookes.

Pridham, K.F. (1995). *Standards and guidelines for pre-*

licensure and early professional education for nursing care of children and their families. Project #MCJ-559327). Washington, DC: Maternal and Child Health Bureau.

Rushton, C.H., Armstrong, L., & McEnhill, M. (1996). Establishing therapeutic boundaries as patient advocates. *Pediatric Nursing, 22*(3), 185–189.

Shelton, T.L., Jeppson, E.S., & Johnson, B.H. (1987). *Family-centered care for children with special health care needs.* Washington, DC: Association for the Care of Children's Health.

Shelton, T.L., & Stepanek, J.S. (1994). *Family-centered care for children needing specialized health and developmental services.* Bethesda, MD: Association for the Care of Children's Health.

Stewart, E. (1995). Family-centered care for the bereaved. *Pediatric Nursing, 21*(2), 181–184.

Wiedenbach, E. (1967). *Family-centered maternity nursing.* New York: Putnam.

Willis-Brandon, C. (1990). *Learning to say no: Establishing healthy boundaries.* Deerfield Beach, FL: Health Communications, Inc.

Acknowledgments

The following parents and professionals graciously shared their thoughts in the development of this chapter: Polly Arango, Family Voices; Laura Bedrossian, Family Consultant, Children's Hospital of Philadelphia; Gayle Brown, Family Voices, Washington DC Liaison; Deborah Dokken, Partners in Intensive Care; Beverley H. Johnson, President, Institute for Family-Centered Care; Mary Lou Kelleher, MS, RN, Massachusetts General Hospital; Tamie Jo Olmstead, Family Voices of NY; Ceci Shapland, RN, Pacer Center, Minneapolis, and Family Voices Regional and State Coordinator; Josie Thomas; Renee Walbert, Parent Advocate; Josie Woll, RN, Director, Sultan Easter Seal School of Honolulu; Jo Yoder, Program Director, Parent to Parent of Vermont.

STUDY QUESTIONS

1. Collaborative relationships are characterized by all of the following EXCEPT:
   a. communication.
   b. dialogue and negotiation.
   c. setting priorities for the family.
   d. active listening.
   e. acceptance of difference.

2. When using a family-centered nursing process, the nurse's primary role in assessment of the family is to:
   a. assess the family's needs formally and informally.
   b. assess the family's strengths and needs.
   c. facilitate the family's self-assessment of needs.
   d. facilitate the family's self-assessment of needs and strengths.
   e. use a variety of tools for a thorough assessment.

3. Tanya is a 4-year-old child with cerebral palsy. She has a 6-year-old brother and 18-month-old twin sisters. Although she would benefit from three sessions of therapeutic exercises each day, her parents tell the nurse that they will only be able to perform the exercises twice a day. This statement likely reflects which of the following circumstances?
   a. Tanya's parents do not understand the importance of the exercises.
   b. Meeting the needs of Tanya's siblings requires a great deal of the parents' time.
   c. Tanya's parents have established as a priority meeting the needs of all the family members to the best of their ability.
   d. Tanya's parents are willing to neglect her.
   e. b and c

4. Symptoms of boundary problems in the nurse-family relationship include all of the following EXCEPT:
   a. an exaggerated sense of responsibility for things beyond one's control.
   b. assuming that parents have the ability to make decisions for their children.
   c. avoiding conflict and confrontation.
   d. giving help when it is not needed or requested.
   e. putting the needs of others above personal needs.

5. Mrs. A. is concerned about leaving her 7-year-old son Jeremy who is hospitalized to attend her daughter's dance recital. Her son's condition is stable, she knows that nurses will be in and out of his room, but she worries that he will be upset during the time she is gone. Which of the following actions indicate empowering behavior on the part of the nurse?
   a. Offering to stay during off-duty time to be with Jeremy
   b. Helping Mrs. A. explore options, such as having a family member, friend, or hospital volunteer stay with Jeremy
   c. Telling Mrs. A. that there will likely be other recitals so she should probably just skip this one
   d. a and b
   e. b and c

6. All of the following are features of a therapeutic relationship EXCEPT:
   a. identification with the patient.
   b. mutual goal setting.
   c. trust.
   d. empathy.
   e. empowerment of both patient and professional.

7. Which of the following practices are appropriate in an emergency department?
   a. Providing a comfortable waiting area
   b. Sharing information with families
   c. Allowing families in the treatment area
   d. a and b
   e. all of the above

8. Sam has been in the intensive care unit for several days following a head injury. His condition is stable, but today he has shown no signs of improvement. Over the past shift, Sam's father has seemed increasingly upset over apparently minor concerns. Toward the end of the shift, he yells at you when the IV alarm goes off. The most appropriate response(s) include:
   a. "You sound upset."
   b. "I am going to get my supervisor for you."
   c. "You need to take a break."
   d. a and c
   e. a and b

9. Which of the following activities are appropriate for siblings in a health care setting?
   a. Accompanying the family to ambulatory care visits
   b. Visiting the sibling in the critical care environment
   c. Participating in sibling support programs
   d. Participating in therapeutic activities with the brother or sister
   e. all of the above

10. Strategies for negotiating disagreements between parents and professionals DO NOT include:
    a. problem identification.
    b. assurance of professional expertise.
    c. noting the risks or drawbacks of the family's suggestion(s).
    d. jointly brainstorming options.
    e. valuing family priorities.

ANSWERS

1.c 2.d 3.e 4.b 5.b 6.a 7.e 8.a 9.e 10.b

Questions 1 and 3 taken, with slight modification from Continuing Education Series Posttest (1994). *Pediatric Nursing, 20*(2), 132–133.

Questions 4–6 taken, with slight modification, from CE Posttest (1996). *Pediatric Nursing 22*(3), 204–205.

Chapter 29

Cultural Influences

Francine Clark Jones, PhD, RN

Concept

◆◆◆◆◆◆◆◆◆◆◆◆◆◆◆◆◆◆◆◆◆◆◆◆◆◆◆

◆ Cultural competence

Objectives

◆◆◆◆◆◆◆◆◆◆◆◆◆◆◆◆◆◆◆◆◆◆◆◆◆◆◆

At the completion of this chapter, the reader will be able to:

◆ Define what culture is and what it is not.

◆ Understand the effects of historical factors on the culture of racial/ethnic groups.

◆ Identify similarities and differences in various ethnic groups' beliefs, values, and health practices.

◆ Examine differences in cultural influences upon utilization of biomedical health care.

◆ Identify aspects of family structure and relationships that affect provision of culturally relevant health care.

◆ Evaluate personal ethnic heritage and its effects upon assumptions, values, and health practices.

Key Points

◆◆◆◆◆◆◆◆◆◆◆◆◆◆◆◆◆◆◆◆◆◆◆◆◆

◆ Knowledge of history of a people provides the nurse with a broader framework from which to view forces that shape culture.

◆ The degree of retention of one's culture of origin is influenced by the individual's level of acculturation and assimilation.

◆ Culture underlies folk theories and explanations of recurrent circumstances, and becomes the basis of an individual's health care practices and health-seeking behaviors.

◆ Recognizing, understanding, and accepting heterogeneity within and between racial and ethnic groups enables the nurse to provide care that the client is more likely to accept.

◆ Knowledge about one's own ethnic heritage adds depth to the nurse's self-understanding about personal practices related to health and illness.

29

Cultural Influences

◆◆◆◆◆◆◆◆◆◆◆◆◆◆◆◆◆◆◆◆◆◆◆◆◆◆◆◆◆◆◆◆◆◆◆◆

I. OVERVIEW

Culture exerts powerful influences in every aspect of our lives. Culture shapes our identity and beliefs about what constitutes health, illness, and disease. Culture provides an explanatory model of health, illness, and disease, how we react to changes in our physical and mental status, and our thoughts about what to do to resolve our health problems. Culture also directs our help-seeking behavior.

A. The American Nurses Association (ANA) Code and the ANA Social Policy statement address the need for nurses to recognize health and illness as unique experiences, the cultural context, and to provide care regardless of social or economic status, personal attributes, or the nature of health problems.

B. As nurses attempt to understand individuals whose cultures vary from their own, generalizations will arise.
 1. These generalizations act as a temporary guide for action and should be constantly checked against observations for accuracy during individual nurse-client encounters.
 2. These actions will enable nurses to provide culturally appropriate and relevant care for children and their families.

II. DEFINITIONS

A. What culture is: beliefs, values, norms, customs, and practices that are learned, shared, active, and identity forming.
 1. Culture is viewed as the lifeways of a particular group with its values, beliefs, norms, patterns, and practices that are learned, shared, and transmitted intergenerationally (Leininger, 1996).
 2. Culture is a patterned behavioral response that develops over time as a result of imprinting the mind through social and religious structures and intellectual and artistic manifestations; culture is acquired and affected by internal and external

environmental stimuli (Giger & Davidhizer, (1995).
 3. In essence, culture acts as an invisible blueprint for living.
  a. Some aspects of culture (diet, behavior, religious practices) are observable.
  b. Others aspects (values and beliefs) are not observable.
   (1) These aspects can only be traced through the observable elements of a culture.
   (2) It is within this area of nurse-client interaction that nurses are most culturally challenged.

B. What culture is not: a number of misconceptions about culture exist. The following concepts represent some influences on culture, but should not to be equated with the term culture.
 1. Culture does not imply ethnic homogeneity or sameness.
  a. Although similarities may exist, each culture has many ethnic groups in which differences can be observed between and within groups (heterogeneity) and different races.
  b. Cultural practices are heterogeneous (e.g., vary in expression of religion, customs) and are based on the degree of acculturation.
 2. Acculturation should not be viewed synonymous with ethnicity.
  a. Acculturation is a process by which groups or individuals change or learn how to take on aspects of another cultural group while simultaneously maintaining their own culture.
  b. For example, an individual from India may wear Western business attire at work in the United States, yet retain other aspects of his or her culture at home (e.g., dress, language, foods, customs, celebrations).
 3. Culture is not assimilation.
  a. Assimilation is the process by which other groups adopt the patterns of the dominant culture.
  b. Examples of assimilation include speaking the language of the dominant culture, intermarriage, having strong friendships with the

dominant culture.
   c. The term *Americanized* can be used to illustrate this concept.
4. Race and culture are not synonymous.
   a. Race is a biologic term usually referring to members sharing distinguishing physical features such as skin color, bone structure, genetic traits, or blood group.
   b. Ethnic and racial groups can and do overlap.
      (1) For example, a black-skinned, Spanish-speaking person from Latin America is identified as a "Latino" rather than an African American.
      (2) Hence, specific cultures may well encompass many races.
5. Ethnicity and culture are not interchangeable with race.
   a. Ethnicity includes more than biologic identification.
   b. Ethnicity refers to groups whose members share a common social and cultural heritage or identity passed on to each successive generation.
6. Minority is not a culture.
   a. A minority can consist of a particular racial, gender, religious, or occupational group that constitutes less than a numerical majority of the population.
   b. Some use the term "minority" to indicate power relationships within a society, not numerical magnitudes within a population (Irish, Lundquist, & Nelsen, 1993).
      (1) Those of the White race actually constitute a distinct minority numerically when one considers the entire world; "people of color" are the vast majority.
      (2) In some instances, for example South Africa, White numerical minorities have maintained power over non-White majorities, controlling the circumstances under which they live.
      (3) In other cases, for instance in the United States and Canada, White majorities have dominated non-White minorities (e.g., American Indians and Africans who were brought to the New World as slaves).
   c. For some, the term *minority* has negative connotations.
      (1) A group designated by the term *minority*, which reflects the concept of "less than," may be assumed to possess inferior traits and/or supposedly undesirable characteristics.
      (2) To address this concern, there is increased use of more descriptive terms, such as *people of color*, in place of *minority*.

7. Poverty and culture are not synonymous.
   a. Cultural variables need to be separated from socioeconomic indicators.
   b. Poor African Americans, Asians/Pacific Islanders, Latinos, and American Indians are people of color, but are not culturally identical.

C. Other definitions.
1. Cultural relativity: the idea that any behavior must be judged first in relation to the context of the culture in which it occurs.
2. Cultural universals: structures or functions found in every extended culture such as a family unit, marriage, parental roles, education, health care, forms of work or endeavors to meet basic physiologic needs, and forms of self-expression that meet psychologic and spiritual needs.
3. Ethnocentrism: the tendency to view one's own cultural group as the center of everything, the standard against which all others are judged; assuming that one's own cultural patterns are the correct and best ways of acting.
4. Racism: a belief that race is the primary determinant of human traits and capacities and that racial differences produce an inherent superiority of a particular race.

III. CULTURAL MODELS
◆◆◆◆◆◆◆◆◆◆◆◆◆◆◆◆◆◆◆◆

A. Sunrise Model (Leininger, 1996).
1. Depicts theory of cultural care diversity and universality.
2. Commonalities among and between cultures are addressed to assist nurses to provide culturally congruent nursing care to improve health or to offer a different kind of nursing care service to people of diverse or similar cultures.
3. Key concepts.
   a. Cultural care.
   b. Cultural care diversity.
   c. Cultural care universality.
   d. Generic care.
   e. Professional care.

B. Culturally Competent Model of Care (Campinha-Bacote, 1994).
1. Assists the provider to move beyond awareness and sensitivity in the provision of care to effectively work within an individual's cultural context.
2. Presents a process model that describes four facets of becoming a culturally competent professional. The process of becoming culturally

competent is both interactive and cyclic in nature.

3. Key concepts.
    a. Cultural awareness.
    b. Cultural knowledge.
    c. Cultural skill.
    d. Cultural encounter.

C. Culturally Competent System of Care Model (Cross, Bazron, Dennis, & Issacs, 1989).
1. Developed for child protective purposes.
2. Describes six stages of cultural competency at the organizational level, but has been adapted for use at the individual level.
3. Key concepts.
    a. Cultural destructiveness.
    b. Cultural incapacity.
    c. Cultural blindness.
    d. Cultural precompetence.
    e. Basic cultural competency.
    f. Advanced cultural competency.

D. Intercultural Sensitivity Model (Bennett, 1993).
1. Developed primarily with education.
2. Consists of a continuum of six stages moving from ethnocentrism to ethnorelativism.
3. Key concepts.
    a. Denial.
    b. Defense.
    c. Minimization.
    d. Acceptance.
    e. Adaptation.
    f. Integration.

IV. CULTURAL INFLUENCES

◆ ◆ ◆ ◆ ◆ ◆ ◆ ◆ ◆ ◆ ◆ ◆ ◆ ◆ ◆ ◆ ◆ ◆

A. Cultural influences consist of direct and indirect aspects of ones' culture that have an impact on the individual's thinking, doing, and being. These include:
1. History (migration) and demographics.
2. Politics.
3. Degree of acculturation.
4. Assimilation (i.e., intermarriage).
5. Race/racism.
6. Family values.
7. Customs.
8. Health beliefs and practices.
9. Childrearing.
10. Language.
11. Socioeconomic status.
12. Geography.
13. Susceptibility to certain health problems.
14. Special circumstances.

B. History and demographics of racial/ethnic groups in the United States.
1. History, migration, and demographics of a people are central to culture.
    a. Historical events have shaped the way people interpret surroundings and the actions of others, and behave in ways that make sense to them.
    b. History allows individuals to view their own behavior in the context of others.
    c. Ethnic history reveals cultural clashes that can assist nurses to understand and accept peoples' cultural identity, understand customs and traditions, and appreciate heterogeneity within the same cultures.
2. The various cultural groups currently in the U.S. have settled here by way of enslavement, conquest, or immigration.
    a. Many Europeans chose to migrate to the U.S. to escape religious and political oppression, poverty, or for the adventure of coming to a new land; today, people from all over the world continue to choose to come to America for these same reasons.
    b. Others, like African Americans, did not have a choice; they were enslaved and brought here against their will.
    c. American Indians, present before the first Europeans arrived, were forced to take on a different lifestyle, one that was alien and destructive.
    d. The nurse must consider the historical and sociopolitical contexts of individuals as crucial to their perceptions of access utilization and evaluation of health care services and providers.
3. See Table 29-1 for the demographics of major racial/ethnic groups in the United States.

C. Cultural clashes in the history of major racial/ethnic groups in the United States.
1. American Indians.
    a. American Indians had lived in America for thousands of years, possibly migrating from Asia, before the first European explorers arrived.
    b. Indians had bitter experiences of wars, conquest, murder, enslavement, and forced geographic isolation with Europeans.
    c. The U.S. government developed policies aimed at forcible assimilation into the "White man's image" or annihilating the American Indians.
    d. Influences of culture clashes on the health of American Indians include distrust of Euro-American folkways, poverty, smallpox, tuber-

Table 29-1

Demographics of Major Racial/Ethnic Groups in the United States

	Projected % of U.S. Population			Comments
	2000	**2020**	**2050**	
American Indian: persons having origins in any of the original peoples of North America who maintain cultural identification through tribal affiliation or community recognition; includes American Indian, Eskimo, and Aleut; 0.9% of the U. S. population	0.9%	1.0%	1.1%	There are 512 federally recognized American Indian tribal governments (i.e., Shoshone, Blackfoot, Sioux, Cree, Apache Ojebwa, Oneida) and 202 Alaskan native villages. Cultural differences in language, demography, and social and economic variations exist from reservation to reservation. This group is expected to grow steadily.
Whites: persons having origins in any of the original peoples of Europe, North Africa, or the Middle East; 83.0% of the U.S. population	82.1%	79%	74.8%	There are 53 ethnic groups in the U.S. (i.e., Germans, those of English ancestry [British, English, Welsh, and Scottish], Irish Americans, Polish, Greeks, Scandinavians, Russians, Amish). "White ethnic" is also used interchangeably with "European American" to refer to all white families of European heritage who are non-Hispanic. Whites are the slowest growing racial group in the U.S.
Asian and Pacific Islanders: persons having origins in any of the original peoples of the Far East, Southeast Asia, the Indian subcontinent, or the Pacific Islands; 3.6% of the U.S. population.	4.1%	6.1%	8.7%	Group members differ in migration history, language, educational level, socioeconomic status, and degree of acculturation. Asians comprise about 95% of this population and are divided among 17 groups, including Filipinos, Koreans, Asian Indians, Vietnamese, Cambodians, Thai, Hmongs, Hawaiians, Bangladeshis, Burmese, Indonesians, Malayan, Okinawans, Pakistanis, Sri Lankans. Pacific Islanders (API) constitute about 5% of this population and comprise 8 specific groups: Hawaiian, Samoan, Guamanian, Tongan, Taitian, North Marianas, Paiauan, and Fijian. Asian American groups speak 32 different primary languages; sometimes many dialects are spoken within each group. Asians make up the fastest growing group in the U.S.
Hispanic: all individuals with ethnic origins from countries where Spanish is the primary language (i.e., Mexico, Puerto Rican, Cuba, Dominican Republic, Central and South American, and Spain); those from Spain are categorized as "other Hispanics"; 10.2% of the U.S. population.	11.4%	16.3%	24.5%	Although many Brazilians consider themselves Latinos, they are not classified as Hispanics because Portuguese and not Spanish is the primary language of Brazil. The U. S. Bureau of Census' use of the term "Hispanic" has become a political issue and source of conflict among Latinos related to identity and nationalism. Hispanic/Latinos are Mexican, Puerto Rican, Cuban, (the three largest Latino groups) Chicanos, Dominicans, Central or South Americans, Costa Ricans Nicaraguans, Salvadorians, Argentineans, or other Spanish culture or origin, including the Caribbean regardless of race. About 50% of the undocumented immigrants (between 250,000–300,000 per year) in the U.S. are of Hispanic origin (from Mexico, Guatemala, and El Salvador). Hispanics are expected to be the second largest racial group in the country from 2120 to 2050.
Blacks: persons having origins in any of the black racial groups of Africa (i.e., Haitians, Jamaican, Trinidadians, Nigerians, Kenyans, Ethiopians); approximately 12.6% of the U.S. population.	12.9%	14%	15%	Many "Blacks" in the U.S. prefer and use the term "African American" to designate cultural heritage and self-defined identity. By the middle of the next century, the Black population is expected to nearly double its present size to 61 million.

culosis, alcoholism, suicide, and depression.
  e. Today most American Indians hold U.S. and tribal citizenship.
    (1) American Indians living on the reservations obtain health services from the Indian Health Services.
    (2) Those who live in urban areas often lack adequate health insurance and may return to reservations to obtain health care.
2. European Americans.
  a. "In the creation of our national identity, America has been defined as "white" (Tataki, 1993, p. 2).
  b. The immigration law of 1790 allowed only European American immigrants to become U.S. citizens.
  c. The colonial English shaped basic American social and political institutions so that the American culture became the ideal by which all subsequent ethnic groups were judged; acculturation meant acquiring Anglo-Protestant lifestyles, values, and language.
  d. European American culture was derived from the migration of four distinct regional groups developed in England, which became four distinct U.S. regional cultures.
    (1) Puritan New Englanders (1629-1641).
    (2) Anglicans of the South (1645-1676).
    (3) Quakers of the MidAtlantic (1685-1715).
    (4) Appalachians of the Highland South (1717-1775).
  e. Cultural characteristics of each group led to differential adjustment to the dominant European groups.
  f. Anti-Semitism against Jews and racism toward people of color, urban problems, economic repression, and political corruption helped create an extreme nationalism and ethnocentrism, which continues in part today.
  g. Influences of cultural clashes on health are associated with ethnic differences, adjustment to environmental differences, geographic isolation, poverty, poor diet, and communicable diseases.
3. Asian and Pacific Islanders.
  a. The Chinese were the first Asians to immigrate to the U.S. in large numbers.
    (1) Chinese came in 1800s and met the need for cheap labor to build railroads.
    (2) Most were men who left their families behind to find work.
    (3) They clung to their customs and beliefs and resided in their own communities.
  b. Japanese Americans (120,000) were placed in internment during World War II.
  c. Immigration in 1965 brought large numbers of Chinese, Koreans, and Filipinos.
  d. After the Vietnam War ended in 1975, a large number of mostly educated Southeast Asians immigrated to the United States.
  e. Later, Southeast Asian immigrants with little education, mostly Vietnamese, Chinese Vietnamese, Cambodians, Laotians, Hmongs, and Iu Mien came to the U.S. to escape persecution.
  f. Hmong Americans, the largest of the most recent groups to arrive in the U.S., suffered torture, permanent separation from family, traumatic stress, and exposure to chemicals in honor of their agreement to assist the U.S. in the war against Communist domination.
  g. Influences of cultural clashes on health include poverty, inadequate health insurance, posttraumatic stress disorder (PTSD), sudden unexpected nocturnal death syndrome (SUNDS), disruptions due to rapid acculturation, and inability to speak English.
4. Hispanics/Latinos.
  a. The history of Latinos, including those from the Caribbean, Central America, and South America, is one of conquest oppression, defeat, and struggle for liberation.
    (1) The Spaniards and Portuguese took the land, destroyed culture and religion, killed the men, and raped the women.
    (2) Within 50 years after the conquest, Latinos were enslaved and killed in the Caribbean; African, Central, and South American slaves were brought to do the work.
  b. Different historical ties to the U.S. have affected their entrance and acceptance in this country (e.g., Cubans' arrival after the Castro won the revolution in 1959).
  c. Latino groups have had different experiences, which have caused intraethnic distrust as well as distrust for the European American groups.
  d. Influences of cultural clashes upon the health of Latinos include poverty, choosing to retain language of origin, poor housing, unemployment, communicable diseases, alcoholism, and exposure to chronic stressors.
5. Blacks/African Americans.
  a. Migration was not a choice.
    (1) Slave trade of captured Africans grew from the 15th to the 19th century.
    (2) Africans were scattered throughout the hemisphere (to the British Caribbean Islands, Cuba, Central and South America, and Mexico.
  b. Many Africans died on slave ships in their passage to America.

(1) Those who survived were separated from family.
(2) Millions suffered horrendous degradation and died under the hardships of slavery.
c. Efforts to obliterate Africans various ethnicities, cultures, and religious beliefs were commonplace among slaveholders, which led to revolts against the racial and economic injustice and oppression.
d. Differences among people from African descent by regions and the cultural characteristics must be appreciated.
(1) Africans from Spanish colonies of Central and South America and the Caribbean exhibit the influences of Spanish culture.
(2) Africans from French and Dutch colonies of the Caribbean who grew up in the numerical majority are less likely to view themselves as minorities than are African Americans born in the U.S.
e. Influences of cultural clashes on the health of African Americans include poor diet, diet and stress-related diseases, high infant mortality rate, poverty, inadequate health insurance, limited education, unemployment, and poor housing.

D. Family. *See Chapter 7: Home and Family.*
1. The family is culture at its most basic and foundational level.
a. Shared understandings of self and others, identity, prohibitions, and taboos are first learned within the family and among peers, and are then transmitted across successive generations.
b. These culturally constructed beliefs become culture-bound, the foundation of individual and collective responses on conscious and unconscious levels.
2. Structure.
a. Cultural groups differ in the roles and positions taken by members within families, as well as in the way they are structured hierarchically.
b. In many countries distinct lines are drawn between members of society based on family connections, education, and wealth (e.g., the caste system in India).
3. Constitution.
a. The nuclear family concept or some variation thereof is considered the norm in the U.S.
(1) This differs from other countries; approximately 94% of all cultures in the world hold the norm of extended family.
(2) The nuclear family is the perception upon which most U.S. heath care programs are designed.

b. Family types consist of two-parent, extended, or generational living in the same household, blood-related, non-blood-related, and adoptive. An increasing number of children are reared by a single head of household — one parent, divorced, or never-married women.
(1) Families are heterogeneous in race, ethnicity, income, and education.
(2) African Americans and Latinos are disproportionately represented among the one parent, single head of household family structure.
(3) Non-blood-related "kin" relationships may exert a significant influence on health related decisions.
(4) Many two-parent family types of Asian, African American, American Indian, Latino/Hispanic are patriarchal.
(a) Acculturation and economics have modified the dominance and authority of the male as head of the family.
(b) For example, in the U.S. an increasing number of women are working, slowly eroding a patriarchal role and moving to more egalitarian-shared role of the spouses.
4. Family ties/intermarriage.
a. A significant number of children live in households with at least one adult with a different religious identity.
b. The number of children living in families in which one parent is White and the other is Black, Asian, or American Indians tripled from 1970 to 1990.
(1) This figure does not include those living in single or in divorced families.
(2) Families with parents of different races and varying ethnicities will face additional challenges in dealing with both the biracial and bicultural issues with identity, parenting, and family dynamics.
c. Some children are adopted "informally" by biologic relatives such as grandparents, aunts, and uncles, a situation termed "kinship care."
(1) Children are reared to respect these relatives as "mother or father."
(2) Lineage may become confusing within and outside the family and create problems related to obtaining an accurate health care history.

E. Values.
1. The acceptance of values, whether class or culture bound, is not homogenous.
a. Values are often thought of in relation to class (e.g., the dominant middle-class

Table 29-2
Some Fundamental Dimensions of Western vs Non-Western World Views

Western	Non-Western
Individual is most important	Group as "collective" is most important
Achievement reflects the individual	Achievement reflects the group
Must master and control nature	Harmony with nature
Relies on nuclear family	Reliance on extended family
Dualistic thinking	Holistic thinking
Religion distinct from other parts of culture	Religion permeates culture
Feelings that their world view is superior	Acceptance of world views of other cultures
Adherence to rigid time schedule	Time is relative
High reliance on technology of the health care system for treatment	Utilization of known, traditional systems of treatment a priority

Adapted with permission from Anderson, J.A. (1988). Cognitive styles and multicultural populations. *Journal of Teacher Education, 39*(1), pp. 1–9.

European American values).
  b. See Table 29-2 for examples of Western and Non-Western cultural values.
2. Values are learned in childhood, during the process of acculturation, and provide the framework for belief, attitudes, and behavior.
3. Values are standards for guiding action and developing and maintaining attitudes toward situations, morally judging others and self.

F. Communication.
Also see Chapter 30: Communication.
1. Language is characterized by verbal and nonverbal expressions, style, slang, fluency, and varies in relation to physical and emotional health, situations, migration patterns, geography, and level of education.
  a. Persons initially learn ways of speaking through family and community members and peers; the resultant communication reflects intimacy and feelings of solidarity with others who share its use.
  b. Mutual respect for differences in introductions include introducing oneself and requesting the client to indicate how he or she prefers to be addressed.
    (1) Abbreviating names and/or the use of slang or nicknames without permission may be offensive (e.g., the use of the words "boy" or "gal" by others is highly offensive to African Americans).
    (2) Nicknames or slang indicate disrespect or unwarranted intimacy, as well as discredit the professional in the eyes of the client.
2. Nonverbal communication such as eye contact,

nodding affirmatively, body proximity, and touching has cultural implications.
  a. In the U.S., nurses are socialized to maintain eye contact when speaking to clients; however:
    (1) Eye contact may be viewed as a sign ranging from disrespect, to aggression, to desire for intimacy.
    (2) Additionally, staring at the floor or away from the nurse may not indicate a lack of listening but quite the opposite, paying very close attention.
  b. Asian clients may nod affirmatively that they understand and say "yes" when asked if information is understood; however:
    (1) They may be only agreeing with the nurse to preserve dignity and self-esteem (save face).
    (2) They may be too embarrassed to disagree with the nurse, or to admit they do not understand.
3. Personal space.
  a. Individual variations may exist in the amount of personal space required by nurses and clients from different cultures.
  b. Many Latinos, East Indian, and Middle Eastern client may prefer close physical proximity and may perceive European American nurses' distancing behavior as rude.
4. Touch.
  a. The meaning of touch varies among cultures.
  b. Many Asians believe that one's strength is in the head; touching the child's head is a sign of disrespect.
  c. The concept of the evil eye or "mal ojo" is

Table 29-3
Consideration When Using an Interpreter or Translator

1. Use a trained medical interpreter (one who knows terminology, client rights, and interpreting techniques).
2. Give attention to the client, speaking to the client and remembering the degree of eye contact that is culturally appropriate.
3. Use same gender interpreter whenever possible, and usually one that is more mature and experienced.
4. Avoid interpreters from rival tribes, states, regions, or nations. Political and cultural differences can affect relationships.
5. Be aware that socioeconomic differences can affect interpretations.
6. Reinforce information with visual aids or simple written words if the client can read or if his or her language is translated into English.
7. Do not ask children to interpret information for their parents or other family members, especially if that communication is personal, private, or intimate information.

believed by 80% of the world's population and has different definitions (Andrews & Boyle, 1995).
  (1) The "evil eye" is a folk belief that is produced by the eye (sometimes mouth) and strikes the infant or child with injury, illness, or other misfortune.
  (2) The evil eye can be attributed to the nurse who looks at and admires a child without touching the child; this action may be viewed by certain cultures (e.g., Latinos) as a curse or the cause of sickness.
5. Other communication issues.
  a. Silence is valued by many cultures (e.g., American Indians, Asian Americans, some Latino cultures).
    (1) Silence communicates respect and listening.
    (2) Silence is required to contemplate and provide an answer.
    (3) People representing these cultures may not speak unless a question is asked.
  b. People from certain cultures may ask many questions to ascertain the nurse's competency, decrease anxiety around health care situation, and to obtain as much information as possible about an illness.
  c. The family member(s) a family perceives as significant and responsible for health care decisions varies among cultures.
    (1) In many Asian cultures it is the obligation and duty of the eldest son to assume the primary responsibility to make health

care decisions for aging parents.
    (2) Male elders of a Hmong clan or tribe may speak for the child.
    (3) Godparents and female members of an extended family may speak on behalf of the child of Latino and African American heritage.
  d. The use of interpreters or translators should reflect certain considerations (see Table 29-3).

G. Childrearing practices.
  1. Cultural views and the role of children in families influence child rearing.
    a. Many Puerto Ricans view children as a "poor man's wealth."
    b. American Indians and African Americans view children as the "future."
  2. In many cultures the male child is more highly valued than the female (e.g., some Asian, Arab, Latino).
  3. Wide cultural variations exist among cultures regarding the dominant parent in childrearing; however, in most cultural groups, the mother is the care provider.
  4. Behavior of children and adolescents is influenced by childrearing practices, parental beliefs about involvement with children, and type and frequency of disciplinary measures.
    a. Disciplinary practices have changed over time to the use of a more cognitive, permissive style for many groups in the U.S.
    b. Parents may use a number of disciplinary measures that reflect cultural values (e.g.,

Table 29-4
Health Issues Related to Specific Disease of Children and Adolescents by Racial Heritage in United States

African American	Asian/PI American	American Indian	Latino American
Infant mortality	Cardiovascular disease	Pregnancy	Violence
Asthma	Cancer	Otitis media	Depression
Pregnancy	Cerebrovascular disease	Substance/tobacco use	Diabetes
Anemias	Accidents	Fetal alcohol syndrome	Obesity
Psychosis	Pneumonia and influenza	Depression	MVA
Tuberculosis	Tuberculosis	Abuse and neglect	Nutrition
Violence	Stress (PTSD)	Suicide	STDs/HIV/AIDS
Depression (underestimated)		Motor vehicle accidents (MVA)	Infectious disease
			Substance use/abuse
			Suicide

corporal punishment, shame, silence, isolation, and restrictions).

c. Members of certain cultures (e.g., African Americans, American Samoans) use strict childrearing practices that members of other cultures may consider abusive. For example, certain cultures do not view physical punishment as abusive but as a measure of gaining respect and showing concern, and as a matter that belongs within the family who knows and loves the child.

H. Illness susceptibility.
1. Certain health disparities and diseases do not affect all ethnic groups within each race equally, if at all.
2. Poverty is a major determinant of growth and development. See *Chapter 1: Biologic Development* and *Chapter 3: Cognitive and Psychosocial Development.*
   a. Families in poverty may not have resources to provide adequate nutrition.
   b. Adequate nutrition decreases susceptibility to illness.
3. Diabetes mellitus, hypertension, sickle cell disease, systemic lupus erythematosus, and other diseases have a racial/ethnic prevalence.
4. Racism has been considered a factor in a number of stress-related diseases (e.g., mental illness, hypertension, diabetes) found in people of color.

I. Health-related issues affecting children and adolescents of various cultural heritage.

1. Adolescents face many health-related issues and personal concerns such as peer pressure, alcohol and drug use, poor nutrition, violence, and premature sexual activity.
2. Racial heritage is a factor in health issues related to specific diseases (see Table 29-4).

J. Pharmacologic effects/drug interactions.
1. Individuals from different races metabolize drugs in different ways at different rates.
   a. Genetic differences exist within racial and ethnic groups, which can affect metabolism of the most frequently used medications in the treatment of diseases such as depression, hypertension, and infections such as tuberculosis.
   b. Genetic differences cause variations between races in enzyme activity, which can cause a problem with the elimination of drugs such as isoniazid, hydralazine, and procainamide.
2. Asians in general, Chinese in particular, and Latinos require smaller doses of some antidepressants than European Americans.
3. African Americans and European Americans differ significantly in their responses to certain drugs because of the differences in underlying causes(s).
   a. Regarding heart drugs (e.g., beta blockers, ACE inhibitors, diuretics), African Americans respond better to diuretics or calcium blockers because hypertension in this population tends to result from excess fluid; European Americans respond better to ACE inhibitors or beta blockers because hypertension in this population is often the result of chemical imbalances.

b. African Americans show a more rapid therapeutic response but also more toxic side effects from tricyclic antidepressants than do European Americans.

4. Regarding propranolol, a beta blocker used to treat hypertension, angina, heart attacks, and migraine headaches:
   a. Chinese eliminate the drug at double the rate of European Americans.
   b. Many Chinese are more sensitive to propranolol and require only half the blood level as European Americans to achieve therapeutic effect and are more likely to suffer fatigue as a side effect.

K. Specific beliefs and perceptions of health and illness.
1. Religious beliefs influence the lifestyles of most cultures.
   a. A family's religious orientation dictates a code of morality and influences the family's attitudes toward education, male and female role identity, and attitudes regarding their ultimate destiny.
   b. In certain instances (Mennonite and Amish communities), religion is the basis of a common way of life that determines where the children are reared and the lifestyle.
   c. A family's religious affiliation has implications for many health-related functions and procedures (Wong, 1995).
      (1) Dietary restrictions (e.g., certain foods, fasting).
      (2) Baptism (e.g., for Roman Catholics, infant baptism is mandatory).
      (3) Rites or practices related to death (e.g., Muslims have a carefully prescribed procedure for washing and shrouding the dead).
      (4) Other religious rituals (e.g., circumcision, the use of amulets or icons).
      (5) Medical and/or surgical treatment (e.g., for Orthodox and Conservative Jews, donation or transplantation of organs requires rabbinical consent).
   d. Faith healing and religious rituals are closely linked to many folk-healing practices.
2. Differences in health beliefs and perceptions are drawn from a blending of multiple ancestry with regional variations. The following generalizations are made based on composites and similarities:
   a. African Americans view wellness as harmony in nature and oneness with self and environment.
      (1) Illness may be viewed as a punishment

for a misdeed or as an opportunity for growth.
      (2) Religion is interwoven with health care beliefs and practices and involves the whole family in treatment and care.
      (3) God is viewed as the supreme being by most African Americans; some African Americans infuse religious practices such as faith, prayer, fasting, and laying on of hands by local elders, ministers, and congregational members for supernatural healing.
      (4) Wellness can be restored for other African Americans through the use of folk medicines and by practicing the healing methods, rituals, etc., of the community (mostly in the southern regions of the U.S.).
   b. American Indians view wellness as harmony in body, mind, and spirit.
      (1) Disease may be attributed to soul loss, spirit intrusion (i. e., body and mind can not be separated), intrusive objects, sorcery, or violation of ethnic taboos, in addition to symptoms exhibited by the individual.
      (2) Both natural and supernatural forces are believed to cause illness.
      (3) There is a Supreme Creator and there are lesser beings.
      (4) All things in the universe are dependent on each other.
      (5) Unnatural illness is caused by disharmony with nature and witchcraft.
   c. Asian Americans view wellness as a harmonious relationship with nature.
      (1) The universe is linked to individuals and individuals are linked to each other, which requires environmental adjustment.
      (2) The dualistic principles of yin and yang represent the universe and the human body.
      (3) Restoring the balance of yin and yang enhances health.
         (a) The yin is viewed as negative, inactive or female (stores life strength), and yang is viewed as positive, active or male (protects from outside entrance of harmful forces).
         (b) Yin and the yang constitute a power force that controls the body, the consumption of food, and all creation.
         (c) Food (cold and hot), body systems, and diseases are categorized as yin or yang.
   d. European Americans view wellness in a variety of ways such as a result of lifestyle, pun

ishment for sin, genetic origin, and mishap.
  (1) Illness is viewed as maladaptation of bio-
      logic or physical processes in the person
      to treatment and/or cure when the bio-
      medical health care system is used.
  (2) Illness can be interrupted if individuals
      take care of themselves (adapt a healthy
      lifestyle).
  (3) Technology is increasingly viewed as
      synonymous to excellent health care.
  (4) Some European Americans who lack
      access to hospitals or health clinics (e.g.,
      Appalachians) will rely upon folk medi-
      cines.
  (5) Some Irish are fatalistic in their view of
      health, and the ability to effect change in
      their illness is outside their ability to
      control.
  (6) Many Jewish people believe that the
      health of body and soul is required by
      religion; dietary habits and requirement
      for cleanliness are based on the Torah's
      focus on prevention of illness.

**L. Traditional folk medicine and Western modern
medicine.**
  1. The Latino curanderismo is a folk medical sys-
     tem that functions at different levels. The wife,
     mother, grandmother or respected elder in the
     family practices the art of healing; the cuan-
     dero/curandera folk healer takes care of the most
     serious social, emotional, and physical illnesses.
     a. Treatment includes massage, diet, rest,
        indigenous herbs, prayer, magic, and super-
        natural rituals.
     b. The curandera is consulted prior to medical
        treatment or concurrently.
     c. The jerbero is a folk healer who specializes
        in using herbs and spices for preventive and
        curative purposes.
  2. To the American Indian, religion, medicine, and
     healing are inseparable.
     a. Each tribe has its own unique set of beliefs,
        which has been influenced by contact with
        non-Indians and other Indian groups.
     b. Tribes have medicine men and women,
        priests, shamans, and caciques.
        (1) These individuals, who may also have
            titles that are specific to each tribe, are
            responsible for specialized, perhaps
            sacred, knowledge.
        (2) They help pass knowledge and sacred
            practices from generation to generation,
            storing what they know in their memories.
     c. American Indian folk medicine and herbal
        remedies provided the forerunner of many of

today's pharmaceutical remedies.
  (1) Nurses should obtain a list of all folk
      medicines that have been used to try to
      heal the patient.
  (2) Consultation with a tribal medicine man
      or woman may be needed.
  3. African Americans may use special salves, oils,
     and herbs, which arise out of folk medicines.
     a. Astrologers are sometimes consulted.
     b. In some situations, an old woman is brought
        in to undo a perceived spell or magic worked
        by voodoo.
  4. Asian/Pacific Islander healers include shamans
     (among the Southeast Asians) or older women
     who use herbs.
     a. Practices can include herbal medicines, moxi-
        bustion, cupping, skin scrapping, massage,
        and acupuncture.
     b. Chinese use both herbal and western medi-
        cines simultaneously to treat illness; some of
        the herbs and medicines may have additive or
        antagonistic effects.
     c. Southeast Asians may tie a string around the
        wrist, burn incense, or make food offering to
        the spirits; if these practices are not harmful,
        the nurse should respect them.

V. THE NURSE AS A CULTURAL BEING

A. Examining personal beliefs.
  1. Learning about one's personal ethnic heritage
     and belief system will help nurses identify their
     personal assumptions, values, and practices relat-
     ed to health and illness and the role their own
     ethnic heritage has played in their development.
  2. It is important to identify and interpret rituals
     and remedies used by the family of origin to
     prevent illness and maintain health. Self-assess-
     ment of ethnic health practices includes the
     following:
     a. What is your ethnic background(s)?
     b. What did your parents' family, your family of
        origin, do to maintain health?
     c. What did they do to prevent illness?
     d. What particular specific folk or traditional
        home remedies or practices did your family
        use?
     e. Who primarily administered illness care?
     f. From what other people within the family or
        community did your parents seek help to
        treat illness?
     g. At what point in the illness process did your
        parents seek biomedical care?
     h. When biomedical care was delayed, what
        were some of the reasons?

i. To what degree did your parents (and you presently) trust Western modern medicine?
j. How have your own practices changed from those of your family's?

B. Examining assumptions.
1. Both provider and client have cultural assumptions about the other's view of the world, rules of conduct, race, expectations about education, socioeconomic status, and so on. These cultural assumptions are learned and exist on various levels of awareness.
   a. It is important to identify and examine one's own cultural assumptions. Nurses must question their own rules around the following factors:
      (1) Family structure.
      (2) Interpersonal relationships.
      (3) Patterns, nuances and subtleties of communication.
      (4) Factors one considers in solving a problem or making decisions.
      (5) Authority patterns and behavior at home.
      (6) Food.
      (7) Celebrations and holidays.
      (8) Values (desirable and undesirable attributes).
   b. Examples of questions include:
      (1) Are interruptions during conversations usually tolerated?
      (2) Do you view avoidance of direct eye contact a sign of inattentiveness or lack of respect?
      (3) Is the distance between the client and yourself acceptable?
      (4) Is it customary to shake hands with some one of the opposite sex?
      (5) Does a loud, assertive voice signal impending violence?
2. Ethnocentrism is the perception that one's way is the best way and others are inferior.
   a. There is a strong identification with the family of one's own culture and devaluation of the unfamiliar as represented by another cultural group.
   b. This view can lead to covert and/or overt hostility, racism, stereotyping, and unequal treatment of children and their families by the nurse.
3. Racism and discrimination are often subtle and covert. It is important that nurses explore their personal history and experiences and examine ways to overcome prejudice and discrimination.
   a. Although no human being is born with racist, sexist, and other oppressive attitudes, early on, children notice differences and mentally organize these observations into categories to make sense of their ever-expanding world (Rollins & Mahan, 1996).
      (1) Attitudes about "us and them" are learned and reinforced in the home, school, church, and through the media.
      (2) By 3 years, children have learned to categorize people into "good or bad," based on superficial traits such as race or gender.
      (3) Children 2 years or younger learn names of colors, then begin to apply these names to skin color.
      (4) By 3 or even earlier, children can show signs of being influenced by what they see and hear around them; they may even pick up and exhibit "preprejudice" toward others on the basis of race or disability.
      (5) Children of 4 and 5 may use racial reasons for refusing to interact with others who are different from themselves; they may act uncomfortable around or even reject people with disabilities.
      (6) By the time children enter elementary school they may have developed prejudices.
      (7) Stereotypes remain until personal experience or someone attempts to correct them.
   b. Nurses can begin to explore the issues of racism and discrimination by considering their experience as a person having or lacking power in relation to:
      (1) Ethnic identity.
      (2) Racial identity.
      (3) Class identity.
      (4) Sexual identity.
      (5) Professional identity.
      (6) Within the family.
4. Examples of erroneous assumptions by nurses that negatively affect care provision include:
   a. "People from that ethnic group do not have a value toward health and wellness. If they did, they would not wait so long to get treatment."
      (1) The nurse likely did not consider the client's cultural time orientation, perception of what constitute health or illness, symptom-relieving practices previously used by the client, or degree of trust in medical institutions.
      (2) These factors are considered basic to evaluation of utilization of biomedical facilities and preferred culture practices of the client.

b. "Differences in ethnic groups do not matter; my job is to care for all people."
   (1) While this statement basically is true, it occludes the fact that caring constitutes actions that assist, support, or enable another individual or group to ameliorate or improve the human condition or life way.
   (2) To do this, one needs to know how to deliver caring in the context of cultural differences.

C. Examining values.
1. Nurses of varying ethnic backgrounds, socioeconomic status, and educational levels may hold certain values in high esteem, but clients may not hold these values in similar regard.
   a. For example, many Western nurses value assertiveness and egalitarianism; cultures that have strong patriarchal structures may not.
   b. Nurses may unconsciously introduce conflict by regarding the dominant culture's values as preferred.
2. Nurses value compliance or adherence to medical protocols, but clients may not.
   a. Nurses must discover what hinders adherence, and if adherence is appropriate for the client.
   b. For example, the client may have negative side effects from medication and does not want to embarrass the physician, who is viewed as the expert or authority.
3. Some nurses value the power of Western technology; clients from other cultures may not.
   a. Those unfamiliar with technology may be frightened by it.
   b. Additionally, technology does not "cure" the client, whereas confidence in familiar traditional folkways may bring about an abatement of symptoms, which was not achieved by a CT scan.

D. Examining practices.
1. Communication.
   a. Determine the level of fluency with the English language; don't make the assumption that because a person speaks a language he or she can read it.
   b. Be sensitive to use of technical jargon.
      (1) Use of "medicalese" can serve to alienate and humiliate those that do not speak English, and who are unfamiliar with the language of health care providers.
      (2) Hospital language becomes a "foreign language" to the clients and sometimes to nurses who find themselves in the "client role."
      (3) Be empathic, choose easy to understand words, draw diagrams, use pictures from textbooks, ask for return demonstrations and evidence of understanding.
      (4) Learn some common words of the language central to your practice area and use them as a way to indicate your respect for the culture and desire to communicate.
      (5) Check clients' understanding and acceptance of recommendations.
   c. Ask questions to enhance care.
      (1) In some cultures the authority of physicians is unquestionable (i.e., Hmong, Japanese, Asian Indian).
      (2) However, by asking clients many questions, the credibility of the physician may decrease because "good doctors" will know the answers and know what they are doing; in such cases it may be best that the nurse asks the client the necessary questions.
   d. Consider a client's culture as well as individual preferences when providing information.
      (1) Not all clients want to know everything about their illness or its course.
      (2) If there is no cure, or death is impending, it is best to discuss these issues with the head of family before telling the patient.
2. Cultural practices.
   a. When cure is not a reality or consent for certain procedures cannot be obtained, consider bringing in a traditional healer or minister/elder who may promote confidence in health measures through use of alternative, complementary, or integrative measures.
      (1) Traditional healers use treatments and ingredients that have been known to be effective.
      (2) Religious faith and prayers have been shown to be successful; comatose states, complications of surgery, and seemingly hopeless cases have been met with spontaneous recovery.
   b. Build on cultural practices.
      (1) Reinforce those practices that strengthen culture and are positive in outcomes.
      (2) Mutually work toward changing only those practices that are harmful.
   c. Be patient with yourself and the client.
      (1) Remember that not all seeds of knowledge that fall on fertile soil produce immediate change in the nurse or the client.
      (2) Changes in one's view of culture and its importance to health may take years.
   d. Produce positive cultural outcomes. Such

outcomes:
(1) Are culturally appropriate and acceptable to biomedical and health care providers and clients alike.
(2) Have the potential for increased client adherence to therapeutic regimes that result from nurse-client collaboration and mutually derived interventions that lead to constructive changes in the health care delivery system that make it responsive to the cultural dimension of care.
(3) Yield substantive opportunities to further understanding that is grounded in the client's experience.

BIBLIOGRAPHY

Andrews, M.M., & Boyle, J.S. (1995). *Transcultural concepts in nursing.* Philadelphia: Lippincott.

Bennett, M.J. (1993). Toward ethnorelativism: A developmental model of intercultural sensitivity. In A.M. Paige (Ed.), *Education for the intercultural experience* (pp 1–51). Yarmouth, ME: Intercultural Press.

Campinha-Bacote, J. (1994). *The process of cultural competence in health care: A culturally competent model of care* (2nd ed.). Wyoming, OH: Transcultural C.A.R.E. Associates Perfect Printing Press.

Center for the Future of Children. (1994). *Critical health issues for children and youth, 4*(3), 43–72; 134–144.

Cross, T.L., Bazron, B.J., Dennis, K.W., & Issacs, M.R. (1989). *Toward a culturally competent system of care: A monograph on effective services for minority children who are severely emotionally disturbed.* Washington, DC: CASSP Technical Assistance Center, Georgetown University Child Development Center.

Day, J. (1996). *Population projections of the United States by age, sex, race, and Hispanic origin: 1995 to 2050.* U.S. Bureau of the Census, Current Population Reports (P25-1130). Washington, DC: U.S. Government Printing Office.

Davis, G.J., & Voegtle, K.H. (1994). *Culturally competent health care for adolescents: A guide for primary care providers.* Chicago, IL: American Medical Association.

Giger, J.N., & Davidhizer, R.E. (1995). *Transcultural nursing: Assessment and intervention.* St Louis: Mosby.

Irish, D., Lundquist, K., & Nelsen, V. (1993). *Ethnic variations in dying, death, and grief: Diversity in universality.* Washington, DC: Taylor & Francis.

Kafawa-Singer, M., Katz, P.A., & Vanderryn, J.H.M. (1996). *Health issues for minority adolescents.* Lincoln, NE: University of Nebraska Press.

Leininger, M. (1996) Cultural care theory, research, and practice. *Nursing Science Quarterly, 9*(2), 71–78.

McGoldrick, M., Giordano, J., & Pearce, J.K. (1996) *Ethnicity and family therapy* (2nd ed.). New York: Guilford Press.

Purnell, L.D., & Paulanka, B.J. (1997). *Transcultural health care: A culturally competent approach.* Philadelphia: F. A. Davis.

Randall-David, E. (1989). *Strategies for working with culturally diverse communities and clients.* Washington, DC: Association for the Care of Children's Health.

Rollins, J., & Mahan, C. (1996). *From artist to artist-in-residence: Preparing artists to work in pediatric healthcare settings.* Washington, DC: Rollins & Associates, Inc.

Wong, D. (1995). *Whaley & Wong's nursing care of infants and children* (5th ed.). St. Louis: Mosby.

Study Questions

◆◆◆

1. The study of culture acknowledges that:
   a. the nurse use stereotypes as initial basis for practice.
   b. generalizations will occur and become temporary guides for practice.
   c. it is never safe to generalize.
   d. once generalizations are checked they are considered accurate.

2. Characteristics of culture include:
   a. shared, learned, active beliefs, practices, and customs.
   b. homogeneity within families.
   c. members who have assimilated.
   d. similarities in migration history and demography.

3. Nurses use cultural models to guide their care for culturally diverse clients. Cultural models:
   a. emphasize a progression of skill from awareness to competence.
   b. have been developed by nursing professionals only.
   c. are not useful in working with individuals of one's own ethnic group.
   d. increases nurses' ethnocentrism.

4. Cultural clashes with European American cultures influenced the health of racial groups by:
   a. enhancing acculturation of immigrants.
   b. diminishing environmental influences in developing diseases.
   c. increasing use of biomedical facilities.
   d. increasing distrust, poverty, and development of diseases.

5. The fastest growing racial group in the U.S. is:
   a. Latinos.
   b. Asian/PI.
   c. African Americans.
   d. American Indians.

6. Cultural childrearing practices are culture bound and nurses must consider:
   a. the degree of societal commitment.
   b. level of acculturation and assimilation.
   c. the number of relatives living in the same household.
   d. the gender of the primary caretaker.

7. Communication with individuals from various cultures includes which of the following concepts?
   a. Fluency of language spoken and read
   b. Gestures
   c. Use of silence
   d. Use of same gender interpreter
   e. All of the above

8. A value shared by many European Americans is:
   a. harmony.
   b. relative time orientation.
   c. emphasis on the group.
   d. emphasis on the individual.

9. When giving medication to clients of different groups it is important to remember that:
   a. all clients metabolize medications in basically the same manner.
   b. evidence of genetic differences in drug metabolization is inconclusive.
   c. genetic differences are related to variations in the elimination of drugs.
   d. only responses to tricyclic antidepressants have been shown to be different across cultures.

10. For many ethnic groups in the U.S, utilization of the health care system is based on:
    a. health insurance.
    b. access to folk health treatments.
    c. perception of racism.
    d. values regarding Western health care.
    e. all of the above.

Answers

◆◆◆◆◆◆◆◆◆◆◆◆◆◆◆◆◆◆◆◆◆◆◆◆◆◆◆

1.b 2.a 3.a 4 d 5.b 6.b 7.e 8.d 9.c 10.e

Chapter 30

Communication

Carmel C. Mahan, MSEd, CCLS

Concept

◆◆◆◆◆◆◆◆◆◆◆◆◆◆◆◆◆◆◆◆◆◆◆◆

◆ Communication

Objectives

◆◆◆◆◆◆◆◆◆◆◆◆◆◆◆◆◆◆◆◆◆◆◆◆

At the completion of this chapter, the reader will be able to:

◆ Identify sensory modalities for communicating with children and families.

◆ Recognize developmental influences on communication.

◆ Identify several strategies for communicating effectively with children and families.

◆ Recognize considerations for choosing developmentally appropriate language.

◆ Recognize children and families' perspectives on the communication process.

◆ Identify elements of a therapeutic relationship.

◆ Identify available resources for use when communicating in special situations.

Key Points

◆◆◆◆◆◆◆◆◆◆◆◆◆◆◆◆◆◆◆◆◆◆◆◆

◆ Assessment of affect and communication abilities should directly impact choice of language and communication techniques.

◆ Communicating caring and maintaining a therapeutic relationship are essential skills in pediatric nursing care.

◆ Special situations require the use of additional resources to provide clear communication for all members of the healthcare team.

◆ Verbal communication should be appropriate to the developmental level of the child.

◆ Nonverbal communication comprises the largest percentage of any message sent or received.

◆ Written communication should be appropriate to child/parent's reading abilities.

30

Communication

I. OVERVIEW

"The nurse will communicate effectively with child and family and others who participate in the care and the education of the child and family" (Pridham, Broome, & Woodring, 1996, p. 273). Effective communication is an essential component of quality nursing care. It is central to successful assessment, intervention, and outcome, to the entire nursing process.

A. Definition: communication is sending and receiving information through verbal and nonverbal means.

B. Special considerations.
   1. Communicating with children and families in health care settings presents special considerations related to pediatric care (Rollins & Mahan, 1996).
      a. Children are not simply "little adults."
      b. Children are growing and changing almost by the minute.
      c. How children experience health care encounters is very different from how adults experience health care encounters.
      d. Children experience health care encounters differently from one year — or even one week — to the next.
   2. Communicating effectively requires a shift in perceptions.
      a. Adults often forget how children view the world.
      b. Imagining situations through a child's eyes can transform an adult's perceptions.
      c. Similarly, viewing the health care experience of a child through the eyes of a parent can alter perceptions.
      d. Remaining mindful of questions such as: "What does a 5 year old understand about how his/her body works?" or "What do these parents want for themselves and their children?" causes a very basic shift in awareness that affects every nurse who practices this strategy.
      e. Remembering to question assumptions before responding to a child or family member, and attempting to "try on" another's shoes prior to any attempt to assess or meet another's needs are important aspects of communication in pediatric settings.

II. ASSESSMENT

A number of quick, easy, and informal methods exist to assess the effectiveness of communication. Most of them include observation of the child, family, and those with whom they interact in the health care setting.

A. Observation.
   1. Nonverbal communication involves exchange of information between or among participants in an interaction, without or in addition to the use of words.
      a. Nonverbal communication represents a large percentage of the content of any message; this is especially true for children.
      b. From infancy, humans pay closer attention to nonverbal than to verbal messages.
      c. If there is a perceived conflict, the nonverbal message will be believed; actions do speak louder than words.
      d. As infants grow into toddlers, they begin to use words, but gestures and other nonverbal communication still predominate.
      e. In normally developing children, verbal communication becomes increasingly important with age.
      f. Even adults rely heavily on nonverbal cues to interpret messages.
      g. The meanings of nonverbal cues need validation.
   2. Observing and interpreting children's play.
      a. Play is an important means by which children learn about the world.
         (1) Children use their physical and mental capacities to create their own knowledge through play.
         (2) Children interact with their environment to construct their own mental image of

the world by "playing around" with things, people, and ideas.

(3) Most adults think of play as recreational, thereby unimportant. This is not so for the child; child's play is practice in thinking (Beaty, 1994).

b. Children typically use role-play, fantasy, storytelling, music, and art to work with complex emotions they may be unable to name.

(1) These emotions may relate to children's health care experiences, or to any other aspect of their lives.

(2) Frequently, children "depersonalize" strong feelings by attributing them to a character in a song or story rather than "owning" them. This should be viewed as a developmentally appropriate use of play rather than as denial.

c. Observing the child at play and asking open-ended questions will allow the child to explore emotions. For example, if the nurse observes a child playing with a stuffed animal and the child starts to hit a chair with the animal, the nurse could say, "What's happening to your dog?" Possible responses:

(1) The child exclaims, "Nothing!" or remains silent. Possible interpretations:
   (a) The child does not want to speak to the nurse.
   (b) The child is fearful and will not speak to anyone.

(2) The child says, "His mommy is hitting him because he was bad."
   (a) This has many possible interpretations.
   (b) Further assessment is required.

(3) The child responds, "He's jumping around because his fleas are itching." Possible interpretations:
   (a) The child is just playing; no emotional content is evident.
   (b) The child is itching and attributing symptoms to the toy.

d. Numerous opportunities for such observations exist when providing nursing care for children.

(1) Repeated themes and issues should be noted, and not too much emphasis should be placed on any one brief observation.

(2) If something children say or the content of their play causes concern, another member of the team, such as a child life specialist, social worker, psychologist, or pediatrician should be consulted.

e. *See Chapter 15: Acute Illness: Intervention Strategies* and *Chapter 23: Chronic Illness: Intervention Strategies.*

3. Observing parents and children together.

a. Taking advantage of opportunities to observe family members interacting with children provides anecdotal data about:

(1) Parents' expectations of their children.

(2) Communication styles within the family.

(3) Children's developmental level, including language (Beaty, 1994). *Also see Chapter 3: Cognitive and Psychosocial Development.*

   (a) Most children pronounce their first word by the end of the first year or beginning of the second.
   (b) Children between 1 and 2 years of age can use 10 basic sounds and speak in two-word sentences.
   (c) Two- to 3-year-olds use telegraphic speech (e.g., "Mama go work").
   (d) Between 3 and 4, children have mastered most sounds (although they may have difficulty with *s, l, r, th,* and *sk*) and can use proper word order.
   (e) Four- to 5-year-olds may continue to have difficulty with certain sounds; they now can ask questions and produce negative statements using proper word order.
   (f) Most children between the ages of 5 and 6 can use proper grammar and word order.

b. This is valuable information to include in a care plan, which might address a need for parental education about child safety, infant stimulation, or other parenting skills.

4. Observing the parent, child, and nurse interaction.

a. Observations on the impact of a third party on the child and family consider the following issues:

(1) How do their interactions change?

(2) Whose behavior changes? In what ways?

(3) Is there a change in vocalizations, facial expression, or posture?

b. Nurses who seek to answer these questions by close observation are that much nearer to understanding the dynamics of communicating successfully with children and families in health care settings.

c. Practicing these skills incorporates them into existing knowledge of the nursing process, and they soon become a natural part of the assessment process, rather than one more thing to remember.

B. Interview.

1. The standard method of assessment in health

care is the interview.
   a. Called by various names (e.g., admitting history and physical, initial assessment), it is usually a form filled out by the admitting nurse.
   b. For children, the form includes questions about developmental milestones, feeding, toileting, language, and social skills.
   c. If a form does not include these items, it should be revised to include them.
2. Interviewing children.
   a. Too often during admission, children are ignored until it is time for the physical exam.
   b. To promote proactive health behaviors, children should be included in this process to the extent that they are able and willing to participate.
   c. Children can be asked directly about acquired or emerging skills. For example:
      (1) "Can you tie your shoes?"
      (2) "What do you like to be called?" (nickname?)
      (3) "Can you count Mommy's fingers?"
   d. Children may not answer even if the information is known. A child's willingness to cooperate may be affected by one or more factors.
      (1) The nurse is a stranger.
      (2) The interview usually takes place during a stressful experience.
3. Interviewing parents or guardians.
   a. Parents or guardians can supplement a child's incomplete responses, or answer if the child refuses.
   b. Attempts should be made to discourage parents from interrupting children to answer questions for them. For example:
      (1) "Jamie is doing a great job describing how he feels. I'll have some questions for you in a few minutes."
      (2) "Right now I need to hear Kiesha's story. Perhaps you could jot down any questions you have while I finish speaking with her."
   c. Asking about children's attainment of developmental milestones may help to assess a need for family education about child development or parenting skills.
   d. Parents are a tremendous resource for health care professionals. *See Chapter 28: Family-Centered Care.*
      (1) They observe and can share many aspects of the child's baseline behavior, comforting strategies, food preferences, and much more.
      (2) Nurses who offer family members the opportunity to discuss their children as

individuals, and not just the condition or illness they have, go a long way toward building a partnership that will promote good communication and enhance patient care.
4. Discrepancies in verbal and nonverbal communication.
   a. During an interview, any conflict between nonverbal and verbal communication should be noted.
   b. This may signal inaccuracies in or ambivalence about the information.
   c. These areas of conflict should be explored further, either during the interview or at a later time, depending on the circumstances (e.g., lack of privacy).

C. Other resources.
1. Certain circumstances may require the use of other resources.
   a. For example, when children present with developmental delays or language concerns, other resources can be used to provide additional information.
   b. Access to such services varies from one institution to the next, but certain resources are usually readily available.
2. Children's teachers.
   a. Many parents have teacher reports or evaluations available, which may help to clarify the specifics of an individual child's abilities.
   b. The nurse can ask parents for permission to call the teacher if clarification is needed.
3. Developmental evaluation.
   a. Through educational or health care services, most communities have centers for the developmental evaluation of children.
   b. Parents may have the results of a recent evaluation; if not, the physician can order one.
   c. If a child has a chronic condition, or a long admission is anticipated, developmental evaluation is especially important.
   d. Developmental goals can be included in treatment plans so that children do not lose ground developmentally while they are receiving care.
4. Speech and language pathology.
   a. Most hospitals have a Speech Pathology program that provides services that include:
      (1) Speech therapy for existing language problems.
      (2) Programs to help prevent problems or lessen their severity.
   b. For example, a service for an infant may include:
      (1) Developing an oral-motor stimulation

program to help with suck, swallow, and other concerns of feeding or sound production.

(2) Exercises that parents and nurses can perform with children during feeding, bath, or play times.

III. INTERVENTIONS

◆ ◆ ◆ ◆ ◆ ◆ ◆ ◆ ◆ ◆ ◆ ◆ ◆ ◆ ◆ ◆ ◆ ◆ ◆

Throughout their practice, pediatric nurses communicate with patients and families. Children's development influences their communication abilities. Intervention strategies based on these concepts help facilitate successful communication with children and families.

A. Communicating with children.
1. Children's developmental level has an enormous impact on both receptive language (receiving a message) and expressive language (sending a message).
   a. Table 30-1 lists cognitive and emotional development from birth through adolescence.
   b. Cognitive and emotional development affects the child's issues related to health care experiences, potential negative reactions, and appropriate nursing interventions.
2. Working as a team with children, families, and other professionals, nurses can help to facilitate a health care experience that is developmentally growth producing rather than damaging.
3. All health care professionals are charged to "First do no harm." (Hippocratic Oath)

B. Considerations for choosing language.
1. Children pay close attention to nonverbal cues, and also to words.
2. Children below age 8 generally interpret words very literally and concretely.
3. Children frequently misinterpret common medical terms.
   a. Misconceptions can be avoided by choosing more neutral, less threatening language.
   b. Common misconceptions and suggested alternatives are presented in Table 30-2.

C. Communication techniques.
1. Effective communication techniques consider nonverbal and verbal communication and the child's developmental level.
2. Regarding nonverbal communication:
   a. Body language and gestures are important elements of nonverbal communication.
   b. The following are some useful approaches to nonverbal communication with children, cat-

egorized by developmental level (Clutter et al., 1987; 1988):
(1) 0-2 years.
   (a) Pitch, tone of voice, posture and gestures are all noted by infants and toddlers.
   (b) Physical contact, such as gentle patting or stroking, often comforts infants and toddlers.
   (c) Sudden loud noises startle many small children. Reduce volume of unfamiliar noises. Maintain a calm, soothing tone of voice.
   (d) Infants and toddlers feel safer sitting upright, near and in visual contact with a parent.
(2) 3-7 years.
   (a) Avoid sudden approaches; let children make the first move as much as possible.
   (b) Use understated facial expressions. Wide smiles and other facial contortions may appear threatening.
   (c) Approach at child's eye level to de-emphasize the child's small size and to appear less threatening.
   (d) Allow child to remain with parent.
   (e) Use brief eye contact until the child appears comfortable with it.
(3) 8-21 years.
   (a) Continue to use a calm, soothing voice.
   (b) Use an unhurried manner with children or adolescents.
   (c) Avoid facial expressions that convey anger, disappointment, or surprise in response to children's or adolescents' words or behavior.
   (d) Inform adolescents about patient confidentiality policy before asking questions about sexuality, substance abuse, or other sensitive topics.
   c. *See Chapter 29: Cultural Influences* for cultural appropriate nonverbal communication techniques.
3. Regarding verbal communication:
   a. Generally, children of any age respond well to a calm, confident voice and an honest, developmentally appropriate explanation.
   b. Avoid confusing terms or emotionally charged words (see Table 30-2).
   c. The following are some useful techniques to facilitate conversations with children and family members (Clutter et al., 1987; 1988):
   (1) Offer realistic choices, such as:
      (a) "Do you want juice or water with your medicine?"

Table 30-1. Understanding and Communicating with Children Who Are Hospitalized: A Developmental Perspective

Age	Erikson	Piaget	Hospitalization Issues	Possible Troublesome Responses	Interventions
Infant 0–1	Trust vs Mistrust • To get • To give in return	Sensorimotor • Exploration of physical self and environment • Object constancy • Cause and effect	Separation Lack of stimulation Pain	Failure to bond Distrust Anxiety Delayed skills development	Maximize parental information Provide stimulation • Visual • Auditory • Tactile • Kinesthetic • Vestibular
Toddler 1–3	Shame & Doubt • To hold on • To let go	Sensorimotor Preoperational (preconceptual phase) • Can hold and recall images • Increasing use of symbolization • Highly egocentric perception of world	Separation Fear of bodily injury and pain Frightening fantasies Immobility/restriction Forced regression Loss of routine and rituals	Regression (including loss of newly learned skills) Uncooperativeness Protest (verbal and physical) Despair Negativism Temper tantrums Resistance	Maximize parental involvement Maximize parental information Facilitate medical play Promote therapeutic play • Environmental exploration • Freedom within limits • Routine and ritual • Self-expression • Movement activities • Sensory stimulation games
Preschooler 3–6	Initiative vs Guilt • To make (going after) • To "make like" (playing)	Preoperational (preconceptual phase) Preoperational (intuitive phase) • Transition period between depending solely on perception and depending on truly logical thinking • Better able to see more than one factor at a time that influences an event	Separation Fear of loss of control, sense of own power Fear of bodily mutilation or penetration by surgery or injections, castration	Regression Anger toward primary caregiver Acting out Protest (less aggressive than toddler) Despair and detachment Physical and verbal aggression Dependency Withdrawal	Maximize parental involvement Maximize parental information Facilitate medical play Promote therapeutic play • Environmental exploration • Freedom within limits • Routine and ritual • Self-expression • Movement activities • Sensory stimulation games
School-ager 7–12	Industry vs Inferiority • To make things (completing) • To make things together	Concrete operations • Increasing ability to think logically in the physically concrete realm • Understands the meaning of series of actions, of order and sequencing	Separation Fear of loss of control Fear of loss of mastery Fear of bodily mutilation Fear of bodily injury and pain, especially intrusive procedures in genital area Fear of illness itself, disability, and death	Regression Inability to complete some tasks Uncooperativeness Withdrawal Depression Displaced anger and hostility Frustration	Maximize parental involvement Maximize parental information Encourage education/teacher involvement Facilitate medical play/information Promote therapeutic play • Skill building • Meaningful projects • Group activities • Peer support • Freedom within limits • Self-expression
Adolescent 12–18	Identity & Repudiation vs Identity Diffusion • To be oneself (or not to be) • To share being oneself	Formal operations • Deductive and abstract reasoning • Can imagine the conditions of a problem—past, present, and future—and develop hypotheses about what might logically occur under different combinations of factors	Dependence on adults Separation from family and peers Fear of bodily injury and pain Fear of loss of identity Body image/sexuality Concern about peer group status after hospitalization	Uncooperativeness Withdrawal Anxiety Depression	Encourage peer group activities Provide privacy Respect independence (choices) Encourage self-expression Address body image, sexuality, and future concerns Facilitate medical preparation Encourage education/teacher involvement Facilitate visits with peers

Adapted with permission from Rollins, J., & Mahan, C. (1996). *From artist to artist-in-residence: Preparing artists to work in pediatric healthcare settings.* Washington, DC: Rollins & Associates, p. 24.

Table 30-2
Considerations in Choosing Language

Words that have different meanings can be confusing. If it is likely that children will hear the standard medical expressions used, these words should be explained or defined. Ideally, children should be asked if they know what nurses and doctors mean when they say these words. Compare, for example, the phrases in the left column with the suggested alternatives in the right column.

Potentially Ambiguous	**Clearer**
Dressing, dressing change *Why will they undress me?* *Will I be naked?* *Do I have to change clothes?*	Bandages, clean, new bandages
Urine *You're in?*	Ask for the child's familiar term (such as *pee*) and use it.
Shot *With a gun?* *Are they mad at me?* *Did I do something bad?*	Medicine through a (small, tiny) needle
CAT Scan *Cats? Will they scratch me?*	Describe in simple terms; explain what the letters of the common name stand for
P.I.C.U. *Pick you?*	Explain, as above
I.C.U. *I see you? Like peek-a-boo?*	Explain, as above
I.V. *Ivy? Poison Ivy?*	Explain, as above
Stretcher *Stretch her? Who? Why?* *Won't that hurt?*	Bed with wheels
Put you to sleep *My cat was put to sleep. She died.*	Give you medicine (mixed with air or with a needle) that makes you go into a very deep sleep. You won't feel or remember anything until the surgery is over. Then the doctor will stop giving you the medicine, and you will wake up.
Move you to the floor *Why can't I stay in my chair?* *I don't want to sit on the floor!*	Go to a new room (Explain the reason for the move. Reassure that parents will find child; offer concrete solution: "We'll leave a note.")
O.R. (or treatment room) table *I'm not allowed to get on the table.*	A narrow bed
Take your picture (x-ray, CT, and MRI machines are larger than a familiar camera, move differently, and do not yield a familiar end product.)	A picture of the inside of you. The camera can move, but it will not touch you. Describe appearance, sounds, and movement of the equipment.
Flush your IV *Down the toilet?*	Explain. "I need to put medicine in your tube."

Table 30-2 continues on opposite page

Table 30-2 (continued)
Considerations in Choosing Language

Words can be experienced as "hard" or "soft" according to how much they increase the perceived threat of a situation. For example, consider the following word choices.

Harder	Softer
This part will hurt.	It (you) may feel (very): sore, achy, tight, scratchy, snug, full, or... (other manageable, descriptive term.) Children have a small vocabulary for pain. Sometimes "hurt" is the best choice.
The room will be very cold.	Some children say they feel very cool.
Cut, open you up, slice, make a hole	The doctor will make a small opening. (Use a concrete comparison such as, "your little finger" or "a paper clip" if the opening will indeed be small.) Be truthful.
As big as...(e.g., size of incision or catheter)	Smaller than...
As long as...(e.g., duration of a procedure)	For less time than it takes you to...
As much as...	Less than...
(These are open-ended and "extending" expressions.)	(These expressions help to confine, familiarize, and imply the "manageability" of an event or of equipment.)

The unfamiliar usage or complexity of some common medical words or expressions can be confusing and frightening.

Potentially Unfamiliar	Concrete Explanation
Take your vitals (or vital signs)	Measure your temperature; see how warm your body feels; see how your heart is working. (Nothing is "taken" from the child.)
Electrodes, leads	Sticky like a Bandaid, with a small wet spot in the center, and small cords that attach to the snap. Show child electrode and leads before using. Let child handle them and apply to a doll or to self.
Intravenous; IV	Medicine that needs to go into a vein (Intra-Venous). IV stands for "In your Vein." First, ask child if she/he knows what a vein is, and why some medicines are taken by mouth and others need to go into a vein. Explain concept of initials if child is old enough.
Hang your (IV) medication	Bring a new bag of medicine and attach it to the ttube in your arm. I won't touch you, only your tube
NPO	Nothing to eat or drink. Your stomach needs to be empty. (Explain why.) You can eat and drink again as soon as... (Explain using concrete descriptions.)

Table 30-2 continues on next page

Table 30-2 (continued)
Considerations in Choosing Language

Potentially Unfamiliar	Concrete Explanation
Anesthesia	The doctor will give you medicine — you may hear it called "anesthesia." It will make you go into a very deep sleep. You will not feel or remember anything at all. The doctors know just the right amount of medicine to give you so you will stay asleep through your whole operation. When the operation is done, the doctor stops giving you the medicine and that makes you wake up. Your throat may feel sore (after intubation or ENT surgery).
Incision	Small opening. (Follow with discussion of how cuts and scrapes have healed in the past.)

Words have the potential to predispose people's thoughts and perceptions of impending events or experiences, and to cut off or encourage communication and interaction. Compare the impact of the following.

You will have to say goodbye to your parents.	That will be the time when you say "See you later" to your parents.
You are very angry/scared/sad. That was very hard for you.	How was that for you? Was it the way you thought it would be? Is there something else we should tell people about this? (Avoid telling a person what they felt or experienced without first asking them.)

NOTES: Words or phrases that are helpful to one child may be threatening for another. Health care providers must listen carefully and be sensitive to the child's use of and response to language.

    (b) "Shall I measure your blood pressure in your right or left arm?"

(2) Avoid asking a question if there is no choice, for example:
    (a) "I need to measure your temperature, OK?"
    (b) The nurse's "OK" turns a statement into a question.
    (c) Children can then say "no," and a power struggle is created.

(3) Speak to young children's toys or dolls or through a puppet.

(4) Avoid using "good boy" or "good girl" to praise a cooperative child.
    (a) The child may be unclear regarding what he or she did that was "good," and possibly fear being unable to meet expectations the next time.
    (b) Describing behaviors or other attributes of the child are more helpful; for example: "You stayed very still for that x-ray. Good job!"

(5) Replace negative "you" messages with observations that do not blame the child; for example, "The IV is on the floor; it needs to be in your arm" is less accusatory than, "You ripped out your IV!"

IV. COMMUNICATING CARING

◆ ◆ ◆ ◆ ◆ ◆ ◆ ◆ ◆ ◆ ◆ ◆ ◆ ◆ ◆ ◆ ◆ ◆ ◆ ◆

By using the strategies described above, nurses can communicate respect and caring, as well as the literal content of a message. Both children and parents appreciate being treated with honesty, dignity, and compassion, and most will reciprocate such interactions. No one can convey the importance of this nursing role more eloquently than a parent who has experienced months of NICU and PICU care, as well as the death of two infants (Sweeney, 1997, p. 66): "It makes a tremendous difference when staff members take the few minutes needed for a simple introduction and to speak to parents with warmth and compassion, instead of always being in a rush and rattling off a bunch of medical jargon. Courteous, respectful communication is important in any environment, and particularly when a family may be stressed."

A. Context is one more vital cue during communication (Sweeney, 1997).

1. Would the above statement have as much impact if its context were unknown? Perhaps it should, but would it?
2. Awareness of the circumstances of children and families is important when considering possible interpretations of any interaction; doing so may well avert potentially damaging miscommunications.

B. Communicating respect.

1. Many potential power struggles with children can be averted by communicating respect and caring.
2. When nurses listen to children, allow them to express emotions, and offer realistic choices, children's need to protest their situation is minimized.
3. A child who feels respected and cared for often communicates needs and wishes more effectively, enabling nurses to respond to them more efficiently.
4. A child who is offered respect and caring may cooperate with treatment more easily than a child who feels no one is listening.
5. Children who feel no one is listening may feel the need to escalate their protests until caregivers demonstrate understanding of their pain, fear, and/or anger. For example:
   a. Child: "Ow, that hurts! No! Ow, ow, ow! STOP IT! GET AWAY FROM ME!" Nurse: "It didn't really hurt that much, did it? I thought you were a big boy, not a baby!"
   b. Here, pain is clearly expressed by the child, only to be just as clearly negated by the nurse, who also insults the child.
   c. This approach makes it difficult to develop trust and rapport with a child.
6. The following example illustrates a different approach:
   a. Nurse: "I need to take off your bandage now.

Do you want to help me with the tape? I need you to hold still, but you can yell as loud as you want if it hurts." Child: "Do it like Mommy. She does it slow. Ow, ow, ow, ow, OUCH!!" Nurse: "You did a great job holding still! And that was a good, strong shout. I need to put the clean bandage on, and then we're finished. That's when you can go back to your game."
   b. Nurses may believe that they have no time for long explanations.
      (1) Most often, however, the time spent explaining more than makes up for the time spent restraining children, or dodging flying hands, feet, and teeth.
      (2) It is worth the effort, for all concerned.

C. The therapeutic relationship.

1. Caring is an essential component to the nursing role.
   a. The line between therapeutic caring and unprofessional behavior seems fairly clear when patients are adults.
   b. With children, however, the line can become blurred.
2. Families may make requests on behalf of their children that they would never make for themselves.
3. Caring for children often involves hugs, kisses, cuddles, and other comfort measures that are not a part of professional relationships with adults.
4. Advocating for children and families is also a nursing role, but it can become difficult to determine what separates advocacy from favoritism.
   a. An example of advocacy is offering to speak to the doctor (or helping to empower the child or parent to do so) regarding a question about treatment.
   b. An example of favoritism is bringing in a child's favorite food, movies, etc., from one's home.
5. Nurses must take responsibility for structuring the relationship so that boundaries remain intact and the advocacy and caring roles are preserved (Rushton, McEnhill, & Armstrong, 1996).
   a. One measure of success is that children and families feel empowered to care for themselves and to advocate for themselves.
   b. The plan of care should reflect ideas and strategies identified by families, and advocacy may mean supporting children and families in meeting their identified needs.
   c. One danger sign of potential boundary violations is that a care plan reflects the nurses'

needs, and/or encourages families to become or remain dependent on nursing care, instead of progressing towards independence.

6. A therapeutic relations decision making model, the Rainbow Framework, can be used to help the nurse resolve moral dilemmas associated with interactions with children and families (McAliley, Lambert, Ashenberg, & Dull, 1996).
   a. The framework:
      (1) Guides nurses through a process of conscious deliberation when choosing between courses of action that will affect the nature of their relationships with children and families.
      (2) Assesses relationships along a continuum that ranges from disengaged through therapeutic to enmeshed.
      (3) Is built on a utilitarian approach, which assumes that any interaction with a child or family has the potential for producing a variety of both negative and positive consequences.
      (4) Asks nurses to consider potential positive and negative outcomes of an action relative to five different contexts (McAliley et al., 1996, p. 200).
          (a) Philosophy and policy of the organization.
          (b) Impact upon desired child and family outcomes.
          (c) Developmental stage of the relationship.
          (d) Potential negative impact on other children, families, and staff.
          (e) Nurse's philosophy and values regarding role and nature of a therapeutic relationship.
   b. By identifying and weighing the issues in each domain, the nurse is better positioned to determine whether a specific action is likely to foster or detract from a therapeutic relationship.
   c. The nurse then decides to:
      (1) Go ahead with the considered action.
      (2) Forego it.
      (3) Modify it in a manner that avoids or negates the potential hazards.
   d. The use of this framework supports a proactive approach to examining professional relationships.

D. Communicating in special situations.
1. Increasingly, pediatric patients present with developmental or other differences that make coping with a health care encounter even more challenging for children and families.

2. Strategies for communicating with children and families living with hearing impairment include the following:
   a. Use sign language.
   b. Use translators as needed.
   c. Ensure that special teletypewriters, i.e., telecommunications devices for the deaf (TDD), are available in the health care setting.
   d. Post pictures of simple signs that nurses can use to communicate when translators are temporarily unavailable.
   e. Face the person being addressed, and speak clearly to facilitate lip reading.
   f. Use demonstrations and videotapes as teaching aids.
3. Strategies for communicating with children and families living with vision loss include the following:
   a. Use voice and/or touch to inform children and family members of your presence with them.
   b. Contact the Library of Congress for free Braille and audio taped information to provide for families.
   c. Avoid unnecessary bright lights; they are painful to some people who have limited vision.
   d. Avoid using visual cues when asked to describe objects or people (e.g., "It's red with blue spots." Try instead: "It's round like a ball. Do you want to hold it?"
   e. Allow someone with vision loss to place their hand on an escort's arm to enable the individual to feel which way to move with the escort.
4. Strategies for communicating with nonspeakers of the predominant language include the following:
   a. Arrange for translators: minimally once per day for progress updates.
   b. Ascertain whether or not parents can read in their native language.
   c. Provide educational materials (e.g, written, audiotape, videotape) in the family's native language.
   d. Demonstrate procedures, then indicate for child or family to imitate the steps.
   e. Ask to learn words in the family's language and common customs; this conveys respect for another language and culture.
   f. *Also see Chapter 29: Cultural Influences.*
5. Strategies for communicating with children and families with developmental or educational differences include the following:
   a. Use repeated demonstrations to teach care techniques.
   b. Provide readable educational materials.

c. See Hobbie (1995) for more information on readability of parent education materials.

6. Strategies for communicating with the child who is dying include the following:

a. Offer an attentive and reassuring presence; words are not always needed or welcome.

b. Respect family dynamics and preferred comfort measures.

c. Permit children and families to verbalize fears and anxieties.

d. Consistently offer empathy, warmth, acceptance, tenderness, and respect.

e. *See also Chapter 6: Separation, Loss, and Bereavement.*

V. OUTCOMES

The goal of learning to communicate effectively with children and families is to apply these strategies to the task of improving patient outcomes.

A. When nurses use good communication techniques, they gain valuable insight.

B. This insight enables nurses to form partnerships that include children and families in the process of improving and maintaining their health.

C. This, in turn, results in realistic and comprehensive care plans.

D. All children and families deserve the opportunity to participate fully in their care.

1. Adherence to treatment often improves when families feel they have a voice in planning their children's care.

2. According to Sweeney (1997, p. 66):

a. "Ideally, the expertise of parents and of staff complement one another thereby providing the basis for a supportive collaborative relationship."

b. "Caring for children in the context of their families and working together in partnership dramatically improve the [health care] experience for all involved."

c. "Moreover, parental involvement can make a difference in medical outcomes."

E. Incorporating effective communication skills into every aspect of the nursing process gives nurses the tools they need to facilitate those opportunities, and to provide comprehensive, family-centered, child-focused care.

BIBLIOGRAPHY

Beaty, J. (1994). *Observing the development of the young child.* New York: Macmillan Publishing Company.

Brantly, D. (1991). Communicating with children: Age-related techniques. In D. Smith (Ed.), *Comprehensive child and family nursing skills* (pp. 48–53). St. Louis: Mosby Year Book.

Clutter, L., Hess, C., Nix, K., Rollins, J., Smith, D., Stevens, N., & Wong, D. (1987). Communicating effectively with young children. *Children's Nurse, 5*(4) 1–3.

Clutter, L., Hess, C., Nix, K., Rollins, J., Smith, D., Stevens, N., & Wong, D. (1988). Communicating effectively with older children and adolescents. *Children's Nurse, 6*(1) 4, 6, 8.

Gagne, F., & Robichaud-Ekstrand, S. (1995). How to intervene effectively with a dying patient. *Canadian Nurse, 91*(2) 47–51.

Gaynard, L., Wolfer, J., Goldberger, J., Thompson, R., Redburn, L., & Laidley, L. (1990). *Psychosocial care of children in hospitals: A clinical practice manual from the ACCH Child Life Research Project.* Washington, DC: Association for the Care of Children's Health.

Hobbie, C. (1995). Maximizing healthy communication: Readability of parent education materials. *Journal of Pediatric Health Care, 9*(2), 92–3.

McAliley, L., Lambert, S., Ashenberg, M., & Dull, S. (1996). Therapeutic relations decision making: The Rainbow Framework. *Pediatric Nursing, 22*(3) 199–203, 210.

Pridham, K., Broome, M., & Woodring, B. (1996). Standards and guidelines for prelicensure and early professional education. *Journal of Pediatric Nursing, 11*(5) 273–80.

Rollins, J., & Mahan, C. (1996). *From artist to artist in residence: Preparing artists to work in pediatric health care settings.* Washington, DC: Rollins & Associates, Inc.

Rushton, C., McEnhill, M., & Armstrong, L. (1996). Establishing therapeutic boundaries as patient advocates. *Pediatric Nursing, 22* (3) 185–9.

Sweeney, M. (1997). The value of a family-centered care approach in the NICU and PICU: One family's perspective. *Pediatric Nursing, 23*(1) 64–6.

STUDY QUESTIONS

1. ___________ and ___________ are essential components of a therapeutic relationship in nursing.
   a. Caring and curing
   b. Advocacy and caring
   c. Advocacy and curing
   d. Curing and boundaries
   e. Boundaries and favoritism

2. At what age should a child be able to use proper word order consistently in statements?
   a. 4-5 years
   b. 2-3 years
   c. 5-6 years
   d. 3-4 years
   e. 6-7 years

3. Of the following, which is the best strategy for communicating effectively with a young child?
   a. Smile broadly and speak loudly and clearly.
   b. Move quickly and confidently toward the child.
   c. Ask questions that can be answered with "yes" or "no."
   d. Stand and maintain eye contact with child while speaking.
   e. Speak softly and move slowly toward the child.

4. What is the best method for ensuring effective communication with parents and their adolescents?
   a. Arrange a meeting with parents and child to discuss diagnosis and treatment options.
   b. Stand outside child's room to inform parents of diagnosis and treatment plan.
   c. Speak to the child, then inform the parents of the diagnosis and treatment plan.
   d. Inform parents of diagnosis, decide on a treatment plan, then inform the child.
   e. Have a team meeting to decide on treatment plan, then inform the parents.

5. You are describing an IV pump to a visually impaired 9 year old. Which of the following is the most appropriate answer?
   a. It's a blue box with flashing red lights.
   b. The box on this pole controls your IV fluids.
   c. The metal box beeps when we need to add medicine to your IV.
   d. The rectangular box shows us what your IV needs.
   e. The metal box next to your bed beeps when we need to check your IV.

6. Which of the following represents the largest percentage of any message transmitted during communication?
   a. Visual
   b. Verbal
   c. Auditory
   d. Nonverbal
   e. Tactile

7. Which of the following are most helpful to assess when considering appropriate language to use with children?
   a. Communication abilities and affect
   b. Developmental level and gender
   c. Affect and developmental level
   d. Chronologic age and gender
   e. Communication abilities and chronologic age

8. If a parent asks the same question over and over, what is the most likely explanation?
   a. She doesn't believe the answer.
   b. He can't understand what you are saying.
   c. She can't retain the information.
   d. He wants to hear it from as many people as possible.
   e. She is waiting to hear what she wants to hear.

9. Of the following, which is probably not a reason that parents face challenges in communicating with nurses?
   a. Stress due to child's condition
   b. Lack of interest
   c. Family demands
   d. Sleep deprivation
   e. Marital strain

10. At a minimum, what resources should be in place to facilitate communication with people who are hearing impaired?
    a. Telephones and computers
    b. Braille writers and hearing aids
    c. Sign language interpreters and TDD equipment
    d. Books and videos about sign language
    e. Family members and posters

ANSWERS

1.b 2.d 3.e 4.a 5.e 6.d 7.a 8.c 9.b 10.c

Chapter 31

Legal, Moral, and Ethical Issues in Pediatric Nursing

Teresa A. Savage, PhD, RN

Concept

◆ Values and moral and ethical reasoning

Objectives

At the completion of this chapter, the reader will be able to:

◆ Define terms in the language of ethics and law.

◆ Identify and analyze situations for ethical and legal issues.

◆ Facilitate ethical decision making for children.

◆ Employ an ethical decision-making model.

◆ Identify nursing's role and responsibilities in ethical and legal issues.

Key Points

◆ The nurse is a moral agent with multiple and competing obligations to the child, family, employing institution, health care team, and society.

◆ The Code for Nurses with Interpretive Statements (1985) sets forth standards of ethical practice for the pediatric nurse to follow and apply.

◆ Every interaction in the health care relationship is a moral interaction based on respect for persons and occurs with the consent of the parents/guardians and assent of the child, if the child is developmentally capable to assent.

◆ As children mature and develop, increasing weight should be given to their wishes in health care decisions.

◆ Nurses should be mindful of the unique relationship between nurse and child and should maintain professional boundaries that empower the parents and foster family-centered decision making.

◆ The nursing perspective is an essential contribution to ethical decision making for children.

31

Legal, Moral, and Ethical Issues In Pediatric Nursing

◆◆◆◆◆◆◆◆◆◆◆◆◆◆◆◆◆◆◆◆◆◆◆◆◆◆◆◆◆◆◆◆◆◆◆◆

I. OVERVIEW

Health care decisions for children often have legal, moral, and ethical aspects. For example, the decision to have a child immunized is influenced by state law that may mandate immunization before attendance at school is permitted, agency policy that may mandate informed consent before the immunization is administered, and parental prerogative that may accept or reject immunization based on religious or cultural beliefs. In addition to knowing the health history and current clinical condition of the child, the nurse, who would administer the immunization, should be aware of the state laws, agency policy, and process of informed consent that occurred prior to giving the immunization. In pediatric nursing, there are many complex situations that require analysis for the legal, moral, and ethical components.

II. DEFINITION OF TERMS

A. Ethical principles.

1. Autonomy: freedom to choose; parents as surrogate decision makers exercise their child's autonomy prior to their child having legal decisional capacity.
2. Beneficence: promotion of good; determination of what is "good" is part of the ethical decision-making process.
3. Nonmaleficence: prevention of harm; determination of what is a "harm" is also part of the ethical decision-making process.
4. Justice: allocation of benefits and burdens; concept also includes the determination of fairness.

B. Other terms.

1. Advance directive: living will or durable power of attorney for health care; a minor's authorization to have advance directive, as with other issues of informed consent, is not legally recognized.
2. Assent: child's permission or deliberate refusal

to participate in research; parent or guardian may overrule if potential for direct benefit to child exists.
3. Best interests standard: surrogate decision maker (usually the parents) makes a decision that promotes the child's welfare; parents are given wide latitude in determining what is in child's best interests.
4. Brain death: irreversible cessation of whole brain function.
5. Compassionate plea exemption: Institutional Review Board approval to permit experimental treatment for a particular child who otherwise is ineligible to receive treatment; usually requested in studies where randomization into control or experimental groups is required, or child does not meet all the eligibility criteria for inclusion.
6. Confidentiality: protection of information about child and family from unauthorized disclosure.
7. Decisional capacity: cognitive skills to reason and understand the seriousness of the situation, and possession of maturity and judgment needed to weigh consequences; automatically legally recognized at age 18 years unless court has declared person legally incompetent and has appointed a guardian.
8. Do Not Resuscitate (DNR) orders: specific explication of measures to be withheld in the event of patient's need for resuscitation, such as for apnea, bradycardia, or cardiorespiratory arrest.
9. Durable power of attorney for health care: defined by state statute, the designation of an adult to make any and all health care decisions for the patient who is 18 years of age or older when the patient becomes incapacitated to make health care decisions; decision-making authority reverts back to patient should patient regain decisional capacity; allows for refusal of nutrition and hydration.
10. Emancipated minor: legal designation by state statute of a minor who is self-supporting or married (or both) to consent to treatment; the emancipated minor may not, however, refuse

life-sustaining treatment unless the spouse is an adult and concurs or the parents concur.

11. Informed consent: process by which parents or legal guardians give or refuse consent to health care professionals for tests, treatments, or release of information; information is provided to parents in language understandable to them, benefits and risks are explained, and consent is obtained without incentive or coercion.

12. Living will: defined by state statute, describes treatments to be withheld or withdrawn if person is imminently dying and lacks the ability to communicate wishes; may not allow the foregoing of nutrition and hydration.

13. Mature minor: legal designation by state statute and a legal proceeding to satisfy the court that the minor has the cognitive capacity and judgment to make health care decisions.

14. Medical custody: legal authority to make medical decisions for a minor; for example, the court may give medical custody to a guardian when parents who are Jehovah's Witnesses refuse a life-saving blood transfusion.

15. Paternalism: belief that someone other than the patient knows what is best for the patient; parents are expected to be paternalistic when making decisions for their children.

16. Persistent vegetative state: permanent coma characterized by cycles of sleep-wake states, purposeless motor movements, and complete lack of awareness of self or surroundings; usually indicative of global injury to cerebral cortex.

17. Resuscitation: actions to reverse a deteriorating and potentially life-threatening change in the child's condition; for example, artificial ventilation, cardiac massage, cardioversion, administration of cardiotonic medications and/or oxygen.

18. Substituted judgment: surrogate decision maker (usually the parents) makes a decision that reflects the wishes of the child; substituted judgment is usually not employed in pediatrics, although parents of a school age child or adolescent may factor the child's wishes into their decision.

19. Surrogate (or proxy) decision maker: person identified as the legal decision maker for the child, usually the parents; some states have statutes describing process for identifying a surrogate decision maker for purposes of refusing life-sustaining treatment.

III. DECISION-MAKING PROCESS

◆ ◆ ◆ ◆ ◆ ◆ ◆ ◆ ◆ ◆ ◆ ◆ ◆ ◆ ◆ ◆ ◆ ◆ ◆

A. Nurse's role in ethical decision making. The nurse:

1. Examines personal position to recognize potential for influencing parents' decision.

2. Establishes therapeutic relationship with child, parents, with others on health care team.

   a. As case manager, coordinates team to identify goals and develop nursing care plan.

      (1) The case manager may or may not also be the child's primary nurse.

      (2) The care plan establishes goals nursing care will achieve; it may require involving other disciplines to achieve the goals.

   b. As primary nurse, develops and implements nursing care plan through direct care to the child and family and coordination of care within the health care team. The nurse:

      (1) Recognizes power inequity in relationship between parents and health care agency or institution.

      (2) Enacts role as advocate.

         (a) Facilitates parents' decision making through sharing and clarifying information, clarifying their values, rehearsing their questions for others, examining possible options and outcomes, reinforcing their right and responsibility to make decisions for their child.

         (b) Advocates for the child when parental interests conflict with the child's interests or parental decisions do not seem to be in the child's best interests.

3. Identifies ethical and legal issues and seeks assistance from appropriate sources.

4. Verifies relevant information, such as diagnosis, prognosis, consultant's report, and test results.

5. Uses discretion in sharing information with parents; facilitates parents getting accurate and timely information from appropriate sources.

6. Identifies options and possible consequences of each option with parents.

7. Assists parents in assessing benefits and burdens of each option.

8. Assists parents in identifying option consistent with their values.

   a. Assists parents in articulating and clarifying their values.

   b. Clarifies own values and thereby recognizes own biases and potential for influencing parents.

9. Identifies need for additional information.

   a. Advises parents and/or assists them in investigating insurance policies for benefit coverage; may refer to social worker for assistance.

   b. Identifies resources family may wish to use such as speaking with other parents who faced the same decisions.

10. Helps family and health care team establish mutual goals.

11. Articulates and communicates plan of care to the health care team and other parties, with appropriate consents to share information.
12. Implements plan.
13. Evaluates outcome for the child and family.
14. Evaluates process of ethical decision-making for the child, family, and health care team.

B. Advisory resources. The nurse:
1. Determines mechanism in the nurse's institution or agency for assisting nurses in ethical analysis or in facilitating parental decision making.
2. Determines how to access ethics committee.
3. Determines how to access ethics consultants, if available.
4. Uses mechanism within professional nursing association when appropriate.
5. Determines how to access legal consultants to the nurse's institution or agency.
6. Determines how to access risk management in the nurse's institution or agency.
7. Initiates referral for pastoral care or social work when appropriate.
8. Advises parents of availability and accessibility of ad hoc groups such as support groups, specialty groups for specific persons, e.g., Down Syndrome Congress, Spina Bifida Association, Tourette Syndrome Association, American Lung Association, Muscular Dystrophy Association.

IV. SPECIFIC CLINICAL ISSUES IN PEDIATRIC NURSING

◆ ◆ ◆ ◆ ◆ ◆ ◆ ◆ ◆ ◆ ◆ ◆ ◆ ◆ ◆ ◆ ◆

A. Issues with newborns.
1. Informed consent for treatment is obtained from parents/guardian.
   a. Prior to birth: circumcision, routine newborn care in inpatient facility (e.g., blood testing for type, bilirubin levels, glucose, electrolytes, gases).
   b. After birth: institutional policy based on state law indicates what tests or treatments require written informed consent, what tests/treatments can be performed without written consent (e.g., newborn screening mandated by state law), and what tests are mandated to be performed whether or not parent(s) give consent (e.g., urine toxicology screen in infant with symptoms or positive history of maternal substance use, or HIV testing if health care worker occupationally exposed to child's bodily fluids).
2. Treatment/nontreatment decisions for newborns may be based on parents' wishes or federal regulations.

   a. Parents are given wide latitude in deciding best interests of child.
      (1) Parents make decisions in child's best interests, based on their beliefs, values, culture, resources, and resolve.
      (2) Parents weigh potential benefits and burdens of proposed treatment options, based on all available information.
      (3) Parents evaluate possible effect of various treatment options on family and ability to cope with possible outcomes.
   b. Federal regulations initially called Baby Doe regulations influence interactions between parents and health care team.
      (1) Regulations may be interpreted as mandating treatment except in cases where child is in an irreversible, permanent coma, or when treatment would be futile, inhumane, or would only prolong the dying process; interpretation of the regulations vary.
      (2) Parents are informed of child's condition, prognosis, and agree with the treatment (or nontreatment) plan.
      (3) Parents and health care team may disagree on what is futile or inhumane treatment, and/or on plan.
         (a) Health care team advocates nontreatment; parents may not accept prognosis or medical judgment that further treatment would be futile.
         (b) Health care team advocates continued aggressive treatment; parents do not want infant treated if undesirable outcome is more likely than not to occur.
3. Extreme prematurity, defined as the preterm birth of an infant whose viability is dependent upon neonatal intensive care; gestational age is under 25–26 weeks.
   a. Degree of parental involvement in treatment decision making may vary in different Neonatal Intensive Care Units (NICUs).
   b. Parental decision making is dependent upon health care team's philosophy toward neonatal care; application or withdrawal of life-sustaining treatment may not be viewed as parental prerogative, unless outcome for survival is ambiguous or extremely unlikely. *Also see Chapter 28: Family-Centered Care.*
      (1) Interpretation of the child abuse and neglect regulations vary; some institutions interpret regulations as mandating treatment, others interpret them as guidelines to prevent discrimination against infants with a likelihood of being disabled and thereby inappropriately under-

treated, and others may view them as guidelines from when to appropriately limit treatment.

    (2) Some neonatalogists give parents absolute authority to accept or reject life-sustaining treatment.

4. Infants born with life-threatening anomalies (e.g., hypoplastic left heart syndrome, tracheal-esophageal fistula, anencephaly).

    a. Infants with anomalies considered incompatible with life for which there is no known treatment (e.g., anencephaly, some encephaloceles, some cardiac conditions).

        (1) Comfort care, in terms of minimal invasive procedures, analgesia, appropriate nutrition and hydration is provided; attention to grieving process for parents and other family members.

        (2) Life-sustaining interventions may be requested by parents. Court has supported continuing life-sustaining intervention for child with anencephaly at mother's request.

    b. Infants with life-threatening anomalies that can be treated (e.g., gastroschisis, prune belly syndrome, myelomeningocele, tracheo-esophageal atresia)

        (1) Informed consent is sought from parents for surgery and/or life-sustaining treatment (e.g., dialysis, total parenteral nutrition).

        (2) Parents may not be given an option of foregoing life-sustaining treatment.

    c. Infants with multiple anomalies, some that are life-threatening and some that are not (e.g., combination of Down syndrome and cyanotic heart defect, or Trisomy 18 and tracheoesophageal atresia).

        (1) Informed consent is sought from parents for surgery and/or life-sustaining treatment.

        (2) Parents may be given option of forgoing life-sustaining treatment if parents and health care team reach consensus that burden of treatment outweighs benefits; if disagreement exists, the case may be referred to ethics committee or to court.

B. Treatment/nontreatment decisions for children birth to adulthood (age 18 years).

1. Informed consent is sought from parents/guardians for treatment decisions.

    a. Benefits and risks of proposed treatment are explained to parents in understandable terms.

    b. Alternatives to proposed treatment and their benefits and risks are fully explained to parents.

    c. Parents consent voluntarily.

2. Nontreatment decisions can involve either withholding or withdrawing treatment.

    a. Determination is made that child is not responding to treatment or is likely not to respond to treatment; decision to withhold certain treatments, such as surgery, ventilator, dialysis, or resuscitation.

        (1) Resuscitation decisions are considered for children whose survival is unlikely, even with resuscitation, or whose continued existence would be extremely burdensome to the child in terms of pain and suffering.

        (2) A Do Not Resuscitate order may be written in the medical record, according to institution's policy; specific resuscitative measures to be withheld must be clearly documented and communicated.

        (3) Nursing care and treatments for comfort continue.

    b. Decision is made to withdraw certain treatments, such as ventilator or cardiotonic medications because survival with treatment is unlikely.

        (1) Parents and health care team agree with the decision.

        (2) Nursing care and treatments for comfort care continue.

3. Determination of futility of treatment is based on anticipated goal(s).

    a. Goal(s) of treatment are identified.

        (1) The child is cured with minimal adverse sequelae.

        (2) The child is cured with some degree of permanent disability.

        (3) The child's pain and suffering is relieved.

        (4) The child survives.

    b. Treatment is considered futile when goals are unlikely to be met.

    c. Parents and health care team may not agree on futility of continued treatment; consultation from ethics committee is appropriate.

4. The scarcity of organs and tissues for transplantation has led to regulations regarding allocation and donation.

    a. The allocation of organs is governed by United Network for Organ Sharing's (UNOS) oversight of Organ Procurement and Transplantation Network (OPTN), composed of regional organ procurement organizations.

        (1) Organs are distributed according to tissue type and match, medical urgency, length of time on waiting list, size of organ and size of recipient, and geographic close-

ness to origin of donated organ.
(2) Allocation decisions are based on the principle of justice to ensure fairness in distribution of organs.

b. Organs are retrieved from brain-dead donor, non-heart-beating cadaver, or living donor; criteria for procuring organs from brain-dead persons, non-heart-beating cadavers, and living donors is specified by the individual transplant center.

c. Several factors are considered regarding children as organ donors.
(1) Infants with anencephaly legally are not permitted to be used as organ donors; the American Medical Association's Council on Ethical and Judicial Affairs recommended infants with anencephaly be used as organ donors with parental consent, but later rescinded their recommendations.
(2) Other infants who meet brain death criteria, with parental consent, can be organ donors.
(3) Philosophers differ on ethical arguments justifying children as organ donors.
(a) Justification depends on the risk to the donor child, the urgency of need of the organ recipient, the parents' willingness but unacceptability as donors, and the relationship of the donor to the recipient.
(b) Some philosophers support forced altruism for the donor child while others believe there is no justification for forcing a child to donate an organ or tissue to another person.

5. Children, including infants, have the same rights to analgesia and anesthesia as do adults. *See managing pain in Chapter 14: Acute Illness: Symptom Management* and *Chapter 22: Chronic Conditions: Symptom Management.*
a. Historically it was believed that infants could not feel pain, so anesthesia and analgesia were not used.
b. Scientific data confirms that infants, like all children, can experience pain and should receive anesthesia and analgesia.
c. Pharmacologic and nonpharmacologic interventions should be employed with children who are in pain or may experience pain in the course of their health care treatments.
d. Pharmacologic and nonpharmacologic interventions may also be indicated to reduce anxiety, fearfulness, or other suffering while undergoing procedures or treatments.

6. Genetic testing is increasingly spotlighted as an ethical, moral, and legal issue.
a. Testing intended to identify genetic diagnosis in affected child is permissible with parental consent.
b. Linkage testing to assist in diagnosing or counseling a family member is permissible with parental consent.
c. Genetic information about a child may reveal information about parents or grandparents (e.g., child with gene for Huntington's indicates that one parent also has the gene; Huntington Society opposes testing minors under 18 years of age for the Huntington gene).
d. Possible harm to child who undergoes genetic testing exists in the current health care delivery system.
(1) A third party payer can exclude coverage for a preexisting condition.
(2) Parents may forego having their child tested for a genetic condition out of fear that their child would not be able to obtain health insurance because of preexisting conditions if the test is positive.

V. ISSUES WITH CHILDREN WITH CHRONIC CONDITIONS

◆ ◆ ◆ ◆ ◆ ◆ ◆ ◆ ◆ ◆ ◆ ◆ ◆ ◆ ◆ ◆ ◆

A. Confidentiality.
1. Judicious disclosure of information to outside parties is permitted with parental consent.
2. Parents may request information be withheld from other health care practitioners, schools, or other agencies involved with child, out of fear of stigmatizing the child or jeopardizing insurance coverage of the child (e.g., HIV+ status, diagnosis not covered by major medical insurance, attention deficit disorder, genetic diagnosis).
a. This poses a conflict between possibly compromising the child's welfare by withholding information and breaching confidentiality.
b. An adolescent legally can give consent for treatments (dependent upon state statutes) for birth control, pregnancy testing and counseling, treatment of substance abuse, sexually transmitted diseases, or psychiatric conditions.
c. A conflict may arise between respect for adolescent's privacy and parents desire to know.
(1) The nurse should attempt to facilitate communication of sensitive information between adolescent and parent.
(2) In specific situations, the nurse may need to consult the institution's legal adviser to determine parental and adolescent's rights.

Table 31-1
When Parents and the Health Care Team Disagree

1. **Communication between parents and the health care team should be clear, honest, respectful, and timely.** When parents disagree with the health care team it is sometimes assumed that parents are not emotionally capable of understanding the situation, are too inexperienced with the health care environment to understand the ramifications of their decision, are cognitively limited in their ability to understand what they are being told, or are in denial; steps should be taken to dispel these assumptions through improved communication efforts.

2. **A family-centered, culturally respectful approach should be used in identifying the child's best interests.** The health care team has an obligation to advocate for the child's best interests. Deciding what these interests are is often the source of the conflict, especially when life and death choices are involved.

3. **If the health care team believes the parents' decision is not in the child's best interests, they may pursue medical custody through legal channels.** For example, in a situation where parents who are Jehovah's Witness refuse consent for life-saving blood transfusion, the attending physician may petition the court for medical custody for the purposes of consenting to a blood transfusion; custody reverts back to the parents after the transfusion is completed.

   In cases of known effective treatment for life-threatening conditions, the courts are more likely to favor treatment despite parents' refusal.

   When treatment efficacy is unknown, the condition is not life-threatening, the condition is likely to be terminal despite treatment, or the burden of treatment is likely to outweigh the benefit, the courts uphold the parents' right to decide.

4. **Referral to the institution's ethics committee or consultation with an ethicist may be necessary.** This action can be initiated by either a member of the health care team or the parents.

B. Consent.

1. Children who have chronic conditions may have a more mature grasp of their situation beyond their chronologic age.
2. Children as young as 7 years of age should be assessed for decisional capacity regarding their health care, especially if their condition is incurable.
3. Certain factors are considered regarding disagreement between a child and his or her parents about treatment or nontreatment for children with specific conditions.
   a. When parents want treatment and the child does not:
      (1) In terminal conditions (e.g., brain tumor) or chronic, incurable conditions (e.g., muscular dystrophy, cystic fibrosis), a child with decisional capacity should have his or her wishes included in the decision-making process.
      (2) Resources should be made available to the family to mediate disagreement.
   b. When parents refuse treatment but the child wants treatment:
      (1) Parents who belong to specific religious groups, such as Jehovah's Witness, or groups who reject medical treatment may lose medical custody if they refuse life-sustaining, efficacious treatment.
      (2) Through a legal process, medical custody is given to the physician or consenting parent (if parents are in disagreement) to permit life-sustaining treatment or a guardian ad litem (i.e., the guardian has the authority to consent or refuse treatment only for the particular issue in question) for the purposes of determining the best interests of the child.
4. Disagreement about treatment/nontreatment may arise between parents and the health care team.
   a. See Table 31-1: When Parents and the Health Care Team Disagree.
   b. If treatment clearly will benefit the child, risks are relatively low, and delay in the decision may harm the child, the health care team may opt to seek medical custody.
   c. If the benefit of treatment is ambiguous, and risks are relatively high, the health care team will abide by parents' wishes.
   d. If parents request treatment that the health care team believes is futile, court intervention

Table 31-2
Nonemergency Life-Sustaining Interventions

1. Techniques to relieve subglottic stenosis or other partial obstruction
2. Enteral feeding tubes and/or Nissen fundoplication for children unable to receive oral intake, prolonged nasogastric tube feedings not feasible, and multiple episodes of aspiration and pneumonia occurred
3. Organ transplantation to treat irreversible organ failure
4. Surgery, such as amputation for Ewing's sarcoma
5. Chronic pharmacotherapy, such as insulin, anticonvulsants, bronchodilators
    - Foregoing pharmacotherapy could result in life-threatening emergency.
    - Inconsistent administration of medications could result in organ damage, status epilepticus, disability, and discomfort for the child and may be viewed as medical neglect.
6. Dialysis, hemodialysis, or peritoneal dialysis
    - Infants with end-stage renal disease may survive up to 6 months after discontinuing dialysis; older children likely would not survive that long.
    - Children with disabilities, e.g. Down syndrome or cognitive impairment, may not be placed on waiting list for organ transplantation.
7. Long-term oxygen use
    - While not changing the underlying condition, oxygen may relieve child's dyspnea.
    - When relieving dyspnea, oxygen use would be considered primarily a comfort rather than death-delaying measure.
8. Chemotherapy or radiation, palliative
    - Benefits to side effects are evaluated.
    - If benefits outweigh side effects, these can be considered comfort measures.
9. Invasive interventions
    - Certain interventions, such as chest tube, intravenous catheter devices for intravenous fluid administration or blood drawing, intraventricular shunts, bolts, reservoirs, patient-controlled implanted devices for analgesia, insulin, baclofen, are considered invasive.
    - If benefits outweigh side effects, these can be considered comfort measures.

may be sought.

5. Parents may request treatment under experimental protocol or compassionate plea exemption (e.g., non-Food and Drug Administration [FDA] approved medication, chemotherapy available only through protocol). In such cases:
   a. The benefits and risk to the child are evaluated.
   b. If child has decisional capacity, the child's assent or deliberate refusal to treatment is considered.
   c. Parents probably would have to bear costs since insurance usually does not cover experimental treatment and the child is not included in study groups

6. Parents may wish to forego mainstream medical treatment for alternative treatment exclusively. In such cases:
   a. The benefits and risk to the child are evaluated.
   b. Parents are given wide latitude in decisions when risk to child is relatively low.
   c. If child has decisional capacity, the child's assent or deliberate refusal to treatment is considered.
   d. In cases of life-threatening conditions, courts have removed parental custody if the child is forgoing efficacious treatment for unknown efficacy of alternative treatment.

7. Ineffective participation in therapies may occur (e.g., clean intermittent catheterization, irregular medication adherence, improper technique, deviation from prescribed diet [ADA or ketogenic]).
   a. The harm to the child is evaluated.
   b. Parental knowledge of the child's condition and rationale for therapies, their feelings toward therapies, and other lifestyle factors that may influence participation in therapies are assessed.
   c. If harm threatens the child's safety and well-being, the health care team must report as suspected medical neglect.

8. Rejection of nonemergency, life-sustaining interventions may occur.

a. Parents given wide latitude in making decisions; assessment of decisional capacity of the child and his or her preferences should be done.

b. If treatment is viewed as death-prolonging, parents may reject treatment; comfort care should be provided; do not resuscitate order may be appropriate.

c. Table 31-2 lists examples of nonemergency, life-sustaining interventions.

   (1) The parents' decision may be challenged if the health care team believes intervention is in the child's best interests.

   (2) It is ethically permissible for parents to consent or refuse treatment, depending on assessment of benefits and burden of treatment for a specific child.

9. Medication for performance enhancement may bring forth ethical, legal, and moral issues.

a. Stimulant medication, tricyclic antidepressants, or other medications may be used to treat attention deficit disorder with or without hyperactivity.

   (1) The child's condition should be accurately diagnosed.

   (2) The child should be started on a trial of medication to determine responsiveness, adverse reactions, and appropriate dose.

   (3) The parents' decision to accept or reject use of medication should be respected.

   (4) Medication should be a part of a comprehensive program of educational accommodation, home behavioral program, and additional adjunct therapies (psychologic counseling, occupational therapy) as indicated.

b. Other psychoactive medications for treating child's unacceptable symptoms or behaviors (e.g., behaviors associated with autism, Fragile X, obsessive-compulsive disorder).

   (1) The child's condition should be accurately diagnosed.

   (2) The child should be started on a trial of medication to determine responsiveness, adverse reactions, and appropriate dose.

   (3) The parents' decision to accept or reject use of medication should be respected.

   (4) Medication should be a part of a comprehensive program of educational accommodation, home behavioral program, and additional adjunct therapies (psychologic counseling, occupational therapy) as indicated.

c. Athletes or body builders sometimes use anabolic steroids.

   (1) These substances are illegal and potentially harmful to child.

   (2) Nurses should follow institution or agency's policies for managing this issue.

C. Legal issues in childhood education.

1. Relevant federal, state, and local laws pertain to educational rights of children. *See Chapter 9: Influences of Regulatory Mechanisms and Policies of Health Care.*

2. Laws should specify the following:

a. Inclusion of parents in individual family service plan.

b. Intervals between reevaluation.

c. Provision of adjunct services (e.g., nursing care, assistive technology services, transportation, appropriate therapies).

d. Seamless transition from early intervention program to early childhood program in public school.

3. The role of the pediatric nurse in educational settings includes the following:

a. Assessing the impact of the child's health status and developmental condition on learning, family perspective or accommodation to child's needs, and awareness of available resources.

b. Securing relevant physician's orders for management of the child's condition in the setting.

c. Familiarity with policies regarding medication administration in school.

VI. ISSUES WITH CHILDREN WHO ARE DYING

◆ ◆ ◆ ◆ ◆ ◆ ◆ ◆ ◆ ◆ ◆ ◆ ◆ ◆ ◆ ◆ ◆ ◆ ◆

Also see Chapter 6: Separation, Loss, and Bereavement

A. Determination of dying process.

1. The child's condition is deteriorating; he or she is unresponsive to treatment.

2. In the health care team's judgment, the child is dying.

3. Parents may or may not accept assessment that their child is dying. The nurse:

a. Supports parents in the grieving process.

b. Facilitates communication between the child and parents, if needed.

B. Palliative care.

1. The child's comfort is the goal of care.

2. Treatments may be identical to curative treatment, such as chemotherapy and radiation, but the purpose is to promote comfort.

3. Effective pain relief and promotion of comfort is sought through reduction of noxious and/or invasive procedures, and the use of pharmaco-

logic and nonpharmacologic techniques.
a. Nurses may be reluctant to administer adequate doses of analgesia for pain relief for fear of causing respiratory depression and thereby hastening death.
b. Doctrine of double effect holds that it is ethically permissible to administer medication for relief of pain even if secondary effect could be the unintended hastening of death.
   (1) The doctrine pertains only to the ethical justification of giving adequate pain medication.
   (2) If the nurse violates his or her state's practice act in terms of giving medication without orders, giving more than is ordered, or giving it a route other than the ordered one, and the nurse does not have the legal discretion to do this in his/her state, then the nurse is violating state law.
4. Discussion of resuscitation status should occur to clarify plan when death occurs.
a. In an acute care setting, "Do Not Resuscitate" orders should be written on chart.
   (1) Specific measures to be withheld must be clearly listed.
   (2) Progress note should document diagnosis, prognosis, any treatments to be administered (e.g., blood, antibiotics, pressors), and response of parents to plan.
   (3) Institutional policies will specify if ethics consultation is mandatory or advisory when DNR order is written, who may write the order, how often it should be re written in the chart, and what, if any, additional documentation is needed.
b. For the home setting, the physician should draft a letter ordering "Do Not Resuscitate," stating diagnosis, prognosis, specific measures to be withheld, and what should be done in the event of cardiorespiratory arrest.
   (1) Parents and pediatrician (if not the ordering physician) should sign the letter.
   (2) A copy of the letter should be given to the local emergency room and local emergency medical service (EMS) company that would respond to 911; parents should check relevant state or local law that would permit an EMS to respond to call but not resuscitate.
   (3) DNR status should be discussed with all caregivers (professional and lay) who care for child in the home.
c. For the school setting, parents should discuss the plan with child's school administrators and the school nurse.

   (1) Schools are reluctant to honor DNR orders, but may agree to call 911.
   (2) EMS, if previously arranged, will attend to child, but not resuscitate.
5. With some exceptions, advance directives are not legally recognized for minors.
a. State statutes specify details of living will and durable power of attorney for health care.
b. Emancipated minors are legally authorized to draft advance directives.
c. Mature minors, if so designated by the court, are legally authorized to draft advance directives.
d. Even when not legal, advance directives can be respected and used as a communication tool between the minor, parents, and the health care team.
6. Withdrawal of life-sustaining treatment considers certain factors.
a. The child's level of comfort may improve.
b. Withdrawing life-sustaining treatment also can be justified on ethical grounds:
   (1) Promotion of comfort.
   (2) Reduction of painful interventions.
   (3) No obligation to provide futile treatment.
7. The child can be referred to hospice care, if appropriate.

VII. PARTICIPATION OF CHILDREN IN RESEARCH

◆ ◆ ◆ ◆ ◆ ◆ ◆ ◆ ◆ ◆ ◆ ◆ ◆ ◆ ◆ ◆ ◆

A. Therapeutic vs. nontherapeutic research.
1. Institutional Review Board approval is required for the protection of human subjects and requires:
a. Informed consent from parents.
b. Assent of the child.
   (1) This can be overruled by parents if direct benefit to the child is expected and benefit of treatment is greater than risk.
   (2) In nontherapeutic research, the child's deliberate objection to participation in research must be respected despite parental consent.
2. In therapeutic research, the child is likely to receive direct benefit from the treatment, such as through oncology drug protocols.
a. It is ethically permissible for the child to participate if potential direct benefits to the child outweigh potential risks.
b. The child's assent is obtained; however, parents may overrule if the child does not assent but is likely to directly benefit from proposed treatment.
   (1) Emancipated and mature minors can

legally consent without parental consent.
(2) Adolescents can legally consent for inclusion in studies regarding sexually transmitted diseases, birth control, and other conditions for which state law permits treatment without parental consent.
c. Compassionate plea exception permits the child to receive experimental treatment without meeting protocol criteria.
3. Nontherapeutic research, according to some philosophers, is never ethically permissible; others consider it ethically permissible if there is no greater risk of harm to the child than he or she would encounter in everyday life.
4. Informed consent has several requirements.
a. Parents are given information in understandable terms.
(1) Written information is translated into family's language of comfort.
(2) Interpreters are available.
b. The possible benefits and risks are explained.
c. Research concepts such as randomization, double-blind study, and Institutional Review Board approval are explained.
d. Freedom to withdraw from the study and possible consequences of withdrawal are explained.
(1) In therapeutic research, if a child is withdrawn from a study, standard treatment is resumed (or treatment, if deemed futile, may be withdrawn).
(2) In nontherapeutic research, there should be no consequences to the child for withdrawing from study.
e. Parents are free from coercion, either positively, as in monetary incentive for participation, or negatively, as in pressure from attending physician to participate.
(1) Parents may receive money for transportation or time involved in research participation; may also receive "gifts" such as baby formula, diapers, toys; gifts should not be so attractive as to unduly influence parents to participate when they might not otherwise agree.
(2) The researcher assumes the costs of tests in nontherapeutic research; in therapeutic research, the child's insurance pays for tests that are part of treatment and the researcher pays for tests the child undergoes only because child is participant in study.
5. The nurse's role and responsibility in research on children requires:
a. Following institutional policy on research on children.
b. Ensuring that informed consent has been obtained from parents before data are collected or treatment given.
c. Notifying the principal investigator if a child or parent states a desire to withdraw from a study, or has questions the nurse is unable to answer.
d. Referring to the American Nurses Association Ethical Guidelines in the Conduct, Dissemination, and Implementation of Nursing Research.

BIBLIOGRAPHY

American Nurses Association. (1985). *Code for nurses with interpretive statements.* Kansas City, MO: American Nurses Association.

Buchanan, A.E., & Brock, D.W. (1990). *Deciding for others: The ethics of surrogate decision making.* Cambridge, MA: Cambridge University Press.

Cooke, R.E. (1996). Ethics, law, and developmental disabilities. In A.J. Capute, & P. J. Accardo (Eds.), *Developmental disabilities in infancy and childhood* (2nd ed., pp. 511–520). Baltimore: Paul H. Brookes.

Hall, J.H. (1996). *Nursing ethics and law.* Philadelphia: Saunders.

President's Commission for the Study of Ethical Problems in Medicine and Biomedical and Behavioral Research. (1983). *Deciding to forego life-sustaining treatment: Ethical, medical, and legal issues in treatment decisions.* Washington, DC: U.S. Government Printing Office.

Rushton, C.H., & Lynch, M.E. (1992). Dealing with advance directives for critically ill adolescents. *Critical Care Nurse, 12*(5), 31–37.

Rushton, C.H., McEnhill, M., & Armstrong, L. (1996). Establishing therapeutic boundaries as patient advocates. *Pediatric Nursing, 22*(3), 185–189.

Savage, T.A. (1997). Ethical decision making for children. *Critical Care Nursing Clinics of North America, 9*(1), 97–105.

Silva, M.C. (1995). *Ethical guidelines in the conduct, dissemination, and implementation of nursing research.* Washington, DC: American Nurses Association.

Spielman, B. (Ed.). (1996). *Organ and tissue donation: Ethical, legal, and policy issues.* Carbondale, IL: Southern Illinois University.

Thomasma, D.C., & Kushner, T. (Eds.). (1996). *Birth to death: Science and bioethics.* Cambridge, MA: Cambridge University Press.

Weir, R.F. (1984). *Selective nontreatment of handicapped newborns.* New York, NY: Oxford University Press.

Weir, R.F. (1989). *Abating treatment with critically ill patients: Ethical and legal limits to the medical prolongation of life.* New York, NY: Oxford University Press.

Zucker, M. B., & Zucker, H. D. (Eds.). (1997). *Medical futility and the evaluation of life-sustaining interventions.* New York: Cambridge University Press.

STUDY QUESTIONS

◆◆◆◆◆◆◆◆◆◆◆◆◆◆◆◆◆◆◆◆◆◆◆◆◆◆◆◆◆◆◆◆◆◆◆◆

1. The standard used for decision making with children is:
   a. power of attorney.
   b. substituted judgment.
   c. compassionate plea.
   d. best interests.

2. The doctrine of the double effects permits the ethical administration of medication that may hasten death if:
   a. the nurse does not exceed the prescribed dose.
   b. the intent of the person administering the medication is to relieve pain.
   c. the parent has requested that the medication be given.
   d. the patient is Roman Catholic.

3. A "Do Not Resuscitate" order means:
   a. resuscitative measures, as described by the physician, must be withheld.
   b. all treatment must be withheld.
   c. all treatment must be withdrawn.
   d. the nurse at the bedside must decide which resuscitative measures to withhold.

Peter, a 12-year-old with a brainstem glioma, has undergone radiation, chemotherapy, tracheostomy secondary to aspiration, and sensorineural hearing loss from ototoxic medication. His prognosis is grave and he asks not be resuscitated. His parents state that they believe he will "beat the odds" and survive. (For Questions 4 & 5)

4. Peter asks that you not resuscitate him. How do you respond to him?
   a. Explain to him that legally it is not his choice.
   b. Promise him that you won't resuscitate him.
   c. Using a communication board, assist Peter in discussing his wishes with his parents.
   d. Write a DNR order on his chart.

5. You participate in an ethics committee meeting about Peter. The goal of the ethics committee meeting is:
   a. to decide if Peter must legally be resuscitated if he doesn't have a DNR order.
   b. to devise a plan to force Peter's parents to do what he wants.
   c. to discuss how unreasonable everyone thinks Peter's family is.
   d. to analyze the ethical ramifications of resuscitating or not resuscitating Peter.

6. The nurse can facilitate ethical decision making by parents for their children by:
   a. referring the family to an ethics committee or ethics consultant.
   b. exploring with the parents the pros and cons of each option.
   c. assisting the parents in identifying options consistent with their values.
   d. all of the above.

7. Adolescents may legally consent without parental consent or notification to treatment for all of these conditions EXCEPT:
   a. sexually transmitted disease.
   b. birth control and pregnancy counseling.
   c. plastic surgery.
   d. substance abuse.

8. Although philosophers do not agree, children can be organ donors if:
   a. they are born with anencephaly.
   b. they are donating a paired organ (kidney) or lobe (lung or liver) to their sibling.
   c. they have been declared brain dead, and their parents consent to organ donation.
   d. they are in a permanent vegetative state.

9. Children can participate in research if:
   a. they are likely to benefit directly.
   b. they consent.
   c. their parents are paid.
   d. the knowledge to be gained can only be obtained through research on children.

10. The underlying ethical principle in informed consent is:
   a. justice, or fairness.
   b. autonomy, or respect for persons.
   c. loyalty.
   d. fiduciary responsibility.

ANSWERS

◆◆◆◆◆◆◆◆◆◆◆◆◆◆◆◆◆◆◆◆◆◆

1.d 2.b 3.a 4.c 5.d 6.d 7.c 8.c 9.a 10.b

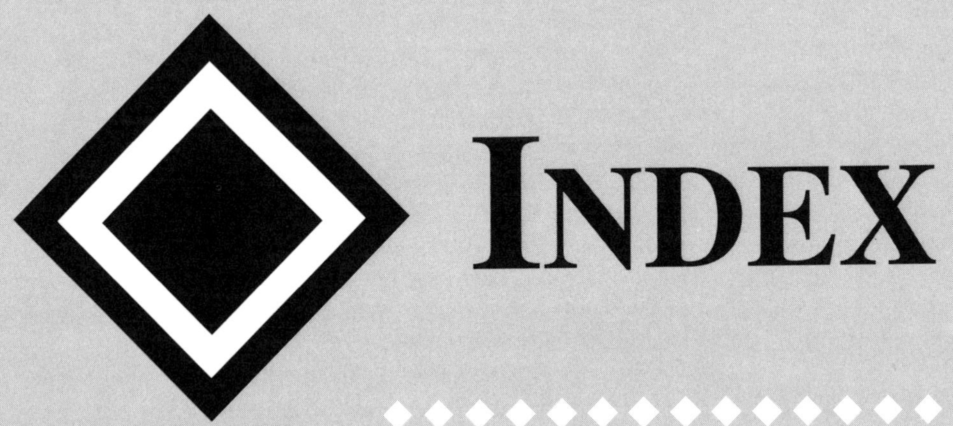

INDEX

A

AAP. *See* American Academy
    of Pediatrics
Abdomen
    injury, from firearm, 240
    physical assessment, 58
Abstract thinking, 35
Accommodation, 34
Acculturation, 395
Acetaminophen poisonings, 234
Acquired immune deficiency
    syndrome (HIV disease), 346
Activated charcoal, for poisoning,
    233
Active listening, 307
Active sleep, 7
Active strategies, for injury
    prevention, 141
Acute illness
    care
        atraumatic, 199, 200
        implementation of, 199
        phases of, 217–218
        planning, 199
        postoperative, 177–178
    catastrophic, impact on family,
        103
    children's views/understanding
        of, 65, 66, 149
    disease processes, 202–203
    environmental safety and
        surveillance, 203–204
    exacerbation to critical condi-
        tion, 322–324
    medications for, 167–169, 203
    nutritional management,
        172–173, 203
    outcomes
        and evaluation, 199, 203
        factors in, 209
        measurement of, 211, 212
        monitoring, 211
        potential, 209–211
        system model for, 212–213
    parental responses to, 157–158
    stress, responses to, 150–151
    as stressor, 149–150
    susceptibility, 403
    symptoms assessment, 183
    teaching principles, 201–202
Acyanotic heart conditions,
    349–350
ADHD (attention-deficit-hyperac-
    tivity disorder), 42, 348

Adhesive otitis media, 227
Adjustment disorder, 41
Adolescents
    behavioral concepts, 40
    with chronic conditions
        developmental aspects of,
            247, 340
        transition to adulthood, 249
    coping strategies, 152
    daily activities, 52
    dying, 88
    illness understanding of, 149
    injury patterns, 137
    linear growth, 6
    nutritional assessment, 51
    physical assessment strategies, 49
    physical growth, 13
    pregnant, 103–104
    preparation for hospitalization, 201
    puberty and, 13
    reproductive development, 13
    response to illness/hospitaliza-
        tion stress, 151
    system maturation, 13–14
    understanding of death, 83
Adrenal cortex, 7
Advance directives, 427
Advocacy
    for child and family, 370
    for family-centered care, 380–381
    by nurse, 428
Affective disorders, 41
Affluence, parenting and, 101
African-Americans, 398, 399–400
    beliefs/perceptions of, 404
    health issues for, 403
    neonatal linear growth, 6
    traditional folk medicine, 405
AGA (appropriate for gestational
    age), 9
Age-related changes, in cognitive
    development, 34
Aid to Families with Dependent
    Children (AFDC), 122
Ainsworth, Mary, 37
Airway adjuncts, 175
Allergies, 346–347
Ambulatory care settings, family-
    centered care in, 387–388
American Academy of Pediatrics
    (AAP)
    neonatal classification, 9
    preventive pediatric health care
        recommendations, 47, 48
American Indians
    beliefs/perceptions, 404

    culture clashes, 397, 399
    demographics, 397
    health issues, 403
    traditional folk medicine, 405
American Medical Association
    Guidelines for Adolescent
    Preventive Services, 47
American Nurses Association
    (ANA)
    Position Statement on Physical
        Violence, 124
    Social Policy statement, 395
Americans with Disabilities, 249
Anabolic steroids, 434
Analgesia, 292, 431
Anesthesia, for infants, 431
Anger, parental grief and, 81
Animal bites, prevention of, 144
Animism, 35
Anorexia, 68, 352
Antibiotics
    infusion pumps for, 279
Anticipatory coping, parental grief
    and, 81, 84
Anticipatory guidance, 60–61, 101,
    219, 369
Antiemetics, 185–186
Antihistamines, for nausea/
    vomiting, 185
Anxiety
    disorder, 41
    of hospitalization, 150
    parental grief and, 81
Apparent life-threatening event
    (ALTE), 281
Appearance, general
    adolescent, 13
    infant, 9
    preschooler, 11
    school-age, 12
    toddler, 11
Approach behaviors, 252
Appropriate for gestational age
    (AGA), 9
Art therapy, 307–308
Asian-Americans
    beliefs/perceptions, 404
    culture clashes, 399
    demographics, 398
    health issues, 403
    traditional folk medicine, 405
Aspirin poisonings, 234
Assent, 427
Assimilation, 34, 395–396
Assist/control ventilation, 176
Associative play, 39